CHANGING TRENDS IN HEALTH AND NUTRITION

CHANGING TRENDS IN HEALTH AND NUTRITION

(In 4 Volumes)

Diet, Nutrition and Changing Style

(Volume 1)

SUJATA K. DASS

ISHA BOOKS
DELHI—110 033

Changing Trends in Health and Nutrition
(Health)

Rs. 3200 (Set in 4 vols.)
Rs. 800 (Each volume)

ISBN: 81-8205-040-5 (Set)
ISBN: 81-8205-041-3 (Vol. 1)

Published in 2004 in India by
Isha Books, D-43, Prithviraj Road
Adarsh Nagar, Delhi-110 033

Lasertypesetting by: Varsha Graphics, Delhi
Printed at: Chawla Offset Press, Delhi

Contents

Preface

Diet and nutrition are important factors in the promotion and maintenance of good health throughout the entire life course. Rapid changes in diets and lifestyles that have occurred with industrialization, urbanization, economic development and market globalisation, have accelerated over the past decade. This is having a significant impact on the health and nutritional status of populations, particularly in developing countries and in countries in transition. While standards of living have improved, food availability has expanded and become more diversified.

Food and food products have become commodities produced and traded in a market that has expanded from an essentially local base to an increasingly global one. Changes in the world food economy have contributed to shifting dietary patterns, for example, increased consumption of energy-dense diets high in fat, particularly saturated fat, and low in unrefined carbohydrates. These patterns are combined with a decline in energy expenditure that is associated with a sedentary lifestyle—motorized transport, labour-saving devices at home, the phasing out of physically demanding manual tasks at work, and leisure time that is preponderantly devoted to physically undemanding pastimes.

Because of these changes in dietary and lifestyle patterns, chronic non-communicable diseases including obesity, diabetes mellitus, cardiovascular disease, hypertension and stroke, and some types of cancer are increasingly significant causes of disability and premature death in both developing and newly developed countries, placing additional burdens on already overtaxed national health budgets.

Promoting healthy diets and lifestyles to reduce the global burden of non-communicable diseases requires a multi-sectoral approach involving the various relevant sectors in societies. The agriculture and food sector figures prominently in this enterprise and must be given due importance in any consideration of the promotion of healthy diets for individuals and population groups.

Editor

1

The Concept of Nutrition and Health

Water, carbohydrate, fat, protein, vitamins, and some of the minerals found in foods are nutrients—substances the body uses for the growth, maintenance, and repair of its tissues. While a look in the mirror would not convince you, a complete chemical analysis of your body would show that it is made of materials similar to those in foods. A healthy 150-pound person's body contains about 90 pounds of water and about 30 pounds of fat. The other 30 pounds are mostly protein and carbohydrate, related organic compounds made from them, and the major minerals of the bones: calcium and phosphorus.

The complete chemical analysis of a food such as the green leafy vegetable spinach shows that it is composed of a number of different kinds of materials but its primary component is water. Most of the solid materials are the compounds carbohydrate, fat, and protein. Vitamins, other minerals, and incidental extras constitute a fraction of a pound. Thus the human body, like spinach, is composed largely of nutrients. If you burn a food such as spinach in air, it seems to disappear. The water evaporates, and all the organic compounds are oxidized to gas and water vapour leaving only a residue of ash. An organic compound contains carbon atoms, usually bounded to other carbon atoms, hydrogen atoms, or both.

The first organic compounds known were natural products synthesized by plants or animals; indeed, it used to be thought that living contributed organic compounds to our world. The term has since been expanded to include all carbon compounds, whatever their origin.

Four of the six classes of nutrients or organic, whereas the other two (minerals and water) are inorganic. During metabolism, three of the four classes of organic nutrients (carbohydrate, fat, and protein) provide energy the body can use. In contrast, vitamins, minerals, and water do not yield energy in the human body.

The energy-yielding nutrients that can break down to yield energy the body can use-are vital to life, for without continual replenishment of the energy you spend daily, you would soon die.

When the body metabolizes the energy-yielding nutrients, the bonds between their atoms break, and the carbon and hydrogen atoms combine with oxygen to yield carbon dioxide and water. As these nutrients break down, they release energy.

Some of this energy is released as heat. Some is transferred into other compounds (including fat) that compose the structures of your body cells, and some is used as fuel for your activities. The amount of energy used as fuel for your activities. The amount of energy the energy-yielding nutrients release can be measured in calories (or more properly, kilocalories or calories), which are familiar to everyone as a measure of food energy and of the energy the body spends during exercise.

People think of 'kcalories' as a constituent of foods, but strictly speaking, they are not; they are a measure of the energy in foods. Thus to speak of the inches in person is incorrect. When completely broken down in the body, a gram of carbohydrate provides about 4 kcalories; a gram of protein also provides; and a gram of fat provides 9 kcalories. The energy content of a food thus depends on how much carbohydrate, fat, and protein it contains.

If your body doesn't use these nutrients to fuel metabolic and physical activities, it rearranges them into storage compounds such as body fat, and puts them away for use between meals and overnight. If you take in more energy than you expend, no matter from which of the three energy-yielding nutrients, the result is a weight gain as body fat. Too much meat is just as fattening as too many potatoes. One other substance contributes food energy: alcohol. Alcohol is not a nutrient, because it supports no growth, maintenance, or repair in the body.

Still, people do consume alcohol, and it shares several characteristics with the energy-yielding nutrients. Like them, alcohol is metabolized in the body to yield energy. When taken in excess of energy need, alcohol, too, is converted to body fat and stored. However, when alcohol contributes a substantial portion of the energy in a person's diet, it is harmful. Practically all foods contain mixtures of all three energy-yielding nutrients, although they are sometimes classified by the predominant nutrient.

Thus it is inaccurate to speak of meat as a protein or of bread as a carbohydrate; they are foods rich in these nutrients. A protein-rich food like beef actually contains a lot of fat as well as portion; a carbohydrate-rich food like bread also contains a trace of fat and a little protein. Only a few foods are exceptions to this rule, the common ones being sugar and oil. The energy-yielding nutrients are (by molecular standards) tremendous in size.

For example, a single molecule of carbohydrate may be composed of 300 smaller molecules, each containing 24 atoms, for a total of some 7,000 atoms. Furthermore, you eat tremendous quantities of the three energy-yielding nutrients-50 to 200 grams or more a day of each. If you could extract and purify the carbohydrate, fat, and protein from your daily diet, they would fill two or three measuring cups.

The foods they come in weigh must more and occupy much more volume. A hundred grams of food may contain only ten or so grams of energy-yielding nutrients, the rest being water, fiber, and other non-kcaloric materials. Your body's use of the energy-yielding nutrients can be summarized, simply, as follows. First, food protein, fat, and carbohydrate, fat, and carbohydrate are broken down to simpler compounds. The process yields energy and small fragments of the original materials.

The vitamins, the next class of nutrients, differ profoundly from the first three classes in almost every way: in their size and shape, in the roles they play, and in the amounts you consume. Perhaps the only characteristics the vitamins share with the first classes of nutrients are that they are vital to life, they are organic, and they are available in food. The vitamins are generally much smaller than energy-yielding nutrients. The body may break them down but does not extract usable energy from them; their role is to serve as helpers, making possible the processes by which the other nutrients are digested, absorbed, and metabolized to body compounds or extracted.

There are 13 different vitamins, each with its own special roles to play. That vitamins are organic has a significant consequence-they are destructible. They can be broken down and altered, and so the body must handle them with care. The body makes special provisions to absorb and transport vitamins, providing many of them with custom-made protein carries.

A vitamin may be useful in one form here and in another there, so special metabolic process subtly alter the characteristics of a vitamin to allow it to perform a particular task. The vitamins are divided into two classes: some are soluble in water and others are soluble in fat (vitamins A, D, E, and K). This fact has many implications for the kinds of foods that contain them; their potential for destruction; and the ways the body absorbs, transports, stores, and excretes them.

Minerals are inorganic elements, even smaller than vitamins. They can occur in the simplest of chemical forms, as single atoms, tiny in comparison with the energy-yielding nutrients, which may be composed of thousands of atoms. Some minerals may be put together into orderly arrays in such structures as bones and teeth-but only with the help of the body's lively metabolic machinery. When minerals float about in the fluids of the body, they give the fluids certain characteristics, but they are not metabolized nor do they yield energy. You consume small amounts of most minerals daily, slightly greater than the amounts of vitamins in your diet.

Some minerals are essential in human nutrition. Other minerals are still being studied; their functions have not yet been determined. Still others are important to nutrition because they are not nutrients, but may displace the minerals needed in the body, causing deranged body functions. The problems caused by one of the containment minerals, lead. The minerals are elements, whereas the other nutrients are all compounds. This means the minerals cannot lose their identity; they exist "forever. When you cook a food containing vitamins and minerals, the elements that make up the vitamins can undergo rearrangement, and so the vitamins can lose their chemical identity; the minerals, however, remain unchanged.

Because they are indestructible, minerals in foods need not be handled with the very special care that vitamins need. They can, however, be bound by substances that make them difficult to absorb or lost in water during cooking. If minerals are scarce in your diet, you have to choose food sources of them with care. Water, indispensable and abundant, forms the major part of almost every body tissue. It is often ignored-because, like air, it is everywhere, and we take it for granted. Water is inorganic, being composed of two atoms of hydrogen bound to one atom of oxygen.

The amounts you must consume relative to the other nutrients are enormous: 2 to 3 liters a day. That's 2,000 to 3,000 grams, compared with 50 or so grams of protein each day, and 200 or so grams of carbohydrate. Water provides the medium in which nearly all the body's activities are conducted. It participates in many metabolic reactions and supplies the medium for transporting vital materials to cells and waste products away from them. In addition to the obvious dietary source-water itself-water comes abundantly in foods and beverages.

In addition, water is generated from the energy-yielding nutrients in foods during metabolism. .Water from these three sources normally balances perfectly with daily water losses. Eating involves more than peoples' simply delivering nutrients to their bodies. Food choices are personal and not always sensible. To a great extent, they resist change. Even people who pride themselves on eating nutritious foods will admit that the other six factors also influence their food choices. No matter how nutritious a meal is, it cannot benefit your health until you eat it.

One reason people like certain foods, of course, is preferences for certain tastes. Two of these preferences are widely shared; the tastes for sugar and salt. People tend to like foods with which they have happy associations-those they eat in the midst of a warm family gathering on traditional holidays, those given to them as children by someone who loved them, or those eaten by people whom they admire.

By the same token, people can attach an intense and unalterable dislike to foods that they ate when they felt sick, or that were forced on them when they weren't hungry, or that are eaten by people they don't respect. Parents may have taught their children to like and dislike certain foods for similar reasons of their own, without even being aware of it. Social pressure is another powerful influence on food behaviour.

An almost necessary element of etiquette and politeness is to accept food or drink being shared by a group or being offered by a host; you are not a member of the social gathering until you do. The influence of availability, convenience, and economy on your food selections is clear. Obviously, you cannot eat foods if they are not available, if you cannot prepare them, or if you cannot afford them. Convenience is a major factor in the purchasing decisions of many people. Consumers look for speed in preparation, recipes with few ingredients, and products that can be cooked in a microwave oven.

Some people are interested in nutrition as a way to avoid illness; others seek nutrition to improve their physical well-being. Food manufacturers have responded to the scientific findings linking health and nutrition with an abundant selection of grocery-store foods and beverages advertised as low-kcalories, low-cholesterol, low-fat, low-sodium, sugar-free, caffeine-free, high-fiber, and calcium-enriched items.

Consumers accept these new, health-promoting foods in their diets, provided that the foods are easy to identity, easy to find in the grocery store, fast and convenient to prepare, and that they taste good-as good as the traditional choices. Sometimes consumers choose products they perceive to offer a benefit-such as an association with luxury and wealth, an image of slimness and weight loss, an association with a concern for health, or with convenience that allows more time for fun and leisure.

With the right image, foods low in fat and high in nutrients would be well-accepted. Foods without labels such as nonfat milk, fruits, vegetables, lean meats, legumes, and whole grains might benefit from some trendy publicity. The revival of the California raisin is an example of just how effective food image campaigns can be, Raisin growers spent millions to change their product's image in 1988, and while the product remained the same, consumers rewarded the growers' efforts with greatly increased sales.

If the deficiency or excess is significant, they get sick, one way or another, and they exhibit signs of malnutrition. Assessment techniques have been developed to detect nutrient imbalances. Malnutrition can be detected by analyzing the combined findings from a number of assessment techniques. One method of evaluating nutrition status is to obtain information about a person's diet. The assessor analyzes a record of an the foods period of days or weeks.

To interpret these exercises correctly, you have to be aware that nutrient values are not absolute and that the exercises assume that reasonable care was taken in the preparation of foods. A second technique that may reveal nutrition problems is the taking of anthropometric measures such as height, weight, and limb circumferences. These measures alert the assessor to such serious problems as growth failure in children, wasting or swelling of body tissue in adults, and obesity-conditions that reflect nutrient deficiencies or excesses.

A third nutrition assessment technique is a physical examination that looks for clues to poor nutrition status. Every part of the body that can be inspected can offer much clues: the hair, eyes, skin, posture, tongue, fingernails, and others. This technique can detect evidence pointing to deficiencies, imbalances, and toxicity states. A fourth way to detect a developing deficiency, imbalance, or toxicity state is to take samples of body tissues and analyze them in the laboratory. The mineral iron can be used to illustrate the stages in the development of a nutrient deficiency. The appearance of an overt iron deficiency is the last of a long sequence of events. First, too little iron gets into the body-either because there is not enough iron in the person's food or because the person's body can't absorb enough of the iron taken in or use it normally.

The body then begins to use up its own stores of iron, so there is a period of declining stores. At this point, the deficiency might be said to be subclinical-that is, to exist already as a covert condition, before outward signs appear. Finally, iron stores are used up, and the body can't make enough of the iron-containing protein hemoglobin to fill the developing new red blood cells that carry oxygen to all the body's cells and enable them to get energy. At this point, the number of red blood cells and enable them to get energy.

At this point, the number of red blood cells declines, the new ones made are smaller than normal and pale, and every part of the body feels the effects of an oxygen lack. The overt symptoms of an iron deficiency-weakness, fatigue, pallor, and headaches-ensure, reflecting the internal state of the blood. This overview of nutrition assessment illustrates the principles that underlie the chapters on the vitamins and minerals. For one, internal changes proceed outward signs of or excesses. As sickness need not appear before a person takes corrective measures. Tests can either reveal that there are problems in the early stages or confirm that nutrient stores are adequate.

One kind of survey-a food consumption survey-determines what foods people eat, calculates or measures the nutrients in them, and compares the amounts of nutrients consumed with a standard such as the Recommended Dietary Allowance, or RDA. Another kind of survey-a nutrition status survey-assesses the nutrition status of the people themselves, using the techniques described in the previous section: a combination of diet histories, anthropo-metric measures, physical examinations, and laboratory tests. Both kinds of surveys have been conducted in the United States and Canada, and the same general impressions have been confirmed. Many people are overconsuming foods, under expending energy, or both.

While the majority of the people are adequately nourished with respect to most individual nutrients, deficiencies and marginal intakes of nutrients do exist. Anyone interested in nutrition needs not only to study nutrients and foods, but also to acquire an understanding of the human body. The interactions among foods, nutrients, and the body are not as simple as one might expect. The highlight introduces the principle of homeostasis, the body's ability to adapt when internal conditions change, and to maintain equilibrium.

The machine has a fabulous central control system-the central nervous system-that can evaluate information about conditions both within the machine and outside it. It machine can call into play whatever parts can best respond to any situation. It gets its information and transmits its instructions by way of a waste system of wiring. The system carries messages in both directions: signals about conditions from the parts to the center, and messages signaling work or rest from the center to the parts.

The smooth functioning that results from the system's adjustments to changing conditions is homeostasis. Homeostasis underlies wise nutrition judgment and competent diet advice; most misguided nutrition behaviour neglects this principle. Throughout all your body systems, all processes are precisely and automatically regulated by hormone and nerve actively, without your conscious efforts. This leaves you free to compose a symphony or to gaze at the stars instead of tying up your energy in worrying about how much calcium to store in your bones or when to contract your heart muscle.

Both physical and psychological stressors elicit the body's stress response Major physical stressors include pain, illness of any kind, surgery, wounds, bounds, burns, infections, a very hot or humid climate, toxic compounds, radiation, and threats constitute psychological stress. The stress response begins when your brain perceives a threat to you equilibrium. The sight of a car hurt lining forward you: the terror that an enemy is concealed around a nearby corner; the excitement of planning for a party, a move, or a wedding; the feeling of pain; or any other such disturbance perceived by the brain serves as an alarm signal.

The effects all favour physical action. Notice the tremendous array of target organs in the description of the stress response that follows. The pupils of your eyes widen so that you can see better; your muscles tense up so that you can jump, run or struggle with maximum strength; breathing quickens to bring more oxygen into you lungs, and your heart races to rush this oxygen to your heart races to rush this oxygen to your muscles so that they can burn the fuel they need for energy. Your liver pours forth the needed fuels from its stored supply, and fat cells release alternative fuels.

Body protein tissues break down to back up the fuel supply and to be ready to heal wounds if necessary. Blood vessels of your muscles expand to feed them better, whereas those of your gastrointestinal track constrict: and gastrointestinal tract constrict: and gastrointestinal tract glands shut down. Less blood follows to your kidney so that fluid is conserved, and less flows to your skin so that blood loss will be minimized at any wound site. More platelets form, to allow your blood to clot faster if need be. Hearing sharpens, and your brain produces local opium like substances, dulling its sensation of pain, which during an emergency might distract you from taking the needed action.

But if the stress is prolonged, and especially if physical action is not a permitted response to the stress, then it can drain the body of its reserves and leave it weakened, worn, and susceptible to illness. Much of the disability imposed by prolonged stress is nutritional: you can't eat, can't digest your food or absorb nutrients, and so can't store them in reserve for periods of need. All three energy fuels carbohydrate, fat, and protein are drawn upon in increased quantities during stress. If the stress requires vigorous physical action, and if there is injury, all three are used.

While the body is busy responding and not eating, the fuels must be drawn from internal sources. The conservation of water at such a time is of utmost importance. The body sends several hormonal messages to conserve water. As for taken from storage for as long as supplies last, but supplies last, but supplies for some are exhausted within a day. Thereafter, body tissues break down to provide energy and needed nutrients. The best nutritional preparation for stress is a balanced and varied diet as part of a lifestyle in which exercise plays a constant part. No supplements or gimmicks will benefit you.

During server stress, the appetite is suppressed. We've already said why: it's an adaptive reaction to a physical threat, the kind of threat that our ancestors experienced during their evolution. Energy at such a time is needed for fight or flight; it would be wasteful and risky to spend energy looking of or eating food. The blood supply has been diverted to the muscles to maximize strength and speed; so even if food is swallowed, it may not be digested or absorbed efficiently. All of this means that to tell people under severe stress to eat is poor advice.

They can't and if they force themselves to eat, they can't assimilate what they've eaten. On the other hand, fasting is itself a stress on the body, and the longer a person goes without eating, the harder it can be to get started again. So it can be a no win situation. It is frightening to see the downward spiral people can get into once they have let stress affect them to the point where they can't eat, and not eating makes it harder for them to handle the stress. It is therefore desirable not to let stress become so overwhelming that eating becomes impossible.

Managing stress so that it does not overwhelm is a psychological task, and may require the help of a counsellor. If you can eat under stress, do so, of course. Take only a little if that's all your can handle, and eat more often to keep meeting your energy and nutrient needs choose a variety of foods. Drink fluids, too. Although the body conserves fluids during stress, it will excrete what it does not need, any by taking in water you enable your kidneys to return blood concentrations of the minerals to their equilibrium.

Diet planning

Knowing the individual nutrients and their recommended intakes, you can now ask how you can juggle the available foods to create a diet that supplies all the needed nutrients in the appropriate amounts for good health. The principle is simple enough l just select a variety of foods that present the nutrients you need.

It helps to keen in mind the basic diet planning principles, listed in the margin in alphabetical order to help you to remember them. Let's begin by discussing dietary balance. The minerals calcium and iron illustrate the importance of dietary balance. Iron is one of the essential nutrients. You can only get it into your body by eating foods that contain it. If you miss out on these foods, you may experience symptoms of iron deficiency. You may feel weak, tired, and unenthusiastic; may have frequent headaches; and can do little muscular work without disabling fatigue. If you had added iron-rich foods to your diet, you might have prevented these symptoms.

Some foods are rich in iron; other are notoriously poor. Meats, fish, poultry, and legumes are in the iron-rich category, and an easy way to obtain the needed iron is to include these foods in your diet regularly. Calcium is another essential nutrient. A diet lacking calcium may result in poor bone development during the growing years and a gradual bone loss in adults that can totally cripple a person in later life.

The iron-rich foods just named are poor sources of calcium; you can get enough calcium only by frequently consuming milk products or carefully selected milk substitutes. Just as foods that are rich in iron are poor in calcium, so is the reverse true, In fact, milk and milk products are so low in iron that the overuse of these foods, by displacing iron-rich foods from the diet, can actually cause iron-deficiency anemia.

And yet no one could accuse milk of being a nutrient-poor food. It is the single most nutritious food for infants and can be an important calcium contributor in the diet of people of all ages. Use enough-but not too many—serving of meat alternates for iron; use enough-but not too many—servicing of milk products for calcium. Save some space for other foods needed for other nutrients. Iron and calcium are only two of some 40-odd essential nutrients, and meat and milk are their most outstanding food sources in most people's diets.

Yet there are other nutrients that are not abundant in either milk or meat; a diet consisting of milk and meat would be far from adequate. To obtain the other nutrients, you have to eat vegetables, fruits, grains, and other foods; variety in the diet helps to ensure adequacy. The task of designing an adequate, balanced diet therefore requires some thought and skilful planning.

The real challenge is to incorporate kcalorie control—to eat an adequate, balanced diet without overeating. Part of secret to eating well without overrating is to select foods that deliver the most nutrients at the lowest kcalorie cost. Take foods containing calcium , for example: 11/2 ounces of cheddar cheese and 8 ounces of nonfat milk each provide about 300 milligrams of calcium but the cheese contributes about twice as many kcalories as the but based on the amount of calcium they offer for a given kcalorie amount, the nonfat milk has higher nutrient density then the cheese.

To evaluate foods this way is to employ the concept of nutrient density. The concept of nutrient density can help the health-conscious consumer make informed choices. The food industry has enthusiastically endorsed the selling of the nutritional adequacy concept. The dairy people proclaim, "Drink milk its good for you". The meat people boast that meat is rich in protein and iron, as indeed it is.

Ware consumers realized, though, that whole milk and meat can also contribute many fat kcalories, and they use those products that are lowest in fat, thereby obtaining more nutrients for the kcalories. By selecting small quantities of low fat foods a person practices moderation, a necessary ingredient to controlling kcalories. Another principle necessary to successful diet planning is variety, it is generally agreed that people should not eat the same foods day after day, except for staple foods such as milk and even for staple foods, some people recommend switching brands from the time to time.

Variety permits you to take advantage of the fact that some foods are better sources of some nutrients than other food are. Also, a monotonous diet may deliver unwanted amounts of undesirable food constituents, such as contaminants. In a diet with variety, each food's ingredients are diluted by the bulk of all the other foods eaten and even further diluted if several days are skipped before it is eaten again. Several approaches to diet planning are possible. Two of the guides most widely used by nutrition- conscious people today are food group plans and exchange patterns.

The person who understands and appreciates both is in a good position to design an optimal diet. One of the most familiar ways of grouping foods in the United States fits the major foods into four groups. Each of the four groups contains food that are similar in origin and nutrient content. The nutrients named in the table are representative of all the nutrients. The assumption is that once you have adequate amounts of these, you will probably have enough of the other two dozen or so essential nutrients as well, because they occur in the same groups of foods.

This is not an entirely safe assumption, but with the precaution that primarily unprocessed foods be used, the Four Food Group Plan provides a reasonable foundation for diet planning. The Four Food Group Plan specifies that a certain quantity of food must be consumed from each group. For the adult, the recommended number of servings from the vegetables and fruits, breads and cereals, milk and milk respectively. Many foods-such as butter margarine cream, sour cream, salad dressing, mayonnaise, potato chips, jelly, broth, coffee, tea, alcoholic beverages, and others—don't fit into any of the four food groups. Some on them do contribute some nutrients, and most contribute energy, to the day's intake.

They are grouped together into a miscellaneous category, because their nutrient content is not significant in the nutrients characteristic of a food group, or their nutrient content has been greatly diluted by fat, sugar, alcohol, or water. The beauty of the Four Food Group Plan lies in its simplicity and ease in learning. It may appear quite rigid, but it can be used with great flexibility once its intent is understood.

For example, cheese can be substituted for milk because both supply protein, calcium, and riboflavin in about the same amounts. Legumes and nuts are alternative choices for meats. The plan can be adapted to casseroles and other mixed dishes, as well as to different national and cultural cuisines. Critics say that half of the food classes are animal products—milk and meat—which leads many people to think that half of the foods they consumer should be milk and meat. Also, a person can follow all of the plan's rules and still fail to meet the day's need for some nutrients-especially vitamin B6 vitamin E, iron, magnesium and zinc.

Some people choose to exclude certain foods or food classes from their diets for religious, philosophical, cultural, or other reasons some exclude red meat only, while eating poultry and fish. Some eat only fish among these foods, some exclude all animal flesh, but eat products produced by animals such as eggs, cheese, and milk. Some are 'pure' vegetarians, eating plant foods only, and some go to the extreme of eating only fruit, not vegetables or grains.

Each of these foodways presents a challenge to the planner-that of obtaining the needed nutrients from fewer foods or food groups. The person who excludes meat and poultry has a nutritionally similar food to rely on fish. In contrast, the person who eats no animal flesh, not even fish, needs an alternative source of iron, zinc, and some of the vitamins offered by meat: for this person, the liberal use of legumes is recommended.

The person who uses only plant foods has to plan with still more care. For example, one nutrient, vitamin B12 is found only in animal foods, so this person has to take a vitamin B12 supplement or use vitamin B12-fortified soy milk or similar products daily. The vegetarian needs to learn much more, and later chapters offer more information. Whereas food group plans help most with dietary adequacy, balance and variety, exchange systems help with kcalorie control and moderation. The person who learns to use an exchange system can gain mastery over food energy intakes, and especially fat kcalories.

Originally developed for people with diabetes, exchange systems proved so useful that they are now in general use for diet planning. Weight Watchers, a well known organization that helps people control their weight while eating a nutritious diet, bases its eating plans on the exchange systems. Food are not always where you might first expect them to be in the exchange system, because they are grouped according to their energy nutrient contents rather than by their outward appearances.

Corn is not a 'vegetable' in the exchange system; it is listed with starch/breads as a 'starchy vegetables'. Similarly, olives are not a 'vegetable': they are classified as a 'fat', and so is bacon. These grouings permit you to see among foods resemblances that are significant to nutrition. The user of the exchange system is encouraged to think of nonfat milk as milk and of whole milk as with added fat. The vegetable list includes only low kcalorie vegetables, so a half cup of any of them will provide about 25 kcalories.

One small banana counts as two fruits. But a cherry pie is not a fruit. It includes a fruit if it contains ten large cherries, but it also includes bread and fat exchanges, and added sugar. The starch/bread, list also clearly specifies portion sizes and makes clear which gain products contain added fat. Lima beans, potatoes, and other starchy vegetables are listed with the breads, not the vegetables, because they are similar to breads in kcalorie and carbohydrate content. Perhaps most important of all meats and cheeses are separated into three categories—lean, medium fat and high-fat—and the fat list by including items lick bacon and avocados, alerts the consumer to foods that are unexpectedly high in fat kcalories.

If you are a diet planner who wants to choose foods that contain all the nutrients you need, you may find both the food group plan and the exchange system useful. The food group plan promotes adequacy and balance, helping you to avoid overemphasizing one class of food. The exchange system provide the lists from which to make your food selections: by following it, your can employ moderation and control kcalories without effort.

Clearly, the person interested in good health, fitness, and weight control will not just eat an adequate diet, but will combine diet and exercise into a daily pattern that supports optimal health. With judicious selections, the diet can meet the need for all the nutrients and provide some luxury items as well. Adequacy and balance would be achieved, not necessarily at each meal, but within each day. The planner could achieve variety by selecting different foods each day from the exchange lists.

Having planned a diet using the principles of adequacy, balance, kcalorie control, moderation, and variety, you can now ask how it compares with recommended nutrient intakes. You will find that the RDA and RNI make specific recommendations for protein, vitamins, and minerals, but only make general statements about energy intakes and do little to protect people from over nutrition. Research has identified excess intakes of sugar, fat, cholesterol, salt, and alcohol as contributing factors to many illnesses, including heart disease, cancer, diabetes, and liver disease.

Many nutrition scientists therefore feel that the public should be urged to curtail their intakes of these substances. However, while some feel justified in offering concrete advice, others feel uncomfortable about offering any advice at all. The two points of view might be characterized as the preventive approach and the medical approach. The preventive approach emphasizes everyone's health, and if it errs, it does so on the side of urging more people to make more changes than may be necessary.

The object is to help everyone forestall or prevent and disease whose onset or severity may be affected by diet. Proponents believe that since we can't predict just which individuals may be responsive to dietary factors related to diseases, we should offer the same advice to all. The medical approach is the more conservative, traditional position. It urges each person who needs to made a dietary change to do so.

The problem is that usually, by the time the person can be identified, symptoms of the disease are already appearing. This approach waits until cure is needed rather than emphasizing prevention, and it puts the physician in the role of treating an already-existing disease rather than promoting health. Choosing the preventive approach, government agencies and other organizations have published dietary guidelines that favour moderation.

Positive Concept of Health

Some countries regard health as a static phenomenon.

Some look on health from a materialistic point of view. Others think health to be mainly a spiritual phenomenon, a matter of attitude, of belief, of self-understanding. With these diverging concepts, it is a challenge to find a basis for a positive, dynamic and holistic understanding of health. This basis can only be found when health is traced back to the very roots of life, so that in the end we can define health as the fulfillment of all basic principles of life. Or negatively expressed, if there is any serious and longlasting violence done against one of the basic principles sooner or later disease will results.

Piaget tried throughout his life to bridge the gaps between biology and psychology. He had a deep feeling for homologies between biological and intellectual structures and a belief that biological principles rule the living world at all level of organization, including the social level and the world of the mind. Normally in biology textbooks we find all or some of the following characteristics of living beings; growth, reproduction, metabolism, irritability, active movement, heredity and mutability. These are found in all organisms, but they are unsuitable for use in the psychological and sociological domains.

We are in need of superordinate terms to describe basic processes underlying any kind of living phenomena, material or spiritual. For this reason the basic principles of life described below are formulated on the abstract level of systems theory so that they may be applied and understood in different disciplines, and, in particular, form a link between science and humanities.

This approach does not mean a fallback reducing humanities to biology, but the attempt to derive both areas of life sciences from the same formalized roots.

Each living phenomenon is continuously counteracting the internal natural increase of entropy by means of energy conversion. Entropy is mainly exported on heat as a carrier, and energy of a higher quality has to be consumed. This high-quality energy yields order to the living phenomenon which in turn, is used to maintain and increase the living order.

This principle is probably not equivalent to the other; it is rather of a higher rank, because the basic structures of a living system and its capability to preserve these structures by continuous reduction of entropy-against the common trend of nature - are the most spectacular and unique properties of such systems. Most of the other principles of life seem to have a serving function only. There is a certain 'conservative trait' innate in all living beings with respect to order, the material basis of which is described by Mandelian genetics.

Health education, however, has not only to develop a positive attitude of children towards maintenance and increase of order, but also to the tolerance or even appreciation of partial disorder. Rigid order, without any flexibility, is as harmful to life as complete chaos; many examples from the history of the biosphere are proving this. It seems that life develops at its best if there is always a small and limited disorder, as a creative element on a strong and reliable basis of order which gives security.

This ambivalence of order/disorder, security/insecurity appears to be most favourable for life and to guarantee maximal reduction of entropy in the biosphere as a whole. Compartments or variables are able to increase or multiply due to a mechanism of positive feedback. However, positive feedback in reverse may also lead to exponential decrease, if a vital variable sinks down. Although living systems may be stabilized as a whole and not grow or reproduce, there are always parts which do so.

There is no cell without plasmatic growth, no organism without growth of certain tissues, no population of a minimum size without children, no economy without growth of capital and/or new technologies, ideas, strategies, etc. and no ecosystem without growing and reproducing populations, as long as these systems behave normally and are healthy. Growth and reproduction are necessary events in order to compensate for the continuous decay of living matter.

In this respect, principle 2 is very closely related to principle 1. However, principle 1 is certainly superordinated to principle 2 as unlimited growth and unlimited reproduction very quickly lead to complete misbalance or disease and finally to death. So each reinforcement of biological substance and structure has to be controlled by regulation mechanisms, keeping the balance which we call 'healthy'.

Each living phenomenon has the capability of self-stabilization. This capability, sometimes called homeostasis, is a general effect of negative feedback functioning in contrast to positive feedback, equally in the opposite direction, to produce stability. Without this ability to stabilize, a living system would be a victim of any kind of disturbance; it would either collapse or explode.

Thus inhibiting processes in our life, although providing negative feedback, should always be acknowledged as making a contribution as they may be vital to the stability of the total system. This aspect has consequences: normally people think predominantly in terms of growth provided it is their own and not the growth of others, and they do not expect to be hindered in this expansion.

It requires an educational effort to make people realize that some amount of self-constraint and even sacrifice is necessary to keep the balance in the community and the ecosystem. Each living phenomenon is able to adjust to its environment by different mechanisms. Either it adjusts external structures to its own structure by means of assimilation, or it adjusts its own structure to the environment by means of accommodation.

In both cases the individuality of the phenomenon is maintained. Adaptation is a variant of elasticity and necessary for health. Any rigidity or lack of flexibility, in body or mind, reduces the chance of finding the optimum of life, and so may lead to permanent stress and eventually disease. Appreciation of this is not self evident, especially as adaptation may often require self-denial and the overcoming of traditional habits.

So health education has to aim at preparing a readiness for a adaptation. However, as for all other principles, there is a limit when a living phenomenon is threatened. Health needs adaptation, but it is not achieved by adaptation alone. Each living phenomenon is delineated from its surroundings by a semi-permeable surface. Furthermore, no living phenomenon is identical to any other each of them is unique in the way that its composition of elements, its structure and its internal an external relationships are not completely reproducible. Denying individuality of human beings by equalizing them in a mass society makes people sick after a while.

Everybody wants to have their own personality, to have a demarcation from others, giving a minimum amount of security for their individual needs. So, supporting individuality means contributing to health. Each living phenomenon has internal borders. However, the borders are not closed, but principally open to matter, energy of information. Living phenomena are characterized by open systems and sub-systems.

All parts within a living phenomenon are related to and dependent on each other. The number of mutual relationships is much greater than the number of parts. If some kind of practised reductionism leads to homogenization of a living system and a diminished complexity, there is always a danger isolation of parts or suppression of individuality. Hence reduced complexity very easily leads to disintegration of the system and thus to disease or even death.

Supporting high complexity in a living system means contributing to the health of the system. The different compartments and relationships within a living phenomenon are not equivalent with respect to survival and development. There are those with high importance, the key parts and key relationships, which can less easily be missed or changed, and those with a lower importance, which can more easily be missed, replaced or changed. There exists a hierarchy.

However, we live in a time of increasing equalisation of people in an industrialized world, despite all that is said about individuals. We experience today attempts to abolish hierarchical structures in societies and to remove any kind of authority. We find unexpected after-effects of monocultures, of mass populations, of vast numbers of substitutes in our markets. People begin to feel ill and they do not know why. Hierarchy in living systems means that there are different priorities. There are organs in our body which need more attention than others; there are in society people who need more attention than others.

There is always a ranking system in any healthy living being, and violation against this or its complete abolition leads to serious damage and disease. Living phenomena have the capability of codifying structures variables by means of signals. They use certain structures or variables as carriers of a meaning. The use of objects as carriers of information is a miraculous phenomenon of life. Their existence may not be essential at the moment, but their existence is vital for the survival of any organism, as they help to recognize dangers in time. Living phenomena store information by codifying it in durable carrier systems.

By this method they are able to make use of present information at later times and thus overcome the "time barrier" to some extent. This principle is strongly connected with 1, the order principle. As information is somehow a spiritual principle in our world which has very precisely to be distinguished from its carriers, information storage means storage of something which is beyond the material world. Positive health education has to take this notion of "inheritance", "continuity", "non-material thinking" into consideration.

It is the author's conviction, born from a long experience with biocybernetic courses, that such a notion is promoting something like a "health of mind", as it is stressing the spiritual side of the world which is the essence of the mind itself. That his attribute has a strong impact on learning needs no explanation. Each living phenomenon is able to move actively either totally or in parts. Movement means translocation in space and time and normally serves principles 1, 2, 3, 4, 7, 8, 9 and 12. How much active movement is necessary for health needs no explanation. Intuitively, all children regard movement as the most characteristic property of living beings and hence very often even do not recognize plants to be alive.

However, when referring to people every child feels the great importance of this principle. It is well-known how many diseases arise from a lack of movement. So a strong encouragement to move should be a vital part of positive health education. Living phenomena, as judged from a human perspective, seem all to have a dimension f subjectivity which transcends the operational possibilities of science.

It is a kind of consciousness, awareness, internal view which we know from ourselves and which to some extent, we must also attribute to other living beings, although we can never prove this. Because of the impossibility of proof, principle 12 is not a scientific part of biology. People have two possible ways of observing themselves; the scientific method, leading to all the disciplines of human biology, and the method of introspection, leading to disciplines like philosophy, the arts, the humanities.

The latter disciplines make statements about feelings, perception, deliberations, sensations. All these are not objects of science as they can only be experienced personally. If we are going to collect principles of life which are relevant for all its manifestations, both the physical and the spiritual ones, we cannot constrain our endeavours to the perspectives of science alone, but have to include the introspective disciplines as well. It seems quite essential for human beings to be acknowledged as subjects with internality and not to be degraded to some kind of machines which just function and are unable to enjoy, to suffer, to love.

With respect to health, it is obvious that people do not feel well for long if they regard themselves as machines or balckboxes. All medical evidence proves the necessity of a psychological view for the maintenance of health. This is the basis for the development of an individual "psychosomatic medicine", and positive health education certainly has to devote much effort to this psychological aspect, as it must also develop something related to the "spiritual aspect". A positive attitude developed in students will manifest itself in a positive form of health care, but also in corresponding ways of treating environmental and other affairs.

Better Environment for Health

The World Health Organization defines health as follows: "Health is a state of complete physical mental, and social well-being, and not merely the absence of disease or infirmity." In order to have a mentally healthful and educational environment, therefore, one should not be concerned merely with providing the proper physical facilities. It is necessary also to take into consideration the administrative practices that play such an important part in providing for the total health of the child. It has been estimated that one of every ten school children is emotionally disturbed. This fact shows the necessity for coming to grips with this problem in every way possible.

Health and physical educators should be especially concerned with mental and emotional health because of their close relationship with physical health and illness. During the last few years psychosomatics in education has increasingly been given more attention. Mental health implies a state of mind which allows the individual to adjust in a satisfactory manner to whatever life has to offer. Good mental health cannot be thought of as a subject that is included in the school curriculum. Instead, it must permeate the total life of the educational institution.

It means that programmes and flexible and geared to individual needs, a permissive climate prevails, children are allowed considerable freedom, and students become self-reliant and responsible for their own actions. It means that the child is recognized and has a satisfying educational experience. The national Association for Mental Health Points out that the well-adjusted person is the one who has the right attitudes and feelings toward himself, other people, and the demands that life places upon him.

A few of the administrative practices that have a bearing upon the mental and emotional health of the students and participants deal with organization of the school day, student achievement, play and reaction, homework, attendance, personnel policies, administrative emphasis, and discipline. The organization of the school day will have a bearing upon whether a healthful environment is provided for the child. The length of the school day must be in conformance with the age of the child.

Classes should be scheduled in a manner that does not result in excessive fatigue. Subjects that require considerable concentration should be scheduled when the individual is more mentally efficient. Usually this is during the early part of the day. Boredom and tension will arise from scheduling similar classes close together, without any breaks. The programme should be flexible to allow for variety, new developments, and the satisfying of children's interests.

Adequate periods rest and play should be provided, not only as a change from the more arduous routine of close concentration but also as a necessity for utilizing the big muscles of the body. "Big-muscle" activity is essential during the growing years. The length of classes should be adequate for instructional purposes but not so excessively long that the law of diminishing returns sets in. Success is an experience that is essential to the development of self-confidence and an integrated person. One who experiences success will be better stimulated to do good work than one who consistently fails.

The child who consistently fails is likely to have behaviour disorders. In view of this, it is important that educational programmes recognize their responsibility for developing each individual. Marks, although supposedly an index quality of work done, are poor guides for such purposes. Many tests that are given as a basis for marks do not measure what they are supposed to measure and have been found to, be unreliable when rated by various persons.

Furthermore, the human element always enters the picture. Marks stimulate competition which is unhealthy in many of its aspects. Too often the underlying reason for such competition is to prove superiority over someone rather than to prove a mastery in a particular subject-matter field or skill. Under such circumstances harm frequently results to the mental health and personalities of students.

Dr. William Menninger and other experts in the field of psychiatry point to the contributions of play and recreation to mental health. Furthermore, to achieve success in the competitive society of today, a person needs a sound body which possesses stamina and endurance and will support long hours of work. Also, the skills in physical activities, music, industrial arts, and allied areas that are learned during the early years of an individual's life will determine to a great degree his hobbies or leisure-time pursuits during adult years.

For these and other reasons, it is important that physical education and other subjects falling into this category be recognized for the contribution they can make to the total growth of the individual. There are many persons in mental institutions today who were capable of working out the most difficult problems in calculus and were expert in their knowledge of geography and other subject.

Educators are increasingly recognizing that homework should be assigned only when it is in the best interest of the whole child. If it is given for the purpose of busy-work, to keep someone occupied during hours after dinner at night, or solely for enabling a person to surpass his classmates, it cannot be justified. Children as well as adults need time for play and recreation. They are entitled to time after school for such purposes. For young children in elementary school there should rarely be any homework because young bodies need great amounts of physical activity. Ample exercise is necessary for body organs and muscles that are developing and gaining strength for future years.

Good mental health in a school programme is tied up very closely with the teacher. The manner in which the teacher and student interact with one another is very important. It is important for the teacher to think of youngsters as living, feeling, and developing human beings who pursue different and varied courses on their ways to inaturity. They are not inanimate objects or receptacles into which the instructor pours knowledge. One of the main responsibilities of any teacher in health or physical education should be student counselling.

Quite frequently specialists in these areas are the ones to whom the child goes in search of information. Anyone who is to perform such an important job as counselling should be well adjusted, understand himself, and get along well with others. The teacher must be in good physical condition in order to do a good job. A teacher may come to a job in excellent physical condition, but if large classes are assigned, the salary is insufficient, and outside work is necessary, physical harm may result.

Furthermore, if there is no provision for sick leave and as a result the teacher must be on the job even when sick or ill, her physical condition will suffer. When this happens, the students also suffer. The teacher's personality has important implication for the mental and emotional health of those with whom he or she comes in contact. The teacher who is happy, wears a smile, is kind, considerate, and likes people in general will impart these qualities to the students. It is bound to "rub off" in the daily interaction that takes place.

Conversely, the teacher or leader who is sarcastic, depressed, prejudiced, and intolerant will also impart these qualities to the children with whom he or she associates. The leader's personality is also reflected in the appearance of the classroom and the teaching methods employed. Administrators should be cognizant of the factors that result in maladjusted personalities for members of their staffs. A few years ago the National Educational Association found that many faculty members were plagued by personnel and working conditions which influenced their mental outlooks.

Some of these were as follows: financial difficulties, economic problems, serious illness of relatives or friends, unsatisfactory progress of pupils, matters of personal health, being unmarried and without normal family relationships, disciplinary problems, an official rating by a superior, possible loss of position, work of a college course, being unhappily married, and religious problems. Many of these frustrating factors could have been eliminated. All teachers should have satisfactory working conditions.

They should receive an adequate salary to eliminate financial worries, be encouraged to develop out-of-school interest in the community, have hobbies in which they can engage after school hours and during vacation periods, and have adequate provisions for sick and sabbatical leaves and leaves of absence so that proper rest and adequate educational standards may be assured. Furthermore, there should be ample opportunities provided for affiliation with professional groups and the development of cultural and other interests conducive to better leadership qualifications.

By provision of such essentials teachers and leaders will be made happier and have better mental and emotional health. In turn, this will be reflected in the total health of the children with whom they come in contact. Human relationships are a most important consideration if one is to grow into a happy, successful, and well-adjusted individual. Of all the traits that should be developed in health and physical education, human relationships rank toward the top of the list. Through counselling, participation in group games and activities under good leadership, and other phases of the programmes, the potentialities are great for developing good human relationships.

Each individual should be made to feel he belongs to the group and has something to contribute in its behalf.There must never be an attempt to make a member of the group feel insignificant and unimportant. More praise should be dispensed than criticism. Every attempt should be made to help each person maintain his self-respect. The atmosphere that pervades the classroom, gymnasium, or recreation center should be relaxed and friendly.

The emotional needs of every individual should be taken into consideration in the class or group activities that are held. The teacher should have good relationships with his or her collegues. Any faculty or staff that is infested with cliques, jealousies, and strife communicates these attitudes to the students. This is just as true here as in the case of quarrelling parents who communicate their feelings to their children. If one is to help others develop good human relationships, one must set an example which is worthy of emulation. There must be good human relationships among the children themselves.

They are dependent upon the feeling of the group toward them and whether or not they are accepted. It is important to have status, among one's associates. The teacher can play an important part in helping to see that everyone gains recognition. This is especially important with such individuals as the dull child in the classroom, the awkward, uncoordinated youngster on the playfield, and the intellectually gifted student in a recreation setting. The teacher should be careful not to accentuate the characteristic which makes a child markedly different from any rest of the group.

2

Diet and Health Control

In the Pacific, over the past 50 years, major changes have occurred in diet and physical activity patterns and that, as a result, overweight and obesity have become public health problems of primary importance. Obesity and pre-obesity (or overweight) are key determinants of chronic noncommunicable diseases (NCDs) such as type 2 diabetes, cardiovascular disease (including hypertension), gall bladder disease and certain types of cancer.

In a workshop on obesity prevention and control strategies in the Pacific, co-organized by the WHO Regional Office for the Western Pacific with the Secretariat of the Pacific Community (SPC), International Association for the Study of Obesity (IASO), International Obesity Task Force (IOTF), the Food and Agriculture Organization of the United Nations (FAO) and International Life Sciences Institute (ILSI).

To improve diets and lifestyles substantially, and thus to control the obesity epidemic effectively, it was decided that a three-pronged strategy is needed:

(1) increase awareness of the problem and promote positive behaviours;

(2) create supportive environments through public health policies that make healthy choices easy choices; and

(3) strengthen the capability and capacity of clinical services to help individuals lose weight and avoid further weight gain.

In 2002, WHO began to formulate a draft Global Strategy on Diet, Physical Activity and Health, to address chronic NCDs such as cardio-vascular disease, cancer and diabetes, which have become the leading causes of death in most parts of both the developed and the developing world. The common risk factors for these diseases include unhealthy diet, physical inactivity, tobacco use and abuse of alcohol.

One key element in developing the strategy is a new joint WHO/FAO expert report, currently being finalized, following extensive consultation with governments, health professional organizations, consumers associations and the private sector. In May 2002, the World Health Assembly adopted a resolution for the formulation of this global strategy and its adoption by May 2004.

The WHO Regional Office for the Western Pacific has addressed the issues and programmes needed to improve diet and physical activity, and thus health, in the Region, through various meetings on nutrition and on NCDs including, in September 2002, in the Ministerial Roundtable held at the Regional Committee in Kyoto, Japan. The Pacific has seen an increase in the rate of obesity of such magnitude over the past 50 years that is has created a major threat not only for the well-being and longevity of the people, but also for the economic prosperity of the Pacific island countries.

Obesity is one of the main determinants of NCDs. The cost of managing diet-related NCDs accounts for about half of health care expenditure in certain Pacific island countries. Lost productivity associated with obesity-related injury and illness among the orkforce adds a further financial burden to the community.

Prevention and Control Strategies in the Pacific, Apia, Western Samoa, 26 to 29 September 2000. The World Health Report 2002 describes in detail how a few risk factors account for a significant proportion of all deaths and disease in most countries. For chronic diseases, the most important include tobacco, several aspects related to food and diet, including low fruit and vegetable intake, high consumption of fatty, sugary and salty foods, excessive alcohol intake and physical inactivity.

Excessive energy intake and limited physical activity result in increased body mass index (BMI). Approximately 58% of diabetes mellitus, 21% of ischaemic heart disease, and 8% to 42% of certain cancers are attributable to BMI above 21 kg/m2 , globally. Low intake of fruits and vegetables is estimated to cause 19% of gastrointestinal cancer, about 31% of ischaemic heart disease and 11% of stroke, worldwide, and 4.9% of total deaths.

Physical activity reduces the risk of cardio-vascular disease, some cancers and type 2 diabetes, through a number of mechanisms: it improves glucose metabolism, reduces body fat and lowers blood pressure. Physical inactivity is estimated to cause, globally, about 10% to 16% of cases each of breast cancer, colon and rectal cancers and diabetes mellitus, and about 22% of ischaemic heart disease.

The effects of exposure to disadvantageous environments accumulate throughout life. Slow growth in childhood (short stature for age) is an indicator of early disadvantage. Some of the highest levels of adult obesity in the world are found in the Pacific islands. Obesity rates vary from around 2% to 3% in the adults living in the highlands of Papua New Guinea to about 80% in Nauru.

In general, obesity is a bigger problem among urban dwellers than among people who live in the countryside and is more prevalent in women than men. Usually, older adults have the highest rates of obesity, however, in some Pacific communities, obesity rates peak at around 35 years of age. This trend has serious consequences for future health.

A major study has shown that women who are obese at 18 years and continue to gain weight in adulthood are 70 times more likely to develop type 2 diabetes than those who remain lean. Information about the status of children's weight in the Pacific is limited.

Surveys that have examined children's growth show that 2% to 23% of children under five years of age in certain Pacific communities have mild to moderate undernutrition and that 2% to 30% of children can be considered overweight or obese.

A survey conducted in 2002 by a team from the WHO Regional Office for the Western Pacific in 27 primary schools of 13 Pacific countries found that prevalence of thinness, or wasting in children >5% was only found in Fiji, while rates of overweight >5% were found in at least one of the schools studied, in nine of 13 countries (70%). There is thus evidence that, at least from school-age, children are already affected by the obesity epidemic in many Pacific countries.

A review of diet, the food supply and obesity in the Pacific was commissioned by the WHO Regional Office for the Western Pacific for a consultation on Food Safety and Quality in the Pacific, held with FAO and SPC in Fiji in November 2002. This review noted that before European contact, the food behaviour of Pacific people may have remained the same for millennia.

Upon European contact, Pacific people were described as strong, muscular and mostly in good health. In recent decades, however, locally produced foods have been largely replaced by foreign imports. Urban families have adopted different cooking methods. The review identified five factors responsible for increasing obesity:

(1) increased urbanization;

(2) higher fat/energy diets;

(3) decreased physical activity levels;

(4) inappropriate government policies; and

(5) new food trade patterns.

The most frequently imported foods providing fat were identified as oil, margarine, butter, meat and chicken, tinned meat and tinned fish. The majority of countries have increased availability of meat, vegetable oils, alcohol and milk. The largest single providers of energy for Pacific countries are cereal products.

However, the largest single increase has been the availability of vegetable oils. The review of dietary studies shows that imported fat has been added to the food supply. The largest single increase in meat products has been the importation of chicken meat. Obesity, consumption of imported foods and reduced physical activity seem to be largely an urban phenomenon in the Pacific.

Diets that consist of locally produced foods have been shown to prevent and reduce obesity. However, Pacific countries have become dependent on food imports, even though most are able to produce a wide variety of food crops. In summary, it appears that the best options to control increasing obesity rates to achieve better local control over the food supply and food distribution through appropriate food policies, regulation and legislation.

Efficient, aggressive and focused marketing, together with better control of the food supply, can increase the market share of local foods and make them the preferred option for consumers. Other issues to be addressed through interventions include cultural factors that favour overeating, such as feasting; for example, in connection with religious services, when large amounts of food are eaten and little or no physical activity occurs. Hunting and gathering, which require physical activity, are perceived by some as being only for the poor.

A common problem in some Pacific islands is the presence of aggressive dogs that discourage walking in the streets. In addition to promoting healthier dietary patterns, it is necessary to explore and promote all opportunities for increasing physical activity in the four main domains of daily life: at work, in transport, domestic duties and leisure time.

Barriers to be overcome in this case relate to changes in lifestyle due to technological advancement, leading to widespread use of labour and energy saving devices in all the above areas of daily life, as well as reduced time and lack of suitable physical spaces for recreation and exercise (parks, pedestrian lanes, etc.), especially in urban environments.

The Roundtable on Diet, Physical Activity and Health held at the WHO Regional Committee Meeting in Kyoto in 2002 discussed in considerable depth the issues, barriers and possible solutions related to nutrition-related NCDs in the Western Pacific Region.

It was recognized that: increasing consumption of vegetables and fruit, reducing salt intake, and decreasing the amount (while improving the quality) of fat consumed are the most important dietary measures for preventing both cardio-vascular diseases and cancers; and.- maintaining normal body weight and engaging in physical activity throughout the life span are the most effective ways of preventing diabetes and other chronic diseases.

Since schools provide unique opportunities to improve knowledge and behaviours, and to reach out to families and communities, Health-Promoting School programmes are proposed as a key channel for action area, "improving the environment to promote healthier diets and lifestyles."

Surveillance is proposed as a fifth action area, cutting across all programmes, to assess the size and distribution of problems and to monitor/evaluate the results of programme implementation. National plans of action for nutrition (NPANs) and national food and nutrition policies (NFNPs) are the main mechanisms through which nutrition programmes are planned and implemented in countries.

Most countries have NPANs and/or NFNPs, however, some lack both the political commitment and human resources to implement them. Only one country has legislation drawn up to enforce nutrition standards on food imports, while other countries have legislation, but often this is not enforced. In general, there is limited coordination among sectors that can play a role in obesity prevention; there are unclear responsibilities and insufficient sharing of experiences.

The Consultation on Food Safety and Quality held in Nadi, Fiji examined opportunities for Pacific island countries to use the existing Agreement on Agriculture, the Agreement on Technical Barriers to Trade and the World Trade Organization (WTO) Agreements to promote and protect national food security and health, by adopting regulatory approaches, including on food import and export, appropriate to the situation of each country.

WHO is considering how this process can be supported. Pricing policies and subsidies can be effective ways of promoting the production and consumption of certain foods and of discouraging the use of others. Similarly, policies can be developed to make environments conducive to healthy lifestyles, by making walking, cycling and exercising easy and safe; ensuring daily physical activity programmes in schools; through workplace policies supporting physical activity breaks; promoting exercise through traditional practices and sports.

Dietary and eating patterns of school-age children should be reviewed to explore how governments can best support programmes that ensure proper food intake at home, through school canteens, healthy tuck shops, community-based feeding programmes or other mechanisms. National policies on health, agriculture, development, education, town planning, housing, transport, tourism, marketing and media use, human resources, should all consider how they could contribute to promoting healthier diets and lifestyles.

Health impact assessment should become an integral policy requirement for all major planning and development processes, correcting the misconception that public health is the concern of health ministries alone. To promote healthy diets and lifestyles, particularly in children and young people, strategic partnerships must be built:

— across all levels of government, industry and other nongovernmental sectors;

— involving grocery organizations, school canteens, fast-food outlets, etc.; and

— especially with the food industry, pointing to common interests and avoiding confrontation, as much as possible.

At the same time, laws and regulations must be created and implemented to restrict commercial food advertising to children. Links with other programme areas should be sought, for example, avoidance of smoking, excessive alcohol consumption and substance abuse. The global drive towards the promotion of healthy lifestyles is certainly making some progress, but not in all societies and across all strata in each society. There are barriers to be overcome to bridge the gap between knowledge and its application.

At the personal level, clearly there are many who do not have about health diets and lifestyles and therefore are not in a position to adopt it. But even for those who have the knowledge needed, there appears to be inertia or lack of motivation to practise it. At the community level, barriers to implementation include lack of conviction, contrarian interests (political and economic), inadequate resources, and criteria used in priority setting for resource allocation.

Health authorities must find strategies to bridge these gaps. A facilitating factor for undertaking positive lifestyle changes is that they can be integrated into the lives of most people by making relatively minor adjustments to daily routines. The World Health Report 2002 emphasizes that much greater benefits in disease reduction derive from small positive changes achieved in a large part of the population, than from large changes achieved in a small proportion of people at higher risk.

At an individual level, what is required is the personal decision to make the change, the commitment to see it through, and the motivation to sustain it. Examples of specific ways and means of raising awareness and providing the conditions needed for change are given below:

Health policy makers should provide living examples of what they are advocating. If important and busy people like them can make the behavioural change, it will certainly motivate others. Other important role models can be sport celebrities, national personalities, etc. Health promotion activities should be integrated into particularly important are because almost the whole population in most countries attends school, and schools can provide not only knowledge but also the environment to practise healthy diets and lifestyles.

Schools can also be a great channel for reaching out to families and the community with messages on health, and of involving them in translating these messages into practice. Creative communication strategies should be developed to promote healthy diets and lifestyle through the mass media; providing awards and prizes, or other incentives for particularly good health promotion programmes and initiatives.

Food labelling and product information should be used extensively to promote consumer education; laws and regulations on food labelling can help ensure that this useful tool is properly used. Traditional healthy cooking techniques and recipes should be promoted and made popular through the use of media, schools and other channels such as religious organizations; cooking demonstrations provide an opportunity to learn to prepare traditional healthy foods as well as suitable new recipes from other parts of the world.

Promoting healthier diets through improved environments means increasing the availability and affordability of healthy foods. The barriers to be overcome in Pacific island countries and areas include:

— The cost of foods that are less healthy (e.g. imported turkey tails, mutton and lamb flaps, canned fish, fried foods) is often lower than that of healthier ones (fresh fish, lean meat, some fruits and vegetables, foods cooked with little or no oil or fat).

— The availability and accessibility of some foods of lower nutritional quality may be greater than those of healthier more nutritious foods.

— The time to prepare some less healthy foods may be shorter than that needed to prepare healthier foods.

— Some less healthy foods are associated in some cultures with higher social status, as is the ability to afford larger portions, to eat more, and to achieve a large body size.

— Some imported foods, though less healthy, are considered desirable because they are the product of technologically more advanced and economically affluent societies (e.g., "fast foods" from Western countries, such as foods produced from highly refined cereals, and foods high in fat, salt, added sugar, and low in micronutrients and fibre) as opposed to traditional foods; and breastmilk substitutes, as opposed to mother's milk; it is thus necessary to change the image and values associated with healthy traditional foods.

Changing the environment with regard to food means adopting agricultural policies, import/export policies, pricing policies that favour the production and consumption of healthy foods over less healthy ones; ensuring the availability of safe water and fresh coconut juice, instead of soft drinks; taxes on soft drinks have been successfully introduced in some countries, and can be applied also to other less nutritionally valuable drinks and foods.

There is evidence that one hour a day or more of physical activity is effective in reducing body fat and improving fitness. These results are maintained when the programme is continued over a two-year period; and academic performance is not adversely affected by the reduction in daily formal teaching time; and establishing or reviewing school lunch and healthy snacks programmes.

Health services have an essential role both in preventing and managing obesity and related NCDs. WHO is supporting programmes for the prevention and control of obesity, initially in two Pacific countries, with plans to progressively support additional countries. Creative strategies for promoting physical activity through clinics and other settings include periodic physical fitness tests (in medical facilities, but also in schools and workplaces) and written prescriptions for physical activity from general practitioners.

Within the lifecycle, key ages for screening need to be identified based on the stage of the "obesity epidemic" and aiming to identify overweight subjects as early as possible. With regard to the assessment and monitoring of food production, food imports/exports and food availability, while some data is available, gaps are widespread: food import data, for example, may be available, but often are not properly collected and collated for easy access.

3

Food and Dietary Suppliments

Nutrient content claims are statements such as "rich in ..." or "low in ...". Such claims can also easily give the impression that use of the product is healthy and reduces the risk of developing certain diseases. Health effects from foods or dietary supplements do not normally occur in everyone. Their occurrence depends partly on factors such as lifestyle, including the consumption of other substances, sex and other genetic factors.

The reporting of a claim that does not specify the target group is incomplete and therefore misleading. In the assessment of claims, account should be taken of any adverse effects that a product may have. It would improve the clarity of the system for the business community, the government and consumers if the same agency were responsible for assessing both the safety and health effects of foods and dietary supplements.

So-called "health products" also fall within the scope of this definition. All foods have some nutritional value or function, and one of the functions of any food is to satisfy the consumer's need to eat. A "functional food" is often defined as a food with a health benefit beyond its nutritional value. However, nutritional value itself also causes health benefits; a distinction is difficult to make. Another phrase in use is "specific health-promoting foods/ingredients".

This is used to refer to a category of specific ingredients with specific health-promoting properties. However, this phrase is also not particularly distinctive, since ingredients such as vitamins and certain fats are also "specific" and have "specific" properties. A claim regarding a health benefit is a commercial translation of (frequently already established) nutritional knowledge.

The precise definition of a "health benefit" is still the subject of some debate. There is scientific evidence to support the contention that the consumption of some foods and dietary supplements can, subject to certain conditions, reduce the risk of particular diseases.

For example, vitamins and minerals can prevent deficiency diseases. Energy intake influences the risk of obesity, and therefore has an effect on the risk of cardiovascular disease, diabetes mellitus and other conditions. Dietary fats and fibres influence the risk of cardiovascular disease.

The use of potassium salt instead of sodium salt can lower blood pressure. Adequate intake of folic acid by pregnant women can reduce the likelihood of foetal neural tube defects. The replacement of sugar by sugaralcohols can reduce the risk of dental caries. Increased calcium and vitamin D consumption can bring down the risk of osteoporosis and bone fracture.

Many people's diets are less than ideal in relation to the consumption of the above-mentioned substances. Under the present circumstances, the greatest public health benefits are likely to be attainable through the consumption of products that utilise these already demonstrated effects of diet on health.

People who start using a product with a health claim may change their consumption of other products. The ultimate effect of using the product with the health claim therefore depends partly on the effects of these other dietary changes.

Some people fear that consumers may feel that, as long as they are using "healthy" products, it does not matter what else they eat. However, there is no evidence that health claims tempt people to adopt "unhealthy" unbalanced diets.

In fact, it appears that the main users of products with health claims are the people who already have "the healthiest" eating habits. The traditional view is that one should not focus on individual products, but always on the overall diet. However, it is only possible to decide whether someone's overall diet is "healthy" by assessing the individual components of that diet and deciding how "healthy" each is.

Consumers are often unaware that the health claims made for food and dietary supplements usually occur only in a - small - part of the population. Beneficiaries may be limited to a group with particular dietary habits or with certain characteristics, of which some may be genetically determined. Products with health claims are more likely to be used by people with relatively healthy lifestyles. These are people who are relatively moderate users of alcohol and tobacco, who exercise more than most, who have relatively healthy diets and whose bodyweight is generally appropriate.

The users of such products also tend to have higher education and higher incomes. The government, healthcare organisations, food producers and retailers all try to encourage consumers to use, or use more of, certain products. One of the conditions for success in this field is a higher level of consumer awareness of the ways that foods and dietary supplements can influence health.

Meanwhile, dieticians - and, to a lesser extent, GPs and other doctors - seek to increase their clients'/patients' understanding of the effects of diet on health. And the producers and retailers of foods and dietary supplements provide product information and create advertising. The use of beneficial substances can also be promoted - or the use of undesirable substances reduced - by modifying industrial food production processes.

Such modifications to industrially produced foods and dietary supplements are desirable only if their effect is beneficial for a substantial proportion of the population. Since 1997, the producers of foods and dietary supplements that meet the definition of a "novel food" have been obliged to demonstrate that their products are safe before introducing them to the European market.

In the Netherlands a Committee of the Health Council assesses such safety dossiers. Some novel foods are accompanied by health claims. The Committee refers to such products as "foods with specific bio-active components". The recommendations of the Committee are as follows:

1) Research into safety biomarkers should be performed.
2) A system for monitoring food-related health symptoms should be developed and implemented.
3) Make it possible to trace genetically modified ingredients and bioactive components down to the level of use by the individual consumer.
4) Food consumption research in Europe should be harmonised.

However, most of the foods and dietary supplements with health claims are not so new that the above-mentioned safety assessment applies. Many of the products with health claims are foods enriched with vitamins or other nutrients (whose properties have long been known), or products in pharmaceutical form that contain such nutrients. When developing a stance on the safety of foods and dietary supplements, it is instructive to consider how the safety of medicinal products is controlled.

Three categories of adverse effect are recognised for medicinal products. First, there are those associated with use that is defined as "normal". Second, there are the consequences of use at a level that is not sufficient to bring about the intended effect of the product. Such consequences are disadvantageous insofar as opportunities for prevention, therapy or cure are missed. Furthermore, "under-dosing" with antibiotics may also cause bacteria to become resistant to the antibiotic. Third, there are the toxic effects of excessive use. It is worth noting in this context that the "therapeutic width" of a medicinal product is typically narrower than the range of intake levels at which a food or food ingredient is both fully effective and safe.

When a medicinal product is assessed, its beneficial effect (efficacy) is weighed up against the risk of adverse effects. In contrast, assessment of the adverse effects of a food or dietary supplement is quite separate from the assessment of any claim that may be made regarding its beneficial effects. The background to this separation is that a food or dietary supplement with a health claim is first and foremost a food or dietary supplement, which must be safe in order to comply with the Commodities Act.

However, it is never possible to exclude the possibility that a - new or established - product has adverse effects. This principle seems to be accepted by the community at large. In the Committee's view, it is acceptable for a food or dietary supplement to have a minorextent) a certain degree of enrichment of a given product is liable to lead to overdosing. One possible way of managing the overdose risk would be to permit successive applicants to enrich their products until a point is reached where estimates suggest that the further availability of enriched products is liable to create an unacceptable overdose risk.

It is also possible to ensure that the packaging of enriched products carries warnings about the danger of consuming multiple products enriched with the same substance. This is already the case with, for example, sorbitol-containing products. A dilemma exists in this field. On the one hand, concentrations of substances foods are enriched with need to be kept low enough to avoid the risk of overdosing. On the other hand, they need to be high enough to sufficiently increase consumption levels and thus to achieve the desired health benefits.

The task of striking the right balance is complicated by great variation between individuals in terms of (a) the amount and dose of enriched products consumed and (b) their nutritional needs and the amount of a nutrient they can safely consume. Furthermore, for many substances the levels of intake at which risks arise are not known.

Market monitoring is another potential approach to detecting adverse effects. As indicated above, it is possible to use food consumption data to estimate the risk of overdosing associated with the proposed enrichment of established food types with familiar nutrients (for which safe upper consumption limits are known). However, where novel ingredients and products are concerned (whether health benefits are claimed or not), it is often unclear how much can be consumed before the risk of adverse effects becomes unacceptable.

Furthermore, the usual small scale and short duration of the pre-market research studies carried out for food products may cause adverse effects to go undetected until after market introduction. After all, there is then a larger group of people using the product, often for an extended period. It is therefore important to monitor the situation carefully following the introduction of a product to market.

By means of market monitoring, it is possible to discern, for example, the effects of the concurrent use of products containing the same ingredient, the effects of interactions, the products' long-term effects and the groups at increased risk of experiencing certain effects.

A health claim is a claim relating to "the promotion or maintenance of health", and is permissible in connection with foods and dietary supplements. Medical claims concern "the prevention, treatment and cure of disease". A medical claim may be made only in connection with a medicinal product; making such a claim for a food or dietary supplement is against the law. Legally speaking, the distinction is clear: if a claim refers to a disease, it is a medical claim. In scientific and practical terms, however, there is overlap.

In the Committee's view, there is no scientific or practical difference between the maintenance of health (the subject of a health claim) and the prevention of disease (which may be the subject of a medical claim only). The view within the business community and the European Commission is that claims regarding the reduction of the risk of disease differ materially from claims regarding the prevention of disease.

However, prevention entails the reduction of risk, and only rarely a reduction to zero. The overlap between foods and medicines has been recognised before. Both foods and medicines can have a beneficial influence on disease risk factors and can therefore reduce the risk of disease (sometimes by the same mechanisms), similar to any effort aimed at disease prevention. There is at best a graduated distinction: the effects of medicines are often stronger than those of foods.

A medical claim would then still be distinct from any other claim in that it refers to the treatment or cure of a disease. However, such a move would have the legal consequence that, for example, vaccines and cholesterol-lowering products no longer come within the scope of medical legislation. According to Kabel, the prohibition on making medical claims for foods or dietary supplements is an extension of the prohibition to mislead.

The underlying logic is that a claim that suggests that an edible or potable commodity is a medicine is inherently misleading, even if otherwise correct, "because a foodstuff is not a medicine". It should always be up to a medical doctor, the argument runs, to determine whether indications are present that make the use of a medicine appropriate and safe.

However, this notion has to some extent been overtaken by the development of non-prescription medicines. The law also prohibits the use of medical claims in marketing on the grounds that it is illegal to play upon fears of disease or infirmity or to give the impression that a product is genuinely curative by making apparently scientific claims. It is common for public information material to draw attention to the influence of certain forms of behaviour - diet, physical exercise and smoking - on the risk of disease, and this is generally considered acceptable.

However, an important difference is that advertising involving health claims has a commercial dimension. Making and being allowed to make a claim in such a context brings a potential commercial benefit; this is not the case where public information material is concerned. Nevertheless, building up and retaining consumer confidence is important both in relation to public information and to product marketing.

A claim to the effect that a product influences a particular factor can give the impression that use of the product reduces the likelihood of developing a certain disease. If this impression is correct, it is better to state explicitly that the product has this health benefit. If this impression is not correct, the claim is irrelevant and therefore misleading.

The Committee shares the view expressed elsewhere that the distinction between the enhancement of bodily functions and the reduction of disease risk is vague. It is likely that disease prevention is the only reason for seeking many functional enhancements. Conversely, any claimed functional enhancement that does not contribute to disease prevention is often of dubious value.

Sometimes, however, a claims made regarding a functional enhancement that is beneficial or desirable in its own right. Examples of this are claims regarding improved mental concentration (e.g. by caffeine), increased endurance, and greater muscle bulk development through strength training.

Nevertheless, it is frequently unclear or at least dubious whether and, if so, to what extent a claimed effect may actually be deemed advantageous. Often, claims regarding functional enhancement give the unspecified impression that the product in question is "healthy", and therefore "healthier" than other - otherwise similar - products.

Depending on how knowledgeable they are, consumers may also obtain the impression that use of such a product reduces a disease risk. This impression is not correct in all cases, and in those cases the claim is misleading. Consideration may be given to allowing claims only concerning products that have a demonstrable advantage over generally similar products for which no such claim is made.

US and Dutch researchers have also found that, depending on the consumer knowledge about nutrition and depending on the substance or foodstuff in question, such claims can give the additional impression that the products reduce the risk of developing a particular disease or condition. Producers have a (commercial) interest in fostering such impressions.

Another US study has shown - consumers tend not to look further than the front of a pack bearing a claim; objective data such as that presented in the table of nutritional information on the back of the pack goes unread. This may - to some extent - be compensated given that many consumers view claims primarily as sales pitches, and place more faith in the table of nutrition content. The situation with regard to "synonym claims" is very similar.

A synonym claim is a variation on the nutrient content claim, utilising the idea that one ingredient is comparable to another, and is therefore expected to have a similar effect. The Committee believes that consumers would be better informed if producers were able to couch claims regarding health benefits in explicit terms, i.e. to state directly that a product can reduce the risk of a particular disease or condition.

The validity of any such claim should of course be scientifically demonstrable. Here applies as well that where no explicit health claim can be made or justified, the Committee believes that a nutrient content claim is misleading. In Sweden, eight claims regarding the reduction of disease risks have been permitted since 1990, on the condition that they are formulated in two steps.

Many diseases are influenced by several risk factors. Whether a given individual actually contracts a disease depends on the combined effect of all these factors. Furthermore, risk factors themselves are usually determined by a number of factors. Coppens et al. asserted that disease risk reduction is essentially different from disease prevention. They argued that disease risk reduction relates to diseases of which the onset is determined by multiple risk factors, and that there is no guarantee that the disease will not occur. The same is true, however, with regard to the "prevention" of a disease by medicinal treatment.

If, for example, one brings down a patient's blood pressure by prescribing medication, his or her risk of suffering a stroke will be reduced. Whether or not the patient eventually suffers from a stroke is, however, uncertain, and does not depend on blood pressure alone but on many other factors as well. However accurate it may be, a claim to the effect that a product influences a factor or function in the body is often irrelevant if it does not - eventually - reduce the risk of developing a disease.

So, for example, reducing a person's cholesterol level is of importance only because scientific data render it sufficiently plausible that this reduces the risk of cardiovascular disease. Similarly, developing and maintaining strong bones is useful only because it reduces the risk of bone fracture. One may consider the evidence to support the effects of cholesterol levels on the risk of cardiovascular disease and of strengthening bones on fracture risk as insufficient.

In that case, the evidence to support the existence of a benefit for consumers would be equally insufficient. Under such circumstances, it would be misleading to refer to cholesterol reduction or bone strengthening as "the maintenance or promotion of health". If, however, one does consider an effect on a disease risk sufficiently plausible, claiming that a product has this effect is - implicitly—claiming that it contributes to disease prevention.

Like a nutrient content claim, a risk factor claim can - depending on how knowledgeable the consumer is - give the impression that the use of a product reduces a disease risk. If this impression can be specified and supported by evidence, it is preferable that the risk-reducing properties of the product be explicitly stated.

The link with disease risk reduction is not relevant in relation to claims regarding effects that may reasonably be supposed to be inherently beneficial or desirable, e.g. increased powers of concentration or the development of greater muscle bulk through strength training.

If a product brings about a very slight reduction in blood pressure in a large number of people, some cases of stroke may be prevented, even though the reduction in risk for the individual consumer is not particularly significant. Where familiar nutrients are concerned, it is important that a producer states on the product packaging what percentage of the recommended daily intake can be obtained from a portion of the product concerned.

A producer should not make a health claim based on the effect of a substance present in the product in small quantities, if a large amount of that substance is required to be effective. Anybody charged with the assessment of claims must consider not only the statistical validity of a claim, but also its practical relevance. However, the situation is complicated by the fact that health benefits are not easy to quantify. Health claims do not remain valid indefinitely and periodic reassessment is therefore desirable.

Nutrition and Population

Health status is a fundamental element of well-being. Health improvements for the poor can improve outcomes for everyone because of the nature of illnesses (widespread communicable diseases among the poor raise risks for everyone) and the nature of interventions, many of which have benefits for everyone (such as immunizations and environmental health interventions).

Health, population, and nutrition inputs can improve outcomes, but so do activities in other sectors. Education, the environment, availability of roads, and safe water supplies also contribute to better health, so achieving goals for the poor depends in part on actions in these other sectors. Within the health sector, appropriate interventions in population and nutrition also contribute independently by increasing the impact and substituting for health service interventions.

The ultimate aim of the health component of the poverty-reduction strategy is to improve health outcomes-especially among the poor and vulnerable. The first stage in formulating such a strategy is an assessment of the current situation.

Population averages often mask large differences within countries between different poverty groups. Bolivia, Kenya and India, for example, all have roughly the same under-five mortality rate-around 108 per 1000 live births.

In Bolivia, the under-five mortality rate among the poorest fifth of households is nearly five times that among the richest fifth. In India, there is a threefold gap between the richest and poorest fifths of households, while in Kenya there is a twofold gap.

In India and Kenya, targeting the bottom two-fifths of the households via a set of interventions appropriate to their main constraints might be effective. The concept of health is a broad one. It embraces not just mortality but also health status, nutritional status, morbidity, management of fertility, and disability. It embraces not just the health of young children but also the health of older children and adults.

It also embraces reproductive health-the health of women during and after pregnancy, and unwanted pregnancies. A useful way of organizing a health assessment is to think in terms of the lifecycle, which starts in pregnancy, and moves through birth, infancy, childhood, the school years, adolescence, adulthood and aging, including the reproductive period.

In the reproductive period, the lifecycle comes full circle, with pregnancy and the birth of a new generation.

A Conceptual Framework for Improving the Health of the Poor

This framework highlights four principles:

— Health interventions have a cumulative impact-the benefit, nature, and cost of interventions at a later age is partially dependent on earlier interventions.

— Prioritizing interventions at several points across the life cycle is necessary for sustaining improvements in health outcomes.

— Interventions in one generation bring benefits to successive generations. The most obvious of these are good prenatal care and programs that help teenage girls delay pregnancy, both of which give babies a healthier start in life,

— The approach also facilitates identification of key risks for families and associated gaps in the health system, where interventions can break the cycle of poverty and ill health.

At each stage of the lifecycle, there are risks to health, and associated with each is a corresponding outcome indicator. For example, during the first year of life (infancy), there are risks of illness, poor nutrition, slow growth and development, and even death. The factors that have a direct influence on health outcomes, such as health service utilization, dietary and sanitary practices, and lifestyle, are not a fixture. They vary widely across countries.

In Uganda 70% of infants are exclusively breastfed; in Senegal only 9% are. The factors influencing health outcomes also vary widely within countries, especially between poor and nonpoor households. In Burkina Faso, for example, poor children are less than a third as likely as rich children to be delivered by a medically trained person.

When they have diarrhea, they are only half as likely to be treated with oral rehydration therapy, and they are less than a third as likely to receive a full course of childhood immunizations. The second stage in understanding poor health outcomes is to measure the factors that have a direct influence on them for different economic groups. For many of the factors directly influencing maternal and child health (MCH) outcomes. Households vary in the resources they have at their disposal, including financial income and assets, and other physical assets (such as land and animals) that together make up their wealth.

Low levels of wealth, but especially of wealth that can easily be converted into cash, are a major constraint for poor households in times of illness and crisis. Also important are the human assets in the household-knowledge, literacy, and education. Knowledge about health issues is especially important.

Lack of knowledge, which is especially common in poor households, often leaves them unaware of available opportunities. In many societies, there is an unequal balance of power within households between men and women. Women may have little control over household finances and play a minor role in decisions concerning the use of contraceptives to prevent unwanted pregnancy and condoms to prevent sexually-transmitted infections. Mothers may be constrained in the household when seeking health care for themselves or their children.

This unequal power, which may be more pronounced in poorer, less educated households, is an important risk factor for poor reproductive health outcomes and the poor diet of many women. One task is to establish, for the country preparing the PRSP, the importance of household-level factors that influence households' utilization of health services, their dietary and sanitary practices, and their lifestyle. Not only do these factors affect the success of interventions, but they may merit being the focus of interventions.

Many surveys also contain some information on health-specific knowledge-e.g. on knowledge of HIV/ AIDS issues. Of special importance here are levels of general education and health-specific knowledge among women and girls. Demographic and Health Surveys (DHS) and knowledge, attitudes, and practices surveys contain a wealth of information about beliefs, behaviours, and formal education.

Community variables, the environment, and infrastructure matter too. Community variables are often bound up in cultural norms and social capital. Environmental influences include indoor and outdoor pollution that damage health. Good sanitary practices, for example, are harder to follow if the water and sanitation conditions in the community are poor.

Respiratory problems are common where fires burn inside poorly ventilated homes for cooking and heat. Infrastructure affects accessibility: getting to a health centre is much harder if the roads are impassible during the rainy season. In these respects, the poor are often disadvantaged. They tend to live in remote areas where the roads become impassable at certain times of the year and on the edges of cities that are not reached by public services.

They are least likely to live in areas with piped water, good sanitary systems, and all-weather roads. In fact, the most binding health constraint might be the lack of infrastructure, especially transport. Management across sectors to coordinate and stage scarce investments-possibly in roads as the highest priority, for example, and health services that conform to the availability of transport-can raise the impact of investments.

Health sector strategies also need to be sensitive to changes in infrastructure. Communities share values and norms that play a large part in shaping health behaviours. Poor communities are often traditional communities, so values, norms, and cultural gaps are key factors affecting their health. Traditional social norms often impede women's access to resources such as land, extension services, credit, and education, which limits their capacity to engage in productive work, to seek health care, and to devote time and energy to child care.

Better reproductive health, along with empowerment of women and their partners to manage fertility, are interventions that must fit into cultural and social norms, but also can help women break through some of the cultural barriers they face. Different ethnic groups have different values, norms, and beliefs. These too often have both poverty and gender dimensions. Female genital cutting, for example, is determined largely by the existence of a cultural norm.

Health programs, however, do not always respond appropriately to differences in norms and values. In the Andes, for example, some poor indigenous populations believe that a child should be born in a warm room; as a result, they are less likely to use modern maternity hospitals. The response of health authorities has often been to teach Indian women the correct modern practices rather than to work with them to make the safer environment more hospitable to them.

Community influences on household behaviours often operate indirectly through the institutions in communities, such as community health services, but also civic associations, such as youth clubs and women's groups that can mobilize community action for better health and nutrition. The term "social capital" is sometimes used to describe the norms and networks that facilitate collective action-such as the setting-up of a community nutrition program.

There are three key layers of social capital: ties within the community ("bonding"), relations between members of different communities ("bridging"), and connections between communities and formal institutions ("linking"). The poor-as both a cause and consequence of their condition-typically have a lot of the first, a moderate amount of the second, and very little of the third.

Health promotion interventions, such as health education units of Ministries of Health and Information, Education and Communication (IEC) components of projects, are not always effectively designed and implemented. These factors operate by altering the utilization of health services or by directly affecting outcomes when services are used. The following are some of the key determinants of health system performance in increasing utilization by the poor:

— *Physical accessibility*: Are the health activities delivered, or are they available, sufficiently close to the poor so that they can make use of them? While this question is usually addressed by measuring the size of the catchment area of health facilities (e.g., the percent of the population living less than 5 or 10 km from a health facility) many other factors can also play a role. Poor households tend to be located at the periphery of the area; if roads are missing a relatively short distance is not always an indication of easy access. In Africa and many other places, to consider the seasonal variation of physical accessibility may also be important.

— *Availability of essential inputs*: Services may be geographically accessible, but essential inputs, such as drugs, vaccines, contraceptives, micro-nutrients or trained staff, may be unavailable or in short supply part of the time.

— *Organizational quality*: The way health services are organized may deter patients from using services. Important characteristics in this respect are the hours of operation and availability to patients, waiting time required to be seen by medical personnel, and the gender of health providers. Other factors affect users' perceptions of the quality of services, including a lack of courtesy on the part of health personnel, conditioning service availability on under-the-table payments, lack of sensitivity to cultural differences, and showing more respect to better off clients.

— *Overcoming household barriers to use*: Typically the needs will be greater among the poor for activities such as outreach services than they are among the better off, to overcome the environmental, infrastructure, and cultural barriers.

— *Timing and continuity*: Certain health services-such as emergency obstetric and surgical care but also epidemic control measures-must be delivered in a timely manner. For other services, such as the completion of tuberculosis treatment or immunizations, continuity is an essential determinant of efficacy and outcome improvement.

— *Technical quality*: If the services are not of good technical quality, either because of the quality of inputs or provider training, health outcomes are not likely to improve despite good utilization and appropriate timing.

— *Social accountability*: Although mechanisms to allow the user to participate in decisions taken in health facilities have been developed, more often than not these are far from perfect, and the poorer client's voice is rarely heard.

The concept of health is a broad one. It embraces not just mortality but also health status, nutritional status, morbidity, management of fertility, and disability. It embraces not just the health of young children but also the health of older children and adults.

It also embraces reproductive health-the health of women during and after pregnancy, and unwanted pregnancies. A useful way of organizing a health assessment is to think in terms of the lifecycle, which starts in pregnancy, and moves through birth, infancy, childhood, the school years, adolescence, adulthood and aging, including the reproductive period.

Some countries have attempted to orient the reform of the health sector towards better serving the poor. They used a matrix of health sector performance. In Benin, for example, reforms in health systems in 1989 provided the basis for a positive trend in most health indicators. Infant mortality dropped from 114 per thousand in 1987 to 88 per thousand in 1996, exceeding the drop in neighbouring countries that were at comparable levels of household consumption.

Many developing and middle-income countries have developed "core packages," which define health interventions to be available at the village (health post), community (health center), and district levels (district hospital). These packages respond in a cost effective manner to the needs of the poorest segments of the population, and represent priority activities for public financing.

The mix of providers-public, private, non-governmental (or charitable)-and their respective policies influence the performance of the sector towards the poor. The poor may use private, traditional, or charitable services as much or more than public services. The availability of drugs affects the clinical quality of health services, costs, and perceptions of clients. Problems with procurement, costly support for local production of pharmaceuticals, and corruption lead many poor countries to pay several times more for drugs, vaccines, and contraceptives than would be paid through international competitive bidding.

Over-prescribing of drugs and poor drug and vaccines stock management lead to wastage, as does inadequate maintenance of equipment and vehicles. Key aspects to be assessed include selection, procurement, distribution, pricing, and quality. Development and management of human resources: The quality, distribution, and responsiveness of health personnel influence availability, quality, and access to interventions by the poor.

In today's mixed public, private, and charitable systems of provision and financing, the government has a central role in using mandates, regulation, incentives, subsidies, and information to influence the behaviour of providers and consumers to achieve better health outcomes. Where public provision has historically been the key public sector role, this powerful tools has been more or less ignored in the past.

For the health system, it will mean moving supply-side subsidies into means-tested subsidies for insurance and prepayment. The entire cost of a well-functioning public system, including public health, preventive services, research, and information; hospital and clinic services, including contracts with other providers; and subsidies for insurance should be explicitly considered in the budget.

Revenues and expenditures in the health sector must be considered jointly. All public health, health education, preventive, and promotive services should be subsidized to the fullest extent possible, given government budget constraints. If they cannot be fully subsidized, policies should be pursued to encourage charitable activities in these areas.

Given the typical resource-constrained public budget, user fees will be necessary for acute services. They should be designed not to create barriers at the point of use for the poor, however, by using waivers, prepayment, credit, or other options. The highest priority should be attached to providing health-specific knowledge through government financing to help the poor prevent and manage health problems.

Knowledge to consumers that can improve their ability to choose providers and consume appropriate services is crucial, given the importance of household behaviour in determining outcomes. Education-especially women's education-is a key of all health, nutrition, and population outcomes. Better educated women, holding constant household income, tend to adopt behaviours that are, on balance, better for these outcomes than less well educated women.

In Cebu, Philippines, for example, it has been estimated that a one-year increase in maternal education reduced the probability of exclusive breast-feeding by 36% and the probability of any breast-feeding by 5%. But it increased the number of calories by 7%, the use of preventive health services by 4%, and the use of soap by 2%. It reduced the probability of poor excreta disposal by 9%.

Overall, these changes were estimated to bring about a 3.2% reduction in the probability of diarrhea at age six months-a 5.2% reduction due to increased calories, preventive care use and better excreta disposal, offset by a 2% increase due to reduced breast-feeding.

In the poorest countries, total government resources spent on health are usually no more than $3 to $5 per capita, and private spending adds roughly the same amount, for a total of $6 to $10 per capita. For the highly indebted countries, debt forgiveness can open some space to add possibly another 20 percent to public health expenditures.

Health system performance issues in the public and private sectors are partially affected by public expenditure policies but also depend on policies that affect the incentive structure for and quality of personnel; the form and use of contracts in the system to deliver services; the institutional environment; the quality of management; and the regulatory regime.

4

Changing Lifestyle and Chronic Diseases

Diet and nutrition are important factors in the promotion and maintenance of good health throughout the entire life course. Their role as determinants of chronic NCDs is well established and they therefore occupy a prominent position in prevention activities. The burden of chronic diseases is rapidly increasing worldwide. It has been calculated that, in 2001, chronic diseases contributed approximately 60% of the 56. 5 million total reported deaths in the world and approximately 46% of the global burden of disease.

The proportion of the burden of NCDs is expected to increase to 57% by 2020. Almost half of the total chronic disease deaths are attributable to cardiovascular diseases; obesity and diabetes are also showing worrying trends, not only because they already affect a large proportion of the population, but also because they have started to appear earlier in life.

The chronic disease problem is far from being limited to the developed regions of the world. Contrary to widely held beliefs, developing countries are increasingly suffering from high levels of public health problems related to chronic diseases. In five out of the six regions of WHO, deaths caused by chronic diseases dominate the mortality statistics.

Although human immunodeficiency virus/acquired immunodeficiency syndrome (HIV/AIDS), malaria and tuberculosis, along with other infectious diseases, still predominate in sub-Saharan Africa and will do so for the foreseeable future, 79% of all deaths worldwide that are attributable to chronic diseases are already occurring in developing countries.

The earlier labelling of chronic diseases as "diseases of affluence" is increasingly a misnomer, as they emerge both in poorer countries and in the poorer population groups in richer countries. This shift in the pattern of disease is taking place at an accelerating rate; furthermore, it is occurring at a faster rate in developing countries than it did in the industrialized regions of the world half a century ago. This rapid rate of change, together with the increasing burden of disease, is creating a major public health threat which demands immediate and effective action.

It has been projected that, by 2020, chronic diseases will account for almost three-quarters of all deaths worldwide, and that 71% of deaths due to ischaemic heart disease (IHD), 75% of deaths due to stroke, and 70% of deaths due to diabetes will occur in developing countries. The number of people in the developing world with diabetes will increase by more than 2. 5-fold, from 84 million in 1995 to 228 million in 2025.

On a global basis, 60% of the burden of chronic diseases will occur in developing countries. Indeed, cardiovascular diseases are even now more numerous in India and China than in all the economically developed countries in the world put together. As for overweight and obesity, not only has the current prevalence already reached unprecedented levels, but the rate at which it is annually increasing in most developing regions is substantial. The public health implications of this phenomenon are staggering, and are already becoming apparent.

The rapidity of the changes in developing countries is such that a double burden of disease may often exist. India, for example, at present faces a combination of communicable diseases and chronic diseases, with the burden of chronic diseases just exceeding that of communicable diseases. Projections nevertheless indicate that communicable diseases will still occupy a critically important position up to 2020.

Another eloquent example is that of obesity, which is becoming a serious problem throughout Asia, Latin America and parts of Africa, despite the widespread presence of undernutrition. In some countries, the prevalence of obesity has doubled or tripled over the past decade.

Chronic diseases are largely preventable diseases. Although more basic research may be needed on some aspects of the mechanisms that link diet to health, the currently available scientific evidence provides a sufficiently strong and plausible basis to justify taking action now. Beyond the appropriate medical treatment for those already affected, the public health approach of primary prevention is considered to be the most cost-effective, affordable and sustainable course of action to cope with the chronic disease epidemic worldwide.

The adoption of a common risk-factor approach to chronic disease prevention is a major development in the thinking behind an integrated health policy. Sometimes chronic diseases are considered communicable at the risk factor level. Modern dietary patterns and physical activity patterns are risk behaviours that travel across countries and are transferable from one population to another like an infectious disease, affecting disease patterns globally.

While age, sex and genetic susceptibility are non-modifiable, many of the risks associated with age and sex are modifiable. Such risks include behavioural factors (e. g. diet, physical inactivity, tobacco use, alcohol consumption) ; biological factors (e. g. dyslipidemia, hypertension, overweight, hyper insulinaemia) ; and finally societal factors, which include a complex mixture of interacting socioeconomic, cultural and other environmental parameters.

Diet has been known for many years to play a key role as a risk factor for chronic diseases. What is apparent at the global level is that great changes have swept the entire world since the second half of the twentieth century, inducing major modifications in diet, first in industrial regions and more recently in developing countries.

Traditional, largely plant-based diets have been swiftly replaced by high-fat, energy-dense diets with a substantial content of animal-based foods. But diet, while critical to prevention, is just one risk factor. Physical inactivity, now recognized as an increasingly important determinant of health, is the result of a progressive shift of lifestyle towards more sedentary patterns, in developing countries as much as in industrialized ones.

Recent data from Sao Paulo, Brazil, for example, indicate that 70—80% of the population are remarkably inactive. The combination of these and other risk factors, such as tobacco use, is likely to have an additive or even a multiplier effect, capable of accelerating the pace at which the chronic disease epidemic is emerging in the developing countries. The need for action to strengthen control and prevention measures to counter the spread of the chronic disease epidemic is now widely recognized by many countries, but the developing countries are lagging behind in implementing such measures.

Encouragingly, however, efforts to counteract the rise in chronic diseases are increasingly being assigned a higher priority. This situation is reflected by the growing interest of Member States, the concerned international and bilateral agencies as well as nongovernmental organizations in addressing food and nutrition policy, health promotion, and strategy for the control and prevention of chronic diseases, as well as other related topics such as promoting healthy ageing and tobacco control.

The 1992 International Conference on Nutrition specifically identified the need to prevent and control the increasing public health problems of chronic diseases by promoting appropriate diets and healthy lifestyles. The need to address chronic disease prevention from a broad-based perspective was also recognized by the World Health Assembly in 1998 and again in 1999. In 2000, the World Health Assembly passed a further resolution on the broad basis of the prevention and control of noncommunicable diseases, and in 2002 adopted a resolution that urged Member States to collaborate with WHO to develop "... a global strategy on diet, physical activity and health for the prevention and control of noncommunicable diseases, based on evidence and best practices, with special emphasis on an integrated approach...".

Several factors have constrained progress in the prevention of chronic diseases. These include underestimation of the effectiveness of interventions, the belief of there being a long delay in achieving any measurable impact, commercial pressures, institutional inertia and inadequate resources. These aspects need to be taken seriously and combated. One example is provided by Finland. In North Karelia, age-adjusted mortality rates of coronary heart disease dropped dramatically between the early 1970s and 1995. Analyses of the three main risk factors (smoking, high blood pressure, raised plasma cholesterol) indicate that diet — operating through lowering plasma cholesterol and blood pressure levels —accounted for the larger part of this substantial decline in cardiovascular disease. The contribution made by medication and treatment (antilipid and hypotensive drugs, surgery) was very small. Rather, the decline was largely achieved through community action and the pressure of consumer demand on the food market.

The Finnish and other experience indicates that interventions can be effective, that dietary changes are important, that these changes can be strengthened by public demand, and finally that appreciable changes can take place very rapidly. The experience of the Republic of Korea is also notable since the community has largely maintained its traditional high-vegetable diet despite major social and economic change. The Republic of Korea has lower rates of chronic diseases and lower than expected level of fat intake and obesity prevalence than other industrialized countries with similar economic development.

There are several opportunities for new global and national actions, including strengthened interaction and partnerships; regulatory, legislative and fiscal approaches; and more stringent accountability mechanisms. The broad parameters for a dialogue with the food industries are: less saturated fat; more fruits and vegetables; effective food labelling; and incentives for the marketing and production of healthier products. In working with advertising, media and entertainment partners, there is a need to stress the importance of clear and unambiguous messages to children and youths.

Global "health and nutrition literacy" requires a vast increase in attention and resources. Many studies show a relationship between health and income, with the poorest sections of the population being the most vulnerable. Poor people are at an increased social disadvantage in terms of the incidence of chronic diseases, as well as access to treatment. They also show lower rates of acceptance of health-promoting behaviours compared with other sectors of society. Thus, policies need to favour the poor and appropriately targeted, as poor people are most at risk and have the least power to effect change.

Hunger and malnutrition remain among the most devastating problems facing the majority of the world's poor and needy people, and continue to dominate the health of the world's poorest nations. Nearly 30% of humanity are currently suffering from one or more of the multiple forms of malnutrition. The tragic consequences of malnutrition include death, disability, stunted mental and physical growth, and as a result, retarded national socioeconomic development. Some 60% of the 10. 9 million deaths each year among children aged under five years in the developing world are associated with malnutrition.

Iodine deficiency is the greatest single preventable cause of brain damage and mental retardation worldwide, and is estimated to affect more than 700 million people, most of them located in the less developed countries. Over 2000 million people have iron deficiency anaemia.

Vitamin A deficiency remains the single greatest preventable cause of needless childhood blindness and increased risk of premature childhood mortality from infectious diseases, with 250 million children under five years of age suffering from subclinical deficiency.

Intrauterine growth retardation, defined as birth weight below the 10th percentile of the birth-weight-for-gestational-age reference curve, affects 23. 8% or approximately 30 million newborn babies per year, profoundly influencing growth, survival, and physical and mental capacity in childhood. It also has major public health implications in view of the increased risk of developing diet-related chronic diseases later in life.

Given the rapidity with which traditional diets and lifestyles are changing in many developing countries, it is not surprising that food insecurity and undernutrition persist in the same countries where chronic diseases are emerging as a major epidemic.

The epidemic of obesity, with its attendant comorbidities —heart disease, hypertension, stroke, and diabetes —is not a problem limited to industrialized countries. Children are in a similar situation; a disturbing increase in the prevalence of overweight among this group has taken place over the past 20 years in developing countries as diverse as India, Mexico, Nigeria and Tunisia. The increasing prevalence of obesity in developing countries also indicates that physical inactivity is an increasing problem in those countries as well.

In the past, undernutrition and chronic diseases were seen as two totally separate problems, despite being present simultaneously. This dichotomy has obstructed effective action to curb the advancing epidemic of chronic diseases. For example, the prevailing approach of measuring child undernutrition on the basis of the underweight indicator (weight-for-age) can lead to gross underestimation of the presence of obesity in populations that have a high prevalence of stunting. Use of this indicator could lead aid programmes to feed apparently underweight people, with the undesirable outcome of further aggravating obesity.

In Latin America, close to 90 million people are beneficiaries of food programmes but that group actually comprises only 10 million truly underweight people (after correcting for height). The two facets of nutrition-related problems need to be brought together and treated in the context of the whole spectrum of malnutrition.

An integrated approach to diet-related and nutrition-related diseases The root causes of malnutrition include poverty and inequity. Eliminating these causes requires political and social action of which nutritional programmes can be only one aspect. Sufficient, safe and varied food supplies not only prevent malnutrition but also reduce the risk of chronic diseases. It is well known that nutritional deficiency increases the risk of common infectious diseases, notably those of childhood, and vice versa. There is, therefore, complementarity in terms of public health approaches and public policy priorities, between policies and programmes designed to prevent chronic diseases and those designed to prevent other diet-related and nutrition-related diseases.

The double burden of disease is most effectively lifted by a range of integrated policies and programmes. Such an integrated approach is the key to action in countries where modest public health budgets will inevitably remain mostly devoted to prevention of deficiency and infection. Indeed, there is no country, however privileged, in which combating deficiency and infection are no longer public health priorities.

High-income countries accustomed to programmes designed to prevent chronic diseases can amplify the effectiveness of the programmes by applying them to the prevention of nutritional deficiency and food-related infectious diseases. Guidelines designed to give equal priority to the prevention of nutritional deficiency and chronic diseases, have already been established for the Latin American region. Recent recommendations to prevent cancer are reckoned also to reduce the risk of nutritional deficiency and food-related infectious diseases, and dietary guidelines for the Brazilian population give equal priority to the prevention and control of nutritional deficiency, food-related infectious diseases, and chronic diseases.

Food consumption trends

Promoting healthy diets and lifestyles to reduce the global burden of noncommunicable diseases requires a multisectoral approach involving the various relevant sectors in societies. The agriculture and food sector figures prominently in this enterprise and must be given due importance in any consideration of the promotion of healthy diets for individuals and population groups.

Food strategies must not merely be directed at ensuring food security for all, but must also achieve the consumption of adequate quantities of safe and good quality foods that together make up a healthy diet. Any recommendation to that effect will have implications for all components in the food chain.

Economic development is normally accompanied by improvements in a country's food supply and the gradual elimination of dietary deficiencies, thus improving the overall nutritional status of the country's population. Furthermore, it also brings about qualitative changes in the production, processing, distribution and marketing of food.

Increasing urbanization will also have consequences for the dietary patterns and lifestyles of individuals, not all of which are positive. Changes in diets, patterns of work and leisure —often referred to as the "nutrition transition"—are already contributing to the causal factors underlying noncommunicable diseases even in the poorest countries. Moreover, the pace of these changes seems to be accelerating, especially in the low-income and middle-income countries.

The dietary changes that characterize the "nutrition transition" include both quantitative and qualitative changes in the diet. The adverse dietary changes include shifts in the structure of the diet towards a higher energy density diet with a greater role for fat and added sugars in foods, greater saturated fat intake (mostly from animal sources), reduced intakes of complex carbohydrates and dietary fibre, and reduced fruit and vegetable intakes. These dietary changes are compounded by lifestyle changes that reflect reduced physical activity at work and during leisure time. At the same time, however, poor countries continue to face food shortages and nutrient inadequacies.

Diets evolve over time, being influenced by many factors and complex interactions. Income, prices, individual preferences and beliefs, cultural traditions, as well as geographical, environmental, social and economic factors all interact in a complex manner to shape dietary consumption patterns.

Data on the national availability of the main food commodities provide a valuable insight into diets and their evolution over time. FAO produces annual Food Balance Sheets which provide national data on food availability (for almost all commodities and for nearly all countries). Food Balance Sheets give a complete picture of supply (including production, imports, stock changes and exports) and utilization (including final demand in the form of food use and industrial non-food use, intermediate demand such as animal feed and seed use, and waste) by commodity.

From these data, the average per capita supply of macronutrients (i. e. energy, protein, fats) can be derived for all food commodities. Although such average per capita supplies are derived from national data, they may not correspond to actual per capita availability, which is determined by many other factors such as inequality in access to food. Likewise, these data refer to "average food available for consumption", which, for a number of reasons, is not equal to average food intake or average food consumption.

Table 1

Global and regional per capita food consumption (kcal per capita per day)

Region	1964—1966	1974—1976	1984—1986	1997—1999	2015	2030
World	2358	2435	2655	2803	2940	3050
Developing countries	2054	2152	2450	2681	2850	2980
Near East and North Africa	2290	2591	2953	3006	3090	3170
Sub-Saharan Africa	2058	2079	2057	2195	2360	2540
Latin America & Caribbean	2393	2546	2689	2824	2980	3140
East Asia	1957	2105	2559	2921	3060	3190
South Asia	2017	1986	2205	2403	2700	2900
Industrialized countries	2947	3065	3206	3380	3440	3500
Transition countries	3222	3385	3379	2906	3060	3180

Actual food availability may vary by region, socioeconomic level and season. Certain difficulties are encountered when estimating trade, production and stock changes on an annual scale. Hence three-year averages are calculated in order to reduce errors. The FAO statistical database (FAOSTAT), being based on national data, does not provide information on the distribution of food within countries, or within communities and households.

Food consumption expressed in kilocalories (kcal) per capita per day is a key variable used for measuring and evaluating the evolution of the global and regional food situation. A more appropriate term for this variable would be "national average apparent food consumption" since the data come from national Food Balance Sheets rather than from food consumption surveys.

Analysis of FAOSTAT data shows that dietary energy measured in kcals per capita per day has been steadily increasing on a worldwide basis; availability of calories per capita from the mid-1960s to the late 1990s increased globally by approximately 450 kcal per capita per day and by over 600 kcal per capita per day in developing countries.

This change has not, however, been equal across regions. The per capita supply of calories has remained almost stagnant in sub-Saharan Africa and has recently fallen in the countries in economic transition. In contrast, the per capita supply of energy has risen dramatically in East Asia (by almost 1000 kcal per capita per day, mainly in China) and in the Near East/North Africa region (by over 700 kcal per capita per day).

The world has made significant progress in raising food consumption per person. The increase in the world average consumption would have been higher but for the declines in the transition economies that occurred in the 1990s. It is generally agreed, however, that those declines are likely to revert in the near future. The growth in food consumption has been accompanied by significant structural changes and a shift in diet away from staples such as roots and tubers towards more livestock products and vegetable oils.

Although the global supply of protein has been increasing, the distribution of the increase in the protein supply is unequal. The per capita supply of vegetable protein is slightly higher in developing countries, while the supply of animal protein is three times higher in industrialized countries. Globally, the share of dietary energy supplied by cereals appears to have remained relatively stable over time, representing about 50% of dietary energy supply.

Recently, however, subtle changes appear to be taking place. A closer analysis of the dietary energy intake shows a decrease in developing countries, where the share of energy derived from cereals has fallen from 60% to 54% in a period of only 10 years. Much of this downwards trend is attributable to cereals, particularly wheat and rice, becoming less preferred foods in middle-income countries such as Brazil and China, a pattern likely to continue over the next 30 years or so.

Consumption of dietary fat

The increase in the quantity and quality of the fats consumed in the diet is an important feature of nutrition transition reflected in the national diets of countries. There are large variations across the regions of the world in the amount of total fats available for human consumption. The lowest quantities consumed are recorded in Africa, while the highest consumption occurs in parts of North America and Europe.

The important point is that there has been a remarkable increase in the intake of dietary fats over the past three decades and that this increase has taken place practically everywhere except in Africa, where consumption levels have stagnated. The per capita supply of fat from animal foods has increased, respectively, by 14 and 4 g per capita in developing and industrialized countries, while there has been a decrease of 9 g per capita in transition countries.

The increase in dietary fat supply worldwide exceeds the increase in dietary protein supply. The average global supply of fat has increased by 20 g per capita per day since 1967—1969. This increase in availability has been most pronounced in the Americas, East Asia, and the European Community. The proportion of energy contributed by dietary fats exceeds 30% in the industrialized regions, and in nearly all other regions this share is increasing.

The fat-to-energy ratio (FER) is defined as the percentage of energy derived from fat in the total supply of energy (in kcal). Country-specific analysis of FAO data for 1988—1990 found a range for the FER of 7—46%. A total of 19 countries fell below the minimum recommendation of 15% dietary energy supply from fat, the majority of these being in sub-Saharan Africa and the remainder in South Asia. In contrast, 24 countries were above the maximum recommendation of 35%, the majority of these countries being in North America and Western Europe.

Table 2. Trends in the dietary supply of fat

Region	*Supply of fat (g per capita per day)*				
	1967—1969	1977—1979	1987—1989	1997—1999	Change between 1967—1969 and 1997—1999
World	53	57	67	73	20
North Africa	44	58	65	64	20
Sub-Saharan Africa	41	43	41	45	4
North America	117	125	138	143	26
Latin America & Caribbean	54	65	73	79	25
China	24	27	48	79	55
East and South-East Asia	28	32	44	52	24
South Asia	29	32	39	45	16
European Community	117	128	143	148	31
Eastern Europe	90	111	116	104	14
Near East	51	62	73	70	19
Oceania	102	102	113	113	11

It is useful to note that limitations of the Food Balance Sheet data may contribute much of this variation in the FER between countries. For instance, in countries such as Malaysia with abundant availability of vegetable oils at low prices, Food Balance Sheet data may not reflect real consumption at the individual household level.

Rising incomes in the developing world have also led to an increase in the availability and consumption of energy-dense high-fat diets. Food balance data can be used to examine the shift in the proportion of energy from fat over time and its relationship to increasing incomes. In 1961—1963, a diet providing 20% of energy from fat was associated only with countries having at least a per capita gross national product of US$1475.

By 1990, however, even poor countries having a gross national product of only US$750 per capita had access to a similar diet comprising 20% of energy from fat. (Both values of gross national product are given in 1993 US$.) This change was mainly the result of an increase in the consumption of vegetable fats by poor countries, with smaller increases occurred in middle-income and high-income countries.

By 1990, vegetable fats accounted for a greater proportion of dietary energy than animal fats for countries in the lowest per capita income category. Changes in edible vegetable oil supply, in prices and in consumption equally affected rich and poor countries, although the net impact was relatively much greater in low-income countries. An equally large and important shift in the proportion of energy from added sugars in the diets of low-income countries was also a feature of the nutrition transition.

Examinations of the purchasing habits of people, aimed at understanding the relationship between level of education or income and the different amounts or types of commodities purchased at different times were also revealing. Research conducted in China shows that there have been profound shifts in purchasing practices in relation to income over the past decade. These analyses show how extra income in China affects poor people and rich people in a differential manner, enhancing the fat intake of the poor more than that of the rich.

A variable proportion of these fat calories are provided by saturated fatty acids. Only in the two of the most affluent regions (i. e. in parts of North America and Europe) is the intake of saturated fat at or above 10% of energy intake level. In other less affluent regions, the proportion of dietary energy contributed by saturated fatty acids is lower, ranging from 5% to 8%, and generally not changing much over time.

National dietary surveys conducted in some countries confirm these data. The ratio of dietary fat from animal sources to total fat is a key indicator, since foods from animal sources are high in saturated fat. Data sets used to calculate country-specific FERs can also be used to calculate proportions of animal fat in total fat. Such analysis indicated that the proportion of animal fat in total fat was lower than 10% in some countries (Democratic Republic of Congo, Mozambique, Nigeria, Sao Tome and Principe, and Sierra Leone), while it is above 75% in some other countries (Denmark, Finland, Hungary, Mongolia, Poland and Uruguay).

These findings are not strictly divided along economic lines, as not all of the countries in the high range represent the most affluent countries. Country-specific food availability and cultural dietary preferences and norms to some extent determine these patterns.

The types of edible oils used in developing countries are also changing with the increasing use of hardened margarines (rich in trans fatty acids) that do not need to be refrigerated. Palm oil is becoming an increasingly important edible oil in the diets of much of South-East Asia and is likely to be a major source in the coming years. Currently, palm oil consumption is low and the FER ranges between 15% and 18%. At this low level of consumption, the saturated fatty acid content of the diet comprises only 4% to 8%.

Potential developments in the edible oil sector could affect all stages of the oil production process from plant breeding to processing methods, including the blending of oils aimed at producing edible oils that have a healthy fatty acid composition.

Olive oil is an important edible oil consumed largely in the Mediterranean region. Its production has been driven by rising demand, which has increasingly shifted olive cultivation from traditional farms to more intensive forms of cultivation. There is some concern that the intensive cultivation of olives may have adverse environmental impacts, such as soil erosion and desertification. However, agricultural production methods are being developed to ensure less harmful impacts on the environment.

Consumption of animal products

There has been an increasing pressure on the livestock sector to meet the growing demand for high-value animal protein. The world's livestock sector is growing at an unprecedented rate and the driving force behind this enormous surge is a combination of population growth, rising incomes and urbanization. Annual meat production is projected to increase from 218 million tonnes in 1997—1999 to 376 million tonnes by 2030.

There is a strong positive relationship between the level of income and the consumption of animal protein, with the consumption of meat, milk and eggs increasing at the expense of staple foods. Because of the recent steep decline in prices, developing countries are embarking on higher meat consumption at much lower levels of gross domestic product than the industrialized countries did some 20—30 years ago.

Urbanization is a major driving force influencing global demand for livestock products. Urbanization stimulates improvements in infrastructure, including cold chains, which permit trade in perishable goods. Compared with the less diversified diets of the rural communities, city dwellers have a varied diet rich in animal proteins and fats, and characterized by higher consumption of meat, poultry, milk and other dairy products.

Table 3 shows trends in per capita consumption of livestock products in different regions and country groups. There has been a remarkable increase in the consumption of animal products in countries such as Brazil and China, although the levels are still well below the levels of consumption in North American and most other industrialized countries. As diets become richer and more diverse, the high-value protein that the livestock sector offers improves the nutrition of the vast majority of the world.

Table 3. Per capita consumption of livestock products

Region	Meat (kg per year)			Milk (kg per year)		
	1964—1966	1997—1999	2030	1964—1966	1997—1999	2030
World	24. 2	36. 4	45. 3	73. 9	78. 1	89. 5
Developing countries	10. 2	25. 5	36. 7	28. 0	44. 6	65. 8
Near East and North Africa	11. 9	21. 2	35. 0	68. 6	72. 3	89. 9
Sub-Saharan Africa	9. 9	9. 4	13. 4	28. 5	29. 1	33. 8
Latin America & Caribbean	31. 7	53. 8	76. 6	80. 1	110. 2	139. 8
East Asia	8. 7	37. 7	58. 5	3. 6	10. 0	17. 8
South Asia	3. 9	5. 3	11. 7	37. 0	67. 5	106. 9
Industrialized countries	61. 5	88. 2	100. 1	185. 5	212. 2	221. 0
Transition countries	42. 5	46. 2	60. 7	156. 6	159. 1	178. 7

Livestock products not only provide high-value protein but are also important sources of a wide range of essential micronutrients, in particular minerals such as iron and zinc, and vitamins such as vitamin A. For the large majority of people in the world, particularly in developing countries, livestock products remain a desired food for nutritional value and taste. Excessive consumption of animal products in some countries and social classes can, however, lead to excessive intakes of fat. Region Meat (kg per year) Milk (kg per year)

The growing demand for livestock products is likely to have an undesirable impact on the environment. For example, there will be more large-scale, industrial production, often located close to urban centres, which brings with it a range of environmental and public health risks.

Attempts have been made to estimate the environmental impact of industrial livestock production. For instance, it has been estimated that the number of people fed in a year per hectare ranges from 22 for potatoes and 19 for rice to 1 and 2, respectively, for beef and lamb. The low energy conversion ratio from feed to meat is another concern, since some of the cereal grain food produced is diverted to livestock production. Likewise, land and water requirements for meat production are likely to become a major concern, as the increasing demand for animal products results in more intensive livestock production systems.

Consumption of fish

Despite fluctuations in supply and demand caused by the changing state of fisheries resources, the economic climate and environmental conditions, fisheries, including aquaculture, have traditionally been, and remain an important source of food, employment and revenue in many countries and communities.

After the remarkable increase in both marine and inland capture of fish during the 1950s and 1960s, world fisheries production has levelled off since the 1970s. This levelling off of the total catch follows the general trend of most of the world's fishing areas, which have apparently reached their maximum potential for fisheries production, with the majority of stocks being fully exploited.

It is therefore very unlikely that substantial increases in total catch will be obtained in the future. In contrast, aquaculture production has followed the opposite path. Starting from an insignificant total production, inland and marine aquaculture production has been growing at a remarkable rate, offsetting part of the reduction in the ocean catch of fish.

The total food fish supply and hence consumption has been growing at a rate of 3. 6% per year since 1961, while the world's population has been expanding at 1. 8% per year. The proteins derived from fish, crustaceans and molluscs account for between 13. 8% and 16. 5% of the animal protein intake of the human population. The average apparent per capita consumption increased from about 9 kg per year in the early 1960s to 16 kg in 1997.

The per capita availability of fish and fishery products has therefore nearly doubled in 40 years, outpacing population growth. As well as income-related variations, the role of fish in nutrition shows marked continental, regional and national differences.

In industrialized countries, where diets generally contain a more diversified range of animal proteins, a rise in per capita provision from 19. 7 kg to 27. 7 kg seems to have occurred. This represents a growth rate close to 1% per year. In this group of countries, fish contributed an increasing share of total protein intake until 1989 (accounting for between 6. 5% and 8. 5%), but since then its importance has gradually declined and, in 1997, its percentage contribution was back to the level prevailing in the mid-1980s.

In the early 1960s, per capita fish supply in low-income food-deficit countries was, on average, only 30% of that of the richest countries. This gap has been gradually reduced, such that in 1997, average fish consumption in these countries was 70% of that of the more affluent economies.

Despite the relatively low consumption by weight in low-income food-deficit countries, the contribution of fish to total animal protein intake is considerable (nearly 20%). Over the past four decades, however, the share of fish proteins in animal proteins has declined slightly, because of faster growth in the consumption of other animal products.

Currently, two-thirds of the total food fish supply is obtained from capture fisheries in marine and inland waters, while the remaining one-third is derived from aquaculture. The contribution of inland and marine capture fisheries to per capita food supply has stabilized, around 10 kg per capita in the period 1984—1998. Any recent increases in per capita availability have, therefore, been obtained from aquaculture production, from both traditional rural aquaculture and intensive commercial aquaculture of high-value species.

Fish contributes up to 180 kcal per capita per day, but reaches such high levels only in a few countries where there is a lack of alternative protein foods grown locally or where there is a strong preference for fish (examples are Iceland, Japan and some small island states). More typically, fish provides about 20—30 kcal per capita per day. Fish proteins are essential in the diet of some densely populated countries where the total protein intake level is low, and are very important in the diets of many other countries.

Worldwide, about a billion people rely on fish as their main source of animal proteins. Dependence on fish is usually higher in coastal than in inland areas. About 20% of the world's population derives at least one-fifth of its animal protein intake from fish, and some small island states depend almost exclusively on fish.

Recommending the increased consumption of fish is another area where the feasibility of dietary recommendations needs to be balanced against concerns for sustainability of marine stocks and the potential depletion of this important marine source of high quality nutritious food. Added to this is the concern that a significant proportion of the world fish catch is transformed into fish meal and used as animal feed in industrial livestock production and thus is not available for human consumption.

Consumption of fruits and vegetables

Consumption of fruits and vegetables plays a vital role in providing a diversified and nutritious diet. A low consumption of fruits and vegetables in many regions of the developing world is, however, a persistent phenomenon, confirmed by the findings of food consumption surveys.

Nationally representative surveys in India, for example, indicate a steady level of consumption of only 120—140 g per capita per day, with about another 100 g per capita coming from roots and tubers, and some 40 g per capita from pulses. This may not be true for urban populations in India, who have rising incomes and greater access to a diverse and varied diet. In contrast, in China, —a country that is undergoing rapid economic growth and transition —the amount of fruits and vegetables consumed has increased to 369 g per capita per day by 1992.

At present, only a small and negligible minority of the world's population consumes the generally recommended high average intake of fruits and vegetables. In 1998, only 6 of the 14 WHO regions had an availability of fruits and vegetables equal to or greater than the earlier recommended intake of 400 g per capita per day.

The relatively favourable situation in 1998 appears to have evolved from a markedly less favourable position in previous years, as evidenced by the great increase in vegetable availability recorded between 1990 and 1998 for most of the regions. In contrast, the availability of fruit generally decreased between 1990 and 1998 in most regions of the world.

The increase in urbanization globally is another challenge. Increasing urbanization will distance more people from primary food production, and in turn have a negative impact on both the availability of a varied and nutritious diet with enough fruits and vegetables, and the access of the urban poor to such a diet.

Nevertheless, it may facilitate the achievement of other goals, as those who can afford it can have better access to a diverse and varied diet. Investment in periurban horticulture may provide an opportunity to increase the availability and consumption of a healthy diet.

Global trends in the production and supply of vegetables indicate that the current production and consumption vary widely among regions. It should be noted that the production of wild and indigenous vegetables is not taken into account in production statistics and might therefore be underestimated in consumption statistics.

In 2000, the global annual average per capita vegetable supply was 102 kg, with the highest level in Asia (116 kg), and the lowest levels in South America (48 kg) and Africa (52 kg). These figures also include the large amount of horticultural produce that is consumed on the farm.

Table 4 illustrate the regional and temporal variations in the per capita availability of vegetables per capita over the past few decades.

Table 4. Supply of vegetables per capita, by region, 1979 and 2000

Region	1979	2000
World	66. 1	101. 9
Developed countries	107. 4	112. 8
Developing countries	51. 1	98. 8
Africa	45. 4	52. 1
North and Central America	88. 7	98. 3
South America	43. 2	47. 8
Asia	56. 6	116. 2
Europe	110. 9	112. 5
Oceania	71. 8	98. 7

Trends in demand, food availability and consumption

In recent years the growth rates of world agricultural production and crop yields have slowed. This has raised fears that the world may not be able to grow enough food and other commodities to ensure that future populations are adequately fed. However, the slowdown has occurred not because of shortages of land or water but rather because demand for agricultural products has also slowed. This is mainly because world population growth rates have been declining since the late 1960s, and fairly high levels of food consumption per person are now being reached in many countries, beyond which further rises will be limited.

It also true that a high share of the world's population remains in poverty and hence lacks the necessary income to translate its needs into effective demand. As a result, the growth in world demand for agricultural products is expected to fall from an average 2. 2% per year over the past 30 years to an average 1. 5% per year for the next 30 years. In developing countries the slowdown will be more dramatic, from 3. 7% per year to 2% per year, partly as a result of China having passed the phase of rapid growth in its demand for food.

Global food shortages are unlikely, but serious problems already exist at national and local levels, and may worsen unless focused efforts are made. The annual growth rate of world demand for cereals has declined from 2. 5% per year in the 1970s and 1. 9% per year in the 1980s to only 1% per year in the 1990s. Annual cereal use per person peaked in the mid-1980s at 334 kg and has since fallen to 317 kg. The decline is not a cause for alarm, it is largely the natural result of slower population growth and shifts in human diets and animal feeds.

During the 1990s, however, the decline was accentuated by a number of temporary factors, including serious economic recessions in the transition countries and in some East and South-East Asian countries. The growth rate in the demand for cereals is expected to rise again to 1. 4% per year up until 2015, slowing to 1. 2% per year thereafter.

In developing countries overall, cereal production is not expected to keep pace with demand. The net cereal deficits of these countries, which amounted to 103 million tonnes or 9% of consumption in 1997—1999, could rise to 265 million tonnes by 2030, when they will be 14% of consumption. This gap can be bridged by increased surpluses from traditional grain exporters, and by new exports from the transition countries, which are expected to shift from being net importers to being net exporters.

Oil crops have seen the fastest increase in area of any crop sector, expanding by 75 million hectares between the mid-1970s and the end of the 1990s, while cereal area fell by 28 million hectares over the same period. Future per capita consumption of oil crops is expected to rise more rapidly than that of cereals. These crops will account for 45 out of every 100 extra kilocalories added to average diets in developing countries between now and 2030.

There are three main sources of growth in crop production: expanding the land area, increasing the frequency at which it is cropped (often through irrigation), and boosting yields. It has been suggested that growth in crop production may be approaching the ceiling of what is possible in respect of all three sources. A detailed examination of production potentials does not support this view at the global level, although in some countries, and even in whole regions, serious problems already exist and could deepen.

Diets in developing countries are changing as incomes rise. The share of staples, such as cereals, roots and tubers, is declining, while that of meat, dairy products and oil crops is rising. Between 1964—1966 and 1997— 1999, per capita meat consumption in developing countries rose by 150% and that of milk and dairy products by 60%.

By 2030, per capita consumption of livestock products could rise by a further 44%. Poultry consumption is predicted to grow the fastest. Productivity improvements are likely to be a major source of growth. Milk yields should improve, while breeding and improved management should increase average carcass weights and off-take rates. This will allow increased production with lower growth in animal numbers, and a corresponding slowdown in the growth of environmental damage from grazing and animal wastes.

In developing countries, demand is predicted to grow faster than production, resulting in a growing trade deficit. In meat products this deficit will rise steeply, from 1. 2 million tonnes per year in 1997—1999 to 5. 9 million tonnes per year in 2030, while in the case of milk and dairy products, the rise will be less steep but still considerable, from 20 million tonnes per year in 1997—1999 to 39 million tonnes per year in 2030. An increasing share of livestock production will probably come from industrial enterprises. In recent years, production from this sector has grown twice as fast as that from more traditional mixed farming systems and more than six times faster than that from grazing systems.

World fisheries production has kept ahead of population growth over the past three decades. Total fish production has almost doubled, from 65 million tonnes in 1970 to 125 million tonnes in 1999, when the world average intake of fish, crustaceans and molluscs reached 16. 3 kg per person. By 2030, annual fish consumption is likely to rise to some 150— 160 million tonnes, or between 19—20 kg per person. This amount is significantly lower than the potential demand, as environmental factors are expected to limit supply.

During the 1990s the marine catch levelled out at 80—85 million tonnes per year, and by the turn of the century, three-quarters of ocean fish stocks were overfished, depleted or exploited up to their maximum sustainable yield. Further growth in the marine catch can only be modest.

Aquaculture compensated for this marine slowdown, doubling its share of world fish production during the 1990s. It is expected to continue to grow rapidly, at rates of 5—7% per year up to 2015. In all sectors of fishing it will be essential to pursue forms of management conducive to sustainable exploitation, especially for resources under common ownership or no ownership.

Diet, nutrition and prevention of chronic diseases

There is a continuity in the influences contributing to chronic disease development, and thus also to the opportunities for prevention. These influences include the life course; the microscopic environment of the gene to macroscopic urban and rural environments; the impact of social and political events in one sphere affecting the health and diet of populations far distant; and the way in which already stretched agriculture and oceanic systems will affect the choices available and the recommendations that can be made.

For chronic diseases, risks occur at all ages; conversely, all ages are part of the continuum of opportunities for their prevention and control. Both undernutrition and overnutrition are negative influences in terms of disease development, and possibly a combination is even worse; consequently the developing world needs additional targeting. Those with least power need different preventive approaches from the more affluent. Work has to start with the individual risk factors, but, critically, attempts at prevention and health promotion must also take account of the wider social, political and economic environment. Economics, industry, consumer groups and advertising all must be included in the prevention equation.

The rapidly increasing burden of chronic diseases is a key determinant of global public health. Already 79% of deaths attributable to chronic diseases are occurring in developing countries, predominantly in middle-aged men. There is increasing evidence that chronic disease risks begin in fetal life and continue into old age. Adult chronic disease, therefore, reflects cumulative differential lifetime exposures to damaging physical and social environments.

Fetal development

The four relevant factors in fetal life are:

(i) intrauterine growth retardation (IUGR);

(ii) premature delivery of a normal growth for gestational age fetus;

(iii) overnutrition in utero; and

(iv) intergenerational factors.

There is considerable evidence, mostly from developed countries, that IUGR is associated with an increased risk of coronary heart disease, stroke, diabetes and raised blood pressure. It may rather be the pattern of growth, i. e. restricted fetal growth followed by very rapid postnatal catch-up growth, that is important in the underlying disease pathways. On the other hand, large size at birth (macrosomia) is also associated with an increased risk of diabetes and cardiovascular disease.

Among the adult population in India, an association was found between impaired glucose tolerance and high ponderal index (i. e. fatness) at birth. In Pima Indians, a U-shaped relationship to birth weight was found, whereas no such relationship was found amongst Mexican Americans. Higher birth weight has also been related to an increased risk of breast and other cancers.

Optimal birth weight and length distribution should be considered, not only in terms of immediate morbidity and mortality but also in regard to long-term outcomes such as susceptibility to diet-related chronic disease later in life.

Infancy

Retarded growth in infancy can be a reflected in a failure to gain weight and a failure to gain height. Both retarded growth and excessive weight or height gain ("crossing the centiles") can be factors in later incidence of chronic disease. An association between low growth in early infancy (low weight at 1 year) and an increased risk of coronary heart disease (CHD) has been described, irrespective of size at birth.

Blood pressure has been found to be highest in those with retarded fetal growth and greater weight gain in infancy. Short stature, a reflection of socioeconomic deprivation in childhood, is also associated with an increased risk of CHD and stroke, and to some extent, diabetes. The risk of stroke, and also of cancer mortality at several sites, including breast, uterus and colon, is increased if shorter children display an accelerated growth in height.

There is increasing evidence that among term and pre-term infants, breastfeeding is associated with significantly lower blood pressure levels in childhood. Consumption of formula instead of breast milk in infancy has also been shown to increase diastolic and mean arterial blood pressure in later life. Nevertheless, studies with older cohorts and the Dutch study of famine have not identified such associations.

There is increasingly strong evidence suggesting that a lower risk of developing obesity may be directly related to length of exclusive breastfeeding although it may not become evident until later in childhood. Some of the discrepancy may be explained by socioeconomic and maternal education factors confounding the findings.

Data from most, but not all, observational studies of term infants have generally suggested adverse effects of formula consumption on the other risk factors for cardiovascular disease (as well as blood pressure), but little information to support this finding is available from controlled clinical trials. Nevertheless, the weight of current evidence indicates adverse effects of formula milk on cardiovascular disease risk factors; this is consistent with the observations of increased mortality among older adults who were fed formula as infants.

The risk for several chronic diseases of childhood and adolescence (e. g. type 1 diabetes, coeliac disease, some childhood cancers, inflammatory bowel disease) have also been associated with infant feeding on breast-milk substitutes and short-term breastfeeding.

There has been great interest in the possible effect of high-cholesterol feeding in early life. Reiser et al. proposed the hypothesis that high-cholesterol feeding in early life may serve to regulate cholesterol and lipoprotein metabolism in later life. Animal data in support of this hypothesis are limited, but the idea of a possible metabolic imprinting served to trigger several retrospective and prospective studies in which cholesterol and lipoprotein metabolism in infants fed human milk were compared with those fed formula.

Studies in suckling rats have suggested that the presence of cholesterol in the early diet may serve to define a metabolic pattern for lipoproteins and plasma cholesterol that could be of benefit later in life. The study by Mott, Lewis & McGill on differential diets in infant baboons, however, provided evidence to the contrary in terms of benefit. Nevertheless, the observation of modified responses of adult cholesterol production rates, bile cholesterol saturation indices, and bile acid turnover, depending on whether the baboons were fed breast milk or formula, served to attract further interest.

It was noted that increased atherosclerotic lesions associated with increased levels of plasma total cholesterol were related to increased dietary cholesterol in early life. No long-term human morbidity and mortality data supporting this notion have been reported.

Short-term human studies have been in part confounded by diversity in solid food weaning regimens, as well as by the varied composition of fatty acid components of the early diet. The latter are now known to have an impact on circulating lipoprotein cholesterol species. Mean plasma total cholesterol by age 4 months in infants fed breast milk reached 180 mg/dl or greater, while cholesterol values in infants fed formula tended to remain under 150 mg/dl.

In a study by Carlson, DeVoe & Barness, infants receiving predominantly a linoleic acid-enriched oil blend exhibited a mean cholesterol concentration of approximately 110 mg/dl. A separate group of infants in that study who received predominantly oleic acid had a mean cholesterol concentration of 133 mg/dl.

Moreover, infants who were fed breast milk and oleic acid-enriched formula had higher high-density lipoprotein (HDL) cholesterol and apoproteins A-I and A-II than the predominantly linoleic acid-enriched oil diet group. The ratio of low-density lipoprotein (LDL) cholesterol plus very low-density lipoprotein (VLDL) cholesterol to HDL cholesterol was lowest for infants receiving the formula in which oleic acid was predominant.

Using a similar oleic acid predominant formula, Darmady, Fosbrooke & Lloyd reported a mean value of 149 mg/dl at age 4 months, compared with 196 mg/dl in a parallel breast-fed group. Most of those infants then received an uncontrolled mixed diet and cow's milk, with no evident differences in plasma cholesterol levels by 12 months, independent of the type of early feeding they had received.

A more recent controlled study suggests that the specific fatty acid intake plays a predominant role in determining total and LDL cholesterol. The significance of high dietary cholesterol associated with exclusive human milk feeding during the first 4 months of life has no demonstrated adverse effect. Measurements of serum lipoprotein concentrations and LDL receptor activity in infants suggests that it is the fatty acid content rather than the cholesterol in the diet which regulates cholesterol homeostasis. The regulation of endogenous cholesterol synthesis in infants appears to be regulated in a similar manner to that of adults.

Childhood and adolescence

An association between low growth in childhood and an increased risk of CHD has been described, irrespective of size at birth. Although based only on developed country research at this point, this finding gives credence to the importance that is currently attached to the role of immediate postnatal factors in shaping disease risk.

Growth rates in infants in Bangladesh, most of whom had chronic intrauterine under-nourishment and were breastfed, were similar to growth rates of breastfed infants in industrialized countries, but catch-up growth was limited and weight at 12 months was largely a function of weight at birth. In a study of 11—12 year-old Jamaican children, blood pressure levels were found to be highest in those with retarded fetal growth and greater weight gain between the ages of 7 and 11 years.

Similar results were found in India. Low birth weight Indian babies have been described as having a characteristic poor muscle but high fat preservation, so-called "thin-fat" babies. This phenotype persists throughout the postnatal period and is associated with an increased central adiposity in childhood that is linked to the highest risk of raised blood pressure and disease (59—61).

In most studies, the association between low birth weight and high blood pressure has been found to be particularly strong if adjusted to current body size — body mass index (BMI) —suggesting the importance of weight gain after birth. Relative weight in adulthood and weight gain have been found to be associated with increased risk of cancer of the breast, colon, rectum, prostate and other sites.

Whether there is an independent effect of childhood weight is difficult to determine, as childhood overweight is usually continued into adulthood. Relative weight in adolescence was significantly associated with colon cancer in one retrospective cohort study. Frankel, Gunnel &Peters, in the follow-up to an earlier survey by Boyd Orr in the late 1930s, found that for both sexes, after accounting for the confounding effects of social class, there was a significant positive relationship between childhood energy intake and adult cancer mortality.

The recent review by the International Agency for Research on Cancer (IARC) in Lyon, France, concluded that there was clear evidence of a relationship between onset of obesity (both early and later) and cancer risk.

Short stature (including measures of childhood leg length), a reflection of socioeconomic deprivation in childhood, is associated with an increased risk of CHD and stroke, and to some extent diabetes. Given that short stature, and specifically short leglength, are particularly sensitive indicators of early socioeconomic deprivation, their association with later disease very likely reflects an association between early undernutrition and infectious disease load. Height serves partly as an indicator of socioeconomic and nutritional status in childhood.

As has been seen, poor fetal development and poor growth during childhood have been associated with increased cardiovascular disease risk in adulthood, as have indicators of unfavourable social circumstances in childhood. Conversely, a high calorie intake in childhood may be related to an increased risk of cancer in later life. Height is inversely associated with mortality among men and women from all causes, including coronary heart disease, stroke and respiratory disease.

Height has also been used as a proxy for usual childhood energy intake, which is particularly related to body mass and the child's level of activity. However, it is clearly an imperfect proxy because when protein intake is adequate (energy appears to be important in this regard only in the first 3 months of life), genetics will define adult height. Protein, particularly animal protein, has been shown to have a selective effect in promoting height growth.

It has been suggested that childhood obesity is related to excess protein intake and, of course, overweight or obese children tend to be in the upper percentiles for height. Height has been shown to be related to cancer mortality at several sites, including breast, uterus and colon. The risk of stroke is increased by accelerated growth in height during childhood.

As accelerated growth has been linked to development of hypertension in adult life, this may be the mechanism (plus an association with low socioeconomic status). There is a higher prevalence of raised blood pressure not only in adults of low socioeconomic status, but also in children from low socioeconomic backgrounds, although the latter is not always associated with higher blood pressure later in life. Blood pressure has been found to track from childhood to predict hypertension in adulthood, but with stronger tracking seen in older ages of childhood and in adolescence.

Higher blood pressure in childhood (in combination with other risk factors) causes target organ and anatomical changes that are associated with cardiovascular risk, including reduction in artery elasticity, increased ventricular size and mass, haemodynamic increase in cardiac output and peripheral resistance (10, 76, 77). High blood pressure in children is strongly associated with obesity, in particular central obesity, and clusters and tracks with an adverse serum lipid profile (especially LDL cholesterol) and glucose intolerance.

There may be some ethnic differences, although these often seem to be explained by differences in body mass index. A retrospective mortality follow-up of a survey of family diet and health in the United Kingdom identified significant associations between childhood energy intake and mortality from cancer.

The presence and tracking of high blood pressure in children and adolescents occurs against a background of unhealthy lifestyles, including excessive intakes of total and saturated fats, cholesterol and salt, inadequate intakes of potassium, and reduced physical activity, often accompanied by high levels of television viewing. In adolescents, habitual alcohol and tobacco use contributes to raised blood pressure.

There are three critical aspects of adolescence that have an impact on chronic diseases:

(i) the development of risk factors during this period;

(ii) the tracking of risk factors throughout life; and, in terms of prevention,

(iii) the development of healthy or unhealthy habits that tend to stay throughout life, for example physical inactivity because of television viewing.

In older children and adolescents, habitual alcohol and tobacco use contribute to raised blood pressure and the development of other risk factors in early life, most of which track into adulthood. The clustering of risk factor variables occurs as early as childhood and adolescence, and is associated with a therosclerosis in young adulthood and thus risk of later cardiovascular disease.

This clustering has been described as the metabolic —or "syndrome X"—clustering of physiological disturbances associated with insulin resistance, including hyper insulinaemia, impaired glucose tolerance, hypertension, elevated plasma triglyceride and low HDL cholesterol.

Raised serum cholesterol both in middle age and in early life are known to be associated with an increased risk of disease later on. The Johns Hopkins Precursor Study showed that serum cholesterol levels in adolescents and young white males were strongly related to subsequent risk of cardiovascular disease mortality and morbidity.

Although the risk of obesity does not apparently increase in adults who were overweight at 1 and 3 years old, the risk rises steadily thereafter, regardless of parental weight. Tracking has also been reported in China, where overweight children were 2. 8 times as likely to become overweight adolescents; conversely, underweight children were 3. 6 times as likely to remain underweight as adolescents.

The study found that parental obesity and underweight, and the child's initial body mass index, dietary fat intake and family income helped predict tracking and changes. However, in a prospective cohort study conducted in the United Kingdom, little tracking from childhood overweight to adulthood obesity was found when using a measure of fatness (percentage body fat for age) that was independent of build. It was also found that only children obese at 13 years of age had an increased risk of obesity as adults, and that there was no excess adult health risk from childhood or adolescent overweight. Interestingly, they found that in the thinnest children, the more obese they became as adults, the greater was their subsequent risk of developing chronic diseases.

The real concern about these early manifestations of chronic disease, besides the fact that they are occurring earlier and earlier, is that once they have developed they tend to track in that individual throughout life. On the more positive side, there is evidence that they can be corrected. Overweight and obesity are, however, notoriously difficult to correct after becoming established, and there is an established risk of overweight during childhood persisting into adolescence and adulthood.

Recent analyses have shown that the later the weight gain in childhood and adolescence, the greater the persistence. More than 60% of overweight children have at least one additional risk factor for cardiovascular disease, such as raised blood pressure, hyperlipidaemia or hyperinsulinaemia, and more than 20% have two or more risk factors.

Habits leading to noncommunicable disease development during adolescence It seems increasingly likely that there are widespread effects of early diet on later body composition, physiology and cognition. Such observations "provide strong support for the recent shift away from defining nutritional needs for prevention of acute deficiency symptoms towards long-term prevention of morbidity and mortality". Increased birth weight increases the risk of obesity later, but children with low birth weight tend to remain small into adulthood.

In industrialized countries there have been only modest increases in birth weight so the increased levels of obesity described earlier must reflect environmental changes. The "obesogenic" environment appears to be largely directed at the adolescent market, making healthy choices that much more difficult. At the same time, exercise patterns have changed and considerable parts of the day are spent sitting at school, in a factory, or in front of a television or computer.

Raised blood pressure, impaired glucose tolerance and dyslipidaemia are associated in children and adolescents with unhealthy lifestyles, such as diets containing excessive intakes of fats, cholesterol and salt, an inadequate intake of fibre and potassium, a lack of exercise, and increased television viewing. Physical inactivity and smoking have been found independently to predict CHD and stroke in later life.

Unhealthy lifestyles do not just appear in adulthood but drive the early development of obesity, dyslipidaemia, high blood pressure, impaired glucose tolerance and associated disease risk. In many countries, perhaps most typified by the United States, changes in family eating patterns, including the increased consumption of fast foods, pre-prepared meals and carbonated drinks, have taken place over the past 30 years. At the same time, the amount of physical activity has been greatly reduced both at home and in school, as well as by increasing use of mechanized transport.

Adulthood

The three critical questions relating to adulthood were identified as:

(i) to what extent do risk factors continue to be important in the development of chronic diseases;

(ii) to what extent will modifying such risk factors make a difference to the emergence of disease; and

(iii) what is the role of risk factor reduction and modification in secondary prevention and the treatment of those with disease?

Reviewing the evidence within the framework of a life-course approach highlights the importance of the adult phase of life, it being both the period during which most chronic diseases are expressed, as well as a critical time for the preventive reduction of risk factors and for increasing effective treatment. The most firmly established associations between cardiovascular disease or diabetes and factors in the lifespan are the ones between those diseases and the major known "adult" risk factors, such as tobacco use, obesity, physical inactivity, cholesterol, high blood pressure and alcohol consumption.

The factors that have been confirmed to lead to an increased risk of CHD, stroke and diabetes are: high blood pressure for CHD or stroke; high cholesterol (diet) for CHD, and tobacco use for CHD. Other associations are robust and consistent, although they have not necessarily been shown to be reversible: obesity and physical inactivity for CHD, diabetes and stroke; and heavy or binge drinking for CHD and stroke. Most of the studies are from developed countries, but supporting evidence from developing countries is beginning to emerge, for example, from India.

In developed countries, low socioeconomic status is associated with higher risk of cardiovascular disease and diabetes. As in the affluent industrialized countries, there appears to be an initial preponderance of cardiovascular disease among the higher socioeconomic groups, for example, as has been found in China. It is presumed that the disease will progressively shift to the more disadvantaged sectors of society. There is some evidence that this is already happening, especially among women in low-income groups, for example in Brazil and South Africa, as well as in countries in economic transition such as Morocco.

Other risk factors are continually being recognized or proposed. These include the role of high levels of homocysteine, the related factor of low folate, and the role of iron. From a social sciences perspective, Losier has suggested that socioeconomic level is less important than a certain stability in the physical and social environment. In other words, an individual's sense of understanding of his or her environment, coupled with control over the course and setting of his or her own life appears to be the most important determinant of health. Marmot, among others, has demonstrated the impact of the wider environment and societal and individual stress on the development of chronic disease.

Ageing

There are three critical aspects relating to chronic diseases in the later part of the life-cycle:

(i) most chronic diseases will be manifested in this later stage of life;

(ii) there is an absolute benefit for ageing individuals and populations in changing risk factors and adopting health-promoting behaviours such as exercise and healthy diets; and

(iii) the need to maximize health by avoiding or delaying preventable disability.

Along with the societal and disease transitions, there has been a major demographic shift. Although older people are currently defined as those aged 60 years and above, this definition of older people has a very different meaning from the middle of the last century, when 60 years of age and above often exceeded the average life expectancy, especially in industrialized countries. It is worth remembering, however, that the majority of elderly people will, in fact, be living in the developing world.

Most chronic diseases are present at this period of life —the result of interactions between multiple disease processes as well as more general losses in physiological functions. Cardiovascular disease peaks at this period, as does type 2 diabetes and some cancers. The main burden of chronic diseases is observed at this stage of life and, therefore, needs to be addressed.

In the 1970s, it was thought that risks were not significantly increased after certain late ages and that there would be no benefit in changing habits, such as dietary habits, after 80 years old as there was no epidemiological evidence that changing habits would affect mortality or even health conditions among older people.

There was also a feeling that people "earned" some unhealthy behaviours simply because of reaching "old age". Then there was a more active intervention phase, when older people were encouraged to change their diets in ways that were probably overly rigorous for the expected benefit.

More recently, older people have been encouraged to eat a healthy diet —as large and as varied as possible while maintaining their weight —and particularly to continue exercise. Liu et al. have reported an observed risk of atherosclerotic disease among older women that was approximately 30% less in women who ate 5—10 servings of fruits and vegetables per day than in those who ate 2—5 servings per day. It seems that, as elderly patients have a higher cardiovascular risk, they are more likely to gain from risk factor modification.

Although this age group has received relatively little attention as regards primary prevention, the acceleration in decline caused by external factors is generally believed to be reversible at any age. Interventions aimed at supporting the individual and promoting healthier environments will often lead to increased independence in older age. Interactions between early and later factors throughout the life course Low birth weight, followed by subsequent adult obesity, has been shown to impart a particularly high risk of CHD, as well as diabetes.

Risk of CHD

Impaired glucose tolerance and an adverse lipid profile are seen as early as childhood and adolescence, where they typically appear clustered together with higher blood pressure and relate strongly to obesity, in particular central obesity. Raised blood pressure, impaired glucose tolerance and dyslipidaemia also tend to be clustered in children and adolescents with unhealthy lifestyles and diets, such as those with excessive intakes of saturated fats, cholesterol and salt, and inadequate intake of fibre.

Lack of exercise and increased television viewing add to the risk. In older children and adolescents, habitual alcohol and tobacco use also contribute to raised blood pressure and to the development of other risk factors in early adulthood. Many of the same factors continue to act throughout the life course. Such clustering represents an opportunity to address more than one risk at a time. The clustering of health-related behaviours is also a well described phenomenon.

Young girls who grow poorly become stunted women and are more likely to give birth to low-birth-weight babies who are then likely to continue the cycle by being stunted in adulthood, and so on. Maternal birth size is a significant predictor of a child's birth size after controlling for gestational age, sex of the child, socioeconomic status, and maternal age, height and pre-pregnant weight.

There are clear indications of intergenerational factors in obesity, such as parental obesity, maternal gestational diabetes and maternal birth weight. Low maternal birth weight is associated with higher blood pressure levels in the offspring, independent of the relation between the offspring's own birth weight and blood pressure. Unhealthy lifestyles can also have a direct effect on the health of the next generation, for example, smoking during pregnancy.

There is good evidence that nutrients and physical activity influence gene expression and have shaped the genome over several million years of human evolution. Genes define opportunities for health and susceptibility to disease, while environmental factors determine which susceptible individuals will develop illness. In view of changing socioeconomic conditions in developing countries, such added stress may result in exposure of underlying genetic predisposition to chronic diseases. Gene—nutrient interactions also involve the environment.

The dynamics of the relationships are becoming better understood but there is still a long way to go in this area, and also in other aspects, such as disease prevention and control. Studies continue on the role of nutrients in gene expression; for example, researchers are currently trying to understand why omega-3 fatty acids suppress or decrease the mRNA of interleukin, which is elevated in atherosclerosis, arthritis and other autoimmune diseases, whereas the omega-6 fatty acids do not.

Studies on genetic variability to dietary response indicate that specific genotypes raise cholesterol levels more than others. The need for targeted diets for individuals and subgroups to prevent chronic diseases was acknowledged as being part of an overall approach to prevention at the population level. However, the practical implications of this issue for public health policy have only begun to be addressed.

For example, a recent study of the relationship between folate and cardiovascular disease revealed that a common single gene mutation that reduces the activity of an enzyme involved in folate metabolism (MTHFR) is associated with a moderate (20%) increase in serum homocysteine and higher risk of both ischaemic heart disease and deep vein thrombosis. Although humans have evolved being able to feed on a variety of foods and to adapt to them, certain genetic adaptations and limitations have occurred in relation to diet.

Understanding the evolutionary aspects of diet and its composition might suggest a diet that would be consistent with the diet to which our genes were programmed to respond. However, the early diet was presumably one which gave evolutionary advantage to reproduction in the early part of life, and so may be less indicative of guidance for healthy eating, in terms of lifelong health and prevention of chronic disease after reproduction has been achieved.

Because there are genetic variations among individuals, changes in dietary patterns have a differential impact on a genetically heterogeneous population, although populations with a similar evolutionary background have more similar genotypes. Most are polygenic in nature and rapidly escalating rates suggest the importance of environmental change rather than change in genetic susceptibility.

There is a vast volume of scientific evidence highlighting the importance of applying a life-course approach to the prevention and control of chronic disease. The picture is, however, still not complete, and the evidence sometimes contradictory. From the available evidence, it is possible to state the following:

— Unhealthy diets, physical inactivity and smoking are confirmed risk behaviours for chronic diseases.

— The biological risk factors of hypertension, obesity and lipidaemia are firmly established as risk factors for coronary heart disease, stroke and diabetes.

— Nutrients and physical activity influence gene expression and may define susceptibility.

— The major biological and behavioural risk factors emerge and act in early life, and continue to have a negative impact throughout the life course.

— The major biological risk factors can continue to affect the health of the next generation.

— An adequate and appropriate postnatal nutritional environment is important.

— Globally, trends in the prevalence of many risk factors are upwards, especially those for obesity, physical inactivity and, in the developing world particularly, smoking.

— Selected interventions are effective but must extend beyond individual risk factors and continue throughout the life course.

— Some preventive interventions early in the life course offer lifelong benefits.

— Improving diets and increasing levels of physical activity in adults and older people will reduce chronic disease risks for death and disability.

— Secondary prevention through diet and physical activity is a complementary strategy in retarding the progression of existing chrcnic diseases and decreasing mortality and the disease burden from such diseases.

As well as preventing chronic diseases, there are clearly many other reasons to improve the quality of life of people throughout their lifespan. The intention of primary prevention interventions is to move the profile of the whole population in a healthier direction. Small changes in risk factors in the majority who are at moderate risk can have an enormous impact in terms of population-attributable risk of death and disability.

By preventing disease in large populations, small reductions in blood pressure, blood cholesterol and so on can dramatically reduce health costs. For example, it has been demonstrated that improved lifestyles can reduce the risk of progression to diabetes by a striking 58% over 4 years. Other population studies have shown that up to 80% of cases of coronary heart disease, and up to 90% of cases of type 2 diabetes, could potentially be avoided through changing lifestyle factors, and about one-third of cancers could be avoided by eating healthily, maintaining normal weight and exercising throughout life.

For interventions to have a lasting effect on the risk factor prevalence and the health of societies, it is also essential to change or modify the environment in which these diseases develop. Changes in dietary patterns, the influence of advertising and the globalization of diets, and widespread reduction in physical activity have generally had negative impacts in terms of risk factors, and presumably also in terms of subsequent disease. Reversing current trends will require a multifaceted public health policy approach.

While it is important to avoid inappropriately applying nutritional guidelines to populations that may differ genetically from those for whom the dietary and risk data were originally determined, to date the information regarding genes or gene combinations is insufficient to define specific dietary recommendations based on a population distribution of specific genetic polymorphisms.

Guidelines should try to ensure that the overall benefit of recommendations to the majority of the population substantially outweighs any potential adverse effects on selected subgroups of the population. For example, population-wide efforts to prevent weight gain may trigger a fear of fatness and, therefore, undernutrition in adolescent girls.

The population nutrient goals recommended by the Joint WHO/FAO Expert Consultation at the present meeting are based on current scientific knowledge and evidence, and are intended to be further adapted and tailored to local or national diets and populations, where diet has evolved to be appropriate for the culture and local environment.

The goals are intended to reverse or reduce the impact of unfavourable dietary changes that have occurred over the past century in the industrialized world and more recently in many developing countries. Present nutrient intake goals also need to take into account the effects of long-term environmental changes, i. e. those that have occurred over time-scales of hundreds of years. For example, the metabolic response to periodic famine and chronic food shortage may no longer represent a selective advantage but instead may increase susceptibility to chronic diseases. An abundant stable food supply is a recent phenomenon; it was not a factor until the advent of the industrial revolution.

A combination of physical activity, food variety and extensive social interaction is the most likely lifestyle profile to optimize health, as reflected in increased longevity and healthy ageing. Some available evidence suggests that, within the time frame of a week, at least 20 and probably as many as 30 biologically distinct types of foods, with the emphasis on plant foods, are required for healthy diets.

The implications of the recommendations would be to increase the consumption of fruits and vegetables, to increase the consumption of fish, and to alter the types of fats and oils, as well as the amount of sugars and starch consumed, especially in developed countries.

The current move towards increasing animal protein in diets in countries in economic transition is unlikely to be reversed in those countries where there are increased consumer resources, but is unlikely to be conducive to adult health, at least in terms of preventing chronic diseases.

Preventing Diet-related Diseases

Consistent with the concept of a safe range of nutrient intakes for individuals, there is often a range of population averages that would be consistent with the maintenance of health. If existing population averages fall outside this range, or trends in intake suggest that the population average will move outside the range, health concerns are likely to arise. Sometimes there is no lower limit; this implies that there is no evidence that the nutrient is required in the diet and hence low intakes should not give rise to concern.

The definition of an increased or a decreased risk should be based on a relationship that has been established by multiple randomized controlled trials of interventions on populations that are representative of the target of a recommendation, but this type of evidence is often not available. The recommended dietary/ nutrition practice should modify the attributable risk of the undesirable exposure in that population.

The following criteria are used to describe the strength of evidence. They are based on the criteria used by the World Cancer Research Fund, but have been modified by the Joint WHO/FAO/UNU Expert Consultation to include the results of controlled trials where relevant and available. In addition, consistent evidence on community and environmental factors which lead to behaviour changes and thereby modify risks has been taken into account in categorizing risks.

Convincing evidence: Evidence based on epidemiological studies showing consistent associations between exposure and disease, with little or no evidence to the contrary. The available evidence is based on a substantial number of studies including prospective observational studies and where relevant, randomized controlled trials of sufficient size, duration and quality showing consistent effects. The association should be biologically plausible.

Probable evidence: Evidence based on epidemiological studies showing fairly consistent associations between exposure and disease, but where there are perceived shortcomings in the available evidence or some evidence to the contrary, which precludes a more definite judgement. Shortcomings in the evidence may be any of the following: insufficient duration of trials (or studies); insufficient trials (or studies) available; inadequate sample sizes; incomplete follow-up.

— *Possible evidence*: Evidence based mainly on findings from case— control and cross-sectional studies. Insufficient randomized controlled trials, observational studies or non-randomized controlled trials are available. Evidence based on non-epidemiological studies, such as clinical and laboratory investigations, is supportive. More trials are required to support the tentative associations, which should also be biologically plausible.

— *Insufficient evidence*: Evidence based on findings of a few studies which are suggestive, but are insufficient to establish an association between exposure and disease. Limited or no evidence is available from randomized controlled trials. More well designed research is required to support the tentative associations.

The strength of evidence linking dietary and lifestyle factors to the risk of developing obesity, type 2 diabetes, CVD, cancer, dental diseases, osteoporosis, graded according to the above categories.

The population nutrient intake goals for consideration by national and regional bodies establishing dietary recommendations for the prevention of diet-related chronic diseases are presented in Table 5.

Table 5
Ranges of population nutrient intake goals

Dietary factor	Goal (%of total energy, unless otherwise stated)
Total fat	15—30%
Saturated fatty acids	<10%
Polyunsaturated fatty acids	6—10%
n-6 Polyunsaturated fatty acids	5—8%
n-3 Polyunsaturated fatty acids	1—2%
Trans fatty acids	<1%

Monounsaturated fatty acids	By difference
Total carbohydrate	55—75%
Free sugars	<10%
Protein	10—15%
Cholesterol	<300 mg per day
Sodium chloride (sodium)	<5 g per day (<2 g per day)
Fruits and vegetables	5 400 g per day
Total dietary fibre	From foods
Non-starch polysaccharides (NSP)	From foods

These recommendations are expressed in numerical terms, rather than as increases or decreases in intakes of specific nutrients, because the desirable change will depend upon existing intakes in the particular population, and could be in either direction.

In Table 1, attention is directed towards the energy-supplying macronutrients. This must not be taken to imply a lack of concern for the other nutrients. The recommendations for total fat are formulated to include countries where the usual fat intake is typically above 30%as well as those where the usual intake may be very low, for example less than 15%. Total fat energy of at least 20%is consistent with good health. Highly active groups with diets rich in vegetables, legumes, fruits and wholegrain cereals may, however, sustain a total fat intake of up to 35%without the risk of unhealthy weight gain. For countries where the usual fat intake is between 15%and 20%of energy, there is no direct evidence for men that raising fat intake to 20% will be beneficial. For women of reproductive age at least 20%has been recommended by the Joint FAO/WHO Expert Consultation on Fats and Oils in Human Nutrition that met in 1993.

Recommendations for total fat

The recommendations for total fat are formulated to include countries where the usual fat intake is typically above 30%as well as those where the usual intake may be very low,for example less than 15%.Total fat energy of at least 20%is consistent with good health.Highly active groups with diets rich in vegetables,legumes,fruits and wholegrain cereals may,however,sustain a total fat intake of up to 35%without the risk of unhealthy weight gain.

For countries where the usual fat intake is between 15%and 20%of energy,there is no direct evidence for men that raising fat intake to 20% will be beneficial. For women of reproductive age at least 20%has been recommended by the Joint FAO/WHO Expert Consultation on Fats and Oils in Human Nutrition that met in 1993.

Free sugars

Higher intakes of free sugars threaten the nutrient quality of diets by providing significant energy without specific nutrients. The Consultation considered that restriction of free sugars was also likely to contribute to reducing the risk of unhealthy weight gain, noting that: Free sugars contribute to the overall energy density of diets.

Free sugars promote a positive energy balance. Acute and short-term studies in human volunteers have demonstrated increased total energy intake when the energy density of the diet is increased, whether by free sugars or fat. Diets that are limited in free sugars have been shown to reduce total energy intake and induce weight loss. Drinks that are rich in free sugars increase overall energy intake by reducing appetite control.

There is thus less of a compensatory reduction of food intake after the consumption of high-sugars drinks than when additional foods of equivalent energy content are provided. A recent randomized trial showed that when soft drinks rich in free sugars are consumed there is a higher energy intake and a progressive increase in body weight when compared with energy-free drinks that are artificially sweetened. Children with a high consumption of soft drinks rich in free sugars are more likely to be overweight and to gain excess weight.

The Consultation recognized that a population goal for free sugars of less than 10%of total energy is controversial. However, the Consultation considered that the studies showing no effect of free sugars on excess weight have limitations. The CARMEN study (Carbohydrate Ratio Management in European National diets) was a multicentre, rando-mized trial that tested the effects on body weight and blood -lipids in overweight individuals of altering the ratio of fat to carbohydrate, as well as the ratio of simple to complex carbohydrate per se.

A greater weight reduction was observed with the high complex carbohydrate diet relative to the simple carbohydrate one; the difference, however was not statistically significant. Nevertheless, an analysis of weight change and metabolic indices for those with metabolic syndrome revealed a clear benefit of replacing simple by complex carbohydrates.

The Consultation also examined the results of studies that found an inverse relationship between free sugars intakes and total fat intake. Many of these studies are methodologically inappropriate for determining the causes of excess weight gain, since the percentage of calories from fat will decrease as the percentage of calories from carbohydrates increases and vice versa. Furthermore, these analyses do not usually distinguish between free sugars in foods and free sugars in drinks. Thus, these analyses are not good predictors of the responses in energy intake to a selective reduction in free sugars intake.

Non-starch polysaccharides (NSP)

Wholegrain cereals, fruits and vegetables are the preferred sources of non-starch polysaccharides (NSP). The best definition of dietary fibre remains to be established, given the potential health benefits of resistant starch. The recommended intake of fruits and vegetables and consumption of wholegrain foods is likely to provide >20 g per day of NSP (>25 g per day of total dietary fibre).

Fruits and vegetables

The benefit of fruits and vegetables cannot be ascribed to a single or mix of nutrients and bioactive substances. Therefore, this food category was included rather than the nutrients themselves. The category of tubers (i. e. potatoes, cassava) should not be included in fruits and vegetables. Body mass index (BMI).

The goal for body mass index (BMI) follows the recommendations made by the WHO Expert Consultation on Obesity that met in 1997. At the population level, the goal is for an adult median BMI of 21--23 kg/m. For individuals, the recommendation is to maintain a BMI in the range 18. 5--24. 9 kg/mand to avoid a weight gain greater than 5 kg during adult life.

Physical activity

The goal for physical activity focuses on maintaining healthy body weight. The recommendation is for a total of one hour per day on most days of the week of moderate-intensity activity, such as walking. This level of physical activity is needed to maintain a healthy body weight, particularly for people with sedentary occupations.

The recommendation is based on calculations of energy balance and on an analysis of the extensive literature on the relationships between body weight and physical activity. This recommendation is also presented elsewhere. Obviously, this quantitative goal cannot be considered as a single "best value" by analogy with the nutrient intake goals. Furthermore, it differs from the following widely accepted public health recommendation:

For better health, people of all ages should include a minimum of 30 minutes of physical activity of moderate intensity (such as brisk walking) on most, if not all, days of the week. For most people greater health benefits can be obtained by engaging in physical activity of more vigorous intensity or of longer duration. This cardio respiratory endurance activity should be supplemented with strength-developing exercises at least twice a week for adults in order to improve musculo skeletal health, maintain independence in performing the activities of daily life and reduce the risk of falling. The difference between the two recommendations results from the difference in their focus.

A recent symposium on the dose—response relationships between physical activity and health outcomes found evidence that 30 minutes of moderate activity is sufficient for cardiovascular/metabolic health, but not for all health benefits. Because prevention of obesity is a central health goal, the recommendation of 60 minutes a day of moderate-intensity activity is considered appro-priate. Activity of moderate intensity is found to be sufficient to have a preventive effect on most, if not all, cardiovascular and metabolic diseases considered.

Higher intensity activity has a greater effect on some, although not all, health outcomes, but is beyond the capacity and motivation of a large majority of the population. Both recommendations include the idea that the daily activity can be accomplished in several short bouts. It is important to point out that both recommendations apply to people who are otherwise sedentary. Some occupational activities and household chores constitute sufficient daily physical exercise.

In recommending physical activity, potential individual risks as well as benefits need to be assessed. In many regions of the world, especially but not exclusively in rural areas of developing countries, an appreciable proportion of the population is still engaged in physically demanding activities relating to agricultural practices and domestic tasks performed without mechanization or with rudimentary tools. Even children may be required to undertake physically demanding tasks at very young ages, such as collecting water and firewood and caring for livestock.

Similarly, the inhabitants of poor urban areas may still be required to walk long distances to their jobs, which are usually of a manual nature and often require a high expenditure of energy. Clearly, the recommendation for extra physical activity is not relevant for these sectors of the population.

Preventing excess weight gain and obesity

Almost all countries are experien-cing an obesity epidemic, although with great variation between and within countries. In low-income countries, obesity is more common in middle-aged women, people of higher socioeconomic status and those living in urban communities.

In more affluent countries, obesity is not only common in the middle-aged, but is becoming increasingly prevalent among younger adults and children. Furthermore, it tends to be associated with lower socioeconomic status, especially in women, and the urban—rural differences are diminished or even reversed. It has been estimated that the direct costs of obesity accounted for 6. 8% of total health care costs, and physical inactivity for a further US$24 billion, in the United States in 1995.

Although direct costs in other industrialized countries are slightly lower, they still consume a sizeable proportion of national health budgets. Indirect costs, which are far greater than direct costs, include workdays lost, physician visits, disability pensions and premature mortality. Intangible costs such as impaired quality of life are also enormous.

Because the risks of diabetes, cardiovascular disease and hypertension rise continuously with increas-ing weight, there is much overlap between the prevention of obesity and the prevention of a variety of chronic diseases, especially type 2 diabetes. Population education strategies will need a solid base of policy and environment-based changes to be effective in eventually reversing these trends.

The increasing industrialization, urbanization and mechanization occurring in most countries around the world is associated with changes in diet and behaviour, in particular, diets are becoming richer in high-fat, high energy foods and lifestyles more sedentary. In many developing countries undergoing economic transition, rising levels of obesity often coexist in the same population (or even the same household) with chronic undernutrition. Increases in obesity over the past 30 years have been paralleled by a dramatic rise in the prevalence of diabetes.

Diet, physical activity and excess weight gain and obesity Mortality rates increase with increasing degrees of overweight, as measured by BMI. As BMI increases, so too does the proportion of people with one or more comorbid conditions. In one study in the USA, over half (53%) of all deaths in women with a BMI>29 kg/m could be directly attributed to their obesity. Eating behaviours that have been linked to overweight and obesity include snacking/eating frequency, binge-eating patterns, eating out, and (protectively) exclusive breast-feeding. Nutrient factors under investigation include fat, carbohydrate type (including refined carbohydrates such as sugar), the glycaemic index of foods, and fibre. Environmental issues are clearly important, especially as many environments become increasingly "obesogenic" (obesity-promoting).

Physical activity is an important determinant of body weight. In addition, physical activity and physical fitness (which relates to the ability to perform physical activity) are important modifiers of mortality and morbidity related to overweight and obesity. There is firm evidence that moderate to high fitness levels provide a substantially reduced risk of cardiovascular disease and all-cause mortality and that these benefits apply to all BMI levels. Furthermore, high fitness protects against mortality at all BMI levels in men with diabetes. Low cardiovascular fitness is a serious and common comorbidity of obesity, and a sizeable proportion of deaths in overweight and obese populations are probably a result of low levels of cardio-respiratory fitness rather than obesity per se. Fitness is, in turn, influenced strongly by physical activity in addition to genetic factors. These relationships emphasize the role of physical activity in the prevention of overweight and obesity, independently of the effects of physical activity on body weight.

There is convincing evidence that regular physical activity is protective against unhealthy weight gain whereas sedentary lifestyles, particularly sedentary occupations and inactive recreation such as watching television, promote it. Most epidemiological studies show smaller risk of weight gain, overweight and obesity among persons who currently engage regularly in moderate to large amounts of physical activity. Studies measuring physical activity at baseline and randomized trials of exercise programmes show more mixed results, probably because of the low adherence to long-term changes. Therefore, it is ongoing physical activity itself rather than previous physical activity or enrolment in an exercise programme that is protective against unhealthy weight gain.

The recommendation for individuals to accumulate at least 30 minutes of moderate-intensity physical activity on most days is largely aimed at reducing cardiovascular diseases and overall mortality. The amount needed to prevent unhealthy weight gain is uncertain but is probably significantly greater than this. Preventing weight gain after substantial weight loss probably requires about 60--90 minutes per day. Two meetings recommended by consensus that about 45--60 minutes of moderate-intensity physical activity is needed on most days or every day to prevent unhealthy weight gain. Studies aimed at reducing sedentary behaviours have focused primarily on reducing television viewing in children. Reducing viewing times by about 30 minutes a day in children in the United States appears feasible and is associated with reductions in BMI.

A high dietary intake of non-starch polysaccharides (NSP) /dietary fibre (protective). The nomenclature and definitions of NSP (dietary fibre) have changed with time, and many of the available studies used previous definitions, such as soluble and insoluble fibre. Nevertheless, two recent reviews of randomized trials have concluded that the majority of studies show that a high intake of NSP (dietary fibre) promotes weight loss.

There is convincing evidence that a high intake of energy-dense foods promotes weight gain. In high-income countries (and increasingly in low-income countries) these energy-dense foods are not only highly processed (low NSP) but also micronutrient-poor, further diminishing their nutritional value. Energy-dense foods tend to be high in fat (e. g. butter, oils, fried foods), sugars or starch, while energy-dilute foods have a high water content (e, g. fruits and vegetables). Several trials have covertly manipulated the fat content and the energy density of diets, the results of which support the view that so-called "passive over consumption" of total energy occurs when the energy density of the diet is high and that this is almost always the case in high-fat diets.

A meta-analysis of 16 trials of ad libitum high-fat versus low-fat diets of at least 2 months duration suggested that a reduction in fat content by 10%corresponds to about a 1 MJ reduction in energy intake and about 3 kg in body weight. At a population level, 3 kg equates to about one BMI unit or about a 5% difference in obesity prevalence. However, it is difficult to blind such studies and other non-physiological effects may influence these findings. While energy from fat is no more fattening than the same amount of energy from carbohydrate or protein, diets that are high in fat tend to be energy-dense. Animportant exception to this is diets based predominantly on energy-dilute foods but which have a reasonably high percentage of energy as fat from added oils.

The effectiveness over the long term of most dietary strategies for weight loss, including low-fat diets, remains uncertain unless accompanied by changes in behaviour affecting physical activity and food habits. These latter changes at a public health level require an environment supportive of healthy food choices and an active life. High quality trials to address these issues are urgently needed. A variety of popular weight-loss diets that restrict food choices may result in reduced energy intake and short-term weight loss in individuals but most do not have trial evidence of long-term effectiveness and nutritional adequacy and therefore cannot be recommended for populations.

Despite the obvious importance of the roles that parents and home environments play on children's eating and physical activity behaviours, there is very little hard evidence available to support this view. It appears that access and exposure to a range of fruits and vegetables in the home is important for the development of preferences for these foods and that parental knowledge, attitudes and behaviours related to healthy diet and physical activity are important in creating role models.

Some studies, but not all, have shown an effect of school-based interventions on obesity prevention. While more research is clearly needed to increase the evidence base in both these areas, supportive home and school environments were rated as a probable etiological influence on obesity.

Part of the consistent, strong relationships between television viewing and obesity in children may relate to the food advertising to which they are exposed. Fast-food restaurants, and foods and beverages that are usually classified under the "eat least" category in dietary guidelines are among the most heavily marketed products, especially on television.

Young children are often the target group for the advertising of these products because they have a significant influence on the foods bought by parents. The huge expenditure on marketing fast-foods and other "eat least" choices was considered to be a key factor in the increased consumption of food prepared outside the home in general and of energy-dense, micronutrient-poor foods in particular.

Young children are unable to distinguish programme content from the persuasive intent of advertisements. The evidence that the heavy marketing of these foods and beverages to young children causes obesity is not unequivocal.

Diets that are proportionally low in fat will be proportionally nigher in carbohydrate (including a variable amount of sugars) and are associated with protection against unhealthy weight gain, although a high intake of free sugars in beverages probably promotes weight gain. The physiolo-gical effects of energy intake on satiation and satiety appear to be quite different for energy in solid foods as opposed to energy in fluids. Possibly because of reduced gastric distension and faster transit times, the energy contained in fluids is less well "detected" by the body and subsequent food intake is poorly adjusted to account for the energy taken in through beverages. This is supported by data from cross-sectional, longitudinal, and cross-over studies.

The high and increasing consumption of sugars-sweetened drinks by children in many countries is of serious concern. It has been estimated that each additional can or glass of sugars-sweetened drink that they consume every day increases the risk of becoming obese by 60%. Most of the evidence relates to soda drinks but many fruit drinks and cordials are equally energy-dense and may promote weight gain if drunk in large quantities.

Classically the pattern of the progression of obesity through a population starts with middle-aged women in high-income groups but as the epidemic progresses, obesity becomes more common in people (especially women) in lower socioeconomic status groups. The relationship may even be bi-directional, setting up a vicious cycle (i. e. lower socioeconomic status promotes obesity, and obese people are more likely to end up in groups with low socioeconomic status). The mechanisms by which socioeconomic status influences food and activity patterns are probably multiple and need elucidation. However, people living in circumstances of low socioeconomic status may be more at the mercy of the obesogenic environment because their eating and activity behaviours are more likely to be the "default choices" on offer. The evidence for an effect of low socioeconomic status on predisposing people to obesity is consistent across a number of cross-sectional and longitudinal studies, and was thus rated as a "probable" cause of increased risk of obesity.

Breastfeeding as a protective factor against weight gain has been examined in at least 20 studies involving nearly 40 000 subjects. Five studies (including the two largest) found a protective effect, two found that breastfeeding predicted obesity, and the remainder found no relationships. There are probably multiple effects of confounding in these studies; however, the reduction in the risk of developing obesity observed in the two largest studies was substantial. Promoting breastfeeding has many benefits, the prevention of childhood obesity probably being one of them.

Several other factors were defined as "possible" protective or causative in the etiology of unhealthy weight gain. Low-glycaemic foods have been proposed as a potential protective factor against weight gain and there are some early studies that support this hypothesis. More clinical trials are, however, needed to establish the association with greater certainty. Large portion sizes are a possible causative factor for unhealthy weight gain. The marketing of "supersize" portions, particularly in fast-food outlets, is now common practice in many countries. There is some evidence that people poorly estimate portion sizes and that subsequent energy compensation for a large meal is incomplete and therefore is likely to lead to overconsumption. In many countries, there has been a steady increase in the proportion of food eaten that is prepared outside the home. In the United States, the energy, total fat, saturated fat, cholesterol and sodium content of foods prepared outside the home is significantly higher than that of home-prepared food. People in the United States who tend to eat in restaurants have a higher BMI than those who tend to eat at home. Certain psychological parameters of eating patterns may influence the risk of obesity. The "flexible restraint" pattern is associated with lower risk of weight gain, whereas the "rigid restraint/periodic disinhibition" pattern is associated with a higher risk.

Several other factors were also considered but the evidence was not thought to be strong enough to warrant defining them as protective or causative. Studies have not shown consistent associations between alcohol intake and obesity despite the high energy density of the nutrient. There are probably many confounding factors that influence the association. While a high eating frequency has been shown in some studies to have a negative relationship with energy intake and weight gain, the types of foods readily available as snack foods are often high in fat and a high consumption of foods of this type might predispose people to weight gain. The evidence regarding the impact of early nutrition on subsequent obesity is also mixed, with some studies showing relation-ships for high and low birth weights.

Strategies for obesity prevention

The prevention of obesity in infants and young children should be considered of high priority. For infants and young children, the main preventive strategies are:

— the promotion of exclusive breastfeeding;

— avoiding the use of added sugars and starches when feeding formula;

— instructing mothers to accept their child 's ability to regulate energy intake rather than feeding until the plate is empty;

— assuring the appropriate micronutrient intake needed to promote optimal linear growth.

For children and adolescents, prevention of obesity implies the need to:

— promote an active lifestyle;

— limit television viewing;

— promote the intake of fruits and vegetables;

— restrict the intake of energy-dense, micronutrient-poor foods;

— restrict the intake of sugars-sweetened soft drinks.

Additional measures include modifying the environment to enhance physical activity in schools and communities, creating more opportu-nities for family interaction, limiting the exposure of young children to heavy marketing practices of energy-dense, micronutrient-poor foods, and providing the necessary informa-tion and skills to make healthy food choices.

In developing countries, special attention should be given to avoidance of overfeeding stunted population groups. Nutrition programmes designed to control or prevent undernutrition need to assess stature in combination with weight to prevent providing excess energy to children of low weight-for-age but normal weight-for-height. In countries in economic transition, as populations become more sedentary and able to access energy-dense foods, there is a need to maintain the healthy components of traditional diets. Education provided to mothers and low socioeconomic status communities that are food insecure should stress that overweight and obesity do not represent good health.

Low-income groups globally and populations in countries in economic transition often replace traditional micronutrient-rich foods by heavily marketed, sugars-sweetened beverages and energy-dense fatty, salty and sugary foods. These trends, coupled with reduced physical activity, are associated with the rising prevalence of obesity. Strategies are needed to improve the quality of diets by increasing consumption of fruits and vegetables, in addition to increasing physical activity, in order to stem the epidemic of obesity and associated diseases.

Body mass index

BMI can be used to estimate, albeit crudely, the prevalence of overweight and obesity within a population and the risks associated with it. It does not, however, account for the wide variations in obesity between different individuals and populations. In recent years, different ranges of BMI cut-off points for overweight and obesity have been proposed, in particular for the Asia-Pacific region. At present available data on which to base definitive recommenda-tions are sparse. Nevertheless, the consultation considered that, to achieve optimum health, the median BMI for the adult population should be in the range 21--23 kg/m, while the goal for individuals should be to maintain BMI in the range 18. 5--24. 9 kg/m.

Table 6
Classification of overweight in adults according to BMI

Classification	BMI (kg/m2)	Risk of comorbidities
Underweight	<18.5	Low
Normal range	18.5—24.9	Average
Overweight	≥ 25.0	
Pre-obese	25.0—29.9	Increased
Obese class I	30.0—34.9	Moderate
Obese class II	35.0—39.9	Severe
Obese class III	≥ 40.0	Very severe

Waist circumference

Waist circumference is a convenient and simple measure which is unrelated to height, correlates closely with BMIand the ratio of waist-to-hip circumference, and is an approximate index of intra-abdominal fat mass and total body fat. Furthermore, changes in waist circumference reflect changes in risk factors for cardiovascular disease and other forms of chronic diseases, even though the risks seem to vary in different populations. There is an increased risk of metabolic complications for men with a waist circumference 5,102 cm, and women with a waist circumference 5, 88 cm.

Physical activity

A total of one hour per day of moderate-intensity

activity, such as walking on most days of the week, is probably needed to maintain a healthy body weight, particularly for people with sedentary occupations.

Total energy intake

The fat and water content of foods are the main determinants of the energy density of the diet. A lower consumption of energy-dense (i. e. high-fat, high-sugars and high-starch) foods and energy-dense (i. e. high free sugars) drinks contributes to a reduction in total energy intake. Conversely, a higher intake of energy-dilute foods (i. e. vegetables and fruits) and foods high in NSP (i. e. wholegrain cereals) contributes to a reduction in total energy intake and an improvement in micronutrient intake. It should be noted, however, that very active groups who have diets high in vegetables, legumes, fruits and wholegrain cereals, may sustain a total fat intake of up to 35%without the risk of unhealthy weight gain.

Preventing diabetes

Type 2 diabetes, formerly known as non-insulin-dependent diabetes (NIDDM), accounts for most cases of diabetes worldwide. Type 2 diabetes develops when the production of insulin is insufficient to overcome the underlying abnormality of increased resistance to its action. The early stages of type 2 diabetes are characterized by overproduction of insulin. As the disease progresses, process insulin levels may fall as a result of partial failure of the insulin producing b cells of the pancreas.

Complications of type 2 diabetes include blindness, kidney failure, foot ulceration which may lead to gangrene and subsequent amputation, and appreciably increased risk of infections, coronary heart disease and stroke. The enormous and escalating economic and social costs of type 2 diabetes make a compelling case for attempts to reduce the risk of developing the condition as well as for energetic management of the established disease.

Lifestyle modification is the cornerstone of both treatment and attempts to prevent type 2 diabetes. The changes required to reduce the risk of developing type 2 diabetes at the population level are, however, unlikely to be achieved without major environmental changes to facilitate appro-priate choices by individuals. Criteria for the diagnosis of type 2 diabetes and for the earlier stages in the disease process—impaired glucose tolerance and impaired fasting glucose—have recently been revised. Type 1 diabetes, previously known as insulin-dependent diabetes, occurs much less frequently and is associated with an absolute deficiency of insulin, usually resulting from autoimmune destruction of the b cells of the pancreas.

Environmental as well as genetic factors appear to be involved but there is no convincing evidence of a role for lifestyle factors which can be modified to reduce the risk. Although increases in both the prevalence and incidence of type 2 diabetes have occurred globally, they have been especially dramatic in societies in economic transition in much of the newly industrialized world and in developing countries.

Worldwide, the number of cases of diabetes is currently estimated to be around 150 million. This numberis predicted to double by 2025, with the greatest number of cases being expected in China and India. These numbers may represent an underestimate and there are likely to be many undiagnosed cases. Previously a disease of the middle-aged and elderly, type 2 diabetes has recently escalated in all age groups and is now being identified in younger and younger age groups, including adolescents and children, especially in high-risk populations.

Age-adjusted mortality rates amongpeople with diabetes are 1. 5--2. 5 times higher than in the general population. In Caucasian populations, much of the excess mortality is attributable to cardiovascular disease, especially coronary heart disease; amongst Asian and American Indian populations, renal disease is a major contributor, whereas in some developing nations, infections are an important cause of death.

It is conceivable that the decline in mortality due to coronary heart disease which has occurred in manyaffluent societies maybe halted or even reversed if rates of type 2 diabetes continue to increase. This may occur if the coronary risk factors associated with diabetes increase to the extent that the risk they mediate outweighs the benefit accrued from improve-ments in conventional cardiovascular risk factors and the improved care of patients with established cardiovascular disease.

Type 2 diabetes results from an interaction between genetic and environmental factors. The rapidly changing incidence rates, however, suggest a particularly important role for the latter as well as a potential for stemming the tide of the global epidemic of the disease. The most dramatic increases in type 2 diabetes are occurring in societies in which there have been major changes in the type of diet consumed, reductions in physical activity, and increases in overweight and obesity.

The diets concerned are typically energy-dense, high in saturated fatty acids and depleted in NSP. In all societies, overweight and obesity are associated with an increased risk of type 2 diabetes, especially when the excess adiposity is centrally distributed. Conventional (BMI) categories may not be an appropriate means of determining the risk of developing type 2 diabetes in individuals of all population groups because of ethnic differences in body composition and because of the importance of the distribution of excess adiposity.

While all lifestyle-related and environmental factors which contribute to excess weight gain may be regarded as contributing to type 2 diabetes, the evidence that individual dietary factors have an effect which is independent of their obesity promoting effect, is inconclusive. Evidence that saturated fatty acids increase risk of type 2 diabetes and that NSP are protective is more convincing than the evidence for several other nutrients which have been implicated.

The presence of maternal diabetes, including gestational diabetes and intrauterine growth retardation, especially when associated with later rapid catch-up growth, appears to increase the risk of subsequently developing diabetes. The association between excessive weight gain, central adiposity and the development of type 2 diabetes is convincing.

The association has been repeatedly demonstrated in longitudinal studies in different populations, with a striking gradient of risk apparent with increasing levels of BMI, adult weight gain, waist circumference or waist-to-hip ratio. Indeed waist circumference or waist-to-hip ratio (reflecting abdominal or visceral adiposity) are more powerful determinants of subsequent risk of type 2 diabetes than BMI (16--20). Central adiposity is also an important determinant of insulin resistance, the underlying abnormality in most cases of type 2 diabetes.

Voluntary weight loss improves insulin sensitivity and in several randomized controlled trials has been shown to reduce the risk of progression from impaired glucose tolerance to type 2 diabetes. Longitudinal studies have clearly indicated that increased physical activity reduces the risk of developing type 2 diabetes regardless of the degree of adiposity. Vigorous exercise (i. e. training to an intensity of 80--90%of age-predicted maximum heart rate for at least 20 minutes, at least five times per week) has the potential to substantially enhance insulin sensitivity.

The minimum intensity and duration of physical activity required to improve insulin sensitivity has not been established. Offspring of diabetic pregnancies (including gestational diabetes) are often large and heavy at birth, tend to develop obesity in childhood and are at high risk of developing type 2 diabetes at an early age. Those born to mothers after they have developed diabetes have a three-fold higher risk of developing diabetes than those born before.

In observational epidemiological studies, a high saturated fat intake has been associated with a higher risk of impaired glucose tolerance, and higher fasting glucose and insulin levels. Higher proportions of saturated fatty acids in serum lipid or muscle phospholipid have been associated with higher fasting insulin, lower insulin sensitivity and a higher risk of type 2 diabetes.

Higher unsaturated fatty acids from vegetable sources and polyunsaturated fatty acids have been associated with a reduced risk of type 2 diabetes and lower fasting and 2-hour glucose concentrations. Furthermore, higher proportions of long-chain polyunsaturated fatty acids in skeletal muscle phospholipids have been associated with increased insulin sensitivity. In human intervention studies, replacement of saturated by unsaturated fatty acids leads to improved glucose tolerance and enhanced insulin sensitivity.

Long-chain polyunsaturated fatty acids do not, however, appear to confer additional benefit over monounsaturated fatty acids in intervention studies. Furthermore, when total fat intake is high (greater than 37%of total energy), altering the quality of dietary fat appears to have little effect, a finding which is not surprising given that in observational studies a high intake of total fat has been shown to predict development of impaired glucose tolerance and the progression of impaired glucose tolerance to type 2 diabetes.

A high total fat intake has also been associated with higher fasting insulin concentrations and a lower insulin sensitivity index. Considered in aggregate these findings are deemed to indicate a probable causal link between saturated fatty acids and type 2 diabetes, and a possible causal association between total fat intake and type 2 diabetes.

The two randomized controlled trials which showed a potential for lifestyle modification to reduce the risk of progression from impaired glucose tolerance to type 2 diabetes included advice to reduce total and saturated fat, but in both trials it is impossible to disentangle the effects of individual dietary manipulation. Research relating to the association between NSP intake and type 2 diabetes is complicated by ambiguity with regard to the definitions used (the term dietary fibre and NSP are often incorrectly used interchangeably), different methods of analysis and, consequently, inconsistencies in food composition tables.

Observations by Trowell in Uganda more than 30 years ago suggested that the infrequency of diabetes in rural Africa may be the result of a protective effect of substantial amounts of NSP in the diet (referred to as dietary fibre) associated with a high consumption of minimally-processed or unprocessed carbohydrate.

Three cohort studies have shown a protective effect of NSP which was independent of age, BMI, smoking and physical activity. In many controlled experimental studies, high intakes of NSP (dietary fibre) have repeatedly been shown to result in reduced blood glucose and insulin levels in people with type 2 diabetes and impaired glucose tolerance.

Moreover an increased intake of wholegrain cereals, vegetables and fruits (all rich in NSP) was a feature of the diets associated with a reduced risk of progression of impaired glucose tolerance to type 2 diabetes in the two randomized controlled trials previously described. Thus the evidence for a potential protective effect of NSP (dietary fibre) appears strong.

However, the fact that the experimental studies suggest that soluble forms of NSP exert benefit whereas the prospective cohort studies suggest that it is the cereal-derived insoluble forms that are protective explain the "probable" rather "convincing" grading of the level of evidence. Many foods which are rich in NSP (especially soluble forms), such as pulses, have a low glycaemic index. Other carbohydrate-containing foods (e. g. certain types of pasta), which are not especially high in NSP, also have a low glycaemic index.

Low glycaemic index foods, regardless of their NSP content, are not only associated with a reduced glycaemic response after ingestion when compared with foods of higher glycaemic index, but are also associated with an overall improvement in glycaemic control in people with diabetes. A low glycaemic index does not, however, per se, confer overall health benefits, since a high fat or fructose content of a food may also result in a reduced glycaemic index and such foods may also be energy-dense.

Thus while this property of carbohydrate-containing foods may well influence the risk of developing type 2 diabetes, the evidence is accorded a lower level of strength than the evidence relating to the NSP content. Similarly, the level of evidence for the protective effect of n-3 fatty acids is regarded as 'possible' because the results of epidemiolo-gical studies are inconsistent and the experimental data inconclusive.

There is insufficient evidence to confirm or refute the suggestions that chromium, magnesium, vitamin Eand moderate intakes of alcohol might protect against the development of type 2 diabetes. Anumber of studies, mostly in developing countries, have suggested that intrauterine growth retardation and low birth weight are associated with subsequent development of insulin resistance.

In those countries where there has been chronic undernutrition, insulin resistance may have been selectively advantageous in terms of surviving famine. In populations where energy intake has increased and lifestyles have become more sedentary, however, insulin resistance and the consequent risk of type 2 diabetes have been enhanced. In particular, rapid postnatal catch-up growth appears to further increase the risk of type 2 diabetes in later life.

Appropriate strategies which may help to reduce type 2 diabetes risk in this situation include improving the nutrition of young children, promoting linear growth and preventing energy excess by limiting intake of energy-dense foods, controlling the quality of fat supply, and facilitating physical activity. At a population level, fetal growth may remain restricted until maternal height improves. This may take several generations to correct.

The prevention of type 2 diabetes in infants and young children may be facilitated by the promotion of exclusive breastfeeding, avoiding overweight and obesity, and promot-ing optimum linear growth. The strength of evidence on lifestyle factors is summarized in Table 3.

Table 7
Summary of strength of evidence on lifestyle factors and risk of developing type 2 diabetes

Evidence	Decreased risk	No relationship	Increased risk
Convincing	Voluntary weight loss in overweight and obese people		Overweight and obesity Abdominal obesity
	Physical activity		Physical inactivity Maternal diabetes[a]
Probable	NSP		Saturated fats

			Intrauterine growth retardation
Possible	n-3 fatty acids Low glycaemic index foods Exclusive breastfeeding[b]		Total fat intake Trans fatty acids
Insufficient	Vitamin E Chromium Magnesium Moderate alcohol		Excess alcohol

[1]NSP,non-starch polysaccharides.
[a]Includes gestational diabetes.
[b]As a global public health recommendation,infants should be exclusively breastfed for the first six months of life to achieve optimal growth,development and health.

Measures aimed at reducing overweight and obesity, and cardiovascular disease are likely to also reduce the risk of developing type 2 diabetes and its complications. Some measures are particularly relevant to reducing the risk for diabetes; these are listed below:

— Prevention/treatment of overweight and obesity, particularly in high-risk groups.

— Maintaining an optimum BMI, i. e. at the lower end of the normal range. For the adult population, this meansmaintaining a meanBMIin the range 21--23 kg/ m and avoiding weight gain (>5 kg) in adult life.

— Voluntary weight reduction in overweight or obese individuals with impaired glucose tolerance (although screening for such individuals may not be cost-effective in many countries).

— Practising an endurance activity at moderate or greater level of intensity (e. g. brisk walking) for one hour or more per day on most days per week.

— Ensuring that saturated fat intake does not exceed 10%of total energy and for high-risk groups, fat intake should be <7%of total energy. Achieving adequate intakes of NSP through regular consumption of wholegrain cereals, legumes, fruits and vegetables. A minimum daily intake of 20 g is recommended.

Preventing cardiovascular diseases

The second half of the 20th century has witnessed major shifts in the pattern of disease, in addition to marked improvements in life expectancy, this period is characterized by profound changes in diet and lifestyles which in turn have contributed to an epidemic of noncommunicable diseases. This epidemic is now emerging, and even accelerating, in most developing countries, while infections and nutritional deficiencies are receding as leading contributors to death and disability.

In developing countries, the effect of the nutrition transition and the concomitant rise in the prevalence of cardiovascular diseases will be to widen the mismatch between health care needs and resources, and already scarce resources will be stretched ever more thinly. Because unbalanced diets, obesity and physical inactivity all contribute to heart disease, addressing these, along with tobacco use, can help to stem the epidemic.

A large measure of success in this area has already been demonstrated in many industrialized countries. Cardiovascular diseases are the major contributor to the global burden of disease among the noncommunicable diseases. WHOcurrently attributes one-third of all global deaths to CVD, with developing countries, low-income and middle-income countries accounting for 86% of the DALYs lost to CVDworldwide in 1998.

In the next two decades the increasing burden of CVD will be borne mostly by developing countries. The 'lag-time' effect of risk factors for CVD means that present mortality rates are the consequence of previous exposure to behavioural risk factors such as inappropriate nutrition, insufficient physical activity and increased tobacco consumption.

Overweight, central obesity, high blood pressure, dyslipidaemia, diabetes and low cardio-respiratory fitness are among the biological factors contributing principally to increased risk. Unhealthy dietary practices include the high consump-tion of saturated fats, salt and refined carbohydrates, as well as low consumption of fruits and vegetables, and these tend to cluster together. Convincing associations for reduced risk of CVD include consumption of fruits (including berries) and vegetables, fish and fish oils (eicosapentae-noic acid (EPA) and docosahexaenoic acid (DHA)), foods high in linoleic acid and potassium, as well as physical activity and low to moderate alcohol intake.

While vitamin E intake appears to have no relationship to risk of CVD, there is convincing evidence that myristic and palmitic acids, trans fatty acids, high sodium intake, overweight and high alcohol intake contribute to an increase in risk. A 'probable' level of evidence demonstrates a decreased risk for a -linolenic acid, oleic acid, NSP, wholegrain cereals, nuts (unsalted), folate, plant sterols and stanols, and no relationship for stearic acid. There is a probable increase in risk from dietary cholesterol and unfiltered boiled coffee.

Possible associations for reduced risk include intake of flavonoids and consumption of soy products, while possible associations for increased risk include fats rich in lauric acid, b -carotene supplements and impaired fetal nutrition. The relationship between dietary fats and CVD, especially coronary heart disease, has been extensively investigated, with strong and consistent associations emerging from a wide body of evidence accrued from animal experiments, as well as observational studies, clinical trials and metabolic studies conducted in diverse human populations.

Saturated fatty acids raise total and low-density lipoprotein (LDL) cholesterol, but individual fatty acids within this group, have different effects. Myristic and palmitic acids have the greatest effect and are abundant in diets rich in dairy products and meat. Stearic acid has not been shown to elevate blood cholesterol and is rapidly converted to oleic acid in vivo.

The most effective replacement for saturated fatty acids in terms of coronary heart disease outcome are polyunsaturated fatty acids, especially linoleic acid. This finding is supported by the results of several large randomized clinical trials, in which replacement of saturated and trans fatty acids by polyunsaturated vegetable oils lowered coronary heart disease risk. Trans fatty acids are geometrical isomers of cis-unsaturated fatty acids that adapt a saturated fatty acid-like configuration.

Partial hydrogena-tion, the process used to increase shelf-life of polyunsaturated fatty acids (PUFAs) creates trans fatty acids and also removes the critical double bonds in essential fatty acids necessary for the action. Metabolic studies have demonstrated that trans fatty acids render the plasma lipid profile even more atherogenic than saturated fatty acids, by not only elevating LDL cholesterol to similar levels but also by decreasing high-density lipoprotein (HDL) cholesterol.

Several large cohort studies have found that intake of trans fatty acids increases the risk of coronary heart disease. Most trans fatty acids are contributed by industrially hardened oils. Even though trans fatty acids have been reduced or eliminated from retail fats and spreads in many parts of the world, deep-fried fast foods and baked goods are a major and increasing source. When substituted for saturated fatty acids in metabolic studies, both monounsaturated fatty acids and n-6 polyunsaturated fatty acids lower plasma total and LDL cholesterol concentrations; PUFAs are somewhat more effective than monounsaturates in this respect.

The only nutritionally important monounsaturated fatty acids is oleic acid, which is abundant in olive and canola oils and also in nuts. The most important polyunsaturated fatty acid is linoleic acid, which is abundant especially in soybean and sunflower oils. The most important n-3 PUFAs are eicosapentaenoic acid and docosahexaenoic acid found in fatty fish, and a -linolenic acid found in plant foods.

The biological effects of n-3 PUFAs are wide ranging, involving lipids and lipoproteins, blood pressure, cardiac function, arterial compliance, endothelial function, vascular reactivity and cardiac electrophysiology, as well as potent anti-platelet and anti-inflammatory effects. The very long chain n-3 PUFAs (eicosapentaenoic acid and docosahexaenoic acid) powerfully lower serum triglycerides but they raise serum LDL cholesterol.

Therefore, their effect on coronary heart disease is probably mediated through pathways other than serum cholesterol. Most of the epidemiological evidence related to n-3 PUFAs is derived from studies of fish consumption in populations or interventions involving fish diets in clinical trials (evidence on fish consumption is discussed further below). Fish oils have been used in the Gruppo Italiano per lo Studio della Sopravvivenza nell 'Infarto Miocardico (GISSI) trial involving survivors of myocardial infarction.

After 3. 5 years of follow-up, the group that received fish oil had a 20%reduction in total mortality, a 30%reduction in cardiovascular death and a 45% decrease in sudden death. Several prospective studies have found an inverse association between the intake of a -linolenic acid, (high in flaxseed, canola and soybean oils), and risk of fatal coronary heart disease.

Cholesterol in the blood and tissues is derived from two sources: diet and endogenous synthesis. Dairy fat and meat are major dietary sources. Egg yolk is particularly rich in cholesterol but unlike dairy products and meat does not provide saturated fatty acids. Although dietary cholesterol raises plasma cholesterol levels, observational evidence for an association of dietary cholesterol intake with CVDis contradictory.

There is no requirement for dietary cholesterol and it is advisable to keep the intake as low as possible. If intake of dairy fat and meat are controlled, there is no need to severely restrict egg yolk intake, although some limitation remains prudent. Dietary plant sterols, especially sitostanol, reduce serum cholesterol by inhibiting cholesterol absorption.

The cholesterol-lowering effects of plant sterols has also been well documented and commercial products made of these compounds are widely available, but their long-term effects remain to be seen. Dietary fibre is a heterogeneous mixture of polysaccharides and lignin that cannot be degraded by the endogenous enzymes of vertebrate animals. Water-soluble fibres include pectins, gums, mucilages and some hemicelluloses. Insoluble fibres include cellulose and other hemicellu-loses.

Most fibres reduce plasma total and LDL cholesterol, as reported by several trials. Several large cohort studies carried out in different countries have reported that a high fibre diet as well as a diet high in wholegrain cereals lowers the risk of coronary heart disease. Even though antioxidants could, in theory, be protective against CVD and there is observational data supporting this theory, controlled trials employing supplements have been disappointing.

The Heart Outcomes Prevention Evaluation trial (HOPE), a definitive clinical trial relating vitamin E supplementation to CVD outcomes, revealed no effect of vitamin E supplementation on myocardial infarction, stroke or death from cardiovascular causes in men or women. Also, the results of the Heart Protection Study indicated that no significant benefits of daily supplementation of vitamin E, vitamin C and b -carotene were observed among the high-risk individuals that were the subject of the study. In several studies where dietary vitamin Creduced the risk of coronary heart disease, supplemental vitamin Chad little effect.

Clinical trial evidence is lacking at present. Observational cohort studies have suggested a protective role for carotenoids but a meta-analysis of four randomized trials, in contrast, reported an increased risk of cardiovascular death. The relationship of folate to CVD has been mostly explored through its effect on homocysteine, which may itself be an independent risk factor for coronary heart disease and probably also for stroke. Folic acid is required for the methylation of homocysteine to methionine.

Reduced plasma folate has been strongly associated with elevated plasma homocysteine levels and folate supplementation has been demonstrated to decrease those levels. However, the role of homocysteine as an independent risk factor for CVD has been subject to much debate, since several prospective studies have not found this association to be independent of other risk factors.

It has also been suggested that elevation of plasma homocysteine is a consequence and not a cause of atherosclerosis, wherein impaired renal function resulting from atherosclerosis raises plasma homocysteine levels. Data from the Nurses 'Health Study showed that folate and vitamin B6, from diet and supplements, conferred protection against coronary heart disease. Arecently published meta-analysis concluded that a higher intake of folate (0. 8 mg folic acid) would reduce the risk of ischaemic heart disease by 16%and stroke by 24%.

Flavonoids are polyphenolic compounds that occur in a variety of foods of vegetable origin, such as tea, onions and apples. Data from several prospective studies indicate an inverse association of dietary flavonoids with coronary heart disease. However, confounding maybe a major problem and may explain the conflicting results of observational studies.

High blood pressure is a major risk factor for coronary heart disease and both forms of stroke (ischaemic and haemorrhagic). Of the many risk factors associated with high blood pressure, the dietary exposure that has been most investigated is daily sodium intake. It has been studied extensively in animal experimental models, in epidemiological studies, controlled clinical trials and in population studies on restricted sodium intake. All these data show convincingly that sodium intake is directly associated with blood pressure.

Diastolic blood pressures are reduced by about half as much, but the association increases with age and magnitude of the initial blood pressure. It was estimated that a universal reduction in dietary intake of sodium by 50 mmol per day would lead to a 50%reduction in the number of people requiring antihypertensive therapy, a 22%reduction in the number of deaths resulting from strokes and a 16%reduction in the number of deaths from coronary heart disease. The first prospective study using 24-hour urine collections for measuring sodium intake, which is the only reliable measure, demonstrated a positive relationship between an increased risk of acute coronary events, but not stroke events, and increased sodium excretion. The association was strongest among overweight men.

Several clinical intervention trials, conducted to evaluate the effects of dietary salt reduction on blood pressure levels, have been systematically reviewed. Based on an overview of 32 methodologically adequate trials, Cutler, Follmann &Allender concluded that a daily reduction of sodium intake by 70--80 mmol was associated with a lowering of blood pressure both in hypertensive and normotensive individuals, with systolic and diastolic blood pressure reductions of 4. 8/1. 9 mmHg in the former and 2. 5/1. 1 mmHg in the latter. Clinical trials have also demonstrated the sustainable blood pressure lowering effects of sodium restriction in infancy, as well as in the elderly in whom it provides a useful non-pharmacological therapy. The results of a low-sodium diet trial showed that low-sodium diets, with 24-hour sodium excretion levels around 70 mmol, are effective and safe. Two population studies, in China and in Portugal, have also revealed significant reductions in blood pressure in the intervention groups.

A meta-analysis of randomized controlled trials showed that potassium supplements reduced mean blood pressures (systolic/diastolic) by 1. 8/1. 0 mmHg in normotensive subjects and 4. 4/2. 5 mmHg in hypertensive subjects. Several large cohort studies have found an inverse association between potassium intake and risk of stroke. While potassium supplements have been shown to have protective effects on blood pressure and cardiovascular diseases, there is no evidence to suggest that long-term potassium supplements should be administered to reduce the risk for CVD.

While the consumption of fruits and vegetables has been widely believed to promote good health, evidence related to their protective effect against CVD has only been presented in recent years. Numerous ecological and prospective studies have reported a significant protective association for coronary heart disease and stroke with consumption of fruits and vegetables.

The effects of increased fruit and vegetable consumption on blood pressure alone and in combination with a low-fat diet, were assessed in the Dietary Approaches to Stop Hypertension (DASH) trial. While the combination diet was more effective in lowering blood pressure, the fruit and vegetable diet also lowered blood pressure (by 2. 8 mmHg systolic and 1. 1 mmHg diastolic) in comparison to the control diet. Such reductions, while seeming modest at the individual level, would result in a substantial reduction in population-wide risk of CVD by shifting the blood pressure distribution.

Most, but not all, population studies have shown that fish consumption is associated with a reduced risk of coronary heart disease. A systematic review concluded that the discrepancy in the findings may be a result of differences in the populations studied, with only high-risk individuals benefiting from increasing their fish consumption. It was estimated that in high-risk populations, an optimumfish consumption of 40--60 g per day would lead to approximately a 50%reduction in death from coronary heart disease.

In a diet and reinfarction trial, 2-year mortality was reduced by 29%in survivors of a first myocardial infarction in persons receiving advice to consume fatty fish at least twice a week. Arecent study based on data from 36 countries, reported that fish consumption is associated with a reduced risk of death from all causes as well as CVD mortality.

Several large epidemiological studies have demonstrated that frequent consumption of nuts was associated with decreased risk of coronary heart disease. Most of these studies considered nuts as a group, combining many different types of nuts. Nuts are high in unsaturated fatty acids and low in saturated fats, and contribute to cholesterol lowering by altering the fatty acid profile of the diet as a whole.

However, because of the high energy content of nuts, advice to include them in the diet must be tempered in accordance with the desired energy balance. Several trials indicate that soy has a beneficial effect on plasma lipids. A composite analysis of 38 clinical trials found that an average consumption of 47 g of soy protein a day led to a 9%decline in total cholesterol and a 13%decline in LDL cholesterol in subjects free of coronary heart disease.

Soy is rich in isoflavones, compounds that are structurally and functionally similar to estrogen. Several animal experiments suggest that the intake of these isoflavones may provide protection against coronary heart disease, but human data on efficacy and safety are still awaited. There is convincing evidence that low to moderate alcohol consumption lowers the risk of coronary heart disease. In a systematic review of ecological, case—control and cohort studies in which specific associations were available between risk of coronary heart-disease and consumption of beer, wine and spirits, it was found that all alcoholic drinks are linked with lower risk.

However, other cardiovascular and health risks associated with alcohol do not favour a general recommendation for its use. Boiled, unfiltered coffee raises total and LDL cholesterol because coffee beans contain a terpenoid lipid called cafestol. The amount of cafestol in the cup depends on the brewing method: it is zero for paper-filtered drip coffee, and high in the unfiltered coffee still widely drunk in, for example, in Greece, the Middle East and Turkey.

Intake of large amounts of unfiltered coffee markedly raises serum cholesterol and has been associated with coronary heart disease in Norway. A shift from unfiltered, boiled coffee to filtered coffee has contributed significantly to the decline in serum cholesterol in Finland.

Dietary intake of fats strongly influences the risk of cardiovascular diseases such as coronary heart disease and stroke, through effects on blood lipids, thrombosis, blood pressure, arterial (endothelial) function, arrythmogenesis and inflammation. However, the qualitative composi- tion of fats in the diet has a significant role to play in modifying this risk. The evidence shows that intake of saturated fatty acids is directly related to cardiovascular risk.

The traditional target is to restrict the intake of saturated fatty acids to less than 10%, of daily energy intake and less than 7%for high-risk groups. If populations are consuming less than 10%, they should not increase that level of intake. Within these limits, intake of foods rich in myristic and palmitic acids should be replaced by fats with a lower content of these particular fatty acids.

In developing countries, however, where energy intake for some population groups may be inadequate, energy expenditure is high and body fat stores are low. The amount and quality of fat supply has to be considered keeping in mind the need to meet energy requirements. Specific sources of saturated fat, such as coconut and palm oil, provide low-cost energy and may be an important source of energy for the poor.

Not all saturated fats have similar metabolic effects; those with 12--16 carbons in the fatty acid chain have a greater effect on raising LDL cholesterol. This implies that the fatty acid composition of the fat source should be examined. Aspopulations progress in the nutrition transition and energy excess becomes a potential problem, restricting certain fatty acids becomes progressively more relevant to ensuring cardiovascular health.

To promote cardiovascular health, diets should provide a very low intake of trans fatty acids (hydrogenated oils and fats). In practice, this implies an intake of less than 1%of daily energy intake. This recommendation is especially relevant in developing countries where low-cost hydrogenated fat is frequently consumed.

The potential effect of human consumption of hydrogenated oils of unknown physiological effects (e. g. marine oils) is of great concern. Diets should provide an adequate intake of PUFAs, i. e. in the range 6-- 10%of daily energy intake. There should also be an optimal balance between intake of n-6 PUFAs and n-3 PUFAs, i. e. 5--8%and 1--2%of daily energy intake, respectively. Intake of oleic acid, a monounsaturated fatty acid, should make up the rest of the daily energy intake from fats, to give a daily total fat intake ranging from 15%up to 30%of daily energy intake.

Where obesity is prevalent, for example, an intake in the lower part of the range is preferable in order to achieve a lower energy intake. While there is no evidence to directly link the quantity of daily fat intake to an increased risk of CVD, total fat consumption should be limited to enable the goals of reduced intake of saturated and trans fatty acids to be met easily in most populations and to avoid the potential problems of undesirable weight gain that may arise from unrestricted fat intake.

It should be noted that highly active groups with diets rich in vegetables, legumes, fruits and wholegrain cereals will limit the risk of unhealthy weight gain on a diet comprising a total fat intake of up to 35%. These dietary goals can be met by limiting the intake of fat from dairy and meat sources, avoiding the use of hydrogenated oils and fats in cooking and manufacture of food products, using appropriate edible vegetable oils in small amounts, and ensuring a regular intake of fish (one to two times per week) or plant sources of a - linolenic acid. Preference should be given to food preparation practices that employ non-frying methods.

Fruits and vegetables contribute to cardiovascular health through the variety of phytonutrients, potassium and fibre that they contain. Daily intake of fresh fruit and vegetables (including berries, green leafy and cruciferous vegetables and legumes), in an adequate quantity, is recommended to reduce the risk of coronary heart disease, stroke and high blood pressure.

Dietary intake of sodium, from all sources, influences blood pressure levels in populations and should be limited so as to reduce the risk of coronary heart disease and both forms of stroke. Current evidence suggests that an intake of no more than 70 mmol or 1. 7 g of sodium per day is beneficial in reducing blood pressure. The special situation of individuals (i. e. pregnant women and non-acclimated people who perform strenuous physical activity in hot environments) who may be adversely affected by sodium reduction needs to be kept in mind.

Limitation of dietary sodium intake to meet these goals should be achieved by restricting daily salt (sodium chloride) intake to less than 5 g per day. This should take into account total sodium intake from all dietary sources, for example additives such as monosodium glutamate and preservatives. Use of potassium-enriched low-sodium substitutes is one way to reduce sodium intake.

The need to adjust salt iodization, depending on observed sodium intake and surveillance of iodine status of the population, should be recognized. Adequate dietary intake of potassium lowers blood pressure and is protective against stroke and cardiac arrythmias. Potassium intake should be at a level which will keep the sodium to potassium ratio close to 1. 0, i. e. a daily potassium intake level of 70--80 mmol per day.

This may be achieved through adequate daily consumption of fruits and vegetables. NSP (dietary fibre). Fibre is protective against coronary heart disease and has also been used in diets to lower blood pressure. Adequate intake may be achieved through fruits, vegetables and wholegrain cereals. The serving should provide an equivalent of 200--500 mg of eicosapentaenoic and docosahexaenoic acid. People who are vegetarians are recommended to ensure adequate intake of plant sources of a -linolenic acid.

Although regular low to moderate consumption of alcohol is protective against coronary heart disease, other cardiovascular and health risks associated with alcohol do not favour a general recommendation for its use. Physical activity is related to the risk of cardiovascular diseases, especially coronary heart disease, in a consistent inverse dose—response fashion when either volume or intensity are used for assessment. These relationships apply to both incidence and mortality rates from all cardiovascular diseases and from coronary heart disease.

At present, no consistent dose— response relationship can be found between risk of stroke and physical activity. The lower limits of volume or intensity of the protective dose of physical activity have not been defined with certainty, but the current recommendation of at least 30 minutes of at least moderate-intensity physical activity onmost days of the week is considered sufficient. Ahigher volume or intensity of activity would confer a greater protective effect.

The recommended amount of physical activity is sufficient to raise cardio-respiratory fitness to the level that has been shown to be related to decreased risk of cardiovascular disease. Individuals who are unaccustomed to regular exercise or have a high-risk profile for CVDshould avoid sudden and high-intensity bursts of physical activity.

Preventing cancer

Cancer is caused by a variety of identified and unidentified factors. The most important established cause of cancer is tobacco smoking. Other important determinants of cancer risk include diet, alcohol and physical activity, infections, hormonal factors and radiation. The relative importance of cancers as a cause of death is increasing, mostly because of the increasing proportion of people whoare old, and also in part because of reductions in mortality from some other causes, especially infectious diseases.

Theincidence of cancers of the lung, colon andrectum, breast and prostate generally increases in parallel with economic development, while the incidence of stomach cancer usually declines with development. Cancer is now a major cause of mortality throughout the world and, in the developed world, is generally exceeded only by cardiovascular diseases.

As developing countries become urbanized, patterns of cancer, including those most strongly associated with diet, tend to shift towards those of economically developed countries. Between 2000 and 2020, the total number of cases of cancer in the developing world is predicted to increase by 73%and, in the developed world, to increase by 29%, largely as a result of an increase in the number of old people.

Dietary factors are estimated to account for approximately 30%of cancers in industrialized countries, making diet second only to tobacco as a theoretically preventable cause of cancer. This proportion is thought to be about 20%in developing countries, but may grow with dietary change, particularly if the importance of other causes, especially infections, declines.

Cancer rates change as populations move between countries and adopt different dietary (and other) behaviours, further implicating dietary factors in the etiology of cancer. Body weight and physical inactivity together are estimated to account for approximately one-fifth to one-third of several of the most common cancers, specifically cancers of the breast (postmenopausal), colon, endometrium, kidney and oesophagus (adenocarcinoma).

Dietary factors for which there is convincing evidence for an increase in risk are overweight and obesity, and a high consumption of alcoholic beverages, aflatoxins, and some forms of salting and fermenting fish. There is also convincing evidence to indicate that physical activity decreases the risk of colon cancer. Factors which probably increase risk include high dietary intake of preserved meats, salt-preserved foods and salt, and very hot (thermally) drinks and food.

Probable protective factors are consumption of fruits and vegetables, and physical activity (for breast cancer). After tobacco, overweight and obesity appear to be the most important known avoidable causes of cancer.

Cancers of the oral cavity, pharynx and oesophagus. In developed countries the main risk factors for cancers of the oral cavity, pharynx and oesophagus are alcohol and tobacco, and up to 75%of such cancers are attributable to these two lifestyle factors. Overweight and obesity are established risk factors specifically for adenocarcinoma (but not squamous cell carcinoma) of the oesophagus.

In developing countries, around 60%of cancers of the oral cavity, pharynx and oesophagus are thought to be a result of micronutrient deficiencies related to a restricted diet that is low in fruits and vegetables and animal products. The relative roles of various micronutrients are not yet clear. There is also consistent evidence that consuming drinks and foods at a very high temperature increases the risk for these cancers.

Nasopharyngeal cancer is particularly common in South-East Asia, and has been clearly associated with a high intake of Chinese-style salted fish, especially during early childhood, as well as with infection with the Epstein-Barr virus. Until about 20 years ago stomach cancer was the most common cancer in the world, but mortality rates have been falling in all industrialized countries and stomach cancer is currently much more common in Asia than in North America or Europe.

Infection with the bacterium Helicobacter pylori is an established risk factor, but not a sufficient cause, for the development of stomach cancer. Diet is thought to be important in the etiology of this disease; substantial evidence suggests that risk is increased by high intakes of some traditionally preserved salted foods, especially meats and pickles, and with salt per se, and that risk is decreased by high intakes of fruits and vegetables, perhaps because of their vitamin C content.

Further prospective data are needed, in particular to examine whether some of the dietary associations may be partly confounded by Helicobacter pylori infection and whether dietary factors maymodify the association of Helicobacter pylori with risk. Colorectal cancer. Colorectal cancer incidence rates are approximately ten-fold higher in developed than in developing countries, and it has been suggested that diet-related factors mayaccount for up to 80%of the differences in rates between countries.

The best established diet-related risk factor is overweight/obesity and physical activity has been consistently associated with a reduced risk of colon cancer (but not of rectal cancer). These factors together, however, do not explain the large variation between populations in colorectal cancer rates. There is almost universal agreement that some aspects of the 'westernized' diet are a major determinant of risk; for instance, there is some evidence that risk is increased by high intakes of meat and fat, and that risk is decreased by high intakes of fruits and vegetables, dietary fibre, folate and calcium, but none of these hypotheses has been firmly established.

International correlation studies have shown a strong association between per capita consumption of meat and colorectal cancer mortality, and a recent systematic review concluded that preserved meat is associated with an increased risk for colorectal cancer but that fresh meat is not. However, most studies have not observed positive associations with poultry or fish. Overall, the evidence suggests that high consumption of preserved and red meat probably increases the risk for colorectal cancer. As with meat, international correlation studies show a strong association between per capita consumption of fat and colorectal cancer mortality.

However, the results of observational studies of fat and colorectal cancer have, overall, not been supportive of an association with fat intake. Many case-control studies have observed a weak association between the risk of colorectal cancer and high consumption of fruits and vegetables and/or dietary fibre, but the results of recent large prospective studies have been inconsistent. Furthermore, results from randomized controlled trials have not shown that intervention over a 3--4 year period with supplemental fibre or a diet low in fat and high in fibre and fruits and vegetables can reduce the recurrence of colorectal adenomas.

It is possible that some of the inconsistencies are a result of differences between studies in the types of fibre eaten and in the methods for classifying fibre in food tables, or that the association with fruits and vegetables arises principally from an increase in risk at very low levels of consumption. Onbalance, the evidence that is currently available suggests that intake of fruits and vegetables probably reduces the risk for colorectal cancer.

Recent studies have suggested that vitamins and minerals might influence the risk for colorectal cancer. Someprospective studies have suggested that a high intake of folate from diet or vitamin supplements is associated with a reduced risk for colon cancer. Another promising hypothesis is that relatively high intakes of calcium may reduce the risk for colorectal cancer; several observational studies have supported this hypothesis, and two trials have indicated that supplemental calcium may have a modest protective effect on the recurrence of colorectal adenomas.

Approximately 75%of cases of liver cancer occur in developing countries, and liver cancer rates vary over 20-fold between countries, being much higher in sub-Saharan Africa and South-East Asia than in North America and Europe. The major risk factor for hepatocellular carcinoma, the main type of liver cancer, is chronic infection with hepatitis B, and to a lesser extent, hepatitis C virus. Ingestion of foods contaminated with the mycotoxin, aflatoxin is an important risk factor among people in developing countries, together with active hepatitis virus infection.

Excessive alcohol consumption is the main diet-related risk factor for liver cancer in industrialized countries, probably via the development of cirrhosis and alcoholic hepatitis. Pancreatic cancer. Cancer of the pancreas is more common in industrialized countries than in developing countries. Over-weight and obesity possibly increase the risk. Some studies have suggested that risk is increased by high intakes of meat, and reduced by high intakes of vegetables, but these data are not consistent.

Lung cancer is the most common cancer in the world. Heavy smoking increases the risk by around 30-fold, and smoking causes over 80%of lung cancers in developed countries. Numerous observational studies have found that lung cancer patients typically report a lower intake of fruits, vegetables and related nutrients (such as b -carotene) than controls. The only one of these factors to have been tested in controlled trials, namely b -carotene, has, however, failed to produce any benefit when given as a supplement for up to 12 years.

The possible effect of diet on lung cancer risk remains controversial, and the apparent protective effect of fruits and vegetables may be largely the result of residual confounding by smoking, since smokers generally consume less fruit and vegetables than non-smokers. In public health terms, the overriding priority for preventing lung cancer is to reduce the prevalence of smoking.

Breast cancer is the second most common cancer in the world and the most common cancer among women. Incidence rates are about five times higher in industrialized countries than in less developed countries and Japan. Much of this international variation is a result of differences in established reproductive risk factors such as age at menarche, parity and age at births, and breastfeeding, but differences in dietary habits and physical activity may also contribute.

In fact, age at menarche is partly determined by dietary factors, in that restricted dietary intake during childhood and adolescence leads to delayed menarche. Adult height, also, is weakly positively associated with risk, and is partly determined by dietary factors during childhood and adolescence. Estradiol and perhaps other hormones play a key role in the etiology of breast cancer, and it is possible that any further dietary effects on risk are mediated by hormonal mechanisms.

The only dietary factors which have been shown to increase the risk for breast cancer are obesity and alcohol. Obesity increases breast cancer risk in postmenopausal women by around 50%, probably by increasing serum concentrations of free estradiol. Obesity does not increase risk among premenopausal women, but obesity in premenopausal women is likely to lead to obesity throughout life and therefore to an eventual increase in breast cancer risk. For alcohol, there is now a large body of data from well-designed studies which consistently shows a small increase in risk with increasing consumption, with about a 10%increase in risk for an average of one alcoholic drink every day. The mechanism for this association is not known, but may involve increases in estrogen levels.

The results of studies of other dietary factors including fat, meat, dairy products, fruits and vegetables, fibre and phyto-estrogens are incon-clusive. Endometrial cancer risk is about three-fold higher in obese womenthan in lean women, probably because of the effects of obesity on hormone levels. Some case-control studies have suggested that diets high in fruits andvegetables mayreduce risk andthat diets high in saturated or total fat may increase risk, but the amount of available data is limited.

Prostate cancer incidence rates are strongly affected by diagnostic practices and therefore difficult to interpret, but mortality rates show that death from prostate cancer is about 10 times more common in North America and Europe than in Asia. Little is known about the etiology of prostate cancer, although ecological studies suggest that it is positively associated with a "westernized" diet. The data from prospective studies have not established causal or protective associations for specific nutrients or dietary factors.

Diets high in red meat, dairy products and animal fat have frequently been implicated in the development of prostate cancer, although the data are not entirely consistent. Randomized controlled trials have provided substantial, consistent evidence that supplements of b - carotene do not alter the risk for prostate cancer but have suggested that vitamin E and selenium might have a protective effect. Lycopene, primarily from tomatoes, has been associated with a reduced risk in some observational studies, but the data are not consistent.

Hormones control the growth of the prostate, and diet might influence prostate cancer risk by affecting hormone levels. Overweight and obesity are established risk factors for cancer of the kidney, and may account for up to 30%of kidney cancers in both men and women. The Consultation recognized the problems posed by the lack of data on diet and cancer from the developing world. There are very limited data from Africa, Asia and Latin America, yet these regions represent two-thirds or more of the world population.

There is thus an urgent need for epidemiological research on diet and cancer in these regions. The need to evaluate the role of food processing methods, traditional and industrial, was also identified. Microbiological and chemical food contaminants may also contribute to carcinogenicity of diets. The nutrition transition is accompanied by changes in prevalence of specific cancers. For some cancers, such as stomach cancer, this may be beneficial while for others, such as colorectal and breast cancers, the changes are adverse.

The main recommendations for reducing the risk of developing cancer are as follows:

— Maintain weight (among adults) such that BMI is in the range of 18. 5-- 24. 9 kg/m and avoid weight gain (>5 kg) during adult life.

— Maintain regular physical activity. The primary goal should be to perform physical activity on most days of the week; 60 minutes per day of moderate-intensity activity, such as walking, may be needed to maintain healthy body weight in otherwise sedentary people. More vigorous activity, such as fast walking, may give some additional benefits for cancer prevention.

— Consumption of alcoholic beverages is not recommended: if con-sumed, do not exceed two units per day.

— Chinese-style fermented salted fish should only be consumed in moderation, especially during childhood.

— Overall consumption of salt-preserved foods and salt should be moderate.

— Minimize exposure to aflatoxin in foods.

— Have a diet which includes at least 400 g per day of total fruits and vegetables.

— Those who are not vegetarian are advised to moderate consumption of preserved meat (e. g. sausages, salami, bacon, ham).

— Do not consume foods or drinks when they are at a very hot (scalding hot) temperature.

Preventing dental diseases

Oral health is related to diet in many ways, for example, through nutritional influences on cranio-facial development, oral cancer and oral infectious diseases. The purpose of this review, however, is to focus on the nutritional aspects of dental diseases. Dental diseases include dental caries, developmental defects of enamel, dental erosion and periodontal disease.

Dental diseases are a costly burden to health care services, accounting for between 5%and 10%of total health care expenditures and exceeding the cost of treating cardiovascular disease, cancer and osteoporosis in industrialized countries. In low-income countries, the cost of traditional restorative treatment of dental disease would probably exceed the available resources for health care. Dental health promotion and preventive strategies are clearly more affordable and sustainable.

Although not life-threatening, dental diseases have a detrimental effect on quality of life in childhood through to old age, having an impact on self-esteem, eating ability, nutrition and health. In modern society, a significant role of teeth is to enhance appearance; facial appearance is very important in determining an individual's integration into society, and teeth also play an essential role in speech and communication.

Oral diseases are associated with considerable pain, anxiety and impaired social functioning. Dental decay may result in tooth loss, which reduces the ability to eat a nutritious diet, the enjoyment of food, the confidence to socialize and the quality of life. The amount of dental decay is measured using the dmf/DMF index, a count of the number of teeth or surfaces in a person's mouth that are decayed, missing or filled as a result of caries in primary dentition/ permanent dentition.

An additional dental status indicator is the proportion of the population who are edentulous (have no natural teeth). In most low-income countries, the prevalence rate of dental caries is relatively low and more than 90%of caries are untreated. Many developing countries have low decayed, missing, filled primary teeth (dmft) values but a high prevalence of dental caries in the primary dentition. The WHOguidelines on oral health state that at age 35--44 years a DMFT score of 14 or above is considered high.

The number of edentulous persons has declined over the past 20--30 years in several industrialized countries. Despite overall gains however, there is still a large proportion of older adults who are edentulous or partially dentate and as the population continues to age tooth loss will affect a growing number of persons worldwide. Dental erosion is a relatively new dental problem in many countries throughout the world, and is related to diet. There is anecdotal evidence that prevalence is increasing in industrialized countries, but there are no data over time to indicate patterns of this disease.

There are insufficient data available to comment on worldwide trends; in some populations, however, it is thought that approximately 50%of children are affected. Nutritional status affects the teeth pre-eruptively, although this influence is much less important than the post-eruptive local effect of diet on the teeth. Deficiencies of vitamins D and A and protein— energy malnutrition have been associated with enamel hypoplasia and salivary gland atrophy, which render the teeth more susceptible to decay. In developing countries, in the absence of dietary sugars, undernutrition is not associated with dental caries.

Undernutrition coupled with a high intake of sugars may exacerbate the risk of caries. There is some evidence to suggest that periodontal disease progresses more rapidly in undernourished populations; the important role of nutrition in maintaining an adequate host immune response may explain this observation. Apart from severe vitamin C deficiency, which may result in scurvy-related periodontitis, there is little evidence at present for an association between diet and periodontal disease.

Some study is investigating the potential role of the antioxidant nutrients in period-ontal disease. Poor oral hygiene is the most important risk factor in the development of periodontal disease. Undernutrition exacerbates the severity of oral infections (e. g. acute necrotizing ulcerative gingivitis) and may eventually lead to their evolution into life-threatening diseases such as noma, a dehumanizing oro-facial gangrene. Dental caries occur because of demineralization of enamel and dentine by organic acids formed by bacteria in dental plaque through the anaerobic metabolism of sugars derived from the diet.

Organic acids increase the solubility of calcium hydroxyapatite in the dental hard tissues and demineralization occurs. Saliva is super-saturated with calcium and phosphate at pH 7 which promotes remineralization. If the oral pH remains high enough for sufficient time then complete remineralization of enamel may occur. If the acid challenge is too great, however, demineralization dominates and the enamel becomes more porous until finally a carious lesion forms.

The development of caries requires the presence of sugars and bacteria, but is influenced by the susceptibility of the tooth, the bacterial profile, and the quantity and quality of the saliva. There is a wealth of evidence from many different types of investigation, including human studies, animal experiments and experimental studies in vivo and in vitro to show the role of dietary sugars in the etiology of dental caries.

Collectively, data from these studies provide an overall picture of the cariogenic potential of carbohydrates. Sugars are undoubtedly the most important dietary factor in the development of dental caries. Here, the term "sugars" refers to all monosaccharides and disaccharides, while the term 'sugar' refers only to sucrose. The term 'free sugars' refers to all monosaccharides and disaccharides added to foods by the manufacturer, cook or consumer, plus sugars naturally present in honey, fruit juices and syrups.

The term 'fermentable carbohydrate' refers to free sugars, glucose polymers, oligosaccharides and highly refined starches; it excludes non-starch polysaccharides and raw starches. Worldwide epidemiological studies have compared sugar consumption and levels of dental caries at the between-country level. Sreebny correlated the dental caries experience (DMFT) of 12-year-olds with data on sugar supplies of 47 countries and found a significant correlation (+0. 7); 52%of the variation in the level of caries was explained by the per capita availability of sugar.

Isolated communities with a traditional way of life and a consistently low intake of sugars have very low levels of dental caries. As economic levels in such societies rise, the amount of sugar and other fermentable carbohydrates in the diet increases and this is often associated with a marked increase in dental caries. Examples of this trend have been reported among the Inuit in Alaska, USA, as well as in populations in Ethiopia, Ghana, Nigeria, Sudan, and on the Island of Tristan da Cunha, St Helena. There is evidence to show that many groups of people with high exposure to sugars have levels of caries higher than the population average.

Examples include children with chronic diseases requiring long-term sugar-containing medicines, and confectionery workers. Likewise, experience of dental caries has seldom been reported in groups of people who have a habitually low intake of sugars, for example, children of dentists and children in institutions where strict dietary regimens are inflicted.

Studies have shown that people with HFI have a low intake of sugars and a higher than average intake of starch, but have a low dental caries experience. Human intervention studies are rare, and those that have been reported are now decades old and were conducted in the pre-fluoride era before the strong link between sugars intake and dental caries levels was established. It would not be possible to repeat such studies today because of ethical constraints.

The Vipeholm study, conducted in an adult mental institution in Sweden between 1945 and 1953, investigated the effects of consuming sugary foods of varying stickiness and at different times throughout the day on the development of caries. It was found that sugar, even when consumed in large amounts, had little effect on caries increment if it was ingested up to a maximum of four times a day at mealtimes only.

Increased frequency of consumption of sugar between meals was, however, associated with a marked increase in dental caries. It was also found that the increase in dental caries activity disappears on withdrawal of sugar-rich foods. Despite the complicated nature of the study the conclusions are valid, although they apply to the pre-fluoride era. The Turku study was a controlled dietary intervention study carried out on adults in Finland in the 1970s which showed that almost total substitution of sucrose in the diet with xylitol (a non-cariogenic sweetener) resulted in an 85%reduction in dental caries over a 2-year period.

Numerous cross-sectional epidemiological studies have compared sugars intake with dental caries levels in many countries of the world. Those conducted before the early 1990s have been summarized by Rugg-Gunn. Nine out of 21 studies that compared amount of sugars consumed with caries increment found significant associations, while the other 12 did not. When the effects of oral hygiene and fluoride were kept constant, the children with a low intake of sugars between meals had up to 86%less caries than those with high intakes of sugars.

Some studies have found fluoride exposure and oral hygiene to be more strongly associated with caries than sugars consumption. A recent study in the United Kingdom of a representative sample of children aged 4--18 years showed no significant relationship between caries experience and level of intake of free sugars; in the age group 15--18 years, however, the upper band of free sugars consumers were more likely to have decay than the lower band.

Many other cross-sectional studies have shown a relationship between sugars consumption and levels of caries in the primary and/or permanent dentitions in countries or areas throughout the world, including China, Denmark, Madagascar, Saudi Arabia, Sweden, Thailand and the United Kingdom. When investigating the association between diet and the development of dental caries it is more appropriate to use a longitudinal study design in which sugars consumption habits over time are related to changes in dental caries experience.

Such studies have shown a significant relationship between caries development and sugars intake. In a comprehensive study of over 400 children in England aged 11---12 years, a small but significant relationship was found between intake of total sugars and caries increment over 2 years. The Michigan Study in the United States investigated the relationship between sugars intake and dental caries increment over 3 years in children initially aged 10---15 years.

A weak relationship was found between the amount of dietary sugars consumed and dental caries experience. In a review of longitudinal studies, Marthaler analysed the relationship between dietary sugars and caries activity in countries where the availability of sugars is high and the use of fluoride is extensive. He concluded that in modern societies that make use of prevention, the relationship between sugars consumption and dental caries was still evident. He also concluded that many older studies had failed to show a relationship between sugars intake and development of dental caries because they were of poor methodological design, used unsuitable methods of dietary analysis or were of insufficient power.

Correlations between individuals' sugars consumption and dental caries increments may be weak if the range of sugars intake in the study population is small. That is to say, that if all people within a population are exposed to the disease risk factor, the relationship betv'een the risk factor and the disease will not be apparent. Frequency and amount of sugars consumption. Several studies, including the above-mentioned Vipeholm study in Sweden, have indicated that caries experience increases markedly whenthe frequency of sugars intake exceeds four times a day.

The importance of frequency versus the total amount of sugars is difficult to evaluate as the two variables are hard to distinguish from each other. Data from animal studies have indicated the importance of frequency of sugars intake in the development of dental caries. Some human studies have also shown that the frequency of sugars intake is an important etiological factor for caries development.

Manystudies have related the frequency of intake of sugars or sugars-rich food to caries development but have not simultaneously investigated the relationship between amount of sugars consumed and dental caries, and therefore no conclusion regarding the relative importance of these two variables can be drawn from these studies. Animal studies have also shown a relationship between amount of sugars consumed and the development of dental caries.

Several longitudinal studies in humans have indicated that the amount of sugars consumed is more important than the frequency, while Jamel et al. found that both the frequency and the amount of sugars intake are important. The strong correlation between both the amount and frequency of sugars consumption has been demonstrated by several investigators in different countries. It is therefore highly likely that, in terms of caries development, both variables are potentially important. Relative cariogenicity of different sugars and food consistency.

Therelative acidogenicity of different monosaccharides and disaccharides has been investigated in plaque pH studies, which have shown that lactose is less acidogenic than other sugars. Animal studies have provided no clear evidence that, with the exception of lactose, the cariogenicity of monosaccharides and disaccharides differs. The above-mentioned study in Turku, Finland, found no difference in caries development between subjects on diets sweetened with sucrose compared with those whose diet had been sweetened with fructose.

The adhesiveness or stickiness of a food is not necessarily related to either oral retention time or cariogenic potential. For example, consumption of sugars-containing drinks (i. e. non-sticky) is associated with increased risk of dental caries. Potential impact of sugars reduction on other dietary components. It is important to consider the potential impact of a reduction in free sugars on other components of the diet. Simple, cross-sectional analysis of dietary data from populations has shown an inverse relationship between the intake of free sugars and the intake of fat, suggesting that reducing free sugars might lead to an increase in fat intake.

There is, however, a growing body of evidence from studies over time that shows that changes in intake of fat and free sugars are not inversely related, and that reductions in intake of fat are offset by increases in intakes of starch rather than free sugars. Cole-Hamilton et al. found that the intake of both fat and added sugars simultaneously decreased as fibre intake increased. Overall dietary goals that promote increased intake of wholegrain staple foods, fruits and vegetables and a reduced consumption of free sugars are thus unlikely to lead to an increased consumption of fat.

Fluoride undoubtedly protects against dental caries. The inverse relationship between fluoride in drinking-water and dental caries, for instance, is well established. Fluoride reduces caries in children by between 20%and 40%, but does not eliminate dental caries altogether. Over 800 controlled trials of the effect of fluoride administration on dental caries have been conducted; collectively these studies demonstrate that fluoride is the most effective preventive agent against caries.

Several studies have that indicated that a relationship between sugars intake and caries still exists in the presence of adequate fluoride exposure. In two major longitudinal studies in children, the observed relationships between sugars intake and development of dental caries remained even after controlling for use of fluoride and oral hygiene practices.

As mentioned earlier, following a review of available longitudinal studies, Marthaler concluded that, even when preventive measures such as use of fluoride are employed, a relationship between sugars intake and caries still exists. He also stated that in industrialized countries where there is adequate exposure to fluoride, no further reduction in the prevalence and severity of dental caries will be achieved unless the intake of sugars is reduced.

A recent systematic review that investigated the importance of sugars intake in caries etiology in populations exposed to fluoride concluded that where there is adequate exposure to fluoride, sugars consumption is a moderate risk factor for caries in most people; moreover sugars consumption is likely to be a more powerful indicator for risk of caries in persons who do not have regular exposure to fluoride. Thus, restricting sugars consumption still has a role to play in the prevention of caries in situations where there is widespread use of fluoride but this role is not as strong as it is without exposure to fluoride.

Despite the indisputable preventive role of fluoride, there is no strong evidence of a clear relationship between oral cleanliness and levels of dental caries. Excess ingestion of fluoride during enamel formation can lead to dental fluorosis. This condition is observed particularly in countries that have high levels of fluoride in water supplies.

Epidemiological studies have shown that starch is of low risk to dental caries. People who consume high-starch/low-sugars diets generally have low levels of caries, whereas people who consume low-starch/high-sugars diets have high levels of caries. In Norway and Japan the intake of starch increased during the Second World War, yet the occurrence of caries was reduced.

The heterogeneous nature of starch (i. e. degree of refinement, botanical origin, raw or cooked) is of particular relevance when assessing its potential cariogenicity. Several types of experiment have shown that raw starch is of low cariogenicity. Cooked starch is about one-third to one-half as cariogenic as sucrose. Mixtures of starch and sucrose are, however, potentially more cariogenic than starch alone. Glucose polymers and pre-biotics are increasingly being added to foods in industrialized countries.

Evidence on the cariogenicity of these carbohydrates is sparse and comes from animal studies, plaque pH studies and studies in vitro which suggest that maltodextrins and glucose syrups are cariogenic. Plaque pH studies and experiments in vitro suggest that isomalto-oligosaccharides and gluco-oligosaccharides may be less acidogenic than sucrose. There is, however, evidence that fructo-oligosaccharides are as acidogenic as sucrose.

As habitually consumed, there is little evidence to show that fruit is an important factor in the development of dental caries. A number of plaque pHstudies have found fruit to be acidogenic, although less so than sucrose. Animal studies have shown that when fruit is consumed in very high frequencies it may induce caries, but less so than sucrose. In the only epidemiological study in which an association between fruit consumption and DMFT was found, fruit intakes were very high and the higher DMFT in fruit farm workers compared with grain farm workers arose solely from differences in the numbers of missing teeth.

Some dietary components protect against dental caries. The cariostatic nature of cheese has been demonstrated in several experimental studies, and in human observational studies and intervention studies. Cow's milk contains calcium, phosphorus and casein, all of which are thought to inhibit caries. Several studies have shown that the fall in plaque pH following milk consumption is negligible. The cariostatic nature of milk has been demonstrated in animal studies.

Rugg-Gunn et al. found an inverse relationship between the consumption of milk and caries increment in a study of adolescents in England. Wholegrain foods have protective properties; they require more mastication thereby stimulating increased saliva flow. Other foods that are good gustatory and/or mechanical stimulants to salivary flow include peanuts, hard cheeses and chewing gum.

Both organic and inorganic phosphates (found in unrefined plant foods) have been found to be cariostatic in animal studies, but studies in humans have produced inconclusive results. Both animal studies and experimental investigations in humans have shown that black tea extract increases plaque fluoride concentration and reduces the cariogenicity of a sugars-rich diet.

In line with the positive health effects of breastfeeding, epidemiological studies have associated breastfeeding with low levels of dental caries. A few specific case studies have linked prolonged ad libitum and nocturnal breastfeeding to early childhood caries. Breastfeeding has the advantage that it does not necessitate the use of a feeder bottle, which has been associated with early childhood caries.

A breastfed infant will also receive milk of a controlled composition to which additional free sugars have not been added. There are no benefits to dental health of feeding using a formula feed. Dental erosion is the progressive irreversible loss of dental hard tissue that is chemically etched away from the tooth surface by extrinsic and/or intrinsic acids by a process that does not involve bacteria.

Extrinsic dietary acids include citric acid, phosphoric acid, ascorbic acid, malic acid, tartaric acid and carbonic acid found, for example, in fruits and fruit juices, soft drinks and vinegar. Erosion in severe cases leads to total tooth destruction. Human observational studies have shown an association between dental erosion and the consumption of a number of acidic foods and drinks, including frequent consumption of fruit juice, soft drinks (including sports drinks), pickles (containing vinegar), citrus fruits and berries.

Age-related increases in dental erosion have been shown to be greater in those with the highest intake of soft drinks. Experimental clinical studies have shown that consumption of, or rinsing with, acidic beverages significantly lowers the pHof the oral fluids. Enamelis softened within onehour of exposure to cola but this may be reversed by exposure to milk or cheese. Animal studies have shown that fruit and soft drinks cause erosion, although fruit juices are significantly more destructive than whole fruits.

The strength of the evidence linking dietary sugars to the risk of dental caries is in the multiplicity of the studies rather than the power of any individual study. Strong evidence is provided by the intervention studies but the weakness of these studies is that they were conducted in the pre-fluoride era. More recent studies also show an association between sugars intake and dental caries albeit not as strong as in the pre-fluoride era.

However, in many developing countries people are not yet exposed to the benefits of fluoride. Cross-sectional studies should be interpreted with caution because dental caries develop over time and therefore simultaneous measurements of disease levels and diet may not give a true reflection of the role of diet in the development of the disease. It is the diet several years earlier tha' may be responsible for current caries levels. Longitudinal studies that have monitored a change in caries experience and related this to dietary factors provide stronger evidence. Such studies have been conducted on popula-tions with an overall high sugars intake but a low interindividual variation; this may account for the weak associations that have been reported. The studies that overcome the problem of low variation in consumption of sugars are studies that have monitored dental caries following a marked change in diet, for example, those conducted on populations during the Second World War and studies of populations before and after the introduction of sugars into the diet. Such studies have shown clearly that changes in dental caries mirror changes in economic growth and increased consumption of free sugars. Sometimes changes in sugars consumption were accompanied by an increase in other refined carbohydrates. There are, however, examples where sugars consumption decreased and starch consumption increased yet levels of dental caries declined. Strong evidence of the relationship between sugar availability and dental caries levels comes from worldwide ecological studies. The limitations of these studies are that they use data on sugar availability and not actual intake, they do not measure frequency of sugars intake, and they assume that level of intake is equal throughout the population. Also, the values are for sucrose, yet many countries obtain a considerable amount of their total sugars from other sugars. These studies have only considered DMFT of 12-year-olds, not always from a representative sample of the population.

Caution needs to be applied when extrapolating the results of animal studies to humans because of differences in tooth morphology, plaque bacterial ecology, salivary flow and composition, and the form in which the diet is provided (usually powdered form in animal experiments). Nonetheless, animal studies have enabled the effect on caries of defined types, frequencies and amounts of carbohydrates to be studied.

Plaque pH studies measure plaque acid production, but the acidogeni-city of a foodstuff cannot be taken as a direct measurement of its cariogenic potential. Plaque pH studies take no account of protective factors in foods, salivary flow and the effects of other components of the diet. Many of the plaque pH studies that show falls in pH below the critical value of 5. 5 with fruits and cooked starchy foods have been conducted using the indwelling electrode technique.

This electrode is recognized as being hypersensitive and non-discriminating, tending to give an 'all or nothing' response to all carbohydrates. Research has consistently shown that when annual sugar consumption exceeds 15 kg per person per year dental caries increase with increasing sugar intake. When sugar consumption is below 10 kg per person per year, levels of dental caries are very low. Exposure to fluoride increases the safe level of sugars consumption.

Population goals enable the oral health risks of populations to be assessed and health promotion goals monitored. The best available evidence indicates that the level of dental caries is low in countries where the consumption of free sugars is below 15--20 kg per person per year. This is equivalent to a daily intake of 40--55 g per person and the values equate to 6--10%of energy intake. It is of particular importance that countries which currently have low consumption of free sugars do not increase consumption levels.

In addition to population targets given in terms of the amount of free sugars, targets for the frequency of free sugars consumption are also important. The frequency of consumption of foods and/or drinks containing free sugars should be limited to a maximum of four times per day. Manycountries that are currently undergoing nutrition transition do not have adequate exposure to fluoride. There should be promotion of adequate fluoride exposure via appropriate vehicles, for example, affordable toothpaste, water, salt and milk. It is the responsibility of national health authorities to ensure implementation of feasible fluoride programmes for their country.

Elimination of undernutrition prevents enamel hypoplasia and the other potential effects of undernutrition on oral health (e. g. salivary gland atrophy, periodontal disease, oral infectious diseases) Osteoporosis is a disease affecting many millions of people around the world. It is characterized by low bone mass and micro-architectural deterioration of bone tissue, leading to bone fragility and a consequent increase in risk of fracture.

The incidence of vertebral and hip fractures increases exponentially with advancing age (while that of wrist fractures levels off after the age of 60 years).

Osteoporosis fractures are a major cause of morbidity and disability in older people and, in the case of hip fractures, can lead to premature death. Such fractures impose a considerable economic burden on health services worldwide.

Worldwide variation in the incidence and prevalence of osteoporosis is difficult to determine because of problems with definition and diagnosis. The most useful way of comparing osteoporosis prevalence between populations is to use fracture rates in older people. However, because osteoporosis is usually not life-threatening, quantitative data from developing countries are scarce.

Despite this, the current consensus is that approximately 1. 66 million hip fractures occur each year worldwide, that the incidence is set to increase four-fold by 2050 because of the increasing numbers of older people, and that the age-adjusted incidence rates are many times higher in affluent developed countries than in sub-Saharan Africa and Asia. In countries with a high fracture incidence, rates are greater among women (by three-to four-fold).

Thus, although widely regarded in these countries as a disease that affects women, 20%of symptomatic spine fractures and 30%of hip fractures occur in men. In countries where fracture rates are low, men and women are more equally affected. The incidence of vertebral and hip fractures in both sexes increases exponentially with age. Hip-fracture rates are highest in Caucasian women living in temperate climates, are somewhat lower in women from Mediterranean and Asian countries, and are lowest in women in Africa.

Countries in economic transition, such as Hong Kong Special Administrative Region (SAR) of China, have seen significant increases in age-adjusted fracture rates in recent decades, while the rates in industrialized countries appear to have reached a plateau. Diet appears to have only a moderate relationship to osteoporosis, but calcium and vitamin Dare both important, at least in older populations. Calcium is one of the main bone-forming minerals and an appropriate supply to bone is essential at all stages of life.

In estimating calcium requirements, most committees have used either a factorial approach, where calculations of skeletal accretion and turnover rates are combined with typical values for calcium absorption and excretion, or a variety of methods based on experimentally-derived balance data. There has been considerable debate about whether current recommended intakes are adequate to maximize peak bone mass and to minimize bone loss and fracture risk in later life, and the controversies continue.

Vitamin D is obtained either from the diet or by synthesis in the skin under the action of sunlight. Overt vitamin Ddeficiency causes rickets in children and osteomalacia in adults, conditions where the ratio of mineral to osteoid in bone is reduced. Poor vitamin Dstatus in the elderly, at plasma levels of 25-hydroxyvitamin D above those associated with osteomalacia, has been linked to age-related bone loss and osteoporotic fracture, where the ratio of mineral to osteoid remains normal.

Many other nutrients and dietary factors may be important for long-term bone health and the prevention of osteoporosis. Among the essential nutrients, plausible hypotheses for involvement with skeletal health, based on biochemical and metabolic evidence, can be made for zinc, copper, manganese, boron, vitamin A, vitamin C, vitamin K, the B vitamins, potassium and sodium.

Evidence from physiological and clinical studies is largely lacking, and the data are often difficult to interpret because of potential size-confounding or bone remodelling transient effects. For older people, there is convincing evidence for a reduction in risk for osteoporosis with sufficient intake of vitamin D and calcium together, and for an increase in risk with high consumption of alcohol and low body weight.

Evidence suggesting a probable relationship, again in older people, supports a role for calcium and vitamin D separately, but none with fluoride. In countries with a high fracture incidence, a minimum of 400--500 mg of calcium intake is required to prevent osteoporosis. When consumption of dairy products is limited, other sources of calcium include fish with edible bones, tortillas processed with lime, green vegetables high in calcium (e. g. broccoli, kale), legumes and by-products of legumes (e. g. tofu).

The interaction between calcium intake and physical activity, sun exposure, and intake of other dietary components (e. g. vitamin D, vitamin K, sodium, protein) and protective phytonutrients (e. g. soy compounds), needs to be considered before recommending increased calcium intake in countries with low fracture incidence in order to be in line with recommendations for industrialized countries.

With regard to calcium intakes to prevent osteoporosis, the Consultation referred to the recommendations of the Joint FAO/WHO Expert Consultation on Vitamin and Mineral Requirements in Human Nutrition which highlighted the calcium paradox. The paradox (that hip fracture rates are higher in developed countries where calcium intake is higher than in developing countries where calcium intake is lower) clearly calls for an explanation.

The report of the Joint FAO/WHOExpert Consultation on Vitamin and Mineral Requirements in Human Nutrition made it clear that the recommendations for calcium intakes were based on long-term (90 days) calcium balance data for adults derived from Australia, Canada, the European Union, the United Kingdom and the United States, and were not necessarily applicable to all countries worldwide. The report also acknowledged that strong evidence was emerging that the requirements for calcium might vary from culture to culture for dietary, genetic, lifestyle and geographical reasons.

5

Nutrition Transition and Prevention of Diseases

Food preferences and dietary habits, which affect energy consumption and nutrient intake, are generally developed over a period of time and particularly during adolescence. Two major factors affect food choices during adolescence. The first is a greater quest for independence; as in earlier periods of life, one of the ways independence is exhibited is through eating, or not eating. It is often a time for making rebellious or nonconformist statements and adopting social causes.

This, coupled with a lack of knowledge and experience necessary to make adequate evaluations of dietary practice, may lead to the adoption of ill-conceived diets . The second factor is greater purchasing power to obtain meals, snacks and beverages. Rather than relying solely on family foods, sources of food may include food outlets, vending machines and school canteens.

There are many other factors noted to influence the food choices and nutritional intake in this age group, including general nutrition knowledge, socioeconomic status, urban or rural residence, family composition, cultural and religious events, participation in sport and food advertising. However, the living situation during adolescence is noted as an important influence on food choice during this period, with families serving as role models that reinforce and support the acquisition and maintenance of eating behaviour.

Some individuals in the adolescent age group live independently with little or no family contact. However, there is a lack of research about the dietary practices of independent adolescents in New Zealand. Peer influence through increased social activity also affects food choices of adolescents. Loss of appetite or refusing to consume food, overeating, eating whatever is available and eating convenience or junk foods are some of the food-related responses to the stress of teenage lifestyle.

Alcohol, tobacco and drug use can also affect nutrition status and food choice in the adolescent, and they also need to be considered. Research into the eating behaviours and patterns of adolescents indicate the unique lifestyle of this age group that creates a particular context for nutrition education and intervention. Also, it must be noted that the onset of the pubertal growth spurt varies for individuals and thus, any advice given to adolescents as a group must consider the wide variation in individual needs.

It is also important to consider cultural-specific dietary practices when evaluating and promoting nutrition education for this age group. The period of adolescence has wide cultural and individual variation. The World Health Organization (WHO) defines 'young people' as those aged between 10 and 24 years. Adolescents of a given chronological age usually vary in their physiological development. Because of this variability among individuals, age is often a poor indicator of physiological maturity and nutritional needs.

Physiologically, adolescence can be defined as the period between pubescence (the time of initial physiological development during which the reproductive organs mature) and the time when the changes are complete. While the dietary recommendations are expressed by chronological age, the information in this paper will encompass adolescence as defined physiologically.

Absolute energy needs for growth are higher during adolescence compared to earlier in childhood, though they rarely exceed 10 percent of the total energy requirements. Even during the adolescent growth spurt, the energy needed for maintenance is greater than the need for growth. However, if the energy needs are not met, the pubescent growth spurt can be delayed or decreased. Thus, energy requirements for adolescence may be best estimated as kJ/cm of height varying with sex and age.

Adolescents who tend to be overweight grow taller during the growth spurt than those adolescents who are underweight. Energy requirements vary with physiological state, and the need for energy increases as body weight increases. Variation between individuals in requirements also exists due to variable levels of physical activity. Adolescents involved in higher levels of physical activity generally have a higher requirement than those who are inactive.

The maintenance of all body functions requires a constant supply of energy. Energy in the diet is provided by carbohydrates, fats and proteins: one gram of carbohydrate (sugars and starches) provides 17 kJ of energy, one gram of fat provides 37 kJ of energy and one gram of protein provides 17 kJ of energy. There is a wide individual variation in energy intake for both sexes.

A US study showed that female adolescents generally did not tend to increase energy intake with increasing age. Consequently, many female adolescents were unable to meet the energy and nutrient requirements for optimal growth at this crucial part of their life. The study showed that for male adolescents, there was a gradual increase in food intake with age, and most were able to meet their energy and nutritional requirements throughout the adolescent period.

Obesity is body fatness significantly in excess of that consistent with optimal health. There are no agreed national standards for assessing overweight or obesity in New Zealand adolescents. The issue of defining overweight and obesity in this age group is problematic and controversial. Height and weight percentile charts can be useful to assess changes in weight with respect to height over time.

Inactivity is considered one of the determinants of obesity. It has been suggested that the recommended energy intake in adolescents should be reduced to take into account that most in this age group do not expend more than 10 percent of energy for physical activity. In the US, television viewing rather than excessive dietary energy intake is considered a leading determinant associated with early life obesity. Other contributing factors to the sedentary lifestyle are increased use of cars and lifts.

In New Zealand, both girls and boys have similar participation rates in physical activity until the age of 10 years, but from 11 years onwards, males show a slight increase and females a decrease in physical activity. The trend observed may be of concern given that the lifestyle established during adolescence may influence lifestyle displayed as an adult.

Diet composition independent of total energy intake, resting energy expenditure and physical activity have been shown to be important in contributing to childhood and adolescent obesity. In diets of the same energy content, high-fat diets promoted more weight gain than low-fat diets. However, results from studies in the adult population show that despite reductions in total fat in the diet, the prevalence of obesity has increased, which suggests that obesity is a complex problem that will not be solved by solely reducing the percentage of fat in the diet.

Diet, exercise and behavioural approaches to the treatment of adolescent obesity have shown no significant long-term effectiveness. However, the family-based treatment of obesity has demonstrated remarkable long-term maintenance of weight loss. Food intake will need to be increased in order to meet the requirements for energy and nutrients of these individuals. The best way to ensure that the individual adolescent is meeting their energy needs is to assess the adolescent regularly using a standardised weight for height chart.

Protein is an essential nutrient for growth and maintenance of tissues. During the adolescent growth spurt, protein needs are high and utilisation of protein is dependent on adequate energy intake. Even if the protein intake is sufficient, it cannot be utilised for growth unless energy requirements are met. Some female adolescents may be at risk of developing protein deficiency due to their low energy intake.

Data from the Australian Bureau of Statistics showed that the contribution of protein to energy intake was approximately 15 percent for Australian adolescents. A cohort study of 4760 teenagers in the UK reported the contribution of protein to energy intake was 12.5 percent: the largest contribution of protein was from meat and meat products (33 percent) followed by cereals and cereal products (24 percent) and milk and milk products (15 percent). The Australian recommendations for adolescents include safe levels of intake that take into consideration growth and maintenance rates. They suggest further allowance to be made if the protein source is of predominantly low quality.

The US-recommended daily allowance (RDA) is based on similar considerations but also expresses the RDA for protein in relation to height, with the daily protein recommendations for adolescents being approximately 0.3 g/cm height. The New Zealand Nutrition Taskforce recommended that the total protein intake not exceed twice the recommended dietary intake for each age group. Peak requirements of protein will coincide with peak energy requirements and therefore can be summarised as 12-14 percent of energy requirements.

Dietary fat is found in both animal and vegetable foods. Saturated fats are commonly found in meat, such as beef, mutton, poultry, and animal products like egg yolks and dairy products (cheese, butter and whole milk). Polyunsaturated fats are found in plant oils, such as peanut, soybean, cotton seed, corn, safflower and those used in margarines.

Monounsaturated fatty acids present in olives, olive oil, canola oil, peanuts, peanut oil, almonds, pecans and avocadoes. Essential fatty acids are linolenic acid and linoleic acid fatty acids, which must be obtained from the diet, as they cannot be produced by the body. Docosohexanoic acid is synthesised from linolenic acid and plays an essential role in brain and retinal visual function.

Fat in food can be divided into two components.

— The visible component, which is butter, margarine, lard, vegetable oils and visible fat on meat.

— This is easy to measure and is easier to restrict in a dietary intervention.

— The invisible component, the fat closely associated with foods includes the fat in cakes, biscuits, cream, pastries and snack foods. The invisible component is variable and harder to measure and its restriction is dependent on food selection.

A high level of low density lipoprotein (LDL) cholesterol has been shown to be the most significant risk factor for coronary heart disease. The other risk factors - for example, physical inactivity, obesity, cigarette smoking, high blood pressure - tend to influence the occurrence of cardiovascular disease only when people have high plasma cholesterol levels.

Coronary mortality has fallen in the US, Australia and New Zealand. Diet has been identified as one of the environmental factors most likely to be responsible for this trend. The largest change of any dietary component is the increase in polyunsaturated fat intake and in the polyunsaturated/saturated fat ratio.

Meta-analysis of controlled experiments confirm saturated fatty acids raise total and LDL cholesterol, polyunsaturated fats lower total and LDL cholesterol and monounsaturated fats are neutral when compared to carbohydrate. The aetiology of coronary heart disease is multifactorial and fat can clearly not be the only determinant.

Foods with a high carbohydrate content, for example, breads, rice, pasta, cereals, beans and potatoes are not only important sources of energy that can replace saturated fatty acids in the diet but they also contain vitamins, minerals and are rich sources of dietary fibre. The main components of dietary fibre come from plant cell walls and are made up of cellulose, hemicellulose and pectin (the non-starch polysaccharides (NSP)).

Lignin, a non-carbohydrate component of the cell wall, is often included. The precise definition of dietary fibre is controversial. There is general agreement that the main component of dietary fibre is NSP, but there is no agreement on whether the other components should be included in the definition. It has been proposed at the joint Food and Agriculture Organization (FAO)/WHO expert consultation that the term dietary fibre be gradually phased out.

Water-insoluble NSP found in wheat bran, cereals and vegetables may increase stool weight and normalise bowel transit time. As a result, insoluble NSP can appreciably reduce the problem of constipation. On a long-term basis, insoluble NSP may be useful in preventing and managing a range of bowel diseases such as diverticular disease, irritable bowel syndrome and gall stones.

Water-soluble NSP found in peas, oats, dried beans, lentils, barley, pasta and fruits, delays gastric emptying and increases the viscosity of the contents of the small intestine. Soluble NSP reduces the glycaemic index of the carbohydrate foods, increases bile acid excretion and may reduce low-density lipoprotein cholesterol levels.

Resistant starch is resistant to small bowel digestion. In the colon both resistant starch and some NSP are fermented to short-chain fatty acids. The profile of fatty acid production depends on the nature of the substrate fibre. These short chain fatty acids provide energy both locally for the lining of the intestine and also energy for the general metabolism.

Most of the health benefits of resistant starch relate to its impact on the colon. It increases bowel action with its mild laxative effect, increases the bowel's beneficial microflora, reduces the secondary bile acids in the faeces, beneficially lowers faecal pH and increases the level of short-chain fatty acids, in particular proprionate and butyrate.

Depending on the method used to determine dietary fibre intakes, the description of dietary fibre intake differs according to the component of dietary fibre measured, that is, dietary fibre and/or NSP and resistant starch. In New Zealand, dietary fibre intake has been reported to be 31 g/day and 17 g/day in males and females respectively, with the fibre/energy ratio being similar for both sexes.

Breads and cereal foods (other than rice and pasta) were the major contributors to fibre intake. Resistant starch intakes have been approximated to be 8.5 g/day and 5.2 g/day in 15-18 year old males and females respectively. Carbohydrate intake of adolescents in New Zealand contributes to approximately half the daily energy intake.

While New Zealand adolescents appear to have intakes within the recommended range for carbohydrate, a high proportion of the carbohydrates are from refined sugars, especially sucrose. The major contributors of sucrose are sugary products, many of which are consumed as snacks -for example, sweet biscuits, cakes, confectionery and carbonated drinks.

Since sucrose can be cariogenic and may lead to accumulation of excess adipose tissue, there needs to be a restriction in the frequency of eating foods high in added sugars. Sugary foods should be taken during meal times instead of as snacks. The major sources of dietary fibre in the adolescent age group are breads and cereals followed by fruits and vegetables.

Iron needs are greatest in the first six months of life and during the pubertal growth spurt. Iron is required for expanding cell mass and growing body tissues in adolescents and, in female adolescents, iron is also required to replace that which is lost through menstruation. The level of physiological requirement varies between individuals.

The iron absorption from food is dependent on a number of factors, including the iron status, the dietary iron intake of the individual and the individual iron requirement. Iron absorption is increased when the iron stores are low. Iron absorption also increases when the need is high, for example, during adolescence. The iron absorbed by the individual depends on the iron content of the diet and on the bioavailability of iron from the diet.

The haem form of iron found in meat, seafood and chicken is more readily absorbed than non-haem iron found in cereals, vegetables and fruit. Non-haem iron absorption is dependent on the presence of promotors and inhibitors. The major promotors of non-haem iron absorption from the common food pool are meat and organic acids, including citric acid, lactic acid and particularly ascorbic acid.

Meat has a twofold beneficial effect on iron nutrition. Not only is it a good source of the bio-available haem iron, but it also promotes absorption of non-haem iron from the common pool. As a result, the absorption of non-haem iron from a variety of staple foods is substantially improved in the presence of meat.

Ascorbic acid is the most powerful promotor of non-haem iron absorption. The inhibitory effect of phytate and tannic acid can be overcome by ascorbic acid. Prolonged heating of foods causes destruction of ascorbic acid, thus affecting the bioavailability of non-haem iron. Inhibitors of non-haem iron absorption include polyphenols (from tea, vegetables, legumes and condiments), phyates (from cereals, nuts and legumes), the dietary fibre complex (wheat), calcium and phosphorus.

Iron-deficiency anaemia is defined as a haemoglobin below a standard cut-off point based on race, age and sex. However, before iron-deficiency anaemia is reached, there are interim stages of iron deficiency. Therefore, a combination of biochemical measures is used as an index of biological iron status. The level of these parameters reflects different stages of iron status, but it must be noted that they can also be affected by dehydration, recent strenuous exercise, and the presence or absence of pathological conditions such as infection, inflammation or malignancy.

While iron deficiency is associated mainly with iron deficiency anaemia (low haemoglobin level), there is abundant evidence to suggest that unsatisfactory iron status can produce pathological effects in the presence of haemoglobin and haemotocrit being within the normal range. Iron deficiency and low iron stores have been associated with problems in both humoral and cellular response to infection, decreased work capacity and specific cognitive learning effect.

Adolescents are vulnerable to low iron stores and iron deficiency due to the high physiological requirements for growth, high losses which accrue in menstruating female adolescents, and diets which are often low in haem iron. Iron is found in many foods. About 40 percent of the total dietary iron is available as haem iron which is found in animal tissues: meat, liver, fish and poultry. The remaining 60 percent of iron and all the iron in plant foods such as cereals, vegetables, legumes, nuts and fruits is non-haem.

The absorption of non-haem iron is increased when raw fruit or vegetables (sources of vitamin C) are eaten at the same time as non-haem iron foods and is further enhanced by a small piece of fish or meat. To meet their high requirements, adolescents are not only encouraged to consume adequate amounts of iron-rich food (meat, chicken, seafood) but also to have appropriate combinations of food, particularly when the iron is in the non-haem form.

Non-muscle protein - for example, egg and cheese - do not have the enhancing effect of meat on iron absorption and good sources of plant protein, for example, soy bean and nuts have a negative effect on iron availability. Therefore, adolescents on these diets need to make use of vitamin C to improve iron availability. Raw fruits, fruit juice or vegetables should be eaten with all meals.

Rapid expansion of the red cell mass during adolescence and the typically iron-poor diet that female adolescents consume put adolescents at increased risk of iron-deficiency anaemia during pregnancy. Since the pre-menarcheal growth spurt can deplete endogenous iron stores, it is suggested that adolescents who conceive soon after menarche may need to meet a greater proportion of their pregnancy-related requirements for iron from exogenous sources.

Thus, pregnant adolescents should be encouraged to increase their intake of iron-rich foods, and health professionals must be aware of the importance of regularly checking maternal iron stores during pregnancy. Supplementation is usually necessary in the adolescent who has conceived soon after her pre-menarcheal growth spurt but must always be in conjunction with the appropriate dietary advice and under medical supervision.

Iron supplements are only necessary when there is evidence of iron-deficiency or depletion. While it has been stated that iron deficiency is common in the exercising population, to date there is no large-scale study that has compared the iron status of those who exercise with those who do not. Although increased iron loss due to haemolysis, increased faecal and urinary excretion and sweat may occur in some athletes, these losses tend to be insignificant. Inadequate iron intake is in general the main cause of deficiency in adolescent athletes. Thus, adolescent athletes need to maintain adequate iron intake and to utilise food iron efficiently.

The period between nine and 20 years seems to be critical for achievement of peak bone mass. Since the contribution of the third decade to peak bone mass is relatively small, the critical period for the maximal bone mass formation is during puberty and early adolescence. Peak bone mass is probably the result of the interaction between endogenous (heredity and endocrine) and exogenous (nutrition, physical activity) factors.

Among nutritive factors, calcium seems to be the most important determinant of peak bone mass in young adults. Calcium deficiency or factors which interfere with calcium intake may be crucial at this time of life. Many female adolescents may be at increased risk for the development of skeletal inadequacy due to an imbalance between calcium intake and high requirements for calcium during this period of increased bone modelling and skeletal consolidation.

It is also possible that anorexic females may have low bone mineral density due to low food intakes and amenorrhoea. Improvements in bone mass have been demonstrated in a number of calcium intervention trials. However, other cross-sectional studies have not found an association between current calcium intake and bone mass. Although osteoporosis generally appears later in life in both sexes or after the menopause in women, chronic deficiency in calcium intake starting early in life is responsible for osteoporotic development.

Adolescents have higher rates of calcium absorption than children and young adults. The major determinants of calcium absorption are the amount of bio-available calcium in the diet and the vitamin D status of the individual. The absorption of calcium may increase with lactose, protein and calcium to phosphorus ratio of 0.6 to 1.0. Under normal circumstances, the efficiency of intestinal calcium absorption is carefully regulated to meet the body's need for calcium.

Negative imbalances can be caused by caffeine and alcohol consumption. High caffeine intake and high alcohol consumption are two potential areas of concern with respect to adolescent bone. Calcium requirements during adolescence are associated with growth of lean body mass and mineral skeleton.

During adolescence approximately 45 percent of the total adult skeleton is laid down. Variation between individuals is due to sex, physiological age as well as body size. Average daily increments of body calcium are still debatable since values differ according to the method of measurement. At the peak of the adolescent growth spurt, the calcium increment can be two to three times greater than normal states of growth. A positive correlation exists between positive calcium balance and calcium intake.

There is still international debate in the literature concerning the effect of sodium intake on normotensive individuals. A meta-analysis of controlled clinical trials provides evidence that sodium restriction in normotensive individuals is unnecessary. However, hypertensive individuals appear to benefit from sodium restriction. Adolescents who present with hypertension usually have mild to moderate hypertension associated with overweight or obesity.

Urinary calcium is dependent on protein and salt intake. Therefore the high sodium intake of adolescents and low calcium intake seen in the two New Zealand surveys is of concern. Since foods popular with adolescents are often high in sodium, some adolescents may be placed at risk of developing negative calcium balance. There are no accurate data on the sodium intakes of New Zealand adolescents, however, foods such as potato crisps, pies and savoury biscuits are popular and contribute to the adolescent's sodium intake.

Therefore, encouraging foods such as fruit, low fat dairy products and bread- based products will help in ensuring a nutrient-dense diet, which may also assist in weight control and therefore may reduce the risk of hypertension. Folate in foods is easily destroyed during storage and cooking, so careful food preparation is necessary. Leafy vegetables, fruits, beans, peanuts, bran, and yeast are good sources of folate, with liver and kidney being the richest sources.

Adolescents may be at risk of low intakes due to low popularity of the folate-rich foods. Folate is important in early pregnancy. Studies have found that periconceptional supplementation of folic acid reduces the reoccurrence and occurrence of neural tube defects. Low blood folic acid concentrations have been associated with high blood homocysteine levels in adults.

Zinc is integral in the synthesis of protein and essential for normal growth and development. The Life in New Zealand Survey found the mean zinc intake of 15-18 year old males to be 14 mg per day and females 9 mg per day. Vegan adolescents may be at greater risk of zinc deficiency since absorption of zinc is inhibited by high fibre foods, phytates and iron. Meat, poultry and fish are good sources of bioavailable zinc.

It is possible that adolescents on vegan diets are at risk of developing vitamin A deficiency because the main sources of vitamin A are dairy products, eggs, liver, meats and fatty fish. Alternatively, vegetable sources of provitamin A include, carrots, pumpkin and dark green leafy vegetables, such as silverbeet and broccoli, and should be encouraged for this group. Vitamin C Vitamin C acts as a co-substrate in hydroxylations requiring oxygen and is a powerful antioxidant.

Vitamin B6 is involved in a large number of enzyme systems associated with nitrogen metabolism. On the other hand, the UK is concerned about toxicological evidence which shows the consumption of high doses of vitamin B6, usually as supplements, over a period of time is harmful to health and may cause sensory peripheral neuropathy. The UK is currently consulting on draft regulations for dietary supplements which propose a maximum daily dose of 10 mg of vitamin B6 sold under food law.

Adolescents should be encouraged to include whole grain cereals, poultry, fish, eggs, green and leafy vegetables and fruit in their diet to ensure an adequate dietary intake of vitamin B6. Vitamin B12 is required for rapid growth of cells. Adolescents would appear to have an increased need for vitamin B12, particularly during the growth spurt. Animal products are the only sources of vitamin B12, adolescents on a vegan diet may be at risk.

Niacin, riboflavin, thiamin These vitamins are involved in energy metabolism, so there is an increase in requirements for these vitamins during adolescence. Niacin, riboflavin, thiamin should be met through increased food intakes, thus supplying both the necessary energy and the vitamins. This is best achieved by encouraging increased dietary intakes of bread, cereal, fruit and vegetables low-fat dairy products and meat.

The water requirement is the amount of water necessary to: balance the insensible losses which varies both within and between individuals maintain a tolerable solute load for the kidneys which may vary with dietary composition and other factors.

Very physically active adolescents need more water to replace fluids lost through perspiration. Young adolescents should be reminded to drink water. A loss of as little as 3 percent of body water could result in exhaustion and dehydration or, less dramatically, cause a person to become tired and less effective during activity. As the level of dehydration increased so did the sensation of thirst. Sports drinks, advertised as a way to replace water and electrolytes lost during exercise, are not generally recommended for non-endurance activities.

Plain water is the most economical source of fluid. Young athletes can use sports drinks, especially if they exercise for more than 90 minutes. Although water is adequate, greater overall fluid intake may be achieved if it is flavoured. Some of these drinks are high in sugar, which may cause cramps, nausea and diarrhoea in some individuals. Lost electrolytes are usually replaced upon eating.

Alcohol dependence is of major concern. Alcohol dependence was the second most prevalent psychiatric disorder found in 18 year olds in the Dunedin Health and Development Study. Prevalence was greater in males, at 12.7 percent, with an overall prevalence of 10.4 percent. Family and peer influences, rather than personality characteristics, are believed to be influential in the establishment of substance abuse in adolescence.

The factors that initiate alcohol consumption during adolescence are stress, peer pressure, rejection of parental authority, deviant behaviour and sensation seeking, ease of access to alcohol at home and working greater than 20 hours per week while studying . Exposure to alcohol before age six and positive parental attitudes to alcohol are also considered to increase vulnerability to frequent heavy drinking in adolescence.

The effect of chronic alcohol abuse on nutritional status during adolescence is not known. However, a high consumption of alcohol can replace calcium intake and contribute to obesity. Poor nutrition can result from impaired nutrient absorption and inadequate dietary intake over a period of time. A number of studies in the UK have shown that alcohol is consumed on a regular basis by over 40 percent of 17 year olds and contributes on average 2 percent of daily energy intakes.

Water intake should be encouraged during adolescence. Milk, especially reduced fat milks, are also recommended. While alcohol intake is not recommended for adolescents, alcohol consumption cannot be completely avoided. Advice for adolescent consumers is:

— limit intake of alcohol

— discourage binge drinking

— eat some food when you drink

— dilute alcoholic beverages and keep count of the number of drinks consumed

— do not drink alcoholic beverages if you intend to drive a car or operate machinery or undertake difficult tasks.

The best nutrition strategy for promoting optimal health and reducing risk of chronic disease is by obtaining adequate nutrients from a wide variety of foods as recommended in the Food and Nutrition Guidelines. Vitamin and mineral supplementation is only appropriate in specific circumstances.

In July 1996, the joint food standards setting system between Australia and New Zealand was introduced. Until a single set of food standards is developed for both countries, New Zealand allows food products to comply either with the New Zealand Food Regulations 1984 or with the Australian Food Standards Code. The Regulations list which foods can be fortified, what nutrients can be added and the quantities of nutrients which can be added to the food.

Food standards need to be reviewed regularly in response to a population's changing nutritional needs and to any emerging health risk which may arise from foods. It is reported that there are no known safety concerns in the UK resulting from the consumption of foods with added nutrients. Vegetarian diets in the context of ecological, environmental, philosophical and health concerns provide a ready focus for adolescents.

It is possible to obtain all essential nutrients without eating animal products. Eating a wide variety of different foods will ensure a good balance of nutrients. A considerable body of scientific data suggest positive relationships between vegetarian lifestyles and risk reduction for several chronic degenerative diseases such as obesity, coronary artery disease, hypertension, diabetes mellitus, colon cancer, osteoporosis and others.

The term vegetarianism encompasses a wide range of dietary practices that can be divided into a number of sub-groups. Lacto-ovo-vegetarians (LOV) exclude meat, fish and poultry from their diet but they do consume dairy products and eggs. Lacto-vegetarians eat no meat, fish, poultry or eggs but they do include milk and milk products (butter, cheese) in their diet. Vegans adopt the strictest form of vegetarianism, as they exclude all animal-derived food from their diet.

The UK is considering developing separate nutrient recommendations for vegetarians. Nutritional adequacy of lacto-ovo-vegetarian diets LOV diets which contain milk products and eggs are generally satisfactory for children and adolescents. They also conform closely with adolescent recommendations for promoting health and reducing the risk of chronic degenerative diseases.

Protein quality may be compromised by limited variety or improper combination of plant sources of protein. Care must be taken to offer the vegan adolescent ample sources of protein and to ensure that energy intakes are adequate. It is important that vegetarians and vegans consume protein from a variety of sources. For vegan diets, it is necessary to consume both grains - which are high in methionine and threonine and low in lysine - and legumes - which are foods high in lysine but low in sulphur-containing amino acids. This will ensure all essential amino acids are provided.

Foods commonly consumed in a vegetarian and vegan diet contain large amounts of fibre, phytate and oxalate. These substances are known to bind minerals such as calcium, iron and zinc and reduce their bioavailability. There is no evidence that this binding will cause deficiency syndromes in an otherwise adequate diet.

Fruits and vegetables are important foods in the vegetarian diet, as they contribute a large quantity of vitamin C. Calcium intake is not affected in LOVs as they consume milk and dairy products. Absence of milk products may influence peak bone mass acquisition in adolescents because of inadequate intakes of dietary vitamin D, calcium and phosphorus.

Sources of calcium in vegan diets include legumes, tofu, oranges, almonds, figs and some leafy vegetables. Calcium-fortified soy beverages is recommended. Zinc is needed for growth and development and the maintenance of body tissues. LOV and vegan diets can be low in zinc due to the dietary exclusion of meats, poultry and seafood, and the binding of zinc by fibre, phytate and oxalate.

Developing adolescents, especially females, are particularly concerned about their body image and excessive weight (either real or perceived) and are under constant pressure to enhance their body image. It has been reported that concerns and dissatisfaction with one's body has become so prevalent that 'it can be considered to be a normal part of the female experience'.

Adolescence is thought to be the period during which distortions of body image may be initiated. Therefore adolescence is a critical time for the development of a realistic body image. There is a correlation between weight and dissatisfaction with body image in females. Most female adolescents tend to associate weight with fatness, which is considered undesirable, while male adolescents tend to associate weight with muscle and bone, which is desirable.

However, the majority of females admitted that they were not happy with their bodies, and that most females felt some social pressure, and consequently compared themselves to the 'ideal' body image. One study has shown that there is a possibility of a causal relationship between regular participation in a fitness programme and excessive concern with dieting and weight, especially in people with bulimia nervosa.

Eating disorders may include a variety of conditions but in particular the clinical syndromes of anorexia nervosa and bulimia nervosa. Anorexia nervosa is a potentially life-threatening illness. Sufferers exhibit an extreme psycho-physiological aversion to food. The disease is characterised by an obsessive compulsion to keep body weight below 85 percent of what would be expected based on age and height. Bulimia nervosa is characterised by repeated binge and purge sessions.

Increased fat laid down during puberty is negatively viewed by most girls, and as puberty progresses the desire to be thinner increases. Preoccupation with dieting is higher in girls than in boys and increases with age. There is a strong association between the dietary concerns of girls and those of their mothers.

Parental beliefs and behaviours are likely to be major influences on a child's and adolescent's view of their own body size. It is important that parents, significant others, and the media do not promote inappropriate body size and shape values. Several overseas studies show that many girls aspire to attain a body shape which is thinner than their current shape. Body shape satisfaction (or the point at which preferred shape is equal to current shape) for girls was met at 11 percent below their mean weight.

Boys desire a more athletic and muscular build and have a body shape satisfaction at 12 percent above their mean weight. A small study based in Hamilton showed that approximately half of the female adolescents sampled had a preoccupation with weight and most desired a reduction in their weight to 'feel better about themselves'. In this study, more than half of those sampled had dieted at some time. Increased awareness of the health hazards associated with being overweight, the pursuit of thinness or distortions in body image perceptions were contributors to the high statistics of dieting.

The major nutritional problem in these disorders is the lack of food consumption. Energy, vitamins, and mineral intakes are inadequate and malnutrition develops. Therefore development of eating disorders during the adolescent years is nutritionally and psychologically devastating. Pre-adolescence is the period when the body lays down fat reserves for the following growth spurt of adolescence. During adolescence there is a dramatic increase in nutrient requirements to sustain growth and maturation.

Therefore, children and adolescents who self-impose energy restriction have a retarded growth rate and puberty is usually delayed. Anorexia nervosa and bulimia nervosa are complex disorders that are multifactorial in aetiology and pathology. The cluster of symptoms and signs often begins in adolescence. Clinicians, health care providers and teachers should be well informed and sensitive to early detection and intervention.

Treatment of eating disorders is usually a long-term, complex process and is best provided by a psychiatrist and dietitian with specialist training and experience in this area. Pregnancy The nutritional recommendations for the pregnant adolescent need to take into account both the health of the mother and the infant. The pregnant adolescent is at risk if she has not completed her growth. Because of the increased nutritional needs of her own growth, as well as foetal growth, the nutritional requirements are higher than for adult women.

Weight gain is very important during pregnancy, since inadequate weight gain of the mother is associated with low birth-weight in the infant. The incidence of low birth-weight infants is higher for adolescents than adult women. Since body image is important to adolescent females and many initially deny a pregnancy, nutritional counselling may be required to assist in the process of gaining appropriate weight.

Several studies in the US have focused on the dietary habits of pregnant adolescents and indicate that intakes of some nutrients may be below recommendations, particularly intake of iron, zinc, calcium, magnesium, folate, vitamin B6 and vitamin A. It does appear that adolescents may make some appropriate dietary changes during pregnancy, skip fewer meals and substitute fewer snacks for meals. However, nutrition education should aim to improve adolescents' knowledge on how to increase their intakes of nutrient-rich foods instead of snacking on less nutritionally valuable foods.

Unfortunately for many pregnant adolescents, pregnancy is a time of great stress and there is usually a complex mix of social, emotional and physical factors complicating the situation. It is necessary that adequate emotional support be given to the adolescent and close contact be maintained to ensure adequate nutrition. Regular assessment of nutritional status is also important. This should include assessment of maternal weight gain, dietary intake and assessment of iron status.

Adolescence is also an important time for developing the values, habits and behaviours of adulthood and as such it becomes an important period for developing a habit of participation in physical activity that can be transferred into adulthood. An international consensus conference on physical activity guidelines for adolescents established recommendations for physical activity for this age group. These guidelines are:

— All adolescents should be physically active daily, or nearly every day, as part of play, games, sport, work, transportation, recreation, physical education or planned exercise, in the context of family, school and community activities.

— Adolescents should engage in three or more sessions per week of activities that last 20 minutes or more at a time and that require moderate to vigorous levels of exertion.

The intent of the first guideline is to encourage adolescents to adopt and maintain an active lifestyle into adulthood. It also aims for adolescents to incorporate weight-bearing activities in order to enhance bone density, daily energy expenditure and to reduce the risk of obesity. The international consensus conference recommended that a minimum of 30 minutes of physical activity be accumulated daily.

The second recommendation aims to maintain cardiovascular fitness in adolescents and to increase HDL cholesterol and improve psychological health.

A demographic transition, from rural societies with low life expectancy at birth and families with many children, to urban societies with higher life expectancy at birth and fewer children, has been well documented. The epidemiological transition that follows the demographic transition is also fairly well understood: a shift from endemic deficiency and infectious diseases, mostly of early life, to epidemic chronic diseases, generally of later life.

There is now sufficient evidence to propose a general theory for this causally and chronologically linked demographic, nutrition, and epidemiological transi-tion. When populations undergo massive social and technological change that includes increasing urbanization, their food supplies and therefore their diets change. Consequently, disease patterns also change. This can be traced in countries that are now economi-cally developed; for example, Britain between the sixteenth and eighteenth centuries, following the agrar-ian and industrial revolutions.

In Africa, Asia, Latin America, and in the Small Island .Developing States (SIDS) of the Pacific, such transitions are taking place very much faster and, in some cases, with extreme rapidity. Current evidence suggests that some diet-related diseases become epidemic at a speed that is a func-tion of the velocity of demographic and nutrition transition, and that they emerge as epidemics in a predictable sequence.

The nutrition transition in Asia and in the SIDS of the Pacific is a central part of a sequence of transi-tions. These begin with the demographic transition. Increased urbanization and technological change lead to a shift from physically active to sedentary occupa-tions, less walking and cycling, more use of cars and television, increased use of labor saving devices at work and home, and changes in income profiles.

The nutrition transition itself is marked by a shift from relatively monotonous diets based on indigenous staple grains or starchy roots, locally grown legumes, other vegetables and fruits, and (except for prosperous subpopulations) limited foods of animal origin, toward more varied diets that include more preprocessed food, more foods of animal origin, more sugar and fat, especially in processed drinks and foods, and often more alcohol.

The most immediate result of the combination of such relatively energy-dense diets with physically inactive lives, is a rapid increase in overweight and obesity. This is a usual, though not inevitable, consequence of urbanization. The consequent epidemiological transition is from a predominance of endemic deficiency and infectious diseases, often caused or exacerbated by poor nutrition, to epidemic, chronic diseases.

Diet-related chronic diseases include tooth decay, gastrointestinal disorders, obesity, adult-onset diabetes, hypertension, peripheral vascular disease and stroke, hyperlipidemia, angina and ischemic heart disease (IHD), and certain cancers. Most of these diseases also have nondietary causes; for example, the use of tobacco with lung cancer. There is also genetic predisposition to some of these diseases. The risk of this eventuating in overt clinical symptoms is increased by inappropriate environmental factors, including diet.

These changes include, among others, fetal and infant nutrition insults, and poor dietary and activity patterns. Other behavioral changes that also contribute to these diseases, such as increased tobacco use and air pollution, are not discussed. First, the chronic diseases affected by dietary and related lifestyle changes are reviewed, and then their health and economic consequences, intervention options, and policy are examined.

Countries in the Asia-Pacific region are at very different stages in the nutrition transition. Moreover, large subpopulation groups, within even the poorest countries, already face a heavy burden from diet-related chronic diseases. In India, for example, urban residents in general, and other residents in wealthy areas such as the Punjab, have very different diets, body composition, and chronic disease profiles than residents in other areas.

Obesity and cardiovascular diseases (CVDs) are prevalent at very high rates in urban India. In most Asian and Pacific countries, there are subpopulations that face food insecurity and undernutrition. There are also significant differ-ences in the undernutrition profiles of Asian men and women. However, in the countries studied here, gender differences in obesity are smaller than those of other regions of the developing world.

Many studies have shown the nutrition transition in Asia and the Pacific, as well as the developing world in general. Typically, there are dramatic increases in overall fat intake and a corresponding reduction in the proportion of dietary energy from starchy staple foods, accompanied by a shift from coarse grains and legumes toward more refined grains (mainly rice and wheat), a greater intake of meat, fish, dairy products, and edible oils, and a reduction in fruit and vegetable intake.

The general effect is to make diets less bulky, and more energy-dense. There are, however, important variations among these countries. For example, the increase in fat intake and decrease in vegetable intake in the Republic of Korea are far less than might be expected from its development status.

Some of the factors that predict high levels of chronic disease: low birthweight (LBW) and stunting, inappropriate diets, low levels of physical activity, and urbanization. The analyses are mainly at country level, with some household and individual level studies. This broad approach, using averages, inevitably obscures varia-tions within countries. A growing set of studies suggests that fetal and infant nutrition insults affect predisposition to CVDs, obesity, hypertension, and adult-onset diabetes. These same insults also may compromise immune function.

These early nutrition-related insults contribute to later, diet-related chronic diseases. LBW (associated with thinness) and stunting, have both been linked with these adverse risk profiles, but the mechanisms for this are unclear and this leads to uncertainty about appropriate interventions. High rates of LBW and stunting, accompanied by concurrent rapid shifts in diets and activity patterns and increased obesity, are of special importance in rapidly developing countries, such as those of Asia and the SIDS of the Pacific.

There are very high inci-dences of LBW in the lower low-income countries, particularly in Bangladesh, India, Nepal, Pakistan, and Sri Lanka and in the Lao PDR. There is, however, enormous variation in LBW rates among countries in the same income groups. There are no systematic data on the proportion of LBW babies who were born with disproportionately retarded intrauterine growth (IUGR) and who were born very thin.

Stunting prevalence is very high in Bangladesh and Indonesia, countries with high LBW rates, but there are high stunting rates in other upper and lower low-income countries, and in the Republic of Fiji Islands, the only SIDS for which we have data. Elsewhere in Asia, researchers have shown a decline in the proportion of children who are stunted, albeit a decline that is slower than declines in wasting and in LBW.

Some countries are dominated by one or two countrieswith large populations, e.g., the high-income group by the Republic of Korea, the middle-income group by Thailand and the Philippines, the SIDS by Papua New Guinea, the upper low-income group by the PRC, and the lower low-income group by India. Three-year averages were calculated for each country and the averages were weighted for 1996 population size within country groups, so that the values would represent the actual population sizes within country groups.

In general, Asia and Pacific SIDS are becoming less dependent on locally produced and frequently monotonous diets based on staple grains and starchy roots. They are being replaced by diets that include much more fat, more foods of animal origin, and often more sugary food and drink, much of which is produced elsewhere in the country or imported. At the same time, the shift toward diets that are notably more energy-dense, that contain much more fat, more added sugar and sometimes more alcohol, with a marked reduction of starchy staples, is increasing the incidence of diet-related chronic diseases, some of which have become epidemic with remarkable speed.

The lowest income countries, dominated by India, show an actual increase in cereal and starchy roots availability and more modest increases in other foods. In contrast, the highest income countries have decreased their supplies of cereals and starchy roots, tripled their fruits and vegetable availability, and increased their dairy and egg, meat and poultry, and added sugar availability.

Apart from increases among lower low-income and a slight increase among upper low-income countries, there is a marked decline in the availability of cereals and starchy roots-items that have provided much of the dietary energy of Asians and Pacific islanders for centuries. These aggregate trends mask a signifi-cant shift away from so-called coarse and higher fiber grains to rice and wheat, which are usually refined.

The highest intakes are in the lower low-income countries. This reflects partially, among the high-income countries, the low importance of dairy products in the Republic of Korea. Hong Kong, China has a high supply of dairy products, but this accounts for little in the total weighted average in the high-income group.

India is predominant in the lower low-income group and is a high consumer of dairy products. This gives the impression that the availability in the lower low-income group is high relative to all other groups. Eggs and dairy products are important sources of saturated fats in the diet. In India, consumption of ghee, a highly saturated fat product, is important because high consumption of saturated fats is closely related to chronic diseases.

Meat and dairy products are also major sources of saturated fats and major contributors to chronic diseases. A very rapid annual growth in consumption of meat and dairy products from 1993 to 2020 has been projected, e.g., for the PRC, consumptionof meat and dairy products is projected to increase at 3.0% and 2.8% per year, respectively, over this period.

Fruit and vegetable availability has increased markedly for the high-income and the upper low-income countries. It is improving slightly for the middle-income and lower low-income countries. It remains very high for the SIDS. However, continuing reductions in fruit and vegetable intake have been indicated by household surveys in the PRC.

The availability of added animal fats and vegetable oils has increased markedly for all the countries stud-ied. Availability is particularly high for edible vegetable oils. These vary in origin from country to country and include red palm, coconut, corn, soybean, and cot-tonseed oils. In Sri Lanka and the Philippines, coconut oil is a major source of saturated fat. In Malaysia, edible oil comes largely from red palm oil, which has a high polyunsaturated to saturated fat ratio and is more healthy than coconut oil.

The processing of these edible oils varies greatly. There is little systematic research on the composition of these oils. One small study has found trans fatty acid levels of about 50% in dalda, a vegetable ghee widely consumed in India. Increased edible oil is a key reason for the marked increases in energy density of Asian diet.

Energy from added sugar was separated from energy from carbohydrates, to describe its energy contribution meaningfully. Energy from sweeteners in food balance sheets was considered to be 'energy from added sugar' and this was subtracted from total carbohydrate energy to get 'energy from carbohydrate excluding added sugar.' This is a roughestimation for both 'energy from added sugar' and 'energy from carbohydrate excluding added sugar,' because energy from sweeteners also comes, though minimally, from other nutrients.

Similarly, 'energy from added animal fat' was considered to be from animal fats such as butter, ghee, and fish liver oil in the food balance sheets. These refer, however, to a limited category of foods including added animal fats, but not any other fats of animal origin, such as those in meats. At the same time,'energy from added animal fat' also includes minimal amounts of energy from other nutrients, similar to the case for added sugar.

A very rough approximation for 'energy from vegetable oil' was made by subtracting 'energy from added animal fats' from 'total fat energy.''Energy from vegetable oil' is, therefore, essentially 'energy from fat excluding added animal fats and therefore differs from the calories from vegetable oil presented in the sources used here, i.e., the food balance sheets.

The high-income countries have shifted from diets dominated by complex carbohydrates to diets with more fats, added sugar, and protein. These countries have per capita available energy for consumption of over 3,000 kcal/day. In general, this change to more diverse diets improves access to adequate micronutrients and decreases the incidence of micronutrient deficiencies. reduced physical activity, at work and at home, for men and women.

In all countreis, men are shifting much more than women from agriculture toward industry and service sector jobs. No Asian or Pacific studies were available for another important determinant of physical activity-modes of transportation. However, there is a shift away from walking and cycling to mass transit and cars-a major change in regular physical activity and thus in energy expenditure. Reduced physical activity outside work also apparent.

One of the most remarkable changes in the Asia-Pacific region is the explosion of new information sources and mechanisms that reach households even in the most isolated villages and towns. The expansion of mass media, such as television, has major influences on consumer knowledge and attitudes, as well as on diets and physical activity.

The percentage of households that own television sets has increased dramatically throughout Asia, particularly in the PRC and higher income countries. In the PRC, the China National Health Surveys showed that television ownershipincreased, even for the lowest income tertile: from 43% of households in 1989 to 76% in 1993, and to 89% in 1997. Habitual television watching affects diet and activity patterns.

Diets can change as a result of exposure to advertising and role models in the television programs. People consume snacks while watching television. Watching television is sedentary and displaces more active leisure activities. There is a vast literature, from high-income countries in other regions, that has linked watching television to greater inactivity and obesity, but no comparable studies have been made yet in the Asia-Pacific region.

During the last half century, there has been a large shift of populations from rural to urban areas throughout the developing world. Urbanization is occurring more slowly in Asia and the Pacific than in Latin America, the Middle East, and Africa. In Asia and the Pacific, however, the rate of increase in urban populations from the 1960s to the present has been more than four times greater than the increase in rural populations.

The urban proportion of Asian-Pacific populations has increased continuously in the past three decades and this trend continues. During the twentieth century, the population in rural Asia decreased, while it increased in urban areas. As people move into cities, their food supplies change, and therefore, so do their diets and body composition. High levels of obesity are particularly apparent in lower- and middle-income countries.

Urban occupations, transportation and food marketing systems, housing markets, and concentration of population, combine to create different patterns of food supply and demand, and of time allocation. The consequence is overnutrition, meaning that people eat more than they need. This causes overweight, obes-ity, and other major chronic diseases, such as CVDs.

In the developing world, rapid urbanization results in the co-existence of malnutrition and obesity within many households. The urban diet, even in very low-income countries and the poorest areas of cities, contains much more energy from fats and sugar than the rural diet. Urban food is more likely to be processed and often contains more highly refined cereals and sugars and fewer unrefined, staple foods than rural diets.

In urban areas, even poor people are able to afford processed foods that are relatively high in fat and also in refined starches and sugars. Edible oils, in particular, can be very cheap. Further, the high intake of processed food in the urban diet greatly increases consumption of salt; a factor linked to hypertension. In Asia and the Pacific, urban diets are generally more diverse than rural diets, contain more animal food and therefore more animal protein, and often contain more micronutrients.

However, the effect ofrelatively energy-dense diets and physical inactivity is to increase the incidence of overweight, obesity, and other diet-related chronic diseases. Diet-related chronic diseases It has been agreed for many years that the nature and quality of diets affect the risk of chronic diseases, including some that for half a century have been the major causes of premature death in the developed world.

Diet-related chronic diseases vary in severity. They include diseases that are disagreeable, notably tooth decay and various gut disorders; others that are disabling, such as adult-onset diabetes, obesity, and osteoporosis; and others that are deadly, notably IHD and other CVDs, with hyperlipidemia and angina or precursors, cerebrovascular disease and its precursor hypertension, and certain cancers.

A major report specifies cancers, the risks for which are modified by food and nutrition (including alcohol), as well as by physical activity and body composition. Some of these cancers have additional nondietary causes, notably the use of tobacco and cancers of the mouth, throat, esophagus, and lung. Severe gut diseases, notably cancers of the colon and rectum, emerge later in the stages of dietary change and economic development. CVDs and breast cancer might take two generations to become epidemic. This hypothesis, based on preliminary observations and anecdotes, is supported by some epidemiological stud-ies but has not yet been rigorously tested.

Diets that increase the risk of chronic diseases are those relatively high in total fat, saturated fat, sugar, salt, alcohol, refined grains, and foods of animal origin. Diets that protect against chronic diseases are relatively high in minimally processed grains, legumes, fiber, vegetables, fruits, and foods of plant origin.

However, plant-based diets that are monotonous, very high in staple grains or starchy roots, and low in vegetables, fruits, and foods of animal origin can increase the risk of deficiency diseases. Such "poverty diets" emphasize the need for plant-based diets to be varied and not too high in grains or roots of any one type. It has been estimated that appropriate diets and lifestyle can reduce cancer risks by 30% to 40%.

It is commonly supposed that infectious and deficiency diseases are the main public health problems through-out Asia and the Pacific but the following review of mortality trends reveals a more complex picture. Infectious and parasitic diseases were the major causes of all deaths in Asia during much of the twentieth century and before. Although they remain very important, they no longer represent the major cause of death in any country studied here.

In the countries that are furthest along in the nutrition transition (such as Singapore, with higher fat diets and higher rates of obesity) cancers and CVD together account for close to 60% of all deaths: a rate similar to those of North America and western Europe. In the PRC and the Republic of Korea, now more than half of all The importance of the nutrition transition for healthcombined with an aging of the population.

Deaths in India from these same NCDs will also increase, reducing the overall decline in deaths. At very early stages of economic development and nutrition transition, when deaths caused by infectious disease and parasitic infections are still very high, the chronic disease that causes much mortality is hemorrhagic stroke. Hypertension and stroke rates increase with economic development. Where resources allow, treatment of hypertension can lead to a decrease in cerebrovascular disease, as in the Republic of Korea.

India and the PRC are vast countries in which different areas, and rural and urban areas in general, are at different stages of transition. A most remarkable epidemic of adult-onset diabetes and related conditions is emerging in urban India. At a later stage of the nutrition transition, CVDs emerge as the primary cause of chronic disease deaths.

In the Republic of Fiji Islands, where major diet andlifestyle shifts have been followed by very high levels of obesity, diabetes, and other causes of CVD, over a third of deaths were caused by CVDs by the 1970s. CVDs were also the most common cause of death in the1990s in the Kyrgyz Republic, a country with very high levels of obesity and also very high consumption of fats. In 1993, over 30.4% of the dietary energy intake of Kyrgyz adults came from fat. The Republic of Korea is at a relatively late stage of transition and its low level of deaths from CVD is remarkable.

At late stages of the nutrition transition, in countries with relatively high average incomes, deaths from certain cancers increase in absolute and relative importance. Deaths from cancers in Singapore and the Republic of Korea account for 21 to 26% of total deaths. In the PRC, cancers cause almost 20% of all deaths. These rates are all similar to those in developed countries.

Elsewhere in Asia, almost 5 to 10% of deaths are caused by cancers. Mortality by site-specific cancers varies among countries.

One chronic disease that is linked directly to obesity and inactivity, and for which there are relatively good Asian and Pacific data, is adult-onset diabetes. From the best available sources on adult-onset diabetes in Asia, the following data and projections were published for total cases in the region: 1994, 51.2 million; 2000, 94.7 million; and 2010, 138.1 million.

Fetal and perinatal insults are combinations of undernutrition of the mother and fetus or child, caused by diets that are low or deficient in key micro- and macronutrients. In the case of obesity in later life, the hypothesis is that fetal growth retardation results in metabolic changes that are adaptive to nutri-tionally stressful circumstances in utero. A similar argument can be made for postnatal growth retarda-tion, manifested as stunting.

As the child grows, the metabolic efficiencies that were necessary to cope with undernutrition become maladaptive to subsequent overnutrition, leading to the development of abnormal lipid profiles, altered glucose and insulin metabolism, and obesity. Such fetal programming does not by itself lead to increased morbidity and mortality. Rather, it shifts metabolism such that LBW infants become more susceptible to obesity, adult-onset diabetes, and CVD when faced with a richer, more energy-dense diet, reduced physical activity, and increased adiposity, as children or as adults.

Studies on humans are difficult because they require detailed information about status at birth, early postnatal growth, and health or anthropometric status in later childhood and adulthood. The few studies done have generally relied on current status assessment of children or adults, with data for infancy obtained from medical records linking birth status with later hypertension, diabetes, and CVD.

Moreover, with every decade of age, the reduction in systolic blood pressure with birthweight increases by 0.35 mm of Hg per kg. Fewer studies have examined the relationship between birthweight and adult-onset diabetes. Insulin production and insulin resistance, both impor-tant in the etiology of adult-onset diabetes, appear to be affected by fetal development, but it is hard to select a specific risk ratio (RR).

For CVD, although its Diet-related conditions that increase the risk of chronic diseasesdefinitions have not always been consistent, a general result is clear. LBWs, in particular low PI births, appear to be strongly positively related to CVD. It has been suggested that long-term health risks are greater for disproportionately IUGR infants, i.e., those who are thinner.

Underweight during infancy and stunting in early childhood are risk factors for subsequent obesity. In some cases, infant and early childhood growth retarda-tion result from the same underlying factors that cause IUGR, e.g., poverty, poor maternal nutrition, poor weaning diet, and consequent increased risk of infections. IUGR increases the risk of stunting in infancy and later childhood.

Independent of IUGR, many children in developing countries, and indeed impoverished and undernourished children in North America and other developed regions, become stunted during infancy as the result of inappropriate weaning practices, repeated infections, and poor diet: all in the context of poverty.

The highest incidence of stunting occurs in the weaning period and soon after. Early childhood stunting is not readily reversible when children remain in the same poor environments. Improved diets and other environmental effects will, however, lead to catch-up growth.

In the few longitudinal studies of the role of LBW as a cause of stunting in Asia, for example, half or more of stunted children did not have LBWs. Obesity: the effect of diet and physical activity on the risk of chronic diseases There is a massive and growing literature on the causes of overweight and obesity.

Obesity increases the risk of other major chronic diseases, notably CVD and certain cancers. Approaches to correct obesity in adult life remain a matter for debate, but there is an established consensus, reflecting common sense and known biological mechanisms, that energy-dense diets and physical inactivity increase the risk of overweight and obesity. Therefore, the incidence of overweight and obesity in any country can be seen as a function of the energy density of diets and levels of physical inactivity.

Obesity is now a major public health problem in Asia and the Pacific. A generation ago, it was identified as a major problem perhaps only in some western Pacific islands. National surveys from several Asian countries have since shown that the problem is more widespread. Overweight is a lesser condition than obesity and is usually defined by a body mass index (BMI) between 25 to 30.

BMI is defined as weight in kg divided by height in meters squared (kg/m 2). Overweight is a precursor of obesity and can increase the risk of other diseases such as diabetes, hyperten-sion, and CVD. International standards used to delineate the over-weight and obese are not appropriate for Asia. A BMI of 25 in an Asian adult appears to have a far greater adverse metabolic effect than it would in a Caucasian adult.

WHO and the International Obesity TaskForce (IOTF) formed a group of scientists and agencies in Asia to review this. This group has proposed BMI lower limits of 23 for overweight and 25 for obesity for Asians. The issue is complex, however, as there is extensive racial and ethnic heterogeneity in the Asia-Pacific region. For example, BMI-morbidity relationships for East or South Asians, might not be appropriate for Pacific islanders.

Patterns of metabolic disease vary across Asia and the Pacific. Asians tend to put on more abdominal fat, whereas Pacific islanders tend to suffer overweight- and obesity-related diseases at greater BMIs, but are more prone to diabetes. Hence, approaches to obesity must be considered in a regional, subregional, and national context. This change would affect considerably definitions of over-weight and obesity in different parts of Asia and the Pacific.

In Asia and the Pacific, gender differences in obesity are usually smaller and less consistent than in Africa, the Americas, and Europe. Except for Nauru and the Kyrgyz Republic, higher levels of economic development are linked with high obesity levels. Pacific SIDS, such as Samoa and Nauru have been the subject of many studies related to their high rates of obesity and related chronic diseases.

Obesity levels are not only associated with being wealthy. In Indonesia, there is a pronounced difference in overweight and obesity patterns by income tertile. This pattern is not so clear-cut in the other three countries. In the Kyrgyz Republic, overweight is constant across income groups, though obesity increases slightly with income.

In many households, underweight and overweight persons coexist. As Asian and Pacific populations shift toward more-energy dense and lower fiber diets and lower activity levels, it is predicted that there will be a major problem of coexistence of underweight and overweight persons in the same household.

Households with both underweight and overweight members represent 3 to 15% of all households in these countries, levels that are far above chance. An underweight child coexisting with an overweight, nonelderly adult was the predominant pair combination. As the overall prevalence of undernutrition declines, there appear to be shifts in diet and activity patterns that lead, in many households, to a greater coexistence of obesity with persistent undernutrition.

Diet-related chronic diseases

Cardiovascular disease (CVD) is the term used by the scientific community to embrace not just conditions of the heart [ischemic heart disease (IHD), valvular, muscular, and congenital heart disease] but also hypertension and conditions involving the cerebral, carotid, and peripheral circula-tion. Diabetes is usually placed in a separate category from CVD. It is well recognized that the risk of CVD is related to diet, physical activity, and body.

The patterns of food supplies and of food and nutrition that modify the risk of CVD are also well known. The governments of many developed and many developing countries have issued dietary and other recommendations designed to control the incidence of CVD. The basic agreed finding is that varied diets that are high in vegetables, fruits, and starchy staple foods (preferably in minimally processed form) and that are relatively low in energy density, fats, saturated fats, sugar, and salt, are most protective against CVD.

Such diets approximate those that have been traditional in many countries in Asia and Pacific SIDS, where public health problems have been food insecurity, undernutrition, and monotony of diets. However, when people have enough to eat and when diets are varied, diseases of undernutrition are not major public health problems.

Additionally, there is conclusive evidence that regular physical activity maintained throughout life, together with nutrient-dense diets, protects not only against obesity and therefore indirectly against CVD. This finding has very important implications for developing countries in Asia and the Pacific, where protective diets and lifestyles are not as established as they are in developed countries.

Programs and policies designed to control obesity and CVD in Asia and the Pacific should emphasize what is valuable in traditional and existing agriculture and food systems, food supplies, diets, and activity patterns. Inappropriate diets are a major determinant of the risk of cerebrovascular diseases including hyperten-sion and stroke.

Dietary recommendations for preventing these pathologies are the same as those for obesity and CVD except for an added focus on diets with less salt. There is also now a consensus that, in broad terms, the same diets and associated lifestyles that protect against obesity, diabetes, cerebrovascular diseases, and CVD, also protect against certain cancers, i.e., major cancers of epithelia as well as hormone-related cancers that become or remain epidemic as a consequence of demographic, nutrition transitions.

These cancers include those of the lung, breast, endometrium, colon, and rectum, and also cancers that may be associated with traditional diets, such as those of the mouth, throat, esophagus, and stomach. At 1995 levels, such a reduction would correspond to three to four million cases per year worldwide. Diets and physical activity that protect against cancer also protect against other chronic diseases, and have no deleterious effect on other diseases.

Current diet recommendations, following food science, emphasize food and dietary patterns more than individual macro- and microconstituents. Food-based dietary guidelines are now generally accepted. The diets that are most protective against chronic diseases, especially in sedentary populations, comprise mainly foods of plant origin.

These diets are varied and high in nutrients, but relatively low in energy. They include substantial amounts of legumes and other vegetables, fruit, and minimally processed grains and other starchystaples.

They are also relatively low in fat, especially saturated fat, and in sugar, salt, and alcohol. In general they contain only modest amounts of foods of animal origin. The World Cancer Research Fund (WCRF) emphasized the importance of year-round variety in diets, and also the value of small amounts of meat, fish, poultry, and dairy foods, especially when diets might otherwise be monotonous.

Epidemic, diet-related chronic diseases, entail important human and economic costs. The human costs have been quantified in terms of disability and death. To date, however, there are almost no estimates of the economic costs in developing countries, although a study is in process for the Pacific islands. There have also been studies for the United States, for example.

The five diet-related chronic diseases considered here are CVD (especially IHD), diabetes, hyperten-sion, stroke, and cancers. Among these, CVD, stroke and cancers are major causes of premature death. Hypertension and diabetes, themselves life-threatening diseases at late stages of pathology, also increase the risk of stroke and CVD.

For example, the link between overweight and hypertension, although well established, was not modeled. The effects of overweight on IHD directly were modeled. It is not valid to double count and to add the indirect effects of overweight, via hypertension, on IHD. The focus here is on diet and does not includethe additional effects of physical activity, except in so far as activity has indirect effects, via energy imbalance and overweight status.

However, physical activity is known to have direct effects on hypertension, diabetes, and CVD. Therefore, again, the estimates here are cautious. The effect of inappropriate diets on disease risk is multidimensional. There are potentially overlapping effects, e.g., LBW, via obesity, on CVD; LBW, via hypertension, on CVD; and LBW, via diabetes, on CVD. Therefore, care was taken, when estimating overall effects, not to double count such effects.

The separate effects of different pathways can be added only if the clinical studies, on which the RR estimates are based, also control for confounding effects. For example, in order to be able to add up the effects of LBW, via overweight and via hypertension, on CVD, it is necessary to control for current weight in the link between LBW and hypertension and in the link between hypertension and CVD.

There are enormous potential benefits from poli-cies and programs to control epidemic diet-related chronic diseases. Furthermore, the dietary and other determinants of important chronic diseases are well understood, and preventative lines of approach are already fairly well defined. Approaches that focus on the nutrition of the mother and child, from preconcep-tion to weaning, and thereafter in infants and children throughout preschool and school are strongly recom-mended.

There is limited experience in this area in Asia and in Pacific SIDS. Few large-scale programs and evaluations have been undertaken to date. Moreover, basic data on nutrition and epidemiologic transitions is lacking in most Asian countries and in Pacific SIDS. Without such information, intervention programs will be guesswork to some extent and their results will be hard to assess.

It is, however, encouraging that interventions designed to control other chronic diseases can be efficient and effective, for example, smoking control and low-cost drug therapies for hypertension reduction for stroke prevention. Diet-related programs, designed to control chronic diseases, can and should be highly cost-effective.

In the United States, for example, a government-backed campaign that reduced national fat consumption by between 1% to 3% of total calories, saved, over a 10-year period, US$4.1 to 12.7 billion in medical costs and lost productivity. Increased physical activity, as specified in other US government-backed campaigns could significantly reduce CVD in the United States.

In Asia and in Pacific SIDS, there have been few systematic attempts to use food and nutrition policy to prevent NCDs and to enhance adult health. The focus to date has been on food insecurity. Many programs have been successful, in countries as diverse as the PRC, Sri Lanka, and Thailand. Given a national com-mitment to address a health problem, a number of Asian countries and Pacific SIDS have the ability to make changes.

The PRC is one of the few countries in Asia, indeed in the world, that has addressed nutrition and public health issues in terms of food supply systems on a national level. In 1993, the Government of the PRC organized the National Commission for Food Reform and Development. The State Council issued in 1993 the first document that addressed future food produc-tion and marketing, in terms of its significance for nutritional well-being.

In the Republic of Korea, mass media campaigns, such as television programs, promote local foods, emphasiz-ing their higher quality and the need to support local farmers. In Thailand, maternal and child nutrition are promoted in the context of social marketing of condoms, to protect against sexually transmitted diseases (STD) in general, and HIV-AIDS in particular.

The most important causal agent in the decline of obesity in Brazil was probably the mass media cover-age. The first consistent and publicly directed mass intervention to control obesity in Brazil was launched in 1997, after the recorded decline. In the United States, the 'five-a-day' program has focused on large-scale education, along with intensive local efforts, to increase fruit and vegetable intake. This program is part of a new generation of proactive initiatives by the US National Institutes of Health.

Schools are an excellent setting for programs designed to protect or to improve good nutrition, together with regular physical activity. Singapore has been a leader in promoting experience and weight control in schools. In the early 1990s, Singapore recognized, as central health concerns, a marked reduction in physical fitness and increased obesity among schoolchildren.

Nutrition Security for HIV/AIDS

Livelihoods are being devastated and the food and nutrition security of millions of households seriously undermined. The specific role of food aid is examined, since inadequate access to food is one of the first signs of distress in an HIV/AIDS-impacted household. Over 36 million individuals are currently living with HIV/AIDS, 95 percent of whom are from developing countries. Assuming that each HIV/AIDS case directly influences the lives of four other individuals, a total of more than 150 million people are being affected by the disease.

Sub-Saharan Africa is the region most affected, where HIV/AIDS is now that areas leading cause of adult morbidity and mortality. Most, if not all, of the 25 million people in sub-Saharan Africa who are living with HIV/AIDS will have died by the year 2020, in addition to the 13.7 million Africans already claimed by the epidemic. HIV/AIDS is also spreading dramatically in Asia.

India is estimated to have 3 to 5 million HIV infections and, though national data are not reliable, some Chinese specialists estimate up to 10 million HIV infections in China. Asia will overtake sub-Saharan Africa in absolute numbers before 2010, and by 2020 Asia will be the HIV/AIDS epicentre.

The HIV/AIDS pandemic is transforming the landscape upon which development must take place in much of the developing world. Like other infectious diseases that become epidemic, HIV starts out as an idiosyncratic shock that turns into an aggregate shock. But it is different from other diseases or shocks for the following reasons:

— *It is incurable and fatal*: It kills the most productive members of society, thus increasing household dependency ratios, reducing household productivity and caring capacity, and impairing the inter-generational transfer of local knowledge and skills. The effect on the household may be permanent; certain premature death undermines the incentive to accumulate assets and the very survival of the household unit is threatened.

This bleak prognosis makes intervention efforts (prevention or mitigation) difficult. Most development interventions can offer some hope of some improvement in human welfare. Effective HIV prevention can offer only an absence of decline.

Effective HIV mitigation can offer only a temporary improvement in human welfare from an already HIV/AIDS-lowered level. Life-prolonging treatment is too expensive for most HIV-infected people, although there is significant scope for major cuts in the prices of drugs.

— *It is socially invisible*: The private nature and divergent cultural attitudes towards sex lead to silence, denial, stigma, and discrimination at many levels. This makes effective prevention and mitigation difficult to implement. HIV has a very long incubation period between infection and full-blown symptoms during which individuals are infective.

In the absence of routine HIV testing, infected individuals have less of an incentive to alter risky behavior and a long period over which to undertake those activities. Both invisibility and long duration increase chances of HIV transmission. Individuals who are unaware of their HIV status and their families cannot begin to alter livelihood strategies in response to the coming shock.

— *It has both rural and urban dimensions*: As with poverty, the death of one or more income-earners in rural households often forces survivors to migrate to seek work in cities. A death of an urban worker may force survivors to send children back to rural extended families to be cared for.

— *It affects both the rich and the poor,* though it is the poor who are most severely exposed and most severely impacted.

— *It affects both sexes but is not gender-neutral:* To the extent that women are marginalized and powerless, they are more at risk of being exposed to HIV. Women are also more likely to succumb rapidly to HIV/AIDS, as they are more biologically vulnerable.

— Finally, one of the most disturbing aspects of the pandemic is the fact that, as it intensifies with a parallel need for action, the actual capacity to act is decreasing.

Organizations that are located in areas that are experiencing a high HIV/AIDS prevalence, are characterized by high absenteeism, high turnover, a loss of institutional memory, and reduced innovation. As individuals in government and nongovernmental organizations continue to die, the capacity gap-between what is needed and what can be delivered is becoming an abyss.

HIV/AIDS and poverty (a large part of which relates to food insecurity) interact in a vicious circle. Poverty increases the exposure to, as well as the impact of HIV. It diminishes the perceived value of avoiding HIV, it increases the relative costs of both avoiding and treating the illness, and it exacerbates the impact of weakened immunological integrity as a result of a more hostile bacterial and viral environment.

Poverty also increases the radius of impact of HIV on family and friends (for the poor, informal coping mechanisms are more dependent on family and friends and less so on insurance companies and the state). In the reverse direction, HIV/AIDS also impoverishes. It increases poverty in the short to medium run by stripping assets of many kinds—human, social, financial, physical, natural, informational, and political.

Nevertheless, as with other aggregate shocks, the nonpoor are thought less able to avoid HIV infection and its impacts. While this might generate wider political support to confront AIDS, it undermines the ability of middle-income's taffed governments, private-sector firms and other formal organizations to mobilize human resources to combat it.

There is also a danger that public-sector health budgets will become more skewed towards the wealthier and the more vocal urban HIV/AIDS population to the detriment of the rural poor in general. Primary health care clinics may become increasingly poorly equipped. Waiting and travel times for the poor might also increase as a consequence, further stretching the demands on the remaining able-bodied labour.

Women are biologically, socio-economically, and socio-culturally more at risk of HIV infection than men. Biologically, the risk of becoming infected with HIV during unprotected vaginal intercourse is between two and four times higher for women than for men. Women are also more susceptible to other sexually transmitted diseases (STDs) and less likely to seek treatment. If untreated, STDs may multiply the risk of HIV transmission by 300-400 percent.

Such biological susceptibility further threatens reproductive health status; pregnancy and child-bearing now involve considerably greater risks not only to the women but to their future offspring, while STDs can be potentially life-threatening. HIV/AIDS also exacerbates social, economic, and cultural inequalities that define women's status in society.

Women are often more susceptible to HIV infection and more vulnerable to AIDS impacts than are men for the following reasons: the predominant culture of silence and passivity regarding sex stigmatizes women who try to access STD treatment services; the norm of virginity restricts adolescent girls' access to information about sex, and the risk of sexual coercion; economic vulnerability increases the chance of the exchange of sex for food, money, etc.; male power is often manifested in sexual violence; susceptibility to HIV infection is increased through sexual practices, including genital cutting, dry sex, and ritual cleansing; and finally women are discriminated against with regard to inheritance rights.

Other important changes in gender asymmetries relate to less personal but nonetheless crucial assets. Premature adult male death may deprive the female of the necessary time to build up a set of extrafamily levers, such as access to community land, to community groups, and to microfinance groups—that can be used to exert power within the family.

If property and user rights for a whole range of assets are not clearly and equitably defined or are not enforced, women are likely to become less able to shape their own destinies. This lessening of women's relative power will tend to be reinforced via the subsequent diminished ability to control decisions relating to their own needs and those of their children in terms of health care, food intake, and work time.

HIV/AIDS may have on households and communities with regard to their food and nutrition security, in the context of their livelihoods, particularly with regard to rural populations dependent on agriculture. There are three points to be made at the outset. First, impacts are often revealed through the responses, or "coping strategies" made by households and communities.

The term coping may not always be accurate, simply because many responses are those of distressed households that are not coping. Coping implies a reversible management strategy. It also somehow suggests that the adoption of such strategies is not too costly. The reality is that many households are forced to make distress sales or change livelihood strategies in ways that are irreversible.

The price of such short term coping may be long-term deprivation or even destitution. Second, it is important to differentiate susceptibility to HIV infection—that is, the likelihood of becoming infected with the virus—from the vulnerability to the different types of impacts, once infection has taken place.

Third, it is important to recognize that different stages of the HIV/AIDS epidemic will have different indicators, different impacts and different responses. There are also differences between countries or sub-national regions with regard to the gradient and the peak prevalence of the HIV/AIDS epidemic, relating in part to the velocity of transmission, which itself is related to behaviours and the pathogenicity of the particular HIV strain.

HIV/AIDS has significant impacts on nutrition at the level of the individual, household and community. Malnutrition in turn increases both the susceptibility to

HIV infection and the vulnerability to its various impacts. At an individual level, HIV infection essentially accelerates the vicious circle of inadequate dietary intake and disease that leads to malnutrition, while malnutrition increases the risk of HIV transmission from mothers to babies and the progression of HIV infection.

HIV-infected individuals have higher nutritional requirements than normal, particularly with regard to protein, and energy. They are also more likely to suffer a loss of appetite, even anorexia, thus reducing dietary intake at the very time when requirements are higher. Moreover, such interactions are thrown into starker contrast for the poor, who are more likely to be malnourished prior to becoming infected.

Some study shows that the onset of the disease and even death might be delayed in well-nourished HIV-positive individuals, and diets rich in protein, energy and micronutrients help in building resistance to opportunistic infections in AIDS patients. Mother-to-child transmission (MTCT, or vertical transmission) of HIV is a major nutritional issue. MTCT may occur during pregnancy, at birth, or via breastfeeding.

In a recent study, exclusive breastfeeding has been seen to confer a significantly lower risk of HIV transmission than partial breastfeeding. Observational data have shown that three-month-old infants of HIV-positive women who were breast-fed exclusively have the same risk of contracting HIV as infants who were never breastfed. In contrast, infants who were partially breastfed had a significantly higher risk.

A follow-up prospective study of 551 HIV-infected pregnant women in South Africa has shown that infants exclusively breastfed for 3 months or more had nc excess risk of HIV infection over 6 months than those never breastfed. Several biological mechanisms could explain why exclusive breastfeeding might be protective compared with partial breastfeeding.

These include reduced exposure of the infant to bacterial contaminants and food antigens, thus reducing immune activation, increased integrity of the intestinal wall, development of microflora that limit adhesion and growth of pathogenic organisms and reduced risk of sub-clinical mastitis, which occurs during breast engorgement.

Infants of mothers who have an adequate vitamin A status might have a reduced risk of vertical transmission. In many poor households, even those unaffected by the pandemic, child care may be compromised in the short term to ensure food security in the long term. Any adverse impacts on the quality or quantity of child care of such decisions are likely to be exacerbated by shocks such as HIV/AIDS, which may drastically reduce household caring capacity.

A livelihood represents the interaction between assets and transforming processes and structures that generate a means of living, all conditioned by the context that individuals find themselves in. Agriculture is the main livelihood of most rural populations in sub-Saharan Africa.

Assets are important to livelihoods only if they can be accessed and have an ability to support livelihoods when accessed. The rules governing access and value can be broadly labelled as institutions. Access to assets and the value of the assets tend to be determined by cultural norms and values and by formal laws, policies, and organizations.

Most obviously HIV/AIDS attacks human capital. Infected individuals eventually die prematurely. Living but infected individuals are rendered less productive once AIDS emerges, due to a series of opportunistic infections, of which tuberculosis is the most frequent. A scale of the impact on mortality and morbidity is given by numbers on disability-adjusted life years (or DALYs).

At a global level, HIV/AIDS was 28th in terms of causes of DALYs in 1990, and is projected to be 10th in 2020. In sub-Saharan Africa HIV/AIDS is projected to be the 3rd leading cause of DALYs in 2020 (from 7th in 1990) and for India HIV/AIDS is also projected to be the 3rd leading cause in 2020. These figures, dramatic as they are, do not capture the full impact of HIV on labour in terms of livelihood generation, because the labour of healthy individuals is diverted into other crucial activities such as caring for those infected and attending the funerals of those who have died. The measured impact of these changes in demographic profile on household dependency ratios is inconclusive.

This may reflect the household or community's response to the shock in terms of importing prime-age labour and exporting children via family or informal nonfamily networks. These labour movements may entail costs to the children in terms of the quality of care provision and may exacerbate the spread of HIV/AIDS if the imported labour comes from heavily infected areas.

These are areas for further research. With regard to agriculture, obviously farming systems that are less dependent on labour will be better able to respond to these losses. Studies have investigated the specific characteristics associated with vulnerability and resilience of farming systems in the face of loss of labour.

Replacementls labour can be found either via social networks or via the labour market. Otherwise less labour-intensive, livelihood-sustaining ways of farming land have to be developed. Both types of labour replacement strategy run the risk of new HIV infection. Labour market help might not be affordable for families affected by HIV. Moreover, the low labour intensity strategy is by no means guaranteed to be more livelihood sustaining than the system it replaces.

Other impacts on land and land use include the cultivation of crops that are less labour intensive, but less nutritious (e.g. some tubers) and the fallowing of land. If the family can afford not to use the land, this will improve its quality for future cultivation. On the other hand, non-use of land may make the family vulnerable to loss of land rights.

As highlighted by those with traditionally weaker land rights (e.g. some women and orphans) greater clarity and equity with respect to local property rights is particularly important. Additionally, it is important to take into account the current diversity of livelihoods that farmers exhibit and the potential they have to diversify further into nonfarm activities that are less labour-dependent.

The impacts of HIV/AIDS on the commercial agricultural sector are less well understood. If the commercial sector is dependent on migrant labour it is susceptible to HIV/AIDS, more so if the labourer is resident without his or her family. Social networks will also tend to be weaker for labourers in the commercial sector.

However, the commercial sector can be a force for good in the sense that it can provide information and training for prevention, and it might provide opportunities for AIDS orphans to learn some essential agricultural skills. But human capital is about much more than manual labour. It is also about knowledge.

The striking-down of adults in their prime by HIV/AIDS severely reduces the ability of individuals to transfer knowledge both within their generation and from their generation to the next. Both verbal and role model mechanisms are interrupted by HIV/AIDS. New generations are less able to draw on the body of knowledge that dies along with their parents and they are deprived of learning by doing under the guidance of someone more experienced.

The ability to acquire and use information is also impaired by HIV/AIDS as younger generations are pulled out of school to bolster the family's ability to provide care to the ill and to maintain its current livelihood, or develop new ones. This is an example of an ultimately destructive coping strategy. Tomorrow's livelihoods are being sacrificed in order to hang on to today's.

Financial capital is damaged by HIV/AIDS in a number of ways. Because drug, burial and related transport expenses become major items in budgets, families need to find ways to maintain current consumption levels. In terms of financial capital services (credit, savings, and insurance) poor families either have to sell stores of value (e.g. jewellery and livestock), assets (e.g. equipment or tools), borrow funds in a sustainable manner, or—which seems most unlikely—have access to some kind of insurance, health, or otherwise.

The poor invariably are reliant on informal credit at high interest rates or on group-based microfinance products. Unfortunately both of these types of services tend to be spatially concentrated and hence vulnerable to aggregate shocks. Even when the epidemic is in its early stages, the infected family is less able to avoid default and hence is less attractive to group-based liability schemes.

Social capital—or the strength of associational life, trust, and norms of reciprocity—may be undermined by HIV in several ways. First, social reproduction in terms of the role-modeling of norms of trust and good citizenship is impaired. Future generations not only do not witness farming practices they also do not experience the informal exchanges of knowledge, tools, and animal draught labour that are often embodied in such livelihood activities.

Second, the incentives for coordinated group action may be diminished as a result of the heavy discounting of the future benefits of such action. This has a particularly negative consequence for natural resource management practices that are dependent on collective action such as integrated pest management, social forestry, and watershed development.

Third, the formal institutions that also contribute to social capital formation, such as church groups, sports clubs, and professional associations are likely to be weakened as members die.

Fourth, social networks tend to be spatially concentrated. The networks that are more heterogeneous should have a greater carrying capacity. However, members who are highly mobile or live in urban areas will make a network more susceptible to HIV/AIDS.

Fifth, social capital may be weakened through an increased exclusiveness of network membership. The stigma attached to HIV/AIDS is not conducive to the establishment of crosscutting ties across the different strands of social capital. HIV/AIDS might lead to the generation of a type of social capital formation that is exclusive.

The basic infrastructure and productive equipment that are relied upon for the pursuit of livelihoods also comes under threat as a result of HIV/AIDS. The possible sale of productive equipment or mortgaging of land in response to large health and funeral expenses has been noted as has the possible neglect of health infrastructure for the poor. As time becomes an ever-scarcer commodity in HIV/AIDS areas, access to water and energy sources must be improved, particularly given the fact that such access relates to activities that are socially determined to be the responsibility of women, who most often care for their family members, irrespective of their HIV/AIDS status.

HIV/AIDS might undermine the ability of communities and user groups to pool risk and act collectively to sustainably manage common property including rangeland, cropland, and river basins. Clear and equitable delineation of property and land rights becomes more important as individuals leave their dwellings to search for alternative livelihoods, or to help out friends and families outside their community.

A number of private-sector responses have deliberately reduced the abilities of households with infected members to mitigate the effects of HIV/AIDS. Examples include the capping of medical benefits for HIV-infected employees, reductions in funeral leave, and reductions in company contributions to funeral expenses—all examples from South Africa.

More difficult to detect, but perhaps less difficult to amend are the interventions or policies that inadvertently increase the risk of HIV infection or impair the ability of households and communities to mitigate the effects of AIDS. Actions that reinforce gender imbalances in power or those that displace individuals without adequate HIV monitoring and prevention efforts would fall into this category.

The painfully slow recognition that HIV/AIDS is a major global developmental crisis, and not just an isolated health problem, has finally dawned. Yet strategies, where they exist, tend not to go beyond prevention, and they remain in the domain of the health sector. Very little is happening in mitigation, and very little in reviewing food and nutrition security policies and programmes through an HIV lens.

Many government/public civil servants who work in agriculture or rural development do not understand the link between HIV and food security. Programming is very ad hoc, with different groups intervening in different ways. Effective advocacy is vital to mainstreaming HIV/AIDS.

Advocacy strategies that consider the role of values, attitudes, and interests as well as information per se, undertaken by skilled policy entrepreneurs, ideally backed up by nationally prominent champions, need to be developed. Conventionally the distinction is made between prevention aimed at reducing HIV infection through behavioural change and mitigation aimed at reducing the severity of HIV/AIDS impacts on households, communities, and other institutions.

Care interventions focus on those infected and affected, particularly the children of HIV-infected parents, orphans, widows, etc. The focus on programming for HIV/AIDS has been largely on prevention, with care secondary and, until recently, mitigation relatively neglected. This needs to change.

It is increasingly obvious that not only are all these strategies vital in the long run, but should be integrated as far as possible. This is because the distinctions are actually quite blurred in reality, and the strategies are complementary in their implementation and effects. Successful mitigation efforts, for example, can be preventive.

To the extent that poverty increases HIV/AIDS susceptibility and vulnerability, mitigation that succeeds in alleviating or preventing poverty can reduce HIV exposure and future impacts. Interventions thus need to be designed and assessed not only in terms of their ability to mitigate the current impacts of HIV/AIDS, but also in terms of their ability to reduce susceptibility to future infection and vulnerability to various types of impact.

Care too is inextricably linked with mitigation; care clearly mitigates individual- level impacts, and other forms of mitigation may improve the capacity to care within households and communities. Irrespective of the discovery of an AIDS vaccine, prevention needs to focus on shutting down the engine of growth of the infection, namely by minimizing the risky behaviours of individuals who are most likely to catch and spread the disease.

But changing the behavior of individuals is about more than access to information and services, and cajoling and exhorting. It is also about the incentives—cultural, social, and economic—that lead individuals to a highly risky course of action as opposed to a less risky one. The consensus view now recognizes the importance of poverty as a factor in the implicit cost-benefit calculations made by those contemplating such risky behaviours (e.g. commercial sex).

If we can identify certain types of livelihoods as being more likely to result in HIV infection, and we can begin to understand the constraints to various livelihood options, then policy can begin to provide incentives for individuals to switch to less risky and more sustainable livelihood choices. Mitigation is about creating environments that support those who are affected by but not infected with HIV/AIDS, namely families, households, and communities.

As with HIV prevention, some livelihood strategies are better than others in supporting HIV/AIDS mitigation. As we begin to understand better the social and economic impacts of HIV/AIDS, the features of livelihoods that allow more effective mitigation can be identified. Ideally, mitigation for food and nutrition security would be integrated into a full package of interventions that include awareness-raising, biomedical, psycho-social counselling, testing, care and mitigation.

While this type of package addresses many issues beyond the food security arena, it nevertheless has significant potential for improving food and nutrition security in an HIV/AIDS-impacted household. When, specifically, when do governments, NGOs, communities, and development agencies need to:

(i) improve the performance of existing efforts;

(ii) view HIV-prevention and mitigation interventions through a poverty lens and modify appropriately;

(iii) view agriculture, anti-poverty, and nutrition interventions through an HIV lens and modify appropriately; or

(iv) design completely new interventions to address HIV/AIDS.

One problem here is that food security programming per se is very weak in many countries. Programming for food and nutrition security rather than just agricultural production is difficult due to the multi-sectoral nature of the issues. Linking it with HIV/AIDS complicates the matter even more. This is coupled with the fact that many countries do not include extensive food security policies and programmes in their overall poverty reduction strategy, which marginalizes the issue further.

For those who are poor, HIV/AIDS is just one more event/shock that affects their ability to get ahead and improve their lives. Programming for mitigation needs to look very closely at what all of the other constraints are that impact food security for HIV/AIDS-affected households.

It is often these other constraints that will affect the success of the intervention, and how HIV/AIDS impacts different households and different members of a household. Because of the complexity of these interactions, it can be difficult to identify mitigation activities that are sustainable, address food and nutrition insecurity and contribute to the prevention of HIV infection.

There is a need to recognize the different stages of the disease in different parts of a country. In some areas, the biggest issue is prevention; in others, where there has already been a clear impact on households' ability to ensure their food security, mitigation becomes increasingly important. Different interventions will also be required for different groups.

The impact of HIV/AIDS on food security of a pastoralist group is likely to be different from that on an agriculturalist community. Particularly susceptible and vulnerable are communities affected by complex emergencies, which are usually epicentres for the transmission of the disease. This is because the lethal mix of population displacement, rape, occupying troups, women in desperate circumstances, unsafe blood supplies, drug abuse, unsafe sexual practices and insufficient control activities make HIV transmission highly likely.

There is no need to identify HIV-infected individuals or households. To avoid the stigma attached to HIV, community-based targeting is usually the most appropriate option. If the programme is designed to identify the poorest for safety net schemes or food aid development projects using known community structures appears to be the best way to target. Programmes that target very poor food-insecure households that have been impacted not by HIV but by other factors should not be considered an inclusion error.

Most HIV/AIDS programmes are very small scale in nature, and have been referred to as expensive boutiques available only to a small percentage of the affected population. For example, in Kagera, Tanzania, a highly studied region, only two of five districts are covered by HIV/AIDS services (in this case, preventive), and within these districts, a mere 5 percent of the population has access to services.

Multisectoral top-down coordination of integrated rural development programmes failed in the 1970s and 1980s, and such mistakes should not be repeated. Nonetheless there remains a need for some top-down support of bottom-up processes in the areas of setting of policies and programme parameters, cofinancing programmes, facilitation and training, monitoring, and evaluation.

Effective interventions are rooted in a community response and depend heavily on the participation of local health authorities, community representatives and people living with HIV/AIDS. The greater involvement of people living with HIV/AIDS in all aspects of related programming can be a powerful and influential factor in effective prevention, mitigation and care interventions. The best partner organizations working on HIV/AIDS are community based.

Many of the organizations aiding and supporting people living with HIV/AIDS and their families have religious affiliations. Food security programmes need to work to maximize the inputs of such organizations, while recognizing the possible constraints and gaps left by their involvement. For example, in many areas, religious groups are active in home-based care, but do not promote the use of condoms for HIV prevention.

A monitoring system that is relatively simple but able to track the changing HIV/AIDS situation and its impacts on food and nutrition security, with the required accuracy and reliability to guide timely ameliorative action remains elusive. This is likely to be due both to a weak demand for such information and a weak ability to supply it.

The stigma, denial and silence attached to HIV/AIDS makes the task more difficult than, for example, developing early warning drought indicators. Moreover, the capacity to generate such information is undermined by HIV/AIDS. A balance has to be found between indicators that can be compared across communities and administrative units, and a community-driven process that can generate more context-specific indicators.

Programming in emergencies should focus on controlling HIV/AIDS in the affected population and preventing further spread of the disease. This can be done through the provision of free condoms, provision of information, prevention of HIV transmission through blood transfusions and adherence to universal precautions for all health staff. There are several different approaches to designing and implementing appropriate nutrition-relevant actions aimed at preventing and/or mitigating HIV/AIDS impacts.

A first distinction needs to be made with regard to the objective. For individual persons living with HIV/AIDS (PLWHA), nutritional care and support is critically important in preventing or forestalling nutritional depletion. Relevant specific objectives might include to improve quantity and quality of diet, to build or replenish body stores of micronutrients, to prevent or stabilize weight loss, to preserve (and gain) muscle mass, to prevent diarrhea and other digestive discomforts associated with fat malabsorption, to speed recuperation from HIV-related infections, and to prepare for and manage AIDS-related symptoms that affect food consumption and dietary intake.

Nutritional support has the potential of significantly prolonging the life of individuals for their own benefit and the benefit of those who are dependent on them for care (e.g., young children), thus, in a sense, postponing mitigation and reducing vulnerability to impacts. Such interventions are likely to have the greatest overall impact early in the course of disease by prolonging the period of relative health with asymptomatic infection—the period before metabolic abnormalities are driving the nutritional course of infection, i.e., before AIDS.

Nutrition interventions may also be targeted to communities with the objective of preventing and/or mitigating impacts through reducing the interactions of HIV/AIDS with malnutrition, either upstream or downstream of HIV infection. Any nutrition intervention should take into account the three main preconditions of good nutrition (food security, health and environment services, and care).

For PLWHA, this means that appropriate treatment of opportunistic infections, stress management, physical exercise, and emotional, psychological, and spiritual counseling and support, for example, are all relevant, along with conventional approaches such as home-delivered, ready-to-eat foods for homebound AIDS patients who are unable to prepare their own meals.

Community-level targeting to communities that are found to be significantly affected by HIV/AIDS (using whatever proxy indicators are relevant) is likely to be far more feasible and effective than targeting to individuals or households. A second-stage targeting might be employed with regard to stages in the life cycle that are particularly susceptible and vulnerable (e.g., adolescent girls, pregnant women, and young children).

As also with all nutrition programming, it is important that HIV/AIDS-related programming is not just community based, but also community driven. Process is thus a major consideration. At the community level the key is to create space and develop capacity for an iterative process of assessment, analysis and action. It is also important to build partnerships and foster convergence of relevant programmes.

As a multifaceted subject requiring action from several sectors, nutrition is, and always has been, vulnerable to bureaucratic inertia deriving from compartmentalized organizational structures that offer few incentives for integration or convergence. Magic bullets have generally been the preferred way to go—witness the prominence attached to vitamin A capsule distribution and salt iodization during the 1990s.

There is nothing intrinsically wrong with magic bullets, unless they end up crowding out other important and necessary longer-term holistic approaches to nutrition. This has certainly happened, as borne out by the relative stagnation of child anthropometric outcomes when compared with micronutrient indicators.

While micronutrient supplementation (particularly vitamin A) will have a role in nutritional support to AIDS-affected communities, this mistake should especially not be repeated in the case of HIV/AIDS communities—not least given the significantly raised energy and protein requirements of PLWHA, which cannot be met by pills. The role of food aid in HIV/AIDS mitigation and care has just begun to be explored by field-based organizations.

Food is often cited by poor HIV-impacted families as their greatest need. The biggest challenge for food-assisted interventions is to provide food to meet consumption and/or nutritional needs but also to programme interventions so that family members and communities are left with a means of improving their food and nutrition security after the food assistance stops.

As with any non-emergency food aid intervention, food should be provided only as part of a larger package of assistance. The appropriate package for HIV/AIDS beneficiaries will depend on country- and community-specific conditions. Information, education and awareness (i.e. prevention) are an essential component of both care and mitigation activities.

Combining food with either training or income-generating activities (IGA) appears to be a way both to assist households in dealing with reduced access to food and to build self-sufficiency in those same households struggling with either a chronically ill adult or the death of a family member.

Close consultation with affected communities on how to target and deliver food assistance needs to be an integral part of the project. Considerations concerning the most appropriate types of food need to be discussed with participants, particularly when family members include chronically ill individuals and infants. Appropriateness includes not only issues of taste and nutrition but also preparation, including cooking.

For example, decreased family labour can have an impact on the supply of household energy, such as firewood. Communities often have their own means of identifying the poorest households and selecting those who need food. In order to avoid the stigma, households that are poor and food insecure but that have not been visibly impacted by HIV/AIDS should still be included in the beneficiary group, if selected by the community.

Food-assisted projects present certain challenges. They can, for many reasons, be more complicated for implementing organizations than other types of development projects. Most of the community-based HIV/AIDS organizations, which would assist in the implementation of food aid projects, are very small and operate on minimal funds. They frequently lack the expertise and full capacity to undertake expanded activities and the experience in transporting, storing, handling and distributing food.

Organizations dealing in food-assisted projects need to recognize this capacity gap and plan for capacity-building and training in these areas. Furthermore, many of these organizations have never used food in their programming. Education concerning the role food should play in either a care or mitigation intervention is essential.

Where to concentrate HIV/AIDS food-assisted programmes and projects can also present challenges. Food aid is generally targeted to the geographic areas of a country that are the most food insecure, and then, within those areas, to those communities/families that cannot meet their food needs. In many countries these are not the areas that have the highest prevalence of HIV/AIDS.

Food-insecure areas are often more remote, have low production potential and weak market structures. Areas with high infection rates are often located in or around urban or semi-urban areas, or areas where markets and transportation networks function relatively well and where commercial activities, including agricultural trade, take place.

In order to target food aid effectively in areas considered food secure, food-assisted intervention need to be able to locate and identify those families and communities that have been impacted by AIDS and that are having difficulty meeting household food needs. If local institutions, NGOs, or community-based organizations working with HIV/AIDS-affected populations are not present, then it will be extremely difficult to identify families and populations for whom food aid will make a difference.

Furthermore, food-assisted programmes dealing with HIV/AIDS need to broaden their reach in terms of prevention activities. Many organizations that deal with food aid also transport it within countries. This is done either with their own trucks or through contracting local transportation companies. Because long-haul drivers are a known vector for the spread of HIV, it is important to include this group in education and awareness campaigns and training, including condom distribution.

Organizations that programme food aid should consider targeting transportation personnel, particularly agencies that deal in emergencies where the quantities of food and hence the number of truckers needed are greatly increased. For example, school feeding in particular has potential as a means of encouraging the school attendance of orphans, and to prevent school drop-out.

By providing take-home rations for families fostering orphans as part of a regular school feeding programme, families are encouraged to continue caring for children whose parents have died and orphans are encouraged to attend school. Experience shows that while foster families will continue to send their own children to school when times get difficult, foster children are often pulled out of school. Although food can and should be distributed to and through institutions, caution must be exercised to avoid undermining household and community care strategies.

But perhaps the most profound challenge to the agriculture sector in countries threatened by HIV/AIDS is the need to develop agricultural and natural resource management systems that are more labour-extensive and use less purchased inputs but that support sustainable livelihoods. In the absence of new technology and techniques, farmers are switching to feasible low-input, low-output farming that is preferable to infeasible labour-intensive, higher-input farming.

Yet, in so doing, they run the risk of adopting an ultimately destructive coping strategy. If the loss in agricultural productivity from pre-epidemic levels is sufficiently large, farm and nonfarm incomes will slowly cycle downwards. The move to low-input, low-output farming buys some time but is unlikely to be a sustainable solution.

The challenge for the agricultural community and specifically for the agricultural research community is to develop farming practices that adapt to the reality of HIV/AIDS-affected environments and yet maintain productivity levels. For this to happen, surviving farmers should be ever more closely involved in planning and implementation of supporting research. One simple example of a technological adaptation to an HIV/AIDS environment is the development of lighter ploughs for use by women and youth.

Information losses are also crucial in terms of the role traders play in bridging the gap between farm and market. Recent research has emphasized the important role played by trader-farmer networks of information and social relations that embody reciprocity based on trust. This is one of the forms of social capital that HIV/AIDS is thought to undermine. Mobile traders are thought likely to be relatively susceptible to HIV/AIDS, and given the already thin nature of agricultural markets in many parts of sub-Saharan Africa, the consequences are likely to be serious.

Agriculture does not take place in a vacuum. Successful efforts to strengthen the institutions that support farming in the face of the HIV/AIDS onslaught are difficult to find. An important first step is to improve the access to HIV prevention information and technology for members of that institution. Recent experiences from some of the most badly affected countries have demonstrated the ability of an important rural institution, microfinance, to innovate and develop products that better meet the needs of the emerging clientele—especially as in Uganda where national leadership has openly confronted HIV/AIDS.

The roles of microfinance institutions and the NGO community that helps animate them will be crucial in the prevention and mitigation of HIV/AIDS in the new HIV/AIDS battlegrounds of South and Southeast Asia, where so much microfinance innovation has taken place in general. If such types of innovation are to occur at the intersection between community and institutions that are accountable to them, donors will need to be more creative in the programming of resources.

Bibliography

Adamson A. J et al., "The contribution of foods from outside the home to the nutrient intake of young adolescents", *Journal of Human Nutrition Dietetics* 9:55-68, 1996.

Ahrens E. H., "Obesity and coronary heart disease: new dimensions", Arteriosclerosis 4: 177–9, 1984.

Baghurst P, Baghurst K, Record S., "Dietary fibre, non-starch polysaccharides and resistant starch a review", *Food Australia 48* (3 suppl): S3–35, 1996.

Ballin A, Berar M, Rubinstein E, et al., "Iron state in female adolescence", *American Journal of Dis Child* 146: 803–5, 1992.

Bauman A, Bellow B, Booth M., "Towards Best Practice for the Promotion of Physical Activity in the Areas of NSW", *National Centre for Health Promotion, Centre for Disease Prevention and Health Promotion,* NSW Health: Australia,1996.

Bigler-Doughten S, Jenkins R.M., "Adolescent snacks: nutrient density and nutritional contribution to total intake", *Journal of American Dietetics Association 87*: 1678–9, 1987.

Brady M.C., "Addition of nutrients: current practice in the UK", *British Food Journal* 98(9): 12–9, 1996.

Brinsdon S, George J, Paulin J.A., "Survey of the Nutrient Intakes of a Sample of Form One Children", *A report for the Personal and Public Health Policy Section*, Wellington: Health

Research Services, Department of Health, 1992.

Browne M.E., "The adequacy of vegetarian diets for preschool children, *Thesis*. Dunedin: Department of Human Nutrition, University of Otago, 1991.

Barnett, T. and M. Halswimmer, "The impact of HIV/AIDS on farming systems in Eastern Africa", *Food and Agriculture Organization of the United Nations*, Rome, 1995.

Barnett, T., and Rugalema, G., "HIV/AIDS and Food Security", In: Flores, R. and Gillespie, S. (eds) *Health and Nutrition: Emerging and Reemerging Issues in Developing Countries*, 2020 Focus 5, IFPRI Washington DC, 2001.

Crawley H.F, While D., "Parental smoking and the nutrient intake and food choice of British teenagers aged 16-17 years", *Journal of Epidemiology and Community Health* 50(3): 306–12, 1996.

Czeizel A.E, Dudas I., "Prevention of the first occurrence of neural-tube defects by periconceptional vitamin supplementation", *New England Journal of Medicine* 327: 1832–5, 1992.

Davies D, Apley J, Fill G, et al., "Diet and retarded growth", *British Medical Journal* 1: 539–42, 1978.

Davis C, Fox J, Cowles M, et al., "The functional role of exercise in the development of weight and diet concerns in women", *Journal of Psychosomatic Research* 34(5): 563–74, 1990.

Dietz W, Gordon J., "Obesity in infants, children and adolescents in the United States", II., Causality, *Nutrition Research* 1: 193–208, 1981.

Epstein L. H., "Family based behavioural intervention for obese children", *International Journal of Obesity Related Metabolic Disorders 20* (1 suppl): S14–21, 1996.

Index

CHANGING TRENDS IN HEALTH AND NUTRITION

CHANGING TRENDS IN HEALTH AND NUTRITION

(In 4 Volumes)

Health and Nutrition

(Volume 2)

SUJATA K. DASS

ISHA BOOKS

DELHI—110 033

Changing Trends in Health and Nutrition
(Health)

Rs. 3200 (Set in 4 vols.)
Rs. 800 (Each volume)

ISBN: 81-8205-040-5 (Set)
ISBN: 81-8205-041-3 (Vol. 2)

Published in 2004 in India by
Isha Books, D-43, Prithviraj Road
Adarsh Nagar, Delhi-110 033

Lasertypesetting by: Varsha Graphics, Delhi
Printed at: Chawla Offset Press, Delhi

Contents

Preface

India's health system is at a crossroads. Since independence, there have been significant changes in health conditions and major transformations in knowledge and technology. Today, new health threats are stretching the capacity of the health system to respond. An estimated 3.5 million Indians are living with HIV, and the virus has now spread beyond highly susceptible groups to the general population in some states, threatening to erase much of the social, economic, and health gains since independence. Building robust health systems is a critical part of the response to this and future health threats.

India's health transition is characterized by shifting demographics, altered health behaviours, and changes in disease patterns, with more degenerative and man-made diseases and more polarization of health conditions. A high proportion of the population continues to suffer and die from preventable infections, pregnancy and childbirth-related complications and under nutrition—the 'unfinished agenda' of the health transition. There are also large disparities across India, which places the bulk of the burden of these conditions on the poor, women, and scheduled castes and tribes. The poorest 20 percent of Indians have more than double the mortality rates, malnutrition, and fertility of the richest quintile.

Despite all this, the public remains badly informed about much of the health system. It knows little about whether health services are appropriate, who is benefiting from them, whether quality is sufficient, or whether people are getting good value from public and private spending on health. There are major problems with equity, quality, and accountability in both the public and private health sectors. The time has come to reassess how the Indian health system should function, and retool it for the new millennium.

Improvement in the health status of the population has been one of the major thrust areas in social development programmes of India. This was to be achieved through improving the access to health services with special focus on under-developed and under-privileged sections of the society.

The present book provides a detailed and valuable information about the problems, challenges and development in the India health sector. It proposes that health sector reform is needed, and outlines some broad principles for reform, which should be led by government.

Editor

1

The Indian Health System

Improvement in the health status of the population has been one of the major thrust areas in social development programmes of India. This was to be achieved through improving the access to health services with special focus on under-developed and under-privileged sections of the society. Let us look at some of the important indicators of health status to assess whether this very crucial parameter has shown any signs of improvement. Two basic indicators used in analysing the health status are infant mortality rate and life expectancy at birth.

Infant Mortality Rate

The infant mortality rate (IMR), measured in terms of death per thousand of children below 6 years, is considered to be a sensitive indicator of not only the health status of the population but also the level of human development in the context of education, economic conditions, nutrition etc. Poverty, malnutrition, a decline in breast- feeding, and inadequacy or lack of sanitation are all associated with high infant mortality. High infant mortality and high fertility are related concepts. There is evidence that in the short run infant mortality reduces overall population growth, other things remaining constant. However, the indirect and long run effect of reduced mortality is probably to reduce fertility by more than a compensating amount -as, with greater certainty about child survival, parents reduce "insurance births" and shift to child quality investments. Almost all the States in India have registered declining infant mortality rates over the period 1971 to 1998, yet some States have done better than the others, as may be seen in Table 1.

In 1981, Madhya Pradesh had the highest IMR at 150 followed by Uttar Pradesh at 130. Haryana, Orissa and Arunachal Pradesh also recorded high IMRs. Manipur recorded the lowest IMR at 32. By 1991, the IMR had fallen for almost all the States. But the fall in IMR for males was much higher than for females unlike in 1981, when female IMR was lower. The fall was faster between 1991 and 1998. IMR for all India for 1998 was 71. States with relatively high IMR today are Orissa, Madhya Pradesh, Uttar Pradesh and Rajasthan. The north eastern States of Mizoram at 23 and Manipur at 25 recorded the lowest IMRs amongst all States. There is cause for concern over the higher IMR for females than males in some of the States like Punjab, Uttar Pradesh, Haryana and Bihar, as the status of the female child is considered to be low in these States.

Life Expectancy at Birth

Life expectancy at birth or longevity is an overall indicator of the economic and social well being of the

Table 1 State-wise Infant Mortality Rate

Sl	States/Union	1961			1981			2001
No	Territorries	Male	Female	Person	Male	Female	Person	Person
1	Kerala	55	48	52	45	41	42	16
2	Pondicherry	77	68	73	32	35	34	21
3	Mizoram	73	65	69	51	56	53	23
4	Manipur	31	33	32	29	27	28	25
5	Andaman & Nicobar Islands	78	66	77	71	61	69	30
6	Lakshadweep	124	88	118	100	78	91	30
7	Chandigarh	53	53	53	50	47	48	32
8	Goa	60	56	57	56	48	51	36
9	Arunachal Pradesh	141	111	126	111	103	91	44
10	Jammu & Kashmir	78	78	78	NA	NA	NA	45
11	Maharashtra	96	89	92	72	76	74	49
12	Tripura	106	116	111	81	84	82	49
13	Delhi	66	70	67	55	51	54	51
14	Meghalaya	81	76	79	79	82	80	52
15	Sikkim	105	87	96	58	62	60	52
16	Tamil Nadu	89	82	86	55	51	54	53
17	West Bengal	103	57	95	75	51	62	53
18	Punjab	74	79	77	81	53	74	54

19	Karnataka	87	74	81	74	72	74	58
20	Dadra & Nagar Haveli	102	93	98	84	73	81	61
21	Gujarat	81	84	84	74	82	78	64
22	Himachal Pradesh	101	89	92	84	81	82	64
23	Andhra Pradesh	100	82	91	67	51	55	66
24	Bihar	95	94	94	62	89	75	67
25	Haryana	87	119	94	57	54	52	69
26	**All India**	**122**	**108**	**115**	**74**	**79**	**77**	**71**
27	Assam	NA	NA	NA	96	87	92	78
28	Rajasthan	114	114	114	94	79	87	83
29	Uttar Pradesh	131	128	130	98	104	99	85
30	Madhya Pradesh	158	140	150	131	136	133	97
31	Orissa	119	111	115	129	111	125	98
32	Nagaland	76	58	68	51	52	51	NA
33	Daman & Diu	60	56	57	61	50	56	NA

Note : *a) The estimates for Goa and Daman & Diu are aggregated.*

b) Female and Male Infant Mortality Rate not available from 1998

c) The estimates are not available for smaller States/Union Territories.

d) NA: Not available.

Source : *Office of the Registrar General of India, Ministry of Home Affairs* people. As a society advances, the life expectancy of its people also increases. Kerala, followed by Punjab, had the highest life expectancy rate from among major States right from 1981-85 till 1993-97.

A look at the sectoral composition of Plan expenditure in the last two decades reveals that the allocation to agriculture and irrigation has shown a downward trend for most of the bigger agricultural States between 1981-82 and 1997-98. The percentage declined from 30.17 to 19.05 in Uttar Pradesh and from 25.24 per cent 12.75 per cent in Punjab. Haryana and Madhya Pradesh have also registered falling shares of public expenditure going to agriculture. Karnataka, Gujarat and Maharashtra are the only States in which the share of Plan expenditure going towards agriculture have gone up in this period.

In the case of social sectors, many States have registered increases in percentage of expenditure over this period. Even in less developed States like Orissa and Madhya Pradesh the share of social sectors in Plan expenditure has risen. The trends are similar for Uttar Pradesh, Rajasthan, Assam and Haryana. Kerala, Maharashtra and Jammu and Kashmir however registered a fall in this percentage. An interesting point to note is the high expenditure in the north eastern States in the year 1997-98. All these States spend more than 40 per cent on the social sector.

The expenditure undertaken specifically for human development. The education and health expenditures as a ratio of total public expenditure. Since a large component of public expenditures in these sectors would fall outside the Plan, these ratios may provide a better comparative indicator. It can be seen that most of the States have registered increases in the education expenditure ratios. This implies that they are spending a higher proportion of public spending on education.

The education expenditure ratio has increased from 12.76 in 1980-81 to 26.34 in 1998- 99 for Assam. It increased from 13.19 to 21.16 in Bihar in the same period. However, this increase does not get reflected in corresponding improvements in educational achievements for Bihar, perhaps because of the low absolute levels of Plan expenditure. Kerala, on the other hand, registered a fall in this ratio in spite of the fact that it had registered the highest literacy rate. The expenditure ratio for health has shown a decline for most of the States. The highest fall was registered for Meghalaya where the ratio fell from 15.34 to 7.22 between the two time periods considered. It has also shown a significant decline for Haryana and Madhya Pradesh.

The highest ratio in 1998-99 was for Tamil Nadu at 8.34 per cent. There is probably a case for strengthening relative budgetary support to the health sector in many States. The fact that some States spend a higher proportion than the others on social sectors like health and education should also get reflected in the social sector indicators. States devoting a larger share to education should also register higher literacy rates and those spending higher share on health should have better health indicators. To the extent this outcome is not seen as in the case of Bihar & Assam for Education, it would suggest that the impact of proportionately higher expenditures also depends on the absolute levels per capita of such expenditures, and effective implementation and follow-up on the ground.

Challenges of India's Health System

India's health system is at a crossroads. Since independence, there have been significant changes in health conditions and major transformations in knowledge and technology. Today, new health threats are stretching the capacity of the health system to respond. An estimated 3.5 million Indians are living with HIV, and the virus has now spread beyond highly susceptible groups to the general population in some states, threatening to erase much of the social, economic, and health gains since independence. Building robust health systems is a critical part of the response to this and future health threats.

India's health transition is characterized by shifting demographics, altered health behaviours, and changes in disease patterns, with more degenerative and man-made diseases and more polarization of health conditions. A high proportion of the population continues to suffer and die from preventable infections, pregnancy and childbirth-related complications and under nutrition-the "unfinished agenda" of the health transition. There are also large disparities across India, which places the bulk of the burden of these conditions on the poor, women, and scheduled castes and tribes. The poorest 20 percent of Indians have more than double the mortality rates, malnutrition, and fertility of the richest quintile.

Despite all this, the public remains badly informed about much of the health system. It knows little about whether health services are appropriate, who is benefiting from them, whether quality is sufficient, or whether people are getting good value from public and private spending on health. There are major problems with equity, quality, and accountability in both the public and private health sectors. The time has come to reassess how the Indian health system should function, and retool it for the new millennium.

This review is a product of extensive consultation and research done by over a dozen Indian institutions. It proposes that health sector reform is needed, and outlines some broad principles for reform, which should be led by government. The main message is to raise the sights in four ways:

1. Overseeing the needs of the entire population-by making the health system more pro-poor, gender-sensitive and client-friendly, and by responding to the high burden of preventable diseases borne by the poor, scheduled tribes and castes, and women.
2. Looking forward to the health transition-by preparing for the shift in disease burden and increase in health costs by developing health financing systems.
3. Removing the blind spot to the private sector-by harnessing its energy and countering its failures.
4. Focusing efforts-by emphasizing quality, efficiency, and accountability of health services in both public and private sectors.
5. Ultimately, changing the shape of the health system depends on political decisions at national, state, and local levels-decisions that will be shaped by expressions of political preferences, social expectations, and the positions that leaders take at each level. International experience tells us that there is no single correct answer for shaping a country's

health system. In India, the priority of issues and choice of options should vary according to the conditions in the various states and districts. An explicit approach to policy formulation and implementation will help to continually evolve the health system-and to ensure that the health system is improving the health of all Indians in an accountable, equitable, and affordable manner.

Despite the establishment of a large public network of health providers, public spending on health is very low, stagnant at around 1% of GDP. Such spending puts India among the bottom 20% of countries. It is lower than what most low income countries spend, and is far below what is needed to provide basic health care to the population. The bulk of public spending on primary health care has been spread too thinly to be fully effective, while the referral linkages to secondary care have also suffered. As in other countries, preventive health services take a back seat to curative care. The states, which bear between 75% to 90% of the burden of public health spending, have their funds largely tied up in "non-plan" salary expenditures, leaving little room for essential drugs, supplies, operations and maintenance. The large variance in health financing among Indian states is increasing the gap in public resources for health between rich and poor states, and further threatens to expand existing gaps in health system outcomes. The states of Kerala, Punjab, and Tamil Nadu have double the per capita public health spending of Bihar and Madhya Pradesh.

Using the 1995-96 National Statistics Organization Survey to determine who is benefiting from public spending on health, it was found that curative services are highly pro-rich in distribution. About Rs. 3 is spent on the richest quintile for every Rs. 1 spent on the poorest 20 percent. Yet in three states (Kerala, Tamil Nadu, and Maharashtra), the distribution of public spending on health is nearly uniform across income groups. There are also differences in distribution for different types of services: immunizations and outpatient services at primary health centers are pro-poor, but inpatient services are less likely to reach the poor. Statistically, states with better equality in their public spending have better health status outcomes. 8. Private health spending is another story, accounting for more than 80 percent of all health spending. This is one of the highest proportions of private spending found anywhere in the world. There are only five other countries in the world comparable to India in such dependence on private financing for health services, but unlike India, these are countries with a recent history of civil conflict leading to major breakdowns in public service provision.

Nearly all the private spending in India is out-of-pocket at the point of service use, an inefficient way to finance health care that leaves people highly vulnerable. As in most developing countries, poorer households purchase less curative health care from the private sector than do richer households. Partly because of inability to pay and the lack of risk pooling, the poor are much less likely to get hospitalized. Across India, those above the poverty line have more than double the hospitalization rates of the poor.

Hospitalization frequently results in financial catastrophe, especially in the absence of risk pooling mechanisms. Only 10 percent of Indians have some form of insurance, and most of this is inadequate. Hospitalized Indians spent more than half (58%) of their total annual expenditures on health care. More than 40 percent of hospitalized people borrow money or sell assets to cover expenses. One conservative estimate finds that one quarter of hospitalized Indians fall below the poverty line because of hospital expenses, with the risk varying greatly from state to state. Even at public hospitals, which are intended to protect the poor from financial risks, the poor are vulnerable to health costs. In some states (Uttar Pradesh, West Bengal, Madhya Pradesh, Rajasthan, Haryana, and Bihar), the poor are more likely to borrow money when hospitalized in the public sector than in the private sector.

The private sector accounts for the majority of curative care services in India, thought here is considerable variation across services and states. The public sector accounts for over 80 percent of all hospitalizations in Orissa and the Northeast States, but less than 30 percent in Bihar and Andhra Pradesh. Indians below the poverty line are over 10 times more likely to be hospitalized in Kerala than they are in Bihar, Punjab, Uttar Pradesh, and Rajasthan. Overall, the distribution of private services is even more skewed toward the rich than the public sector. The poor still depend on the public sector for the majority of their health services, with one exception. The private sector provides 79 percent of outpatient care for those below the poverty line, much of which is of low quality and provided by untrained practitioners.

Private health markets differ significantly from state to state, and understanding the sevariations helps government to develop policies to influence private markets. In Uttar Pradesh and Andhra Pradesh, differences were found among private practitioners in the types of cases seen, the therapies offered, consultation charges, incomes, costs of doing business, types of concessions offered to the poor, and interest and participation in national health programs.

Alternative private practitioners (untrained in western, allopathic medicine, or practicing Indian systems of medicine) make up a larger segment of the private ambulatory care market than qualified allopathic doctors who practice western medicine. Irrespective of type of provider, quality assurance is a problem, with poor clinical practices and standards, and inadequate staffing.

Health is a shared responsibility of the central government and the states. How much discretion each state has over the policy options in any given area will vary. In some public health activities, the central government will likely take the lead through centrally sponsored schemes. But in curative services there is already enormous variation in what states attempt to do, and especially in how well they do what they do.

Whereas health status in Kerala compares with upper-middle income countries such as Argentina and Mauritius, most Indian states are comparable to lower-middle income countries. However, the poorest performing states compare with low-income countries such as Sudan and Nigeria.

Because the parts of the health system are related in a variety of complex ways, what happens in one part of the system will affect all other parts. Oversight, in particular, affects all the other dimensions-from public health services to health financing. How the provision of ambulatory curative services is organized will affect how preventive and promotional activities are carried out. Obviously the organization of health financing and the inpatient services are intimately related. But each of these activities has different institutional and organizational conditions for success and raises different policy questions, and so each is treated individually.

The costs of strengthening oversight are small in financial terms, but require are orientation of what governments do, consume considerable time and energy, and depend on the development of new capacities. Yet the benefits are considerable. Oversight activities are prerequisites to improving quality, equity, and being able to use health insurance or strategic purchasing of health services. The potential benefits thus include more efficient health services and greater public accountability. But increasing measurability in the health system may conflict with providers, raise the risk of manipulated results, and require technical expertise that may not be available.

Public action is not synonymous with government action. One cannot assume that creating a government body with responsibilities and powers to have oversight over the health sector will improve matters. Public oversight means empowering people who use the health system. Therefore, a wider variety of potential actions to improve oversight are considered. Each of these approaches are part of a fully functional health system. Given the growing prominence of the private sector, there is now a greater urgency than ever to intervene in oversight functions that address the private sector. International and domestic experience suggests that relying on only one approach is unlikely to be sufficient. One of the first steps that each state can take to better fulfill its oversight functions, is to develop more comprehensive health policies and strategies that outline which of these actions it will pursue. The differences between what states can and should do may depend more on the opportunities available, the leadership that emerges in the states, and the urgency of the issues.

Considering how little formal collaboration there has been to date between the public and private sectors, and the past limitations of the public sector to enforce regulations, it is likely that the most productive strategies are those that take a more balanced approach. In most states, this should begin with steps to bring public and private sector together on developing a common agenda. Using independent organizations as honest brokers to measure performance may also be a better way to start than relying on government or provider organizations, because the problems of credibility and conflict may be larger at the beginning of these reforms. But such steps also depend the development of trust between public and private sector players, which can also be enhanced through involvement of professional organizations. Increasing the role of consumer advocates is another good approach to strengthening oversight, particularly to make health services more directly accountability to the public. Formal public sector regulation will still be needed, but the analysis suggests that these approaches have more potential to be more successful in regulating factor inputs to the health sector, such as drug quality control, than regulating provider and hospital behaviours. In any case, given the limitations in public sector regulatory capacity, it is best to be selective in starting actions to strengthen formal public regulation.

For states mid to late in the transition and with moderate to high capacity, there is a much greater need to use these strategies to institutionalize quality assurance procedures in inpatient and ambulatory services. For other states, earlier in the transition and with less capacity, it maybe more feasible to focus initial activities on expanding public information approaches to empower people to demand better health services-and on initiating steps to bring public and private sector actors together. As experience and confidence is gained, more options could be pursued.

Public Health Service Delivery

Since public health is an area that is particularly under-financed in India, both in relative and absolute terms, the most relevant actions for India involve allocating more resources and effort on public health services. However, simply putting in more money into public health is not considered a sufficient action. Since most of India is still in the early part of the health transition, India ought to redouble its efforts to attack the unfinished agenda as its highest public health priority. Continuing the current approaches across the country is unlikely to suffice, even with additional resources. The success of public health programs usually depend on more than funding the technical interventions, as demonstrated in recent "success stories" in health in low-income countries. In the short term, intensive training and supervision in management, provision of supplies, and stronger and more professional health education that strengthens people's ability to make healthy choices are important measures to make these programs more effective.

The evidence from these studies makes a convincing case to involve private practitioners in these critical programs in most states because of their extensive reach and willingness to participate. Priority programs benefit from central sponsorship in funding, media attention, and guidance, but they are hindered by excessive central planning and rigid management systems. Central and state resources should be even more focused on reproductive and child health interventions, nutrition, and tuberculosis and malaria control, along with investments in sanitation and water, but in ways that will encourage local initiative and use of funds. Attention from national and state leaders is needed, as well as greater autonomy, resources, and flexibility in implementation at local levels. Initiatives that enable ordinary Indians to demand more of their health programs can only help. In some states where there are strong panchayat institutions, they can also play an important role in stimulating good performance of public health personnel if they are given support.

All states need to place additional effort on HIV prevention because of its potential damage and need for timely action, though the balance of interventions may be different from state to state because of differences in social conditions and transmission patterns. The HIV epidemic and the emergence of other diseases have also exposed the weaknesses of the current public health system. In the medium to long term, investing in public health systems is a necessary strategy to provide the personnel and systems needed to carry out the current agenda and respond to future challenges.

There are other state differences that should be considered. Kerala and Tamil Nadu, being further along in the transition and having greater capacity, have more compelling reasons to focus on introducing and expanding public health services for cardiovascular disease, mental health, and injuries, as these are now the prominent conditions facing their populations. Other states such as Maharashtra and Karnataka—in mid-transition and with moderate capacity-are in the position of considering when and how to introduce these programs, as these threats loom large in the near future. Yet there are also states that are earlier in the transition that should also consider selective interventions in these areas. For example, Orissa and West Bengal have very high rates of chewing tobacco and smoking, particularly among their poor. They should consider putting more effort on public health campaigns against tobacco, and ensure that they are not using public funds to subsidize or encourage tobacco production and use.

Ambulatory Curative Services

In the area of ambulatory care, there are some clear choices facing governments. Economic analysis indicates that this is the area where there is the least rationale for direct government provision of services, except that many preventive health programs depend on the opportunities and infrastructure used for outpatient curative care. Outpatient care is also the area where the public has most contact with the health system, and where most private money is spent. It is therefore a public concern, at least from an oversight perspective. The options considered here all involve relatively more resources than oversight and public health actions, though there may also be more scope to make better use of the large private funds already being spent on ambulatory care. Given the large presence of the private sector, its clear that all states need to focus more attention on services provided privately. Partly this can be done by supporting the oversight options. But it also means delivering more credible ambulatory care services through both public and private sectors. Influencing private practice by financing them, and focusing public delivery on areas where the private sector does not reach should be the most logical choice for most states, even though there may be considerable resistance to change. Working first with more well established nongovernmental organizations (NGOs) service providers may be a safer way to begin in many states.

This would also provide a means to increase the scale of some of the more flexible and innovative approaches to providing care that many such NGOs are able to offer. The higher capacity states may wish to move towards something like a combination of revitalizing public facilities in disadvantaged areas and demand-side mechanisms for the poor. In these states, the health sector is well developed so that only in remote areas would the presence or absence of a public facility make a difference, and they would have sufficient capacity to form linkages with the private sector to protect the poor.

In the low and very low capacity states that still have high infant mortality and low coverage of basic public health measures (immunizations, nutrition), a de-emphasis on publicly provided ambulatory curative care would allow a reallocation of effort into the public health activities. This could be done by eliminating public ambulatory curative care from non-hospital facilities in well served areas, and revitalizing public facilities in disadvantaged areas. This option may be more viable in states with higher private provision of outpatient services, although the fear of political repercussions may prevent such approaches.

The states mid way into the health transition and with moderate capacity face the largest strategic questions. Do they want to invest the effort and resources necessary to create a well functioning public ambulatory curative care system, as the private sector may still be underdeveloped and the treatable conditions of the "unfinished agenda" comprising a large component of mortality? Or should they want to skip that effort entirely and move to more links with the private sector, since that's where most people get their ambulatory curative care?

The most expensive option is to try to revitalize the entire network of public facilities. Following such a strategy without a several-fold increase in resources may avoid difficult political decisions, but would lead to little improvement in public services. The resources are spread too thinly, and efforts to improve availability and performance of staff and other resources have made slow progress. Even if a windfall of resources became available, strategies would be still be needed to deal with the much larger private sector that is preferred by the majority of the Indians.

Inpatient Care and Financing

Some unique challenges also face this segment of the health system. Inpatient care is particularly expensive and risky. A "two-tier" system may emerge in which the poor are effectively left out of quality care in the public sector (due to low access and quality) and the private sector (due to cost). Plans for care or insurance that attempt to provide the poor with exactly the same quality and quantity of inpatient care as the rich receive run the risk of cost escalation. Because of the close relationship between financing and high cost per episode inpatient care, consider sets of options for financing and provision of inpatient care together. The reforms proposed are also not cheap, but the costs of not reforming are even greater. Given the high levels of private financing and debt currently caused by inpatient care, methods that are able to capture some of this funding while preventing the hardships of the current situation will have a greater chance of long-term success. Between public and private providers needs to be mended, and steps taken to encourage providers to form networks. Progress is likely to come from those states that have greater administrative capacity, and where governments are able to learn from the experimental and smaller scale community financing schemes being tested by some NGOs. Big experiments are particularly needed to see how to cover the large informal sector, and to gain positive experience in managing health insurance.

Relying on private health insurance is likely to play some role in the short term, since the insurance market has been liberalized, and this consumes little additional public resources. However, it would still be desirable for the central government to play a larger role in actively regulating private insurance, though there is probably scope for states to also contribute to monitoring and regulating health insurance. International experience has shown that the cost of not aggressively regulating private voluntary health insurance is that insurance will become much more difficult to regulate later on, while leading to escalating health costs and increased inequalities.

Pursuing options for reform of hospital provision are complementary to those oriented around financing. For states earlier in the transition and with less capacity, it appears reasonable for governments to spend more effort on improving the quality of existing public first referral hospitals, but to do so in a selective manner that would promote more equitable distribution of public resources. Experience with state health system development projects has shown that such approaches can lead to improved quality of care and greater efficiencies, though it takes several years before many of the benefits are seen. Many countries have tried to make public hospitals autonomous to increase their productivity, but few have been able to obtain the full set of benefits intended at the start of reforms. Even so, given inefficiencies and discontent in public hospitals, some states may find it attractive make hospitals more autonomous in the hope that they can be managed more professionally and made more accountable.

Now is the time to conduct big experiments in India's health sector, particularly since the status quo is leading to a dead end. Either the center or individual states could take the initiative, but new experience is needed to build on what has become an outmoded health system. There now is an opportunity for governments to reform the way they work-and to take on critical oversight functions. Governments also need to consider new public health services and how to implement them differently from the past. New ways of managing ambulatory and inpatient services should be tried, along with a concerted effort to develop a more efficient, equitable, and risk-reducing health financing system.

The new experiments need to build in flexibility to deal with very different conditions in India, and to provide a basis for learning through intensive monitoring and evaluation. It is clear that no single choice is best for India. But there is the opportunity to travel with eyes open, consciously deciding which fork to take. To know which way to go, it is important to consult, analyze, debate, and forge a consensus on key issues. It is also important to try new options not previously considered. In the long run, this approach will best enable India's health system to meet the health needs of its people.

2

Women and Overall Health System

Attention to securing human health and a healthy environment has grown, as governments and people alike struggle with problems of differential access to a diminishing range of environmental resources. While the environmental movement has highlighted aspects of environmental sustainability, changes in the health field have emphasized issues of social justice, equity, and human development. In this spirit significant policy commitments were made to gender, health and environment issues at global meetings since the Earth Summit in 1992.

Prior to this shift environmental health was for many decades associated with a narrow sanitary engineering approach. Characterized by pipes and pumps, sewage and garbage, norms and standards, environmental health research and policy did not lend itself well to either gender or social development perspectives. Only recently have processes of urbanization, industrialization, and globalization prioritized the need to address a broader understanding of health-and-environment issues in the context of sustainability. Within this broader understanding of the 'environment', health, social, and technical dimensions are all equally valued.

Moreover, research and advocacy on women's roles and the gender division of labor, led to the recognition that women - particularly poor women in developing countries - are vulnerable to effects of environmental degradation in ways that differ from men. However, the health sector has not in general been quick to grasp that many health and environment problems have different impacts on men and women. One reason for this is the rather belated acknowledgment by the health sector of development research and policy. Issues long debated in other disciplines are only now being "discovered" by the mainstream health sector, as the need to look beyond the curative medical approach and along the axis of preventive public health is accepted. Despite the growing awareness of the breadth of environmental issues, it is notoriously difficult to arrive at an accurate estimate of the disease-burden of health and environment concerns.

The absence of data is most stark for developing countries and for poor women. While estimates and projections abound, there has been relatively little systematic, rigorous, and clearly articulated research in this field. Reasons for this include the multiple and interconnected nature of many risks which complicates research, a general lack of data in developing countries and fragmented, discipline-oriented data in developed countries. In addition, environmental causes, except for infectious diseases and acute poisonings, are often masked in health statistics. There is, however, agreement that environmentally-related ill-health is broadly underestimated.

Apart from these data gaps, environmental health research methodology tends to privilege pathogens and pollutants while neglecting social determinants linked to poverty and gender discrimination. For these reasons it is difficult to provide scientifically acceptable causal connections in the areas of environment, poverty, and health. Linkages between gender, health and environmental factors remain elusive or often remain implicit. The acquisition of meaningful data in this area, both qualitative and quantitative, is only beginning. Yet between one fifth and one quarter of the world's population live in absolute poverty, of which more than 90% are located in the developing world. Despite aggregate global indications of overall improvements in health and welfare the absolute numbers of poor throughout the world are constantly growing, and are living and working in increasingly unhealthy and unproductive environmental conditions.

While health risks are great for all within this growing number, those most disadvantaged and resource-poor are still predominantly women - particularly rural women. Unsustainability threatens the whole global system, but women feel the first and worst impacts. Women are particularly at risk because their options are doubly restricted. Any meaningful strategy to address environment and health issues must therefore take gender-sensitive poverty alleviation in both rural and urban settings as a central component.

Women and Environmental Health

Many definitions of environment in relation to health exist, ranging from the physiological perspective (dichotomizing between internal and external environment), to the more environmentalist definition (focussing on chemical, biological and physical agents). In its broadest sense environmental health is the segment of public health that is concerned with assessing, understanding, and controlling the impacts of people on their environment and the impacts of the environment on them.

By defining environment as the geographical space sustaining but also limiting human life and health, the environment becomes both a source of hazards and resources. Throughout history, human settlement, organization and technology served to overcome environmental constraints. Economic development in general aims to overcome local environmental resource constraints by better yielding exploitation methods.

Rapid industrialization and scaling up can, however, disrupt existing social arrangements and patterns of resource exploitation. If not carefully checked and accompanied by new institutional and social arrangements, they may increase existing or introduce new inequalities at the same time as introducing a whole range of new environmental hazards. For example, dams may increase water supplies to distant urban centers or for large-scale agriculture, but they also may increase prevalence of waterborne and vector-borne diseases, exposure to pesticides, as well as result in the uprooting or loss of livelihoods of entire communities. Frequently, decisions of those who control resources and policies affect resource accessibility and hazard characteristics of those who don't.

In the glare of publicity surrounding modern environmental hazards, like oil spills, radiation, urban air pollution, pesticide intoxication, climate change, it is easily overlooked that many of the poor continue to struggle with basic issues like access to adequate water and sanitation, safe food, and protection from the infectious diseases. These "traditional" hazards - often associated with lack of development - are sometimes contrasted with the "modern" hazards associated with uncontrolled development patterns. The changing pattern of exposures and health risks over time, and with economic growth, is known as the "risk transition." However for the hundreds of millions confined to the poverty trap the impact of industrialization and globalization may well be simultaneous exposure to both traditional and modern hazards - a phenomenon which has been termed the "risk overlap".

Simultaneous exposure to both traditional and modern environmental risks in many developing countries shows that issues of concern in the North are also relevant to populations of poor countries, as the processes of globalization and unregulated industrialization proceed apace. As there are virtually no data on industrial sources of persistent toxic substances in most of the South, as well as a paucity of detailed data on pesticide use, the following are some brief examples of the nature of problems that exist. Green peace carried out a sampling and analysis program in the heavily industrialized Indian province of Gujarat and found extensive surface water and ground water pollution.

Industrial pollution is also found in ship breaking in Asia. Young men, without any protection, strip asbestos coating from ships with electric drills, exposing not only themselves but the whole neighborhood to dangerous levels of asbestos, apart from other hazardous waste. Apart from the larger, industrial sectors, workers in small enterprises also face a similar range of occupational hazards, but are further at risk by poorer access to clean work places, toilets and water as well as lack of occupational health services. In addition, working and living environment are within close distance, increasing the risks of non-occupational exposure and accidents.

Textile-dying, car painting and repair, small metalry, pottery, shoe-making and carpentry are all examples of small industries that impose physical and chemical hazards and that are also often located within or very close to home. A prime example of exposure to toxic pollution in today's modernizing world is small-scale agriculture. This is the major sector for employment for many of the poor and also the major producer of basic commodities for survival. Small-scale farmers typically use more pesticides and fertilizer for reasons of economic survival. They apply pesticides manually, using old and poorly maintained equipment. Consumption of small-scale sector products is risky, because of pesticide residues as well as mycotoxins from poor storage.

While much has been said here about chemical pollution, it should not be understood that this represents a greater health hazard than the microbiological pollution of food and water which continues to present a major public health risk to hundreds of millions. The difference is that the biology and epidemiology of microbiological contamination, as well as the necessary preventive measures are by now well known. For example, diarrhoeal diseases account for 1.5 billion bouts of illness a year among children under five, with some 2 million resulting in death. This knowledge is not adequately acted upon in the developing world where the bulk of morbidity, mortality, and lost productivity from this cause occur. In contrast, in the case of chemical pollution, science and medicine are still at the threshold of understanding the complex mechanisms and pathways through which exposure and illness occur.

Development should imply the creation of infrastructure like roads, water, electricity and sanitation and public services like transport, immunization and environmental surveillance. Following this the social construct of poverty translates into lacking the means to overcome environmental constraints and to be shielded from environmental hazards. Hence, although the poor in high income countries may be materially better off than the poor in low income countries, they both tend to lack access to public resources that should shield them from modern and traditional environmental hazards. This is particularly the case of high income countries with traditionally weak support for social policies, like the United States, but perhaps less the case of countries with stronger public infrastructure and safety nets, like in Europe.

For example, indigenous peoples in both high and low income countries face high levels of pollution, poor public infrastructure and services, while also still being highly dependent on ever diminishing natural resources. In Mexico, Yaqui rural population revealed alarming rates of impaired neuromuscular and intellectual development compared to a similar community in a less contaminated area. Poor people living in urban environments also face similar problems. This predicament has led to accusations of environmental racism, proven by the empirical finding that the marginalized suffer disproportionately from environmental risks due to industrial pollution, waste dumps and occupational exposure. The resulting controversy and debate about environmental racism and injustice has spread from the US to other industrialized countries and developing countries with the participation of feminists and indigenous peoples.

The greater dependence of the rural poor on natural resources due to the lack of alternatives and public infrastructure affects women disproportionately. Gender differences in time and mobility due to different roles and responsibilities greatly constrain women's economic opportunities and often lead to a high degree of dependence on locally available resources, despite their sometimes lesser quality. Deforestation and unsustainable use of water and marginal land further exacerbate women's heavy workloads and time constraints, as they have to walk longer distances for fuel and water. However even when infrastructure and services exist, they frequently do not meet women's needs. Although large amounts of money have been invested in energy production, poor women's basic fuel needs are still unmet and they continue to toil in smoke filled kitchens. Hence amongst the poor, women are the most environmentally affected by the lack of quality resources and appropriate public infrastructure. As a result, women's personal environment greatly differs from men's, which leads to different environmental hazards and different exposures.

For the poor in general, and particularly for women, the boundary between environmental and occupational health is highly permeable. This is attributable to the undervaluation of women's roles and functions and their high input to domestic or agricultural labor, often unpaid. The overlapping of risks from both inside and outside the formal sector is still under-researched, and is a disadvantage for women who face multiple and often synergistic exposures. Women's health can suffer highly from such work exposures. A marginal farming area in Kenya shows disability levels in women aged 20-60 years approximately double those of men.

Disability was greater for men only from 15-19 years and over 60 years. As women predominantly make up the membership of the poor, it can be argued that poverty as such is a gender issue. However, there are many more justifications for a gendered approach to environment and health. The health risks of poverty are generally far greater for women than for men, because for women poverty is further compounded by gender inequality. Gender discrimination is manifest in women's lack of decision-making power, the invisibility or suppression of their concerns and priorities due to biased cultural norms, their lower levels of education and lower access to health services. Although most gender issues in environmental health are complex and highly interconnected, contributing factors can be grouped under three main categories: biology, gender division of labor and differences in power and status. From a gender equity point of view, differences in biology need to be accounted for in safety standards, work conditions and prevention. Risks derived from the gender division of labor demand more cautious interventions, in order to prevent locking women in socially defined roles. Lastly, lack of power usually translates in female invisibility and neglect of women's needs and concerns. In practice, all three factors may be present.

Even though physiological stress, such as pregnancy and lactation, can affect women's capacity to deal with environmental exposure, toxicological research predominantly uses male subjects in order to avoid variation caused by the female hormonal cycle. However within reproductive health, toxicity is better researched in women than in men, though the latter also run considerable occupational risks to fertility and reproductive health. Consequently little is known about biological differences in environmental health between men and women in areas not linked to reproductive health. Apart from differences in hormonal status, which have hardly been researched, sex-related differences insensitivity to toxic substances might be due to differences in detoxifying activity. Animal research indicates a five times higher detoxifying capacity in males. The challenge in researching chemical effects on health is daunting due to the differing degrees and dimensions of exposure that can occur throughout the life cycle. There may also be variations in the ability to absorb chemicals (children absorb lead twice as fast as adults); and in the susceptibility to damage (greater vulnerability of the fetus to many toxic and mutagenic compounds). For these reasons concentrated research on chemical exposures is needed.

The role of biology in environmental health risk can be more specifically demonstrated through the current widespread attention to endocrine disruptors. These are exogenous chemicals which either "mimic" or "antagonize" the action of endogenous hormones in the human body. Research focuses particularly on processes or tissues affected by estrogens, androgen blocker and thyroid hormones. Sex steroids specifically affect the central nervous system, the immune system, and the reproductive systems, while thyroid hormones affect most tissues in the human body. A gender finding of interest in connection with environmental estrogens is that women are more susceptible than men to autoimmune conditions. Women's heightened immune response to both foreign and self-antigens appears to account for their greater preponderance of autoimmune disease. Quite a few hazardous substances bio-accumulate in adipose tissue, which women typically possess more than men do. Differences in biological susceptibility also threaten men, as shown by the increase in male reproductive cancers, and the decline of male fertility.

Typically, much less is known about the effect of environmental androgens on human health. A common contaminant is the organotin compound TBT (tributyltin), which is used a santifouling agent in ship's paint. It induces masculinization in marine animals and there is every reason to expect similar effects on humans. Exposed groups to organotin compounds include harbor workers, but also farmers and their families as organotin compounds are common ingredients in fungicides.

Most concern however, is about prenatal exposure to endocrine disruptors, as many of these substances pass freely through the placenta, exposing and adversely affecting fetal development. It is estimated that background concentrations of dioxins and PCBs in industrialized areas in North America and Western Europe account for subtle congenital disorders such as hyperactivity and lowered IQ in 10% of the newborn. Other effects include low birth weight, vitamin K deficiency, hypospadia (congenital malformations of the penis), spina bifida and nuerological disorders due to exposure in utero. As for effects on adults, TCDD (tetrachlorodibenzo-p-dioxin) is designated by WHO as a known human carcinogen, and several less potent dioxins as "probable" human carcinogens, although the precise causal mechanisms remain poorly understood.

Breastmilk analysis has become an increasingly common method to monitor body burdens of persistent contaminants. Since many of these substances enter the body through the food chain, it is taken to reflect the background levels of contamination. Breastmilk contamination, particularly in poor populations, is of concern as it may decrease willingness to breastfeed and lead to increased birth rates and infant mortality. It is still unclear at what levels of pollution the advantages of contaminated breastmilk are outweighed by its risks. Any such evaluation would also compare the hygienic condition saffecting the risks of formula feeding. In general breastfeeding is still considered best.

DDT and PCBs in breastmilk is reported to be associated with decreased lactation periods and lesser ability to breastfeed. DDT was phased out in most countries, but stocks of old pesticides form a hazard in all regions. It is still used for pestcontrol in some countries in Latin America, Africa, and Asia, but nobody knows to what extent. Related compounds as chlordane are widely used to control termites. High levels of DDT were reported from rural areas in Venezuela and Sudan and rural/urban are as in Uganda and Zimbabwe. In general DDT breastmilk levels from countries applying DDT are higher than the WHO-standard but it is not too clear from what source, as DDT contamination can occur through the food chain rather than from direct exposure. The presence of DDT was found in breast milk of women from an isolated Papua community, where DDT never has been sprayed. Similarly, high levels of persistent organic pollutants (POPs) have been found in the Arctic food chain. Although they have never been used there, these compounds have settled in the Arctic due to atmospheric transport. Inuit women report increased incidence of cancers by eating fish and game from the region. However in Uganda, urban women had significantly higher breastmilk levels than rural women, but DDT-levels did not relate to vegetarian or non-vegetarian diet, indicating that in this case the food chain was not the primary route of exposure.

Fears about breastfeeding and the safety of the food chain greatly added to the trauma of affected populations in Eastern Europe following the Chernobyl nuclear disaster of 1986. It has been estimated that the psycho social dimensions of the Chernobyl disaster far outweighed the physical disease manifestations for many years afterwards. Women are also disproportionately physically affected in such a situation due to their higher susceptibility to iodine deficiencies and goiter, which can lead to increased uptake of radioactive isotopes. A less publicized but no less extensive environmental catastrophe has been taking place for over 20 years around the Aral Sea, which has shrunk to almost half its original size. Intensive cotton cultivation involving aerial spraying, diversion of feeder rivers for massive irrigation schemes, soil salinization, mineralization and heavy erosion created a series of environmental, health, and social problems from which the region, covering areas of five Central Asian countries, is unlikely to recover. Significant destruction of livelihoods occurred, followed by massive impoverishment and out migration and the weakening of family and social networks.

Breastmilk monitoring in southern Kazakhstan revealed levels of dioxin-like compounds ten times higher than those found in the United States. The levels of concentrations of TCDD (tetrachlorodibenzo-p-dioxin) in the Kazakh women's breastmilk resembled those found in populations exposed to industrial accidents. The data suggest that exposure to these compounds is chronic, environmental and long-term. Cotton defoliants are a likely origin of exposure, with the most likely pathway being contaminated foodstuffs. Similar findings have been reported from Karakalpakstan and Uzbekistan.

At a more general level, when dealing with environmental hardships men have some definite advantages over women. In the case of natural disasters and seasonal hardships, disaster statistics habitually record more female victims than males. Apart from differences in physical strength, social norms restrict women's freedom and independence of movement, which affect their willingness to leave homes and possessions in times of risk.

Indoor air pollution is described as the last major un addressed public health problem and cooking with biomass as "possibly the greatest occupational hazard faced by poor women". There are significant questions linked to exposure to biomass or coal smoke, nutrition, and pregnancy that remain to be researched. Depending on the type of housing, fuel, stove, ventilation, and cooking patterns, exposure to the particulates and gases found in biomass and coal smoke can be very high. The issue can be further compounded through exposure to environmental tobacco smoke. Research in China established that the risk ratio for respiratory symptoms linked to the use of coal as a cooking fuel increased in the presence of environmental tobacco smoke.

It is suggested that exposure to air pollutants hinders uptake of essential nutrients. High prevalence of chronic bronchitis in women in developing countries is associated with exposure to indoor smoke from cooking. A complication of bronchitis in Cor pulmonale, or right-sided heart failure, associated at an uncommonly early age in women with long-term exposure to domestic smoke, particularly in high, cold regions. As women with these conditions are not treated or hospitalized, official statistics still report those mainly affected by chronic lung diseases to be male Pioneering research in India also strongly suggests that use of biomass fuels for cooking substantially increases the risk of active tuberculosis, particularly in rural areas. Armenian women report, that due to prolonged fuel scarcity many urban dwellers took to the burning of municipal waste for cooking and house heating. Burning of plastic, bleached paper, preserved wood and many other modern types of household waste exposed them to heavy loads of dioxin-like substances, PAH and heavy metals. Cooking with biomass fuel or coal generates multiple risks and exposures, which form an intergenerational vicious circle. The health risks to women and infants dependent on low-grade fuel for cooking and heating can be characterized as follows:

— gathering and transporting fuel (time and energy costs, musculoskeletal disorders, falls and fractures, increased risk of prolapsed uterus)

— smoke from biomass/coal burning (respiratory disease, eventually heart disease)

— eye infections and disorders (conjunctivitis, cataract)

— depressed immune response from smoke exposure

— exposure of fetus to CO (affects fetal development and birth weight)

— LBW infant vulnerability to infectious disease

— risk of stunting for infant

Issues of Water Scarcity

Access to and control over environmental resources is of vital importance to those dependent on it. Water scarcity for a large part is human-made, as many irrigation-projects have specifically targeted the larger landholders, assuming 'trickle-down' effects to the poor that never came to pass. Typically women are not acknowledged as stakeholders in irrigation, despite lifelong user rights to land and a willingness to invest in land improvement. Falling ground water tables in India allow those in possession of more expensive equipment, or deep tubewells to keep on extracting water. Meanwhile those with shallow wells and hand pumps, who are more likely to be women, face water shortage with adverse effects on nutritional status, income and workloads. Those who lack good public infrastructure, like many poor urban women, have to pay exorbitant prices to the water sellers. More than a billion people are currently deprived of water of sufficient quantity and quality to meet evenminimal levels of health and well-being. Absolute water scarcity is increasing in many parts of the world, making equitable access a pressing issue. Severe water shortage is predicted for 2.7 billion people, a third of the world population, in the first quarter of this century.

Severe under reporting and lack of research of women's environment-related health problems also relate to power differences. PAN (Pesticide Action Network) Asia and Pacific carried out case studies in eight countries and found that more than 90% of the women involved regularly spray pesticides without adequate protection and know-how. Due to the lack of available childcare, women use pesticides often while carrying a baby on their back. All of them are exposed during weeding, cleaning equipment and clothing, and disposal of leftovers. Many of them cannot read labels or don't follow instructions. Highly toxic pesticides such as parathion, endosulfan, phorate, monocrotophos and phosphamidon were used frequently. Most women reported symptoms of intoxication, which as a rule go untreated. In Sudan, a consistent and significant association between pesticide exposure and perinatal mortality was found, with a 50% higher risk in rural women.

Lack of adequate legislation, ignorance of standards, poor labeling, illiteracy and lack of protective clothing increase the hazards to agricultural workers and environment. While men receive some instructions for pesticide use, no information is given to women. Women buy pesticides at markets that have been repackaged from large containers into smaller containers, frequently lacking labels or instructions for use. Pesticides are transported and stored together with food products and containers are frequently re-used to pack food products for the market. Consumption of small-scale sector products is risky, because of pesticide residues as well as mycotoxins from poor storage.

Worldwide prevalence of acute pesticide poisoningis estimated at 1-3 million, resulting in 220.000 deaths per year, the majority of which occur in the Third World. These figures are probably inaccurate as under reporting is a major problem. Intensification of monitoring pesticide poisoning in South Africa resulted in atenfold increase in the cases reported and a completely inverted picture of the gender profile of poisonings. Routine surveillance suggested that 66% of poisonings involved men, but intensified surveillance found 66% of poisonings in women.

A crucial environmental health problem in developing countries is the use of highly toxic substances that are restricted or banned in industrial countries. Products are used continuously throughout the year, instead of 4-6 months per year in temperate climates. Moreover winters kill many crop pests, leading to lower disease pressure in the temperate zone. Obsolete pesticide stocks are problematic in most regions, but especially so in the South which lacks appropriate disposal methods. The costs of safe disposal amount to $1000-2000 per ton excluding transport, hardly affordable for most developing countries.

Ergonomic Problems

Along with chemical and microbiological exposure in domestic, agricultural, and occupational settings, ergonomic problems are a further category of environmental health hazard for both men and women. Traditionally linked exclusively with occupational health in the formal sector, understanding that ergonomic problems pose health risks in a broader range of settings is growing. Much of this increased awareness is derived from gender debates as well as from more comprehensive definitions of the nature of work. In the traditional view, men were seen as the main victims of occupational hazards and serious injury.

More recently it is being recognized that women suffer many chronic, often undiagnosed and untreated occupational health problems. These include cumulative trauma disorders and specific musculoskeletal disorders in the supposedly "safe" jobs ascribed to them as women's work in both formal and informal sectors. Women's work on conveyer belts, in electronics plants, garment and textile factories, hospitals, and piece-working at home involve speed, repetitive motions and restricted positions. All of these conditions tend to produce these disease patterns which are rarely recognized or compensated in equal proportions to male disability. In recent years, research has called attention to the design and use of equipment, tools, workstations and protective clothing that are inadequate or unsuitable for the users' size and strength. Men are affected mainly when equipment, tools or clothing are imported by foreign-owned enterprises, but women are further disadvantaged as most equipment remains designed around male norms. Failure to take these issues into account results in work inefficiency, accidents, additional energy expenditure, and cumulative trauma in working women .

Rural women's domestic or agricultural tasks often require prolonged work in stooping or squatting positions, or regular weight bearing. Little research has been done on musculoskeletal disorders in women from these causes, although it has been shown that work in awkward positions reduces lifting power and requires greater energy expenditure. Kitchen work is also responsible for extended periods of time spent in stooped and uncomfortable postures, which inconjunction with agricultural tasks may result in several hours daily spent in ergonomically unhealthy postures. The need for attention to multiple exposures is underlined through a Swedish the impact of heavy lifting on birth weight. It found that lifting alone had no negative effect, but in conjunction with other risk factors, for example chemical exposure, heavy lifting could influence pregnancy outcome.

The Indian women found that most were the result of work-related accidents and could be traced to a combination of prolonged unnatural work postures, nutritional deprivation and repeated childbearing. Studies performed in the Gambia and Ethiopia on women's workload and weight-gain during pregnancy found that only half the amount of weight-gain took place in peak agricultural season compared to the low season. It was established that birth weight could be affected by changes in work conditions right up to delivery and that high work intensity was a factor involved in premature delivery. Lower survival rates were detected among infants whose mothers operated heavy farm tools while pregnant.

3

Planning Issues of Health System

India is one of the pioneers in health service planning with a focus on primary health care. In 1946, the Health Survey and Development Committee, recommended establishment of a well-structured and comprehensive health service with a sound primary health care infrastructure.

Improvement in the health status of the population has been one of the major thrust areas for the social development programmes of the country. This was to be achieved through improving the access to and utilization of Health, Family Welfare and Nutrition Services with special focus on under served and under privileged segment of population. Main responsibility of infrastructure and manpower building rests with the State Government supplemented by funds from the Central Government and external assistance. Major disease control programmes and the Family Welfare Programmes are funded by the Centre (some with assistance from external agencies) and are implemented through the State infrastructure. The food supplementation programmes for mothers and children are funded by the State and implemented through the ICDS infrastructure funded by the Central Government. Safe drinking water and environmental sanitation are essential pre-requisites for health. Initially these two activities were funded by the Health Department, but subsequently Dept. of Urban and Rural Development and Dept. of Environment fund these activities both in the State and Centre.

At the time of Independence, the country's health care infrastructure was mainly urban and clinic based. The hospitals and clinics provided curative care to patients who came to them. Out reach of services in the rural areas was very limited; there were very few preventive and rehabilitative services available. From the First five-year Plan, Central and State Governments made efforts to build up primary, secondary and tertiary care institutions and to link them through appropriate referral systems. The private and voluntary sector also tried to cater to the health care needs of the population. Efforts to train adequate number of medical, dental and paramedical personnel were also taken up.

National Programmes for combating major public health problems were evolved and implemented during the last fifty years. Efforts to further improve the health status of the population by optimising coverage and quality of care by identifying and rectifying the critical gaps in infrastructure, manpower, equipment, essential diagnostic reagents, drugs and enhancing the efficiency of the health system are under way.

Improvement in coverage and quality of health care and implementation of disease control programmes resulted in steep decline in the crude death rate (CDR) from 25.1 in 1951 to 9.0 in 1996. Life expectancy rose from 32 years in 1947 to 61.1 years in 1991-96 with female life expectancy (61.7 yr.) higher than the male (60.6 yr.). However, the morbidity due to common communicable and nutrition -related diseases continue to be high. Morbidity due to non-communicable diseases is showing aprogressive increase because of increasing longevity and alterations in life style. During the Ninth Plan efforts will have to be made to tackle this dual disease burden effectively so that there is sustained improvement in the health status of the population.

India today has a vast network of governmental, voluntary and private health infrastructure manned by large number of medical and paramedical persons. Current problems faced by the health care services include:

1. Persistent gaps in manpower and infrastructure especially at the primary health care level.
2. Suboptimal functioning of the infrastructure; poor referral services.
3. Plethora of hospitals not having appropriate manpower, diagnostic and therapeutic services and drugs, in Govt., voluntary and private sector;.
4. Massive interstate/ interdistrict differences in performance as assessed by health and demographic indices; availability and utilisation of services are poorest in the most needy states/districts.
5. Sub optimal intersectoral coordination
6. Increasing dual disease burden of communicable and noncommunicable diseases because of ongoing demographic, lifestyle and environmental transitions,

7. Technological advances which widen the spectrum of possible interventions
8. Increasing awareness and expectations of the population regarding health care services
9. Escalating costs of health care, ever widening gaps between what is possible and what the individual or the country can afford.

The Special Action Plan for Health envisages expansion and improvement of the health services to meet the increasing health care needs of the population; no specific targets have been set.

During the Ninth Plan efforts will be further intensified to improve the health status of the population by optimising coverage and quality of care by identifying and rectifying the critical gaps in infrastructure, manpower, equipment, essential diagnostic reagents and drugs. Efforts will be directed to improve functional efficiency of the health care system through:

a. Creation of a functional, reliable health management information system and training and deployment of health manpower with requisite professional competence
b. Multi professional education to promote team work
c. Skill upgradation of all categories of health personnel, as a part of structured continuing education
d. Improving operational efficiency through health services research.
e. Increasing awareness of the community through health education.

f. Increasing accountability and responsiveness to health needs of the people by increasing utilisation of the Panchayati Raj institutions in local planning and monitoring

g. Making use of available local and community resources so that operational efficiency and quality of services improve and the services are made more responsive to user's needs.

Ninth Plan

The approach during the Ninth Plan will be:

— Horizontal integration of vertical programmes

— Develop Disease Surveillance and Response mechanism with focus on rapid recognition, & response at district level

— Develop & implement integrated Non-Communicable Disease control Programme

— Health Impact Assessment as a part of environmental impact assessment in developmental projects.

— Implement appropriate management systems for emergency,disaster, accident & trauma care at all levels of health care.

— Improve HMIS and logistics of supplies

i. An absolute and total commitment to improve access to, and enhance the quality of, primary health care in urban and rural areas by providing an optimally functioning primary health care system as a part of the Basic Minimum Services;

ii. To improve the efficiency of existing health care infrastructure at primary, secondary and tertiary care settings through appropriate institutional strengthening, improvement of referral linkages and operationalisation of Health Management Information System (HMIS);

iii. To promote the development of human resources for health, adequate in quantity and appropriate in quality so that access to essential health care services is available to all so that there is improvement in the health status of community, periodically organise programmes for continuing education in health sciences, update knowledge and upgrade skills of all workers and promote cohesive team work;

iv. To improve the effectiveness of existing programs for control of communicable diseases to achieve horizontal integration of ongoing vertical programmes at the district and below district level; to strengthen the disease surveillance with the focus on rapid recognition, reporting and response at district level; to promote production and distribution of appropriate vaccines of assured quality at affordable cost; to improve water quality and environmental sanitation; to improve hospital infection control and waste management

v. To develop and implement integrated non-communicable disease prevention and control program within the existing health care infrastructure;

vi. To undertake screening for common nutritional deficiencies especially in vulnerable groups and initiate appropriate remedial measures; to evolve and effectively implement programmes for improving nutritional status, including micronutrient status of the population;

vii. To strengthen programmes for prevention, detection and management of health consequences of the continuing deterioration of the ecosystems; to improve linkage between data from ongoing environmental monitoring and that on health status of the population residing in the area including health impact assessment as a part of environmental impact assessment in developmental projects;

viii. To improve the safety of the work environment and worker's health in organised and unorganised industrial and agricultural sectors especially among vulnerable groups of the population;

ix. To develop capabilities at all levels for emergency and disaster prevention and management; to implement appropriate management systems for emergency, disaster, accident and trauma care at all levels of health care;

x. To ensure effective implementation of the provisions for food and drug safety; strengthen the food and drug administration both at the Centre and in the States;

xi. To increase the involvement of ISM&H practitioners in meeting the health care needs of the population;

xii. To enhance research capability with a view to strengthening basic, clinical and health systems research aimed at improving the quality and outreach of services at various levels of health care;.

xiii. To increase the involvement of voluntary, private organisations and self-help groups in the provision of health care and ensure inter-sectoral coordination in implementation of health programmes and health-related activities;

xiv. To enable the Panchayati Raj Institutions (PRI) in planning and monitoring of health programmes at the local level so that there is greater responsiveness to health needs of the people and greater accountability; to promote inter-sectoral coordination and utilise local and community resources for health care.

Primary Health Care

The primary health care infrastructure provides the first level of contact between the population and health care providers upto and including primary health care physicians and forms the common pathway for implementation of all the health and family welfare programmes in the country. It provides integrated promotive, preventive, curative and rehabilitative services to the population close to their hearth and home. Majority of the health care needs of the population is taken care of by the trained health personnel at the primary health care level. Those requiring specialised care are referred to secondary or tertiary care. Thus, the three-tier system consisting of Primary, Secondary and Tertiary care facilities with adequate referral linkages will provide essential health and family welfare services to the entire population.

At the time of Independence, Health Care services were mainly urban-centered and hospital-based.

Realising the importance of creating a functional Primary Health Care infrastructure, national norms for the primary health care infrastructure were drawn up. These take into account the population, population density and terrain. Earmarked funds were provided under the Minimum Needs Program in the State Plan allocations. The funds received from the Department of Family Welfare and through the Externally Assisted Projects (EAPs) were utilised to build up the Rural Health infrastructure.

At the national level the total number of functional Sub centres and the PHCs nearly meets the set norms (one sub-centre for 3000-5000 population, one Primary Health Centre for 20,000- 30,000 population; one Community Health Centre for four PHCs) for the population in 1991. However, there are marked disparities at the State and district level. It is a matter of concern that many of the districts with poor health indices do not have adequate health infrastructure. There is considerable backlog in terms of construction of the buildings for Sub Centres and PHCs.

Some States have adopted innovative measures including mobilisation of local resources to clear this backlog. Taking cognizance of the widening disparities among the States in the availability of Basic Minimum Services (BMS), the Conference of the Chief Ministers in July 1996, recommended that Additional Central Assistance (ACA) may be provided to the States for correcting the existing gaps in the provision of seven Basic Minimum Services (BMS). The modalities of implementation of the programme are discussed in detail in the section on Basic Minimum Services. Of these, access to primary health care, safe drinking water and primary education were given higher priority with the mandate that universal access to these services is to be achieved by 2000 AD. Increasing involvement of the people's representatives, voluntary organisations and the people themselves in these activities will be further encouraged during the Ninth Plan. Factors responsible for sub-optimal functioning of Primary Health Care Institutions:

— Inappropriate location, poor access, poor maintenance

— Gaps in critical manpower.

— Mismatch between personnel & equipment

— Lack of essential drugs/diagnostics

— Poor referral linkages

— Appropriate remedial measures to improve functional status will be initiated in the Ninth Plan

While computing the requirements for primary health care infrastructure for the growing population, the fact that population increase has occurred in and around the already established centres have to be kept in mind. The already established physical infrastructure cannot be shifted and it will be difficult to add additional centres to serve the population in geographically convenient locations. It might be more feasible to increase the number of functionaries required to cater to the populations need rather than increase the number of centres.

In some areas, the existing Primary Health Care Institutions (PHIs) are functioning sub-optimally because of one or more of the following factors:

i. Inappropriate location, poor access, lack of maintenance;

ii. Lack of professional and para-professional staff at the critical posts;

iii. Mismatch between the requirement and availability of health professionals especially physicians at PHC;

iv. Lack of funds for essential drugs/diagnostics

v. Lack of First Referral Units (FRUs) for linkage of referral services.

These problems need urgent resolution at the local level through adequate provision of resources and intervention of the Panchayati Raj Institutions (PRI).

Unlike the SC and PHCs, the number of functioning CHCs, which form the First Referral Unit (FRU), is far below the projected requirement. This gap should be filled quickly so that the PHCs and Sub Centres do have a nearby referral hospital for the management of 'high-risk patients' who are referred. Inmost of the States there are functioning sub-district and taluk hospitals. With the restructuring of the Primary Health Care Institutions in the Seventh Plan, these institutions were to be re designated as CHCs and suitably strengthened. The Eighth Plan had also reiterated this strategy. States that had implemented this suggestion report that these FRUs are well utilised, as they are located in towns that are well connected with villages by transport and are well known.

During the Ninth Plan, all the States will restructure the existing sub-district, taluk hospitals and block level PHCs into functioning CHCs (FRUs); it is expected that once this restructuring is completed, the current large gaps in functioning CHCs will be narrowed substantially. Similarly existing rural hospital and dispensaries have to be restructured wherever possible to meet the requirements in PHC. Earmarked funds under BMS could be utilised for completing the restructuring and strengthening of these hospitals/dispensaries.

Ninth Plan priorities for Rural Primary Health Care Institutions are:

— Ensure existing SC, PHC are fully operational

— Fill the gaps in CHCs through re-structuring existing block level PHC, Taluk, Sub-divisional hospital

— Establish functional referral linkages

— Provide need based manpower on the basis of distances, difficulties and work load

As per the national norms, one male and one female multi-purpose worker should be available at the Sub-Centre catering to the Health needs of 3000 to 5000 population. The number of sanctioned posts of male multi-purpose workers is only half the number required. This has been cited as one of the major factors responsible for the sub-optimal performance in health sector programmes. There are large numbers of male-workers employed in the malaria, leprosy and TB Control programmes. These workers need be trained and redeployed as male multipurpose workers and given the responsibility of looking after health and family welfare programmes in their sub-centre area. The availability of the female multi-purpose workers in adequate number has been the major factor for the near universal coverage under the immunisation Programme and improvement in ante-natal care; however the quality of care provided needs improvement. The vacancies as well as the lack of sanctioned posts of radiographers, lab-technicians and other para-professionals have adverse impact on ongoing Health and Family Welfare Programmes. These need be rectified as rapidly as possible and funds provided under BMS in 1996-97 have been utilised by some States to fill the critical gaps in health manpower.

During the Ninth Plan, several of the Centrally Sponsored Schemes including Family Welfare Programme, Revised National Tuberculosis Control Programme (RNTCP), National Malaria Eradication Programme (NMEP) will provide funds for recruitment of appropriate manpower. Funds provided under ACA for BMS may also be utilised to fill the critical gaps in health manpower. Every district will undertake district-level manpower survey and planning, so that funds from all these sources are optimally utilised to fill the existing gaps in vital manpower and unnecessary duplication is avoided.

So far, the national norms for manpower requirement have been computed on the basis of the population. During the Ninth Plan the requirement of personnel will be computed not only on the basis of population, but also on the basis of workload, distance to be covered and difficulties in delivery of Health Services. A flexible approach to recruitment of staff, if necessary on part time basis, will be adopted to ensure that the programmes do not suffer due to lack of key personnel.

The number of PHC doctors at the national level exceeds the requirement as per the norms. However, there are marked differences in their distribution. About 10% of the PHCs are without doctors, while a similar number have three or more doctors. The PHCs without doctors are mostly located in remote areas where health care facilities under voluntary or private sector are also limited. The State Governments are taking steps to redeploy the PHC doctors so that the needs of the population in under-served areas are met on a priority basis. Some of the innovative approaches to fill the vacancies in under-served areas currently being tried in some States include:

a. local recruitment of doctors, if necessary on part-time basis;

b. adoption of a village/PHC/district by industrial establishments, cooperatives, self-help groups and religious/charitable institutions;

c. permitting local practitioners to pay a rental and practice in the PHCs after OPD hours.

During the Ninth Plan, the feasibility and usefulness of these approaches will be evaluated and those found useful in any area will be utilised as a part of local area-specific micro planning for effective delivery of essential Primary Health Care.

A substantial proportion of specialist's posts even in the functioning CHCs is vacant. Hence, these CHCs are unable to function as First Referral Units. In view of the serious implications of this lacuna in the establishment of referral system, as well as effective provision of health, MCH/FP care, there is an urgent need to rectify this. Improving the service conditions and providing a conducive environment are essential to ensure that specialists in CHCs do stay and provide the needed services. At the moment, there is no post of Public Health Specialist or Anaesthetist, in the CHCs. Services of Anaesthetist are vital because without an Anaesthetist, emergency/routine surgery in CHCs will not be possible. Efforts will be made to provide this critical manpower, if necessary on part-time basis.

As a long-term measure, sufficient number of in-service candidates may be trained in this speciality. It is vital to provide interlinkage between preventive, promotive and curative services in the CHCs so that health and family welfare programmes, disease surveillance and response mechanisms get strengthened. Until the specialists in public health get posted in CHCs, the existing specialists in these Centres who presently are mainly responsible for curative services, will have to be given Public Health orientation, training in Epidemiology and Health Management so that each one of them assumes the responsibility of looking after the Disease Control Programme in their respective specialities e.g. Immunisation by paediatrician and FP by the obstetrician. This would also improve the linkages between the CHC and the PHCs.

Tribal Health

High disease burden in Tribals is due to :

— Poverty and under nutrition

— Poor sanitation, lack of safe drinking water

— Diseases which are more prevalent in tribals

— Lack of awareness about and access to health care

— Social and economic barriers to utilisation

The Scheduled Castes and Scheduled Tribes constitute 16.48% and 8.08% respectively of the total population of the country as per 1991 census. The highest concentration of tribal population is found in the North Eastern States and also in the UTs of Lakshadweep and Dadra and Nagar Haveli. High concentration of tribal population is also present in the States of Madhya Pradesh, Orissa, Gujarat, Maharashtra and Bihar. The factors that contribute to increased disease burden in these communities include:

a. poverty and consequent under nutrition;

b. poor environmental sanitation, poor hygiene and lack of safe drinking water, leading to increased morbidity from water and vector-borne infections;

c. lack of access to health care facilities resulting in increased severity and/or duration of illness;

d. social barriers preventing utilisation of available health care services;

e. specific diseases they are prone to such as genetic diseases (G-6 PD deficiency), infections etc.

The tribal population is not a homogeneous one. There are wide variations with regard to education and health status, access and utilisation of health services among the tribal populations. The tribal populations in North Eastern States have high literacy levels, they access available health facilities, and hence their health indicators and demographic indices are better than national level inspite of the fact that the region is endemic for malaria. On the other hand, the Onges in Andaman and Nicobar remain a primitive tribe with very little access to either education or health care. Differential area-specific strategies will therefore have to be developed for each of the tribal areas to improve access and utilisation of health Services.

The National Health Policy accorded a high priority to provision of health services to those residing in the tribal, hilly and backward areas as well as to detection and treatment of endemic diseases affecting the tribal population. The strategy adopted for meeting the health care needs during the Eighth Plan period included provision of preventive, promotive and curative services through the primary health care institutions, and at the village level through link health workers and trained Dais. Keeping in view the far-flung areas, forest land, hills and remote villages, where most of the tribal habitations are concentrated, the population coverage norms for PHIs is relaxed to one PHC for every 20,000 population and one Sub Centre for 3,000 population. While choosing the villages for establishments of sub centres the States have been advised to set up at least 15% of these in Scheduled Castes' habitations or villages having 20% or more Scheduled Caste population and 7.5% in tribal areas.

Till June 30, 1996 there were 20097 sub-centres functioning against a requirement of 28383 sub-centres for tribal areas. The number of functioning PHCs were 3260 against a requirement of 4180 and functioning CHCs were 446 against a requirement of 492. There are also 1122 Dispensaries and 120 Hospitals in Modern Medicine, 78 Mobile Clinics in Modern Medicine, 1106 Dispensaries and 24 Hospitals in Ayurveda, 251 Dispensaries and 28 Hospitals in Homeopathy, 42 Unani Dispensaries, 7 Siddha Dispensaries functioning in the tribal areas in the country. As many as 16,845 Sub Centres, 5987 PHCs and 373 CHCs have been established in Scheduled Caste Basties/Villages having 20% or more Scheduled Caste population. In addition 980 Dispensaries in Modern Medicine, 1042 Ayurvedic Dispensaries, 480

Homeopathic Dispensaries, 68 Unani/Siddha Dispensaries are functioning in the Scheduled Caste concentrated areas in the country. Mobile dispensaries and camps were organised to provide health facilities wherever feasible.

Even though efforts have been made to create primary health care infrastructure and sanction necessary manpower both under modern medicine and under ISM&H, there is lack of both professional and para professional manpower, mainly because the State Govt. personnel do not prefer to work in these areas. The State Governments are trying to minimise vacancies by taking even part time staff in tribal areas. A Central Planning Committee has been set up to review the health care activities in 39 districts of 12 States with pockets of extremely backward tribal population.

Strategies for Tribal health:

— Ensuring availability of adequate infrastructure and personnel.

— Area specific RCH programmes.

— 100% central Plan funds for NMEP.

— Effective implementation of the health & FW programmes.

— Close monitoring, early detection of problems in implementation and midcourse correction.

The States have been requested to restructure the existing primary health care institutions, redeploy existing personnel and make them fully operational. After this is done, it will be possible to compute the gaps in manpower/infrastructure and take steps to ensure that these are filled. In addition to State Government funds, allocation from appropriate Centrally Sponsored Schemes will also be available for filling critical manpower gap. For example, under the National Malaria Eradication Programmes 100%. Central assistance is being provided for filling critical manpower gaps, and for drugs and insecticides in North Eastern States many of which have predominantly tribal population. The Tribal sub-project of RCH will also provide funds for manpower, equipment, drugs and training of staff.

Priority was also accorded to research in diseases to which Scheduled Tribes/ Scheduled Castes are prone. The Indian Council of Medical Research has set up five regional medical centres in tribal areas in the country one each at Jabalpur, Bhuvaneshwar, Jodhpur, Dibrugarh and Port Blair to carry out research on health problems of people in these regions, especially the scheduled tribes. The All India Institute of Hygiene and Public Health has also initiated a project "Integrated Health Development of Scheduled Castes and Scheduled Tribes of Sunderbans area of West Bengal." The Central Council for Research in Ayurveda and Siddha has set up research projects, and conducted service- oriented survey to provide medical aid to Scheduled Tribes and Scheduled Castes.

A review of all these activities will be undertaken in the Ninth Plan so that information generated so far is transformed into well-structured action programme. During the Ninth Plan period priority action will be:

a. norms for establishment and staffing pattern of Sub Centres and PHCs will be specifically relaxed in the tribal areas taking into account the difficulty in terrain and problems in health care delivery;

b. implementation of all ongoing programmes will be intensified and closely monitored in these areas;

c. 100% assistance under NMEP to tribal districts in other States will be provided;

d. specific projects will be evolved to meet the requirements for RCH care of the tribal population in the States such as MP, Bihar and Orissa.

States have to prioritise and utilise funds available for primary health care on the basis of the existing infrastructure and the performance indices as follows:

1. States such as Kerala and Tamil Nadu with good infrastructure and good performance require only uninterrupted supply of drugs and devices; management of non communicable diseases should get attention in these states.

2. States like Bihar and Uttar Pradesh with poor infrastructure and poor performance: provision of additional funds to health sector from the states outlay to improve the infrastructure, ensure availability of skilled manpower to effectively manage the programme are critical for improvement of performance.

3. States with below average level of infrastructure but average level of performance such as Himachal Pradesh and Andhra Pradesh: attempt should be made to improve infrastructure through optimal utilisation of funds from all the sources as this may result in rapid improvement in performance.

4. States like Punjab and Haryana with above average level of infrastructure and below average performance in some health indices: specific efforts need be made to identify the factors responsible for the relatively poor performance and correct them.

Rural Primary Health Care

1. Ensure that geographically delineated rural areas are covered by the three tier primary health care institutions as per the norms defined above through integration of the existing hospitals/dispensaries in rural areas into the appropriate tier of the rural primary health care infrastructure.
2. Accord high priority to filling the reported large gap in the vital CHC/FRU by redesignating and appropriately strengthening the existing block level PHCs, subdistrict/ subdivisional hospitals, rural hospitals, subdistrict post partum centres.

Ninth Plan Strategies for improving Urban Primary Health Care:

— Create and strengthen primary health care infrastructure through:

— Re-organisation & restructuring of existing institutions

— Re-deploy existing manpower to operationalise these institutions

— Link primary health care infrastructure with existing secondary and tertiary care institutions in the same geographically delineated areas

— Establish effective referral services

— Involve Nagar Palikas in effective inter-sectoral co-ordination & improving community participation

Ensure that there are no vacancies in the critical para professional posts by skill development and redeployment of already available manpower; where absolutely necessary manpower gaps may be filled through part time appointments.

5. Available funds to be utilised on priority basis for purchase of equipment, consumables, drugs required for improving quality of services; funds may be provided for construction only when absolutely necessary.

Urban Health and Family Welfare Services

Nearly 30% of India's population lives in urban areas. Urban migration over the last decade has resulted in rapid growth of people living in urban slums. The massive inflow of the population has also resulted in the deterioration of living conditions in the cities. From the data it would appear that the urban population has better health facilities and health indices than the rural population. However in many towns and cities the health status of urban slum dwellers is worse than that of the rural population. The urban health facilities provide health care, especially tertiary care to both the urban and rural population. The available urban health care infrastructure is insufficient to meet the health care needs of the growing urban population.

Realising this the municipalities, State Governments and the Central Government have tried to provide funds for building up urban health care. Unlike the rural health services, there have not been any well-planned and organised efforts to provide primary, secondary and tertiary care services in geographically delineated areas in urban health care. As a result, there is either non-availability or substantial under utilisation of available primary care facilities along with an over-crowding at secondary and tertiary care centres.

During the Ninth Plan period, efforts will be made to evolve a well-structured organisation of urban primary health care to remedy the existing situation. A health care delivery system aimed at providing basic health and family welfare services to the population within 1 - 3 kms. of their dwellings will be made available by establishing Urban Health and Family Welfare Centres manned by medical and paramedical persons. These Centres will have:

1. adequate outpatient facility;
2. inpatient facility (at least 10 beds of which four will be for maternity care and the remaining beds will be for medical, surgical and paediatric care);
3. supportive services including laboratory and radiology facilities and pharmacy;
4. provision for referral/ transport of patients.

The essential services, to be provided, will includes are :

1. medical and surgical services including eye and ENT care;
2. obstetric care and new-born care and child health;
3. counselling for reproductive health and contraception
4. dental services;
5. emergency and trauma care;
6. prevention and control of communicable and noncommunicable diseases;

For effective integration of health-related services the urban health centres will co-ordinate with other assigned social sector activities of Nagar Palikas especially for provision of safe drinking water and sanitation.

An overview of all the facilities available in a defined geographical area will be undertaken and appropriate linkages between primary, secondary and tertiary care centres in the area will be established so that provision of basic minimum health services and optimal utilisation of the available health care facilities for referral services will be ensured. Earmarked funds under BMS and the ACA for BMS will be effectively utilised to fill the critical gaps in health manpower and infrastructure in urban areas also so that the performance of both health and family welfare programmes improve.

With the 73rd and 74th Constitutional amendments the Nagar Palikas and Panchayati Raj Institutions, are becoming operational in many States. During the Ninth Plan period, these institutions will play increasing role in ensuring planning, implementation and monitoring of health and family welfare services at the local level. They will also ensure effective coordination of programmes at the local level between related sectors such as sanitation, safe drinking water and women and child development, so that optimal benefit from all these programmes become available to the community and the vulnerable segments receive the attention that they need.

The status of primary health care infrastructure and manpower is being monitored by the Department of Family Welfare; it is also being monitored as a part of the MNP/20 point programme. The Central Bureau of Health Intelligence monitors the health care infrastructure, manpower and health status of the population. Planning Commission monitors the progress in PHC infrastructure/manpower annually during the Annual Plan discussions. These existing mechanisms of monitoring will continue and be strengthened in the Ninth Plan.

Secondary Health Care

The secondary health care infrastructure at the district hospitals today functions both as primary health care infrastructure for taking care of the needs of the population in the city/town in which it is located and as secondary care Centres. This dual role dilutes its effectiveness. To remedy the situation, initiatives were taken during the Eighth Plan to ensure that these hospitals are able to cope with the referred cases. Four States - Andhra Pradesh, Karnataka, West Bengal and Punjab - have initiated Secondary Health System Development Projects with special focus on strengthening the District Hospital and the referral services.

Secondary health care: Priorities in the Ninth Plan

— Provide adequate diagnostics, consumables and drugs

— Strengthen emergency services

— Provide care for high risk cases

— Establish effective, credible linkages with primary and tertiary care facilities in geographically delineated areas.

This step is expected to reduce the burden on the tertiary care hospitals, besides providing a credible and effective linkage with Primary Health Care Institutions. In order to raise resources to meet the recurring costs of good quality diagnostic and curative services, the feasibility of collecting user charges from patients (except those below the poverty line) is also being explored. These experiences will enable the States to evolve and implement appropriate schemes for strengthening these hospitals so that they cater to the increasing need for secondary care services during the Ninth Plan period. Increasing involvement of private and voluntary sector in secondary health care has been reported from many states. The mechanisms by which secondary health care services could be made readily available and affordable through collaboration between Government, private and voluntary sector will be explored during the Ninth Plan period.

Operational Strategy for the Ninth Plan

Nagar Palikas/ State governments will strengthen the primary health care network in urban areas so that the district hospitals act only as referral centre. This step is expected to reduce the burden on the secondary care hospitals and result in creation of a credible and effective linkage with Primary Health Care Institutions. In order to raise resources to meet the recurring costs of good quality diagnostic and curative services, the feasibility of collecting user charges from patients (except those below the poverty line) is being explored by some States. The mechanisms, by which secondary health care services could be made readily available and affordable through collaboration between Government, private and voluntary sector may have to be explored.

Tertiary Health Care

Tertiary health care problems:

— Growing demand for complex, costly diagnostic & therapeutic modalities

— Lack of skilled manpower, equipment & consumables to meet the demand

— Overcrowding

Ninth Plan priorities

— Provide funds for capacity building

— Levy user charges to people above poverty line

— Explore alternative modalities to meet the growing cost of care

Along with the emphasis on enhancing the outreach and quality of primary health care services and the strengthening of linkages with secondary care institutions, there is a need to optimise the facilities available in the tertiary care centres. At this level, there is an ever-widening gap between what is possible and what is affordable either for the individual or for the country. Majority of the tertiary care institutions in governmental sector lack adequate manpower and facilities to meet the rapidly growing demand for increasingly complex diagnostic and therapeutic modalities. Over the last two decades these institutions have been facing increasing resource crunch and have not been able to obtain spares for equipment maintenance, to replace obsolete equipment, to maintain supply of consumables and to upgrade the infrastructure necessary to provide high technology, high quality care at affordable cost to meet the ever increasing needs and rising expectation of the population. Several States have started levying user charges for the diagnostic and curative services offered in these institutions from people above the poverty line, to meet some of the recurring costs in providing such services.

During the Ninth Plan, efforts will be made to provide a one time support to selected tertiary care institutions in each State and Union Territory to update their technical capabilities and to evolve and implement a rational user charge policy that would enable these institutions to provide high quality tertiary care at affordable cost. Some of the States are also taking up experimental projects of establishment of pay clinics/ pay cabins for generating funds required by the institutions. Other States are exploring the feasibility of providing land, water and electricity at lower cost to private entrepreneurs for setting up tertiary care/ super speciality institutions if these entrepreneurs agree to provide 30% inpatient facilities and 40% of the out-patient /diagnostic services free of cost for people below poverty line. Exemption from import duty for import of diagnostic equipment has been given in the past to private/ voluntary agencies that had agreed to provide diagnostic services to poor patients free of cost. The advantages, disadvantages in these experiments need to be documented and those found useful replicated in other settings.

Levying user charges for the diagnostic and curative services offered in these institutions from people above the poverty line, to meet some of the recurring costs in providing such services have to be explored. The feasibility of providing a one time support to selected tertiary care institutions in each State and Union Territory to update their technical capabilities and to evolve and implement a rational user charge policy that would enable these institutions to provide high quality tertiary care at affordable cost may be tested. Some of the States are also taking up experimental projects of establishment of pay clinics/ pay cabins for generating funds required by the institutions. Necessary amendments have to be made to enable these hospitals to retain the funds generated by these activities so that they could be utilised to improve quality of services available. If found successful it might also be possible to use the income from pay clinics as cross subsidy for treatment of patients below poverty line.

Quality and Accountability in Health Care

Ensuring quality and bringing in accountability in health care provided is of utmost importance. In recent years, there has been increasing public concern over these issues because of both increasing awareness of the population and mushrooming growth of institutions providing health care especially in the private sector. The Consumer Protection Act provides one mechanism for redressal of grievances pertaining to quality of care. Some States have attempted to provide a legal framework for the functioning of private health care institutions on the lines of Bombay Nursing Home Registration Act 1949. Until now these legislative measures have not been effectively implemented mainly because of lack of objective criteria for defining 'quality of care' and the possible impact of such regulations on cost of care. The cumulative experience generated thus far will be utilised to evolve norms for quality and cost of health care and ensure accountability in a uniform standardised manner.

Development and utilisation of appropriate technologies for diagnosis and management of patients at primary, secondary and tertiary care is an essential pre-requisite for improvement in quality of health Services without unnecessary escalation in cost of health care. Realising the need for an in-depth review of the requirement for supportive and diagnostic services at primary, secondary and tertiary care a separate Working

Group on this subject was constituted prior to the formulation of the Ninth Plan.

During the Ninth Plan period the recommendations of the Working Group regarding diagnostic and supportive services at each level, technologies and equipment appropriate for each of these levels and maintenance of these will be implemented. In all major institutions, a Technical Appraisal Committee will be constituted to assess the essential requirements and prioritise the same according to funds available. A national mechanism for total quality appraisal of new technologies will be established. Efforts will be made for the development and testing of appropriate inexpensive technologies for:

1. measuring weight and height to facilitate early detection of under nutrition in adults and children;
2. colourimeters for bio-chemical test to improve diagnostic facilities at PHCs;
3. accurate self-recording instruments for measuring arterial blood-pressure for use by ANMs/male multi-purpose workers;
4. hand-held electronic data entry machines for ANM/MMPW to enable record maintenance and updating for Health and Family Welfare Programmes.

Health Insurance

Health insurance to meet the cost of hospitalisation for major illness will ensure that health care costs do not become a major financial burden or cause of indebtedness among these patients or their families. Over the last two decades several health insurance schemes have been introduced. There are individual, family and group insurance schemes for health care, senior citizens insurance and insurance for specific diseases. Some of the currently operationalised insurance schemes include Mediclaim, Group Medical Insurance Scheme, Group Health Insurance Scheme, Bavishya Arogya (Insurance for senior citizens), Senior Citizen UnitPlan, Cancer Insurance, Asha Deep and Jan Arogya Bima Policy.

The experience gained in the implementation of these schemes will provide useful inputs for planning health insurance schemes during the Ninth Plan period. The premium of health insurance may have to be adjusted on the basis of health status of the person and age of the person and his /her family at the time of entry into health insurance. Yearly 'no claim bonus'/ adjustment of the premium could be made on the basis of previous years hospitalisation cost reimbursed by the insurance scheme. This would be a mechanism through which the health education messages regarding the importance of remaining healthy through optimum utilisation of the preventive and promotive services as well as adopting a healthy life style get reinforced by economic incentives. Guidelines regarding what are the services for which reimbursement of treatment cost will be borne by the insurance company may have to be discussed, drawn up and implemented. Appropriate mechanisms through which the insurance premiums for the people below the poverty line are to be met will have to be evolved, tested and implemented.

Development of Human Resources for Health

The outcome and impact of any health programme depends on the competencies and skills of the personnel who implement it. Both in the State and in the Central sector, over 75% of the funds provided are spent to meet the salary of the employees. Personnel costs form a major portion of investment in health service delivery in voluntary and private sector. Unlike health service planning, health manpower planning in India has not received adequate attention. There has been very little attempt to assess the requirement in manpower and to match health manpower production with requirement. While the production of physicians and specialists has been more than the estimated requirement, dental and para-professional manpower production has lagged far behind the present and projected needs.

The curricula have not kept pace with the changing health care requirements of the population or skills and attitudes required for implementation of health and family welfare programmes. Continuous updating of skills and knowledge have not been made an essential mandatory requisite for all practicing health professionals. There are regional disparities both in quantity and quality of available health care professionals. These factors constitute a major impediment to effective implementation of the health and family welfare programmes.

During the Ninth Plan, the objectives will be:

1. to establish an Education Commission of Health Sciences with the assigned responsibility of planning and producing health manpower that is appropriate in quantity to the present and projected needs of the health system;
2. to strengthen the educational process for all categories of health professionals at all levels so that health care professionals possess necessary

knowledge and have appropriate skills, health programme orientation and people orientation;

3. to ensure continuing knowledge and skill upgradation of all health care providers through Continuing Education Programmes with emphasis on multi-professional problem solving learning strategies.

National Education Policy in Health Sciences

The need for National Education Policy in Health Sciences was emphasised in the reports of Medical Education Review Committee 1983 and Expert Committee on Health Manpower Planning, Production and Management 1986. A draft National Education Policy in Health Sciences was prepared by a Consultative Group under the Chairmanship of Member (Health). This draft Policy was adopted in the meeting of the Central Council of Health and Family Welfare held in 1993 and its salient features shall be implemented during the Ninth Plan. The Council recommended urgent action with respect of establishment of Education Commission in Health Sciences.

The Committee on Health Manpower Planning, Production and Management and the Ninth Plan Steering Committee on Human Resource Development for Health recommended that Education Commission in Health Sciences (ECHS) must be established as a Central Organisation on the lines of UGC to provide requisite financial and technical support for professional and para-professional education in health sciences, to provide realistic projection for national health manpower requirement and to establish suitable mechanism to continuously review the projections based on felt needs.

Major functions of the Education Commission to be constituted during Ninth Plan shall include :

1. provision of realistic projections for national health manpower requirements and to recommend the establishment of mechanism(s) through which such projections could be continuously reviewed in the context of evolving social epidemiological and demographic requirements.

2. creation of educational institutions and facilities, or strengthening of such facilities in already existing educational institutions through adequate financial and technical support so as to facilitate the production of projected health manpower, and establishment of one or more Universities of Health Sciences in all States/regions.

3. implementation of desired changes required to be brought about in the curricular contents and training programmes of medical and allied health professionals, at various levels of functioning, to optimise health care delivery system.

4. planning and implementation of appropriate changes in the educational system that would facilitate the establishment of essential inter-linkages between health functionaries of various grades.

5. establishment of a continuing review mechanism for the strengthening of health-related pedagogic communication and information technologies; development of such health- related community educational programmes, using distance education mode that could effectively and optimally utilise these technologies.

6. development of inbuilt mechanism of reviewing, monitoring, and mid-course corrections through financial and technical assistance so as to ensure expeditious implementation of recommendations and decisions.
7. co-ordination of intersectoral health systems research by interlinking the education of suitable manpower with mission oriented research needs.

The Commission will in consultation with the Universities and Professional Councils concerned, take all such steps as they may deem appropriate for the promotion and coordination of Education in health Sciences, including medical sciences at all levels, nursing, pharmaceutical and dental sciences and other categories of health care providers.

The Central Government has already initiated the process for obtaining approval for establishment of the Commission as a statutory body. Due to paucity of funds only a token provision of Rs.1 crore was made for establishment of the Commission during 1996-97. Sufficient funds shall be provided during the Ninth Plan to make the Commission fully operational.

The Universities of Health Sciences will be the implementing arm of ECHS for production, evaluation and sustenance of health manpower policy. The aim of the Universities of Health Sciences is to create a physical and academic environment where all Faculties of Health Sciences can interact together and provide a model for the education and training of health care teams, through multiprofessional and inter-professional education. In order to achieve this it was recommended by the Bajaj Committee that such Universities of Health Sciences be established in the country, one in each region to begin with and subsequently one for each major State. The Universities will affiliate all Medical Colleges, Dental Colleges, Para professional Colleges and Nursing Colleges, besides possibly considering grant of affiliation to Colleges of ISM&H, imparting graduate level education in the State.

These Universities may have one or more constituent professional colleges, and a number of study centres and field project areas. Three Universities have already been established in Andhra Pradesh, Tamil Nadu and Karnataka and another is being started in Punjab. Networking of these Universities with each other and through the ECHS shall be established. Attempts will be made to establish at least one University of Health Sciences in each region during the Ninth Plan period.

Health Manpower Planning

The Bhore Committee was the first to recommend a population-based norm for medical (1/1500) and nursing personnel (1/500). The Mudaliar Committee made realistic recommendations for progressive improvement in health manpower. A comprehensive situation analysis is available in the 1987 Report of the Expert Committee on Health Manpower, Planning Production and Management (Bajaj Committee). This Committee suggested that for assessment of health manpower requirement several parameters including functionary to population ratio, inter-professional ratio and manpower-mix must be considered. It was further emphasised that health manpower requirements would vary depending upon the income-elasticity and the public and private expenditure on health.

During the Ninth Plan, health manpower planning will be linked to the needs and demands of health services. In addition, a fine tuning will be under taken regarding health manpower development required for components of the programme and health

The Eighth Plan clearly stated that "the existing facilities for training of medical graduates has outstepped the needs. No new medical college or an increase in the admission capacity of the existing colleges will be supported during the Eighth Plan". The Indian Medical Council Act was amended in 1993. According to this amendment "no person shall establish a medical college and no medical college shall open a new or a higher course of study or training including a post graduate course of study or training or increase in its admission capacity in any course of study or training, without the prior permission of the Central Government".

The Central Government after due clearance from the Medical Council of India may grant permission for establishment of new Medical Colleges if there was a requirement for manpower in the field of practice of medicine and if other conditions specified in the enabling provisions of the Act are fulfilled. A strict compliance of these provisions is called for.

During the Ninth Plan, no new medical college will be opened nor will there be any expansion in the admission capacity of existing institutions as there are adequate number of doctors in the country. Already, over two third of the doctors are undergoing postgraduate training. Hence there is no need for any addition to existing number of seats in various post graduate institutions, except for identified specialities with un met manpower needs.

There is an acute shortage of dental manpower in the country. There is a need to ensure that adequate number of dental professionals of appropriate quality is trained. The dental colleges are unevenly distributed in the country. As many as 41 out of 96 dental colleges are in one State. The quality of dental education needs to be reviewed and appropriate remedial measures instituted.

Nursing education and nursing services have been given a high priority in order to bridge the large gap between requirement and availability of nurses and ensure quality of nursing training. These efforts will be continued during the Ninth Plan. In addition, efforts will be made to meet the increasing demand for nurses with specialised training in speciality and sub-speciality areas intensive medical and surgical care in hospitals and for public health nurses in health care system.

Many programmes are faltering because of lack of critical para-professional manpower. Over the last three decades, there has been an increasing requirement of several categories of paramedical persons such as male multipurpose worker, laboratory technicians, radiographers. Their availability and requirement vary from State to State and from time to time. Till the Eighth Plan the medical colleges, dental colleges and nursing training institutions have been the major training institutions for para-professionals.

During the Eighth Plan the Open University system and the vocational training courses at 10 + 2 stream have provided two additional mechanisms for education and training of paramedical manpower. During the Ninth Plan the State manpower cells will assess the changing requirements for para-professionals, preferably at the district level and take necessary steps to meet the requirement through all available training channels. The Universities of Health Sciences (UHS) will ensure that appropriate curricula are evolved and followed. The State Governments will make necessary amendments in recruitment rules for these posts so that those who qualify through vocational courses and open university system become eligible for the jobs in Government, voluntary and private sectors. The feasibility of introducing pre-vocational courses at the 9th and 10th standards will be explored.

Ninth Plan priorities for Human Resources Development for Health include:

- Creation of a district data base on requirement, demand and availability for health manpower in the Govt., Private and voluntary sectors
- Periodic updating of information on:
- Requirement of different categories of health manpower
- Availability of health manpower
- Health manpower production based on the needs
- Improvement in quality of undergraduate/ postgraduate education
- Efforts to promote appropriate health manpower distribution
- Continuing medical education for skill upgradation and appropriate people and programme orientation
- Continuing multiprofessional education for promoting team work & intersectoral co-ordination

The health manpower information should encompass all the components of the health manpower management. The Committee recommends development of national health manpower information system as an important support to the health manpower development strategies."

While recommending the establishment of Universities of Health Sciences, it was further emphasized that "it is entirely likely that several new faculties will grow in the University of Health Sciences: It is expected that a faculty of health information systems shall also be established in the Health Science Universities".

In spite of these far reaching recommendations, necessary action plans have yet to the concretised. Information Technology (IT) is now becoming one of the major components of the technological infrastructure for health management. All sub-sectors dealing with the generation, transmission and utilisation of demographic and epidemiological data such as bio-informatics, bio-statistics, health management information system (HMIS) and decision support systems (DSS) are finding increasing use in health planning and management.

With the nation-wide network, NICNET, under the Planning Commission, giving health information support through its MEDLARS, Bio Medical Informatics Programme and Tele-Medicine Programme, a viable nucleus has already been set up which will be enhanced during the Plan period to cover all the Primary Health Centres and district hospitals. MEDNET, when operational, may become a major tool of continuing multiprofessional education and distance learning. Policy initiatives shall be undertaken during the Ninth Plan with the aim of developing clinical leadership, deciding which applications are to be supported, providing the appropriate technology, gaining clinician acceptance, setting up in Universities of Health Sciences one or more clinician-driven academic unit(s) and network(s) that are multidisciplinary and multisite to provide support for new and existing biomedical applications.

Health Manpower Information System

At the moment only infrastructure and manpower at the primary health care institutions are monitored and information periodically updated. There is no mechanism for obtaining and analysing information on health care infrastructure and manpower in private and voluntary sectors in the district.

Unless this information is available it will not be possible to undertake any effective area-specific micro planning so that the health manpower required to meet the local health needs of the population is provided. This exercise becomes even more important in the current context when the population is undergoing a demographic, health and economic transition and there are marked differences in the health profile between States and districts. There is also the need for aggregating this data at the State and Central level so that appropriate policy and programme initiatives can be undertaken and adequate resources allocated.

During the Ninth Plan, attempts will be made to create a district data base on health manpower belonging to various categories (including the ISM&H practitioners) working in Central and State Government, voluntary, private sectors, defense services and Railways and public sector undertakings. The District Manpower Cell will assess district manpower requirement and availability and assist the State in manpower planning at district level. District-based manpower profile data will be updated at least once a year.

Health manpower planning exercise at district, State and regional level by the University of Health Sciences will be carried out utilising this data and the information on the health care needs of the population and health facilities available. The Education Commission for Health Sciences (ECHS) will act as the nodal agency for the exercise at the national level.

The Health Manpower Planning, Production and Management Committee in 1987 recommended that the ECHS must be established as a central organisation on the lines of UGC for professional and para-professional education in health sciences, inter alia to provide realistic projection for national health manpower requirement and suitable mechanism to continuously review the projections based on felt needs.

During the Ninth Plan period, the ECHS will promote all educational activities for all categories of health manpower at all levels. The UHS will develop newer faculties such as health management, health economics, social and behavioural sciences.

UHS will also initiate necessary steps to enhance computer literacy among medical students and expose them to emerging technologies of informatics and telematics which are likely to be the base and basis for 21st century mode of communication through telemedicine and distance learning by open learning system in medicine and health sciences. Health manpower cells in the States will coordinate collection of data on manpower at district level and implement there commendations of UHS for health manpower production.

Quality of Education in Health Sciences

One of the important reasons for the sub-optimal performance of health care institutions is the poor quality and inappropriateness of the education and training of health care providers, resulting in a lack of problem-solving competencies and skills. During the Ninth Plan period, appropriate changes in syllabi, curricula, teaching methods and assessment system will be made through various professional Councils to improve the undergraduate and post-graduate training so that the medical and dental graduates as well as allied health professionals acquire necessary technical knowledge and managerial skills to solve health problems and implement ongoing major national health and family welfare programmes within the existing constraints.

Medical colleges are periodically inspected by the Medical Council of India (MCI) regarding both the physical facilities and training process. During the Ninth Plan, inspection by the MCI will be not only for initial recognition but also for continued recognition as medical colleges and admissions will not be permitted unless the college is recognised. Attempts will be made to reorient education in health sciences so that the health care system becomes more efficient and effective. The existing professional Councils and any other Council which may be established in the future, will be responsible for ensuring the quality of medical and paramedical education, training and ethics of conduct and practices as per the statutory requirements.

In the context of the rapidly evolving technology, demographic transition, changing lifestyles and disease patterns it is imperative that the process of continuing education is internalised throughout the working career of all health professionals so that their knowledge and skills are updated. Currently, in-service training courses in various institutions, thematic CME programmes conducted by National Academy of Medical Sciences, National Board of Examinations, and various professional bodies and associations have played a major role in CME. All these programmes will be expanded and intensified during the Ninth Plan. In addition, Open Universities will play a major role in periodically updating the skills and knowledge of various categories of health personnel.

The Open University mechanism can efficiently and cost effectively provide specific training programmes where there is a major component of didactic learning eg. epidemiology, hospital administration and health management. It is also likely to be one of the most effective, efficient and cost-effective method of CME involving practitioners in Government, private and voluntary sectors and hence requires increased utilisation.

During the Ninth Plan, a major programme of multi-professional and inter-professional education will be initiated for training the members of health care delivery team, so as to enable them to accomplish group tasks in providing health care in the community. At the national level there will be training of the trainers in newer technologies, national programmes on emerging diseases and their management. At the State level there will be a similar training of personnel with special reference to the State's requirement. At the district level two types of training programmes have to be undertaken:

1) the multi- professional health team training in delivery of integrated health and family welfare service at the primary health care level; and
2) the training of the multi-professional team for the delivery of evolving programmes eg. the delivery of RCH care programme.

In addition, there will be training of the health professionals working in the government, voluntary and the private sectors together as a team to tackle the identified health problems in the district. Inter-sectoral training of personnel from related sectors e.g., nutrition, agriculture, water resource management and environmental sanitation will be undertaken as and when necessary.

Operational strategy for ninth plan

1. Attempts will have to be made to create a district data base on health manpower belonging to various categories including ISM&H practitioners working for Govt., voluntary and private sectors. Based on the availability, need and demand appropriate policy and programme initiatives for manpower development have to be made at State/district level.
2. Improvement in quality of pre-service and in-service training for medical and paramedical personnel.
3. Periodic updating of knowledge/skill for all categories of health manpower throughout their working careers so that they are able to provide appropriate quality of health care is essential. In addition to available training programmes increasing use may have to be made of the distance learning.

Control of Communicable Diseases

At the time of independence communicable diseases were the major cause of morbidity and mortality in the country. Efforts were therefore initially directed towards their prevention and control. Small pox, a major killer in pre-Independence era has been eradicated. In 1953, malaria affected over 75 million and killed 0.8 million people.

Strategies to improve performance of Disease Control Programmes during Ninth Plan:

— Rectify identified defects in design and delivery

— Fill critical gaps in infrastructure and manpower

— Make service delivery responsive to user needs

— Ensure skill upgradation, supplies, and referral services

— Improve community awareness, participation and effective utilisation of available services

The National Malaria Control Programme, which was launched in 1953, successfully brought down the incidence of malaria to 0.1 million cases with no death by 1965. Subsequently, there has been a resurgence of malaria. The Modified Plan of Operation has, however, succeeded in keeping morbidity and mortality at relatively low levels. The use of antibiotics has resulted in a substantial reduction in deaths due to common infections. Effective therapy for infections and vaccines for prevention of infection were the major factors responsible for the steep fall in crude death rate from 25.1 in 1951 to 8.9 in 1996.

However, the morbidity due to communicable diseases continues to be high. Deteriorating urban and rural sanitation, poor liquid and solid waste management and overcrowding have resulted in an increasing prevalence of common communicable diseases. The re-emergence of diseases like Kala Azar, and emergence of new infections like HIV have added to the existing disease burden due to communicable diseases. Control of communicable diseases is becoming more difficult because of emergence of drug-resistant pathogens and development of insecticide-resistant vectors.

Even though health is a State subject, the Central Government has over the last forty years provided additional funds through Centrally Sponsored Schemes (CSS) for control of some of the major communicable diseases. Of these, the National Leprosy Eradication Programme is likely to achieve its objective of reduction in leprosy prevalence to below 1 per 10000 by the end of the Ninth Plan. However, malaria, tuberculosis and HIV infection require vigorous and intensified efforts for their containment and control.

The performance in, and shortcomings of, these National Programmes have been evaluated during the Eighth Plan period by Expert Committees. Accordingly, following remedial measures will be taken during the Ninth Plan period to:

1. rectify the identified defects in the design and delivery of these programmes;
2. fill the critical gaps in infrastructure and manpower;
3. improve the operational efficiency and the quality of services;

4. make service delivery system more responsive to users needs;
5. ensure that health care providers have the necessary skills and support, including referral facilities and supplies they need;
6. improve the community awareness of the existing services through IEC efforts so that there is optimal utilisation of available services.

External assistance has been obtained to augment available funds for implementing these programmes. These National Programmes will continue as CSS during the Ninth Plan period.

Initially, when sufficient infrastructure and manpower were not available for management of major health problems, several vertical programmes eg. National Malaria Eradication Programme (NMEP), National Leprosy Eradication Programme (NLEP) were initiated. Subsequently, over the years a three-tier health care infrastructure has been established. During the Ninth Plan period, efforts will be made to integrate the existing vertical programmes at district level and ensure that primary health care institutions will provide comprehensive health and family welfare services to the population.

In order to assist the PHC/ CHCs officers to effectively implement such a horizontal integration, the middle level public health programme managers who are currently heading the vertical programmes at district level will be given the additional task of ensuring coordination and implementation of integrated Health and Family Welfare Programme at Primary Health Care institutions in defined blocks. Involvement of the public health specialists at the subdistrict level will also improve data collection, reporting, strengthening HMIS, improving the supply of essential drugs/devices for all programmes at PHCs/CHCs and enabling operationalisation of the disease surveillance and response at district level.

Given the existing conditions of poor environmental sanitation and the weakness of the public health system it may not be possible to completely prevent outbreaks of communicable diseases in the near future. Delays in recognition and reporting of focal outbreaks, absence of functioning HMIS and disease surveillance system result in delays in implementation of appropriate response and consequent high morbidity and even mortality. The Expert Committee on Public Health System chaired by Member (Health), Planning Commission recommended the establishment of an epidemiological surveillance system.

During the Ninth Plan, establishment of a functioning system for early detection and prompt response for rapid containment and control of the disease outbreak will receive high priority. Disease surveillance and response will be at district level to ensure prompt, effective, efficient remedial action utilising the existing infrastructure. This system will be given the necessary back-up, laboratory and epidemiological support so that containment measures are based on sound data and scientific rationale. This back-up system will be evolved by strengthening and optimal utilisation of the facilities and expertise available in the national institutions/ medical colleges.

The regulations governing notification of diseases vary widely between States. There is an urgent need to develop a uniform regulation for notification of diseases in all States. The diseases that are to be covered under the notification system should consider adequately the problems of new, emerging and re-emerging infections so that appropriate response could be generated to tackle the situation.

Hospital infection control and waste management

Increasing incidence of hospital-acquired infections and accidental infection in health care providers and waste disposers, renders it imperative that efforts are made to improve infection control and waste management through utilisation of appropriate, affordable technology at all levels of health care. During the Ninth Plan period, infection control and waste management in all health care institutions will receive due attention and adequate funding.

National Malaria Eradication Programme (NMEP)

In the early fifties, malaria was not only a major cause of morbidity and mortality in the country but also one of the constraints for ongoing developmental efforts. Illness due to malaria was a major cause of absenteeism in agricultural and industrial labour and in irrigation and construction workers in the fifties. The National Malaria Control Programme, the first of the Health Sector CSS, aimed at reduction of the morbidity and mortality due to malaria, was launched in 1953. It is noteworthy that even though there was no well established health infrastructure in rural areas, the number of cases came down from 70 million in 1950 to 0.1 million by 1965.

However, subsequently, there was a resurgence of malaria. In 1976 over 6.7 million cases were reported. From 1977, the NMEP started implementing a Modified Plan of Operations for control of malaria. After the initial success the number of cases have remained at over 2 million.

Initially, malaria in India was mainly a rural disease. Subsequently, due to major ecological changes five more eco-types have been recognised viz., forest and forest fringe malaria; rural malaria; urban malaria; industrial malaria; border malaria and migration malaria. The North Eastern (NE) States have high incidence of P. falciparum malaria. High morbidity, mortality due to malaria and emerging problem of drug resistance are reported. A major initiative during the Eighth Plan was to provide 100% Central Assistance for NMEP in NE States so that financial constraints do not come in the way of effective implementation of the NMEP. There has been an increase in the number of cases of malaria reported during the Eighth Plan period. The proportion of Pf infection has increased to 40 per cent. Many of the fever patients are not screened, diagnosed and effectively treated primarily because of lack of male multipurpose worker and laboratory technicians. Not all the diagnosed cases are reported to the programme authorities. Residual insecticide spraying is often not done at appropriate.time. Community involvement in spray operations and the bioenvironmental measures for control of mosquito breeding are poor. Some of the vectors of malaria have developed resistance to one, two or three of the currently used insecticides.

There is an urgent need to intensify the malaria control activities during the Ninth Plan period especially in the States which had been reporting large number of malaria cases. The NMEP has, therefore, drawn up a programme for intensive and effective implementation of the Modified Plan of Operation (MPO) in malariogenic areas in the country during the Ninth Plan. Financial assistance has been procured from the World Bank for augmenting domestic funds available for implementation of the programme.

The criteria for selecting the areas for intensive implementation of MPO during the Ninth Plan are: Modified Plan of operation for NMEP during the Ninth Plan Intensification of control activities in areas with:

— API of > 2 in the last three years

— Pf rate of > 30%

— Reported deaths due to malaria

— > 25% of the population is tribal

Components of the Modified Plan of Operation

— Early diagnosis and prompt treatment

— Selective vector control & personal protection

— Prediction , early detection & effective response to out breaks

—IEC

Targets for 2002

— ABER of over 10%

— API <0.5%

— 25% reduction in morbidity and mortality due to malaria

i. annual parasite incidence of more than 2 for the last 3 years;

ii. Pf. rate of more than 30%; deaths due the malaria reported

iii. tribals form more than 25% of the population.

The areas identified on the basis of these criteria are the 7 North Eastern States and 100 districts spread over the States of Andhra Pradesh, Bihar, Gujarat, Madhya Pradesh, Maharashtra, Orissa and Rajasthan.

The ongoing programme with 100 percent Central assistance in the seven North-Eastern States will be continued during the Ninth Plan. Additional inputs will be provided to the 100 hardcore and tribal districts identified on the basis of the above criteria. Enhanced malaria control programme will also be implemented in 19 cities/ towns which have rising slide-positivity rate and in areas where there have been focal outbreaks of malaria in the previous year. The main components of MPO that will be strengthened in these areas are:

1. early diagnosis and prompt treatment, through strengthening of active and passive surveillance and laboratory diagnosis;
2. selective vector control by integrating various vector control approaches and, promotion of personal protection methods;
3. prediction, early detection and effective response to malaria outbreaks;
4. intensified information, education and communication campaign.

In spite of the reported increase in drug resistance, Chloroquin will remain the first line drug for presumptive treatment and Primaquine will be given for radical treatment. Sulpha pyrimethamine drug combination will remain as the second line of treatment especially for Pf cases in areas where drug resistance is reported and selective use of quinine will continue for treatment of severe and complicated malaria.

The village will be the unit for residual insecticide spray operations. DDT will continue to be the insecticide of choice in areas where vector is sensitive because of its efficacy and cost effectiveness. In areas where DDT is ineffective, Malathion may be used. Synthetic pyrethroids will be used only in areas where triple insecticide resistance is reported. Personal protection through use of insecticide impregnatedbed nets will be advocated. In urban areas stringent measures to prevent stagnation of water, ensure covering of overhead tanks and drains and enforcing periodic cleaning will be attempted.

With effective implementation of the Programme, it is expected that by the end of the Ninth Plan the following targets will be achieved in malariogenic areas:

1. ABER of over 10%;
2. API less than 0.5% and
3. 25% reduction in morbidity and mortality due to malaria.

Available data indicates that Kala-azar is endemic in 36 districts in Bihar and 10 districts in West Bengal (population 75 million). Periodic outbreaks of Kala-azar with increase in morbidity and mortality continue to occur in these States. Over 90% of the reported cases and over 95% of the reported deaths are from Bihar. Over two third of the cases in Bihar are reported from 7 districts.

The Government of India is implementing a CSS for control of Kala-azar in Bihar and West Bengal. Following reported increase in the number of cases and deaths due to Kala azar in 1989-91, an intensive programme for containment of Kala-azar was launched in 1992.

The strategy for control of infection includes interruption of transmission through insecticidal spraying with DDT and early diagnosis and treatment of Kala-azar cases. The Government of India is providing insecticides and anti Kala-azar drugs. The State Governments meet the expenses involved in the diagnosis and treatment and insecticide spraying operations.

Effective implementation of the programme resulted in a decline in both Kala-azar cases and deaths during 1993-95. However, there were delays and inadequacy of the insecticidal spray operations during 1995-96 and the decline could not be maintained.

Dengue outbreaks have been reported from urban areas from all States. All the four types of dengue virus exist in India. The vector Aedes Aegypti breeds in peridomestic fresh water collections and is found in both urban and rural areas. Analysis of available data from 54 dengue outbreaks between 1954 and 1995 indicate that:

1. dengue outbreaks occur both in urban and rural areas; and
2. over the years there has been an increase in reported cases of dengue, dengue haemorrhagic fever and dengue shock syndrome.

Diagnostic tests for dengue virus are not readily available in most parts of the country. At present, there is no mechanism for monitoring and surveillance for dengue.

During the Ninth Plan efforts will be made to:

1. establish an organised system of surveillance and monitoring;
2. strengthen facilities for early diagnosis and prompt treatment;
3. intensify IEC efforts to ensure that all households implement peridomestic measures to reduce breeding of Aedes.

Japanese Encephalitis

Japanese Encephalitis (JE) has been reported in the country since mid fifties. With increasing development of irrigation projects and changing pattern of water resource management there has been a progressive increase in number of States reporting cases in India. Twelve States/ UTs have reported outbreaks of JE in the last decade and 378 million population is exposed to risk of JE. The NMEP has been implementing the recommendations of the Expert Committee on JE control. However, implementation of the strategies for improving clinical management, vector control, disease surveillance and health education has been sub-optimal in most States. During the Ninth Plan efforts will be made to intensify all these activities.

Efforts to reduce morbidity and mortality due to vector-borne diseases by appropriate vector control measures aimed at reduction of disease transmission and strengthening of facilities for early diagnosis and treatment of cases in primary and secondary care settings will be continued in the Ninth Plan. Information, education and communication (IEC) activities to ensure community awareness and cooperation, in programmes for prevention, early detection and appropriate treatment of vector borne diseases will be intensified.

National Tuberculosis Control Programme (NTCP)

Tuberculosis is a major health problem in India. The aim of the fight against tuberculosis is at individual level to cure disease, to preserve and quickly restore work capacity, to allow the person to be within the family and community and in this way to maintain their socio-economic status and at the community level, to reduce the risk of tuberculosis infection through case finding and their appropriate management and care. Studies carried out by the Indian Council of Medical Research (ICMR) in the fifties and sixties showed that:

1. unlike the situation in developed countries, BCG did not protect against adult TB and BCG given at/ soon after birth provided some protection against TB in infancy and early childhood.
2. domiciliary treatment with anti TB drugs was safe and effective.

A National Tuberculosis Control Programme was initiated in 1962 as a CSS. The programme was aimed at early case detection in symptomatic patients reporting to the health system through sputummicroscopy and X-ray and effective domiciliary treatment with standard chemotherapy. BCG vaccination at birth was incorporated into the immunisation programme. The Short Course Chemotherapy (SCC) which shortened the duration of treatment to nine months was begun in selected districts in 1983. Over the years, 293 districts were included for SCC.

During the last three decades, because of low case detection, case holding and cure rates, the programme has not succeeded in bringing down the disease burden, in spite of availability of effective chemotherapy. Estimates based on available limited data from small-scale epidemiological studies indicate that the prevalence of active disease continues to be 1.4 per cent. It is estimated that there are about 14 million cases of active tuberculosis. Of these 3.5 million are highly infectious sputum positive tuberculosis cases. With the HIV-TB co-infection the incidence of tuberculosis may increase significantly from the current 1.8 per thousand.

About 1.5 million TB cases are detected and reported by the programme annually. Of these 25% are sputum positive. It is estimated that about 1.5 million cases are detected and treated by the private sector. Both under-diagnosis (missing sputum positive cases) and over-diagnosis (by X-Ray) occur. Under programme conditions completion of therapy is only 30 per cent. Long duration of treatment schedule (especially conventional therapy), irregular supply of drugs, poor follow-up of patients under treatment, lack of counselling regarding adverse consequences of incomplete therapy are some of the major factors responsible for the low treatment completion rates.

A major review of NTCP was undertaken during the Eighth Plan to identify inadequacies in the ongoing programmes and suggest remedial measures. A Revised National Tuberculosis Control Programme (RNTCP) was drawn up with the following aims: (1) to improve cure/completion of therapy rates to 85% by providing drugs for short course chemotherapy (SCC) and strengthening monitoring and supervision of patients under treatment;

and (2) to improve case detection to 70% by providing critical personnel and improving their skills through training.

The RNTCP has been pilot tested in 17 project sites (population of 13.85 million) in different parts of the country during the last three years. The cure rates achieved ranged between 60 and 80%. Encouraged by the results achieved in the pilot projects, it was decided to extend the strategy in a phased manner during the Ninth Plan period. Assistance from the World Bank has augmented the resources available for the Programme during the Ninth Plan period when:

Revised National Tuberculosis Control Programme (RNTCP).

— RNTCP will be implemented in 102 districts

— NTCP will be strengthened in 203 SCC districts

— Strengthening of standard regime in remaining non SCC districts

— Strengthening of Central institutions, State TB Cells & State TB training Institutions

Targets upto 2002

— Enhance case detection to at least 70% of estimated incidence.

— Achieve at least 85% cure rate among smear positive cases in 102 RNTCP districts and 60% cure rate in SCC districts.

— Reduce proportion of smear negative detected to 50% or less of the total cases.

— Ensure no. of TB suspects tested for smear positives is not less than 2.5% of OPD in PHIs and no. of smear tested is at least 3 per suspected patient.

— RNTCP will be implemented in 102 districts;

— NTCP will be strengthened in 203 Short Course Chemotherapy (SCC) districts as a transitional step to adopt the RNTCP;

— Standard regime will be strengthened in the remaining non SCC districts, and the Central Institutions, State TB Cells, & State TB Training Institutions throughout the country will be strengthened.

The targets for the Ninth Plan are:

i. to enhance case detection to at least 70% of the estimated incidence.

ii. to achieve at least 85% cure rate amongst smear positive patients of Tuberculosis in 102 districts implementing RNTCP and 60% cure rates in 203 SCC districts;

iii. to reduce the proportion of smear negatives detected under the programme to 50% or less of the total cases.

iv. to improve the aggregate smear positivity rate at least to 50%.

v. to ensure that the number of TB suspects tested for smear examination is not less than 2.5% of the general OPD attendance of the PHIs and number of smears examined is at least 3 per suspected patient.

It is expected that with the implementation of this Programme over the next 5 years (a) the total number of patients cured will increase to 32.55 lakh (compared to estimated 22.89 lakh who will be curedif NTCP in its original form is continued) and (b) 1.8 lakh deaths will be prevented.

National Leprosy Eradication Programme (NLEP)

Leprosy has been a major public health problem in India. In 1984 it was estimated that there were nearly four million cases of leprosy in the country, 15% of which were children. Recognising that leprosy was a major cause of disability and the infected persons face social ostracism, several non-governmental organisations and social service/voluntary agencies had taken up treatment and rehabilitation of leprosy patients right from the pre-Independence period. However, the outreach of these services was very limited. With the availability of Multi Drug Therapy (MDT) it became possible to cure leprosy cases within a relatively short period (6-24 months) of treatment. The National Leprosy Eradication Programme was launched as a 100% Centrally funded CSS in 1983 with the goal of arresting disease transmission and bringing down the prevalence of leprosy to 1/10000 by 2000 AD. The strategy adopted was:

i. early detection of leprosy cases through active surveillance by trained health workers;

ii. regular treatment of cases with MDT administered by leprosy workers in endemic district and Mobile Leprosy Treatment Units & Primary Health Care Workers in moderate to low endemic areas/ districts;

iii. intensified health education and public awareness campaigns to remove social stigma attached to the disease.

iv. appropriate medical rehabilitation and leprosy ulcer care services.

The programme was initially taken up in endemic districts and was extended to all districts in the country from 1994 with World Bank assistance. The estimated number of persons requiring treatment for leprosy has declined from four million cases in 1984 to 0.54 million cases in March 1996. More than 6.98 million leprosy patients have been cured by MDT and the proportion of registered patients taking MDT treatment has increased from 10% in 1985 to 96% in 1997. The prevalence rate of leprosy has declined from 57.3 per ten thousand population in 1981 to 5.8 per ten thousand population in 1995. However, the number of new leprosy cases detected each year has remained about 0.45 million.

The performance during the Eighth Plan has been satisfactory with respect to new case detection and treatment completion but less than optimal with respect to the reduction in total cases mainly due to treatment of backlog of cases. The incidence of the disease has not shown a marked decline. Earlier 50% of cases were in Andhra Pradesh and Tamil Nadu. Now over 50% of the cases requiring treatment are in UP, MP, Bihar and West Bengal. The laboratory support for diagnosis and assessing the success of treatment is sub-optimal. Available information on recurrence, relapse rates and reactions to drug therapy is inadequate. Even though leprosy infection has been cured, the deformities and disabilities associated with leprosy continue to require treatment and these have not been looked after. During the Ninth Plan the strategy will be:

1. strengthening laboratory services in PHC/CHC, establishing surveillance system for monitoring time

trends in prevalence of the disease throughout the country

2. accelerating the pace of activities, intensifying case detection and MDT coverage in high prevalence States and areas that are difficult to access;

Strategies for NLEP during the Ninth Plan:

— Intensifying case detection and MDT coverage in high prevalence States and areas difficult to access

— Strengthening laboratory services in PHC/CHC, establishing surveillance system for monitoring time trends

— Preparing for & initiating horizontal integration of leprosy programme into primary health care system

— Providing greater emphasis on disability prevention and treatment

— Implementation of Modified Leprosy Elimination campaign

— Ensuring rehabilitation of cured patients.

— Repeal of discriminatory provision under marriage act where leprosy is ground for divorce

Target for Ninth Plan are:

— Reduce prevalence of leprosy to 1/10000.

3. maintaining activities in the previously highly endemic areas;

4. preparing for and initiating horizontal integration of the leprosy programme into the primary health care system.

5. greater emphasis on disability prevention and management through :(a) transfer of knowledge and

technology to affected persons, families, community; (b) strengthening local treatment facilities for ulcers/ leprosy related deformities; © supply of aids and appliances to prevent further impairment; (d) developing trained manpower resources and improving facilities for corrective surgery for deformities

6. implementation of Modified Leprosy Elimination campaign and bringing mass public awareness, training of general health care staff and detection of hidden cases
7. ensuring rehabilitation of cured patients.
8. repeal of discriminatory provision under marriage act where leprosy is one of the grounds of divorce.

National AIDS Control Programme

Sexually transmitted diseases (STD) have been a global problem since time immemorium. Fear of STD and pregnancy had been the major deterrents against promiscuous multi-partner sex and hence, STD levels remained relatively low in general population. With the ready availability of antibiotics for treatment of STD and contraceptives for prevention of pregnancy, sexual mores in most countries underwent a change during the last three decades. Increasing multi partner sex and consequent increase in STD were reported from many countries. Increase in STD rates did not result in rising morbidity or mortality rates because of availability of effective treatment. With the advent of HIV infection the situation underwent a dramatic change because there is no effective drug for treatment or vaccine for protection against HIV infection.

In India, a National STD Control Programme has been in operation since 1967. Its outreach and coverage have been sub-optimal. Available data from small-scale studies indicate that the annual incidence of STD may be about 5% (40 million new cases every year). This however, could be gross underestimate or overestimate. There is no nationwide surveillance system for STD.

The ICMR initiated a National Sero surveillance for HIV infection in 1986 not only among the high-risk groups but also among general population to define the magnitude and major mode of transmission of HIV infection in the country. India was the first country in the world to initiate national sero surveillance in the silent phase of the HIV epidemic. The data from the sero surveillance showed that

1. heterosexual transmission was the major mode of transmission of HIV infection in the country,
2. in the North-Eastern States transmission through contaminated syringes/needles among IV drug users was the major mode of transmission
3. transmission through contaminated blood/blood products and vertical transmission from infected mother to her offspring occur in all States

The apparent differences between States/ districts/ cities might to a large extent be due to differences in the type and number of persons screened. Over the last ten years there has been a progressive rise in the prevalence of infection in all groups. However, the prevalence of infection in the screened population still remains low. Utilising the available data on estimated size of high, intermediate, and low risk groups and available data on sero prevalence in these three groups, ICMR had estimated that the number of HIV infected persons in the country is between 2 and 3 million. More than 50% of them are women and children. Every year approximately 30,000 deliveries in India occur among sero positive women and between 6-8000 infants are perinatally infected with HIV. At present the number of AIDS patients in the country is small. However, over the next decade persons who got infected in the eighties will develop AIDS, resulting in a steep and progressive increase in the number of AIDS patients in India.

Realising the gravity of the HIV epidemic in the country, the Central Government initiated a National AIDS Control Programme in 1992 as a 100% Centrally funded CSS. Adequate funds initially from the national budget, augmented later through Externally Assisted Projects (EAP), were provided for the programme to combat and minimise the magnitude of HIV epidemic. The programme right from its inception has operated through existing health care system at various levels. The major components of the Programme include:

1. obtaining epidemiological data on HIV infection through Sentinel Sero Surveillance and AIDS surveillance;
2. strengthening STD Control including HIV/AIDS control;
3. improving facilities for clinical management of AIDS cases;
4. ensuring safety of blood/ blood products through establishment of comprehensive blood transfusion services. This will also facilitate screening for transfusion transmitted diseases;
5. improving awareness through IEC.

There have been delays in the implementation of the Programme in many States. The performance under STD control and blood banking components had been sub-optimal in all States. The IEC activities had improved awareness in some States; however, the effect, if any, on behavioural change appears to be marginal. Sentinel surveillance, which is an essential component for forecasting the future course of the epidemic in the country has not been carried out according to protocol in most States. Because of this, there is lack of epidemiological database for forecasting the epidemic in the country and evolving appropriate, affordable interventions. Utilisation of funds under the programme has also been sub optimal.

Soon after Independence, the focus of the health sector programme of the Government was on control of communicable diseases. However, the programmes (either Central Sector or Centrally Sponsored) for control of some non-communicable diseases which were perceived as public health problems were also initiated. The National Goitre Control Programme initiated in 1962 is the oldest Central Sector Scheme for control of non-communicable diseases (NCD). The National Blindness Control Programme the first CSS was initiated in 1976. Subsequently, several Central Sector Schemes for control of non-communicable diseases, including the following were taken up:

1. National Cancer Control Programme
2. Programme against micro nutrient malnutrition
3. National Mental Health programme
4. Diabetes Control Programme

5. Cardiovascular Disease Control Programme
6. Prevention of Deafness and Hearing Impairment
7. Oral Health programme
8. Medical Rehabilitation

In addition some of the State Governments have initiated pilot projects for district based integrated non-communicable disease control in some districts.

National blindness control programme

Programme Priorities during Ninth Plan:

— To improve the quality of cataract surgery, clear the backlog of cataract cases

— To improve quality of care by skill upgradation of eye care personnel

— To improve service delivery through NGO and Public sector collaboration

— Increase coverage of eye care delivery among underprivileged population.

Targets for the period 1997-2002

— 17.5 million cataract operations

— 100,000 corneal implants

It is estimated that there are 12.5 million economically blind persons in India. Of these over 50% of blindness is due to cataract. It is estimated that every year about 2 million cases of blindness occur in the country. Most of cataract blind individuals are in their 60s. They may not have the means for cataract surgery. These patients may also have difficulty in accessing services, unless services are available in the vicinity of their house. The National Blindness Control Programme was initiated in 1976 with the objective of providing comprehensive eye care services at primary, secondary and tertiary health care level and achieving substantial reduction in prevalence of eye disease in general and blindness in particular.

The long term objective is to reduce prevalence of blindness from 1.4% to 0.3% by 2000 AD through

a. developing institutional capacity and strengthening of service delivery;

b. development of human resources for eye care;

c. promoting outreach activities and public awareness

The major thrust of the programme during the seventies was to provide ready access to cataract surgery free of charge to the blind persons so that they could regain their vision, enabling them to be independent socially and economically. There had been a gradual rise in cataract surgery from 5.5 lakh in 1950 to 11.34 lakh in 1984-85. However, subsequently there was a plateau in the performance to around 11-12 lakh per year. Surveys carried out in 1986-89 showed that the prevalence of blindness due to cataract and cataract backlog is high in Andhra Pradesh, Jammu and Kashmir, Madhya Pradesh, Maharashtra, Orissa, Rajasthan, Tamil Nadu and Uttar Pradesh. Therefore, a major thrust was given during the Eighth Plan to strengthen the programme in these States and in J & K and Karnataka. Funds from domestic budget as well as EAP were provided for this. District Blindness Control Societies were formed to coordinate the activities of Government voluntary and private sectors and to remove any bottlenecks in the implementation of the Programme. The major objectives of the Programme were :

1. to improve the quality of cataract surgery, to clear the backlog of cataract by performing 11 million operations during a 7-year period
2. to strengthen country's capacity to provide high volume, high quality, low cost eye care by upgrading knowledge and skills of eye care personnel and improve service delivery through non-governmental and public sector collaboration
3. to increase coverage of eye care delivery among the underprivileged population including women, urban slum dwellers and tribals.

The Cancer Control Programme was initiated in 1975-76 as a 100% centrally funded Central Sector project. It was renamed as National Cancer Control Programme in 1985. The objective of the programme were

1. primary prevention of tobacco-related cancers
2. secondary prevention of cancer cervix
3. extension and strengthening of treatment facilities on a national scale.

During the last two Plan periods financial assistance has been provided for the establishment of 12 Regional Cancer Centres and oncology wings in 26 medical colleges. The District Cancer Control Programme for preventive health education, early detection and pain relief was undertaken in collaboration with Regional Cancer Centres in 32 districts. Assistance has been given to 33 voluntary organisations for undertaking health education and early detection. The estimated requirement of cobalt units in the country is 900 (1/1 million). Only

232 cobalt machines are currently available in the country. The focus during the Ninth Plan will be on

1. intensification of IEC activities so that people seek care at the onset of symptoms
2. provision of diagnostic facilities in primary and secondary care level so that cancers are detected at early stages when curative therapy can be administered
3. filling up of the existing gaps in radiotherapy units in a phased manner so that all diagnosed cases do receive therapy without any delay as near to their residence as is feasible
4. IEC to reduce tobacco consumption and avoid life styles which could lead to increasing risk of cancers

National Diabetes Control Programme

The National Diabetes Control Programme was included as a pilot programme in the Seventh Five-Year Plan. The project was initiated in two districts in Tamil Nadu and one district in Jammu &Kashmir during the Seventh Plan. Several States had initiated district diabetes control programme as apart of the State Plan scheme during the Eighth Plan period. Experience gained in implementing the district diabetes control programme during Seventh and Eighth Plans have shown that integrated treatment of diabetes mellitus, hypertension and heart disease within primary and secondary care level is possible provided functional linkages between these and tertiary care centres are developed and utilised. During the Ninth Plan period these experiences will be utilised to develop integrated programme of non-communicable diseases prevention, detection and management programmes at primary and secondary care level in all districts.

National Mental Health Programme

It is estimated that 10 to 15% of the population suffer from mental health problem. Qualified professionals providing mental health care are few and the outreach of services in rural area is very low. The National Mental Health Programme was initiated by the Government of India in 1982 with the objective of improving mental health services at all levels of health care (primary, secondary and tertiary) for early recognition, adequate treatment and rehabilitation of patients with mental health problems with in the community and in the hospitals. However, the Programme did not make much headway either in the Seventh or Eighth Plan. Mental Hospitals are in poor shape. The States have not provided sufficient funds for mentally ill requiring inpatient treatment. The Supreme Court has directed the Centre and the States to make necessary provision for these hospitals so that the inmates do get humane and appropriate care.

The Mental Health Act, 1987, which came into force with effect from April 1993, requires that each State/UT set up its own State level Mental Health Authority as a Statutory obligation. Majority of the States/ UTs have complied with this and have formed a Mental Health Authority.

The Central Council of Health & Family Welfare reviewed the progress and resolved that the National Mental Health Programme should be accorded due priority and full-scale operational support are provided.

During the Eighth Plan, NIMHANS developed a district mental health care model in Bellary district with the following aims;

1. to provide sustainable basic mental health services to the community and to integrate these services with other health services;
2. early detection and prompt treatment of patients;
3. to provide domiciliary mental health care and to reduce patient load in mental hospital;
4. community education to reduce the stigma attached to mental illness;
5. to treat and rehabilitate patient's mental problems within their family setting.

During the Ninth Plan period the experience gained in implementing mental health care both in Central and State Sector will be utilised to provide sustainable mental health services at primary and secondary care levels and to build up community support for domiciliary care. IEC on mental health especially prevention of stress-related disorders through promotion of healthy lifestyle and operational research studies for effective implementation of preventive, promotive and curative programmes in mental health through existing health infrastructure will receive due attention.

National Iodine Deficiency Disorder Control Programme

Iodine deficiency disorders (IDD) have been recognised as a public health problem in India since mid-twenties. Initially, IDD was thought to be a problem in sub-Himalayan region. However, surveys carried out subsequently showed that IDD exists even in riverine and coastal areas. No State in India is completely free from IDD. It is estimated that 61 million population are suffering from endemic goitre and about 8.8 million people have mental/motor handicap due to iodine deficiency. Universal use of iodised salt is a simple inexpensive method of preventing IDD.

The National Goitre Control Programme was initiated in 1962 as a 100% Centrally funded, Central sector programme with the aim of conducting goitre survey supplying good quality iodised salt to areas having high IDD, health education and resurvey after five years. The programme was renamed as the National Iodine Deficiency Disorder Control Programme in 1992. Implementation of the Programme during the initial three decades of operation was sub-optimal and IDD prevalence had remained essentially unaltered. Inadequate production of iodised salt, problems in transport, lack of awareness about the need to take iodised salt are responsible for the poor performance.

During the Eighth Plan period there had been a substantial improvement in the production, quality and transport of iodized salt. The annual production of iodised salt has risen from 5 lakh tonnes in 1985-.86 to 40 lakh tonnes in 1996-97. By mid-1995, a ban on the sale of non-iodised edible salt has been implemented fully or partially in all States/Union Territories except Kerala, Goa and Pondicherry. Currently, it is estimated that about 80% of all edible salt is iodised and the use of iodised salt at household level has increased significantly. However, the target of Universal Iodisation of Salt is yet to be achieved.

During the Ninth Plan period the major thrust of the Programme will be on (a) production of adequate quantity of iodised salt of appropriate quality; (b) appropriate packaging at the site of production to prevent deterioration of quality of salt during transport and storage; (c) facilities for testing the quality of salt not only at production level but also at the retail outlets and household level so that consumers get and use good quality salt (d) IEC to ensure that people consume only good quality iodised salt and (e) survey of IDD and setting up of district level IDD monitoring laboratories for estimation of iodine content of salt and urinary iodine excretion.

Efforts to reduce price differentials between iodised and non-iodised salt and provide ready access to iodised salt through Targeted Public Distribution System will be considered. Integrated Non-Communicable Disease Control Programme

Accelerated economic growth in the nineties does not necessarily imply improvement in health status. Increasing longevity, demographic transition resulting in rapidly rising numbers of aged population, urbanisation, increasing pollution, change from traditional diets, sedentary life style and increase in the stress of day-to-day living have led to an increase in lifestyle-related disorders and noncommunicable diseases. The ongoing change in disease burden is producing a major health transition; over the next two decades, non-communicable diseases are likely to contribute significantly to the total disease burden in the country. Cardio-and cerebro-vascular diseases, diabetes mellitus and malignancies are emerging as major public health problems in the country. It is essential that preventive, promotive, curative and rehabilitative services for NCD are made available throughout the country at primary, secondary and tertiary care levels so as to reduce the morbidity and mortality associated with NCD. However, vertical programmes to control individual non-communicable diseases would neither be feasible nor cost-effective.

Environment and Health

Environment can affect human health in many ways. Deficiency of iodine in soil, water and foodstuffs is the cause of iodine deficiency disorders. Excessive fluoride content in the water is the cause of fluoros is. Environmental degradation may affect air, land and water. Pollutants may enter the food chain. All these may enter human body through various portals and affect the health status.

Rapidly growing population, urbanisation, changing agricultural, industrial and water resource management, increasing use of pesticides and fossil fuels have all resulted in a perceptible deterioration in the quality of environment and attendant adverse health consequences. Environmental pollution due to developmental activities are increasingly becoming the focus of concern. The interactive interdependence of health, environment and sustainable development was accepted as the fulcrum of action under Agenda 21 at the Earth Summit in Brazil in 1992. Environmental health in its broader perspective would have to address the detection, prevention and management of:

i. existing deficiencies or excesses of certain elements in natural environment;

ii. macro environmental contamination of air, land, water and food;

iii. disaster management

Following the suspected plague outbreak in the country during 1994 the Planning Commission constituted a High Power Committee on Urban Solid Waste Management in India under the Chairmanship of Member (Health). This Committee undertook a comprehensive review of current situation of urban solid waste management, specially in cities with one million or more inhabitants and made recommendations for safe methods for collection, transportation of waste and suitable cost-effective, environmentally friendly methods for disposal of these wastes. Pilot projects exploring the dimensions of the problem and aimed at seeking realistic solutions were initiated during the Eighth Plan period. During the Ninth Plan period it is expected that many more cities will initiate programmes for the efficient methods of management of wastes generated and improve environmental sanitation.

So far, the major focus has been on communicable disease burden due to poor environmental sanitation in urban areas and due to improper disposal of human excreta, garbage and waste water in rural areas and methods to tackle these. These efforts will be intensified during the Ninth Plan. In addition, efforts to reduce pollution and related non-communicable disease burden will also be strengthened. Efforts will be made to document the extent of the problem of environmental pollution and its impact on health status of the population through linkages between existing environmental monitoring data and data on health status of population living in these areas. Prevention and management of health consequences of environmental deterioration will receive increasing attention.

The Expert Committee on Public Health System had noted that major developmental activities in any field such as agriculture, industries, urban and rural development may result in environment changes which could have adverse health implications and recommended that health impact assessment may become a part of environmental impact assessment of all large developmental projects. Efforts will be made to implement this recommendation during the Ninth Plan period. The feasibility of making appropriate provision for health care of people involved in developmental activities and prevention and management of health consequences of developmental activities on the population living in the vicinity of the project as a part of the project budget will be explored.

Occupational Health

A healthy work force is an essential pre-requisite for agricultural and industrial development. Efforts to provide health care to workers through schemes such as ESI, creation of health care facilities in industrial towns, arrange for health care services for workers and their families through existing public and private health care services have continued through the last five decades. However, both coverage and quality of care have remained sub-optimal. There is no attempt to link existing data from ongoing work environmental monitoring in the work place with health status of workers and initiate appropriate intervention as and when required. Workers in the agricultural and unorganised sectors have so far not been covered under any programme. Increasing use of mechanisation, induction of poorly trained workers who operate machines with which they are not familiar, use of insecticides, pesticides and chemicals by persons without appropriate knowledge of precautions to be taken are resulting in increasing health hazards to workers in these sectors. During the Ninth Plan continuous monitoring of safety of work environment and workers' health status, both in the organised and unorganised sectors of industry and in agriculture, health problems of vulnerable groups such as women and children with focus on prevention, early detection and prompt treatment of health problems will receive special attention. Documenting the magnitude and types of the occupational health problems, initiating appropriate preventive and remedial measures will be developed into a structured health programme and taken up where ever possible.

Health Management Information System (HMIS)

HMIS is an essential management tool for effective functioning of the health system. Timely reporting and analysis of data from HMIS could also serve as an early warning of focal outbreak of diseases so that appropriate interventions can be initiated. The Central Bureau of Health Intelligence (CBHI) and the States' Bureau of Health Intelligence are nodal agencies for HMIS. During the Eighth Plan period an attempt was made to provide a major thrust for HMIS. The CBHI in consultation with the National Informatics Centre (NIC) and State Health Departments have developed HMIS version 2.0 for sending information through NICNET on essential health indices. This system is being used by 13 States/UTs for sending district level information. The system is still not fully operational in most States. During the Ninth Plan efforts will be made to ensure that the entire country is covered and all the data pertaining to the Health and

Family Welfare Programmes are collected, collated and reported from all the districts through NICNET. The data from HMIS will be utilised not only for improving the efficiency and effectiveness of the health care system but also for effective policy planning.

An Expert group under the chairmanship of Member (Health) undertook a comprehensive review of major problems facing the public health system in the country in ensuring outreach of appropriate services at affordable cost and maintaining quality of services. The Committee recommended several policy and programme initiatives including administrative restructuring, health manpower planning, improving operational efficiency of existing health care services, improving disease surveillance, epidemic control strategy, epidemiological surveillance system and development of appropriate support services. The recommendations of the Committee form the base and basis for the formulation of strategies for revitalisation of the public health system in the country during the Ninth Plan period.

Production and quality control of drugs

Provision of appropriate drugs of good quality at affordable cost is essential for the success of disease control programmes. Equally important is to restrict, and if possible, eliminate, the use of irrational drug formulation, detect and eliminate spurious drugs. The Central Government is responsible for the control over the quality of imported drugs, control over the manufacture and import of new drugs into the country, amendments to the Drugs and Cosmetics (D&A) Act and Rules, coordinate the activities with the State Drug Control Authorities for uniform implementation of D&A

Act and Rules, laying down standards for drugs and updating Indian Pharmacopoeia, training of drugs analysts and drugs inspectors and licensing of whole human blood and blood products, large volume parenterals, sera and vaccines. Provisions for strengthening Drug Control Organisations in the States and the Centre were made in the Eighth Plan. However, the implementation of the scheme has been patchy and tardy. This task will be taken up on a priority basis during the Ninth Plan.

India's need for essential drugs are still not fully met. Patent laws do not cover over 95% of the essential drugs. Bulk manufacture of the generic drug and dispensing them in inexpensive packages to bulk consumers like hospitals will substantially reduce the budget needed to meet the drug cost in public health system. The possibility of providing a dual pricing system for generic and brand drugs will be explored so that essential drugs under generic name are available at affordable cost. This approach can subsequently form the base and basis of "drug cooperatives" as community-managed institutions.

Supply of essential drugs, vaccines/devices holds the key to success in any disease control Programme. Funds for drugs used for primary, secondary and tertiary care centres come partly from the State funds and partly from Central Plan funds (CSS). Procedures for procurement and distribution vary and bottlenecks in these at the national and State level have been a recurrent problem. Inefficient indenting procedures adversely affect drug procurement. Poor inventory management results in unsatisfactory drug procurement and distribution. Some States such as Tamil Nadu have attempted strengthening drug procurement and distribution through formation of a Medical Services Corporation. This Corporation has drawn up an essential drug list, improved purchase and storage of drugs and organised efficient drug distribution within the States and brought about effective inventory control. During the Ninth Plan efforts in improving procurement and inventory control and distribution for drugs at Central and State level will receive priority.

Prevention of Food Adulteration

The Prevention of Food and Drug Adulteration Act, 1954 is aimed at ensuring that consumers get pure and wholesome food of good quality and protecting them from the trade malpractice and frauds in sale of food products. The Act is implemented jointly by the Central and State Government. During the Ninth Plan period, efforts will be made to augment food quality control both at the Central and State levels.

The Indian Council for Medical Research is the nodal organisation for bio-medical research in India. Bio-medical and Health Systems Research is carried out by research institutions, universities, medical colleges and non-governmental organisations and are currently funded by several agencies including ICMR, DST, DBT, CSIR and concerned Ministries. Basic, clinical applied and operational research studies relevant to major health and population problems in the country have been the focus of research programmes during the last fifty years.

The major thrust areas of research include existing problems of communicable diseases, emerging problems of non communicable diseases, improvement of health and nutritional status of women and children and increasing contraceptive acceptance and continuation.

Indigenous development of immuno-diagnostics, research studies on improved drug regimens to combat emerging drug resistance among several bacteria, alternative strategies for vector control in view of the increasing insecticide resistance among vectors, testing innovative disease control strategies through increased community participation have been the major areas of research in communicable diseases.

The ICMR has recently completed a 10-year study on health consequences of Bhopal Gas Disaster providing data base for planning the infrastructure needed to meet the health care requirements of the population exposed to toxic gas over the next decade. Anti-tobacco community education, early detection and prevention of cervical cancer in women and oral cancers in both sexes, lifestyle modification to reduce the rising morbidity due to hypertension and cardiovascular diseases, documenting the health problems associated with lifestyle changes and increasing longevity of life are some of the major research areas in non-communicable diseases. Evaluation of ongoing Mid-day Meal programmes in schools, assessment of changes in dietary intake and nutritional status of urban and rural population indifferent States over the last two decades, investigating the health effects of food contaminants and adulterants are some of the research activities in nutrition research.

Keeping in view the magnitude of the problem of providing effective comprehensive health care to the population, the major research and developmental activities in the country during the Ninth Plan will be directed to applied, operational research for improving quality, coverage, efficiency and the cost-effectiveness of health services. Research studies to test the operational feasibility and economic viability of comprehensive health service schemes similar to National Health Service (NHS) of United Kingdom suitably modified to meet the Indian milieu will be taken up. Multi-disciplinary, multi-centre operational research studies will be carried out by teams with medical scientists, social scientists, health planners and decision-makers, public health experts, health economists, and health managers.

During the Ninth Plan period optimal coordination of the basic and applied research activities will be attempted by networking and if needed by multi-agency funding of important projects. The major thrust areas for basic research will be:

1. immuno diagnostic tests for common infections;
2. development of newer drugs for treatment of common infections in view of the increasing resistance to antibiotics;
3. development of resistance modulating agents to combat the increasing bacterial resistance to antibiotics;
4. development, testing and quality control of newer drugs in the modern system of medicine and ISM&H;
5. newer drug delivery systems for better targeting of drugs and reduction in side effects;
6. development of therapeutic and prophylactic vaccines for infections utilising newer bio-technological tools so that they are thermostable , have long shelf life, free from side effects and are affordable;
7. development of newer vector control measures including testing of bio-pesticides like neem;

Adequate operational research studies do not precede initiation of major national programmes. There are many operational problems in these programmes, which are realised at the time of implementation, and time is lost in rectifying these. During the Ninth Plan, development and testing of alternative strategies for control of communicable and non-communicable diseases will be the focus of operational research. Funds will be made available from ongoing major disease control programmes for Research aimed at improving programme implementation. Operational research for efficient implementation of ongoing health programmes and horizontal integration of the vertical programmes for health and family welfare at the primary health care level are some of the major research initiatives being contemplated during the Ninth Plan period. The mechanisms by which those in the research, service and teaching cadres can move into each other's areas and participate in programme development, testing and implementation will be worked out.

The National Health Policy was formulated and adopted in 1983 providing comprehensive framework for planning, implementation and monitoring of health services. Successive plans have evolved and implemented intervention programmes to achieve the goals set in the National Health Policy. The status for various Health and Family Welfare indices prior to formulation of National Health Policy, goals set in the National Health Policy for 2000 AD.

2000 AD is just two years away. The time is therefore, appropriate for review of achievements against the set goals in the National Health policy. During the last two decades there have been major changes in disease profile, health care infrastructure and health care seeking behaviour of the population. Several newer technologies for diagnosis and management of health problems have become available. These, in turn, have widened the gap between what is possible and what is feasible and affordable at the level of the individual and the country. Increasing expectations of the population, rising cost of diagnosis and treatment and diminishing resources have brought into fore the issue of how to meet the rising health care costs. The essential inter-linkages between health services delivery and health manpower development are still not fully understood and operationalised. Taking all these into consideration it is essential that the National Health Policy undergoes a re-appraisal and re-formulation so that it provides are liable and relevant policy framework not only for improving health care, but also measuring and monitoring the health care delivery systems and health status of the population during the next two decades.

Health is one of the sectors identified under the Special Action Plan. In addition to the funds available from Domestic Budgetary Support, several centrally sponsored disease control programmes are receiving funds from EAPs. Taking all these factors into consideration, the Department of Health has been provided with an outlay of Rs. 5118.19 crores for the ninth plan period. The outlay for the annual plans will be adjusted depending upon the requirements of the department and the availability of funds including reimbursement from EAPs.

Indian Systems of Medicine and Homoeopathy

The Indian Systems of Medicine and Homoeopathy consist of Ayurveda, Siddha, Unani and Homoeopathy, and therapies such as Yoga and Naturopathy. Some of these systems are indigenous and others have over the years become a part of Indian tradition. It is estimated that there are over 6 lakh ISM&H practitioners in the country. Many of them work in remote rural and urban slum areas and thus, could play an important role in improving the quality and outreach of health care. These practitioners are close to the community, not only in the geographical sense but in terms of cultural and social ethos. The cost of care is affordable and hence these systems have wide acceptance among all segments of the population. The National Health Policy visualised an important role for the ISM&H practitioners in the delivery of health services. Measures to popularise and develop Indian Systems of Medicine & Homeopathy have been vigorously pursued during the Eighth Plan. In order to give focussed attention to the development and optimal utilisation of ISM&H for the health care of the population, a separate Department for ISM&H was set up in 1995.

Indian Systems of Medicine & Homeopathy Strengths of the system are:

— There are over 6 lakh ISM&H practitioners

— The practitioners serve in remote rural areas/urban slums

— They are accepted by the community

Problems are:

— Training institutes lack well qualified teachers and quality of training is not of requisite standard

— Lack of essential staff, infrastructure and diagnostic facilities in secondary/tertiary care institutions

— Potential of ISM&H drugs & therapeutic modalities is not fully exploited

— Existing ISM&H practitioners are not fully utilised to improve access to health care

Preservation and Promotion of Cultivation of Medicinal Herbs and Plants

With the new thrust for ISM&H, there will be an increasing demand for drugs used in these systems. Over the last two decades the cultivation of medicinal plants and herbs have been unable to meet the increasing demands. Several medicinal plants are no longer available at affordable cost. Some of the species of medicinal plants are also reported to be endangered because of increasing pressure on the forests.

The Department has initiated a scheme for development and cultivation of medicinal plants. The objective of the scheme is to augment the production of raw herbs of plant origin by providing Central assistance for their cultivation and development . In addition, during the Eighth Plan period several States such as Himachal Pradesh have also set up herbal gardens and linked them to production units of drugs for ISM&H. There is a need to create such herbal farms in public, private and joint sector to ensure that the essential plants and herbs of appropriate quality are produced in adequate quantity to meet the demands and the cost of drugs is maintained at affordable levels. Use of appropriate bio- technological tools for preservation and propagation of important medicinal plants have to be taken up. Inter-sectoral co-ordination with Departments of Biotechnology, Horticulture and Medicinal & Aromatic

Plant Research Institutions are important for ensuring that appropriate herbs are grown taking into account agroclimatic conditions. The Department has utilised three gene banks (at Delhi, Lucknow and Trivandrum) under the Department of Bio- technology to store 2000 species of medicinal plants (Germ plasm) required for ISM&H drugs.

At the village level, cultivation of medicinal plants through appropriate utilisation of waste land will have to be undertaken with active collaboration of agriculture Department, Krishi Vigyan Kendra and Department of Rural Development.

Pharmacopoeial standardisation of Ayurveda, Siddha and Unani Medicine, both for single and compound drugs, is essential. The Department had taken up the task of developing Pharmacopoeial Standards through Pharmacopoeia Committees. Four Pharmacopoeial Committees are working for preparing official formularies/pharmacopoeias to maintain uniform standards in preparation of drugs of Ayurveda, Unani, Siddha and Homoeoapathy and to prescribe working standards for single drug as well as compound formulations. The Pharmacopoeia Committees in Ayurveda, Siddha, Unani and Homoeopathy are headed by experts in their respective fields.

Pharmacopoeial Laboratory for Indian Medicine, Ghaziabad, was established in 1970 as standards setting-cum-drug testing laboratory for ISM at the National level. The standards worked out are published in the form of monographs. During the Ninth Plan period the ongoing pharmacopoeial work, development of pharmacopoeial standards, listing essential drugs and formulations will be completed expeditiously .

The work of pharmacopoeial laboratories attached to the Department will be supplemented by laboratories of CCRAS and university/college departments of Chemistry and Bio-chemistry. Strengthening of State Drug Testing Laboratories will also be taken up to ensure quality of drugs used in ISM&H. In addition GMP for production of drugs of good quality and strengthening of quality control laboratories will be encouraged.

There are four Research Councils in ISM&H; these are Central Council for Research in Ayurveda and Siddha (CCRAS); Central Council for Research in Unani Medicine (CCRUM); Central Council for Research in Homoeopathy (CCRH); and Central Council for Research in Yoga and Naturopathy (CCRYN). They initiate, aid, guide, develop and coordinate basic and applied research, medico-botanical surveys, research on the cultivation of medicinal plants and pharmacognostical studies. These Councils are the apex bodies for research in the concerned systems of medicine and are fully financed by the Government of India.

The Central Research Councils' R&D programmes will be strengthened during the Ninth Plan period, if necessary, by reorganisation and by providing adequate infrastructure and resources. These Councils will also collaborate with outside research institutions and research funding agencies as well as universities. The major focus will be on developing new drug formulations. These, as well as formulations traditionally used in ISM&H for treatment of illnesses for which there is no effective remedy in modern system of medicine will be tested for safety and efficacy. Clinical trials will also be undertaken in formulations traditionally used in tribal societies and reported as being effective.

Formulations found useful will be patented. The Department has established a Patent Cell to keep track of patents being filed in India and other parts of the world with respect to Ayurveda, Siddha, Unani drugs and to extend professional and financial assistance to Government/Private scientists in the ISM&H sector in connection with filing of patents. An Expert Group has been constituted for rendering advise to the Department with regard to the Patent issues relating to ISM&H. This will receive increased attention in the Ninth Plan. The potential contribution of drugs and formulations from ISM&H to meet the national as well as global demands for safe and effective drugs will be fully exploited. Drug safety and pharmacopoieal standards setting will receive due attention. Preventive and curative role of Yoga and Naturopathy in life style related disorders will be fully investigated and utilised. During the initial four years there was underutilisation of the funds provided. However in the last year, after the establishment of the Department of ISM&H, utilisation of funds has markedly improved.

The strength of ISM&H lies in the fact that the practitioners serve in private sector even in remote rural areas and urban slums. Strengthening of undergraduate and post graduate training in ISM&H, establishment of speciality clinics in major hospitals, standardisation of drugs, enhancing availability of raw materials, research and development and IEC are some of the major areas of input by the Deptt of ISM&H at the national level; they will continue to be the focus during the Ninth Plan. Development of human resources and establishment of speciality clinics are activities that take time and have to be achieved in phases. Taking all these factors into consideration an outlay of Rs. 266.35 crore has been provided to the department of ISM&H for the Ninth Plan period. The outlay for the Annual Plans will be adjusted depending upon the requirements of the department and availability of the funds. The State Governments will be making necessary provisions for development of ISM&H in their budget.

4

Basic Nutrition and Community Health

Each human body is built up from food containing these five constituents, and vitamins as well. Food serves mainly for growth, energy and body repair, maintenance and protection. Food also provides enjoyment and stimulation, since eating and drinking are among the pleasures of life everywhere. Truly food nourishes both the body and soul. Even if technology could produce a perfect diet in terms of content, such a diet could still lack, for example, the aroma and flavour of a curry, or the stimulating taste of hot coffee. What controls appetite or the feeling of hunger is not fully understood.

Basic Nutrional Needs

Human beings eat food, and not individual nutrients. Most foods, including staples such as rice, maize and wheat, provide mainly carbohydrate for energy but also significant quantities of protein, a little fat or oil and useful micronutrients. Thus cereal grains provide some of the constituents needed for energy, growth and body repair and maintenance. Breastmilk provides all the macro- and micronutrients necessary to satisfy the total needs of a young infant up to six months of age including those for energy, growth and body repair and maintenance. Cows' milk has the balance of nutrients for all the requirements of a calf.

Water can be considered the most important dietary constituent. A normal man or woman can live without food for 20 to 40 days, but without water humans die in four to seven days. Over 60 percent of human body weight is made up of water, of which approximately 61 percent is intracellular and the rest extracellular. Water intake, except under exceptional circumstances (e.g. intravenous feeding), comes from the food and fluids consumed. The amount consumed varies widely in individuals and may be influenced by climate, culture and other factors. Often as much as 1 litre is consumed in solid food, and 1 to 3 litres as fluids drunk. Water is also formed in the body as a result of oxidation of macronutrients, but the water thus obtained usually constitutes less than 10 percent of total water. Water is excreted mainly by the kidneys as urine. The kidneys regulate the output of urine and maintain a balance; if smaller amounts of fluid are consumed, the kidneys excrete less water, and the urine is more concentrated.

While most water is eliminated by the kidneys, in hot climates as much or more can be lost from the skin (through perspiration) and the lungs. Much smaller quantities are lost from the gut in the faeces. Metabolism of sodium and potassium, which are known as electrolytes, is linked with body water. The sodium is mainly in the extracellular water and the potassium in the intracellular water. Most diets contain adequate amounts of both these minerals. In fluid loss caused, for example, by diarrhoea or haemorrhage, the balance of electrolytes in the blood may become disturbed. Water intake and electrolyte balance are particularly important in sick infants. In healthy infants, breastmilk alone from a healthy mother provides adequate quantities of fluids and electrolytes without additional water for the first six months of life even in hot climates. Infants with diarrhoea and disease, however, may require additional fluids. While food intake is largely regulated by appetite and food availability, fluid intake is influenced by the sensation termed thirst. Thirst may arise for various reasons.

In dehydration it may be caused by drying of the mouth but also by signals from the same satiety centre in the hypothalamus that controls hunger sensations. Dehydration, an important feature of diarrhoea. The phenomenon of water accumulation in the body is manifested in the condition known as oedema, when disease causes an excess of extracellular fluid. Two important deficiency diseases in which generalized oedema is a feature are kwashiorkor and wet beriberi. The excess fluid may result from electrolyte disturbances and accumulation of water in the extracellular compartment. A person can have oedema and still be dehydrated from diarrhoea; this condition is a form of heart failure. Water can also collect in the peritoneal cavity, in the condition known as ascites, which may be caused by liver disease. The human body is sometimes said to be divided into three compartments, accounting for the following shares of the total body weight of a well-nourished healthy adult male:

— body cell mass, 55 percent;

— extracellular supporting tissue, 30 percent;

— body fat, 15 percent.

The body cell mass is made up of cellular components such as muscle, body organs (viscera, liver, brain, etc.) and blood. It comprises the parts of the body that are involved in body metabolism, body functioning, body work and so on. The extracellular supporting tissue consists of two parts: the extracellular fluid (for example, the blood plasma supporting the blood cells) and the skeleton and other supporting structures. Body fat is nearly all present beneath the skin (subcutaneous fat) and around body organs such as the intestine and heart. It serves in part as an energy reserve. Small quantities are present in the walls of body cells or in nerves. Physiologists and those interested in metabolism have developed various ways to estimate body composition, including the amount of fluids in the body and body density.

A common determination is to estimate lean body mass (LBM) or the fat-free mass of the body. These measures vary from the very simple to the very difficult. The simpler ones are of course less precise. Anthropometry using weight, height, skinfold thickness and body circumferences is relatively easy and very cheap to undertake, and does provide some estimate of LBM and body composition. In contrast, methods using, for example, bioelectrical impedance, computerized axial tomography (CAT scans) and nuclear magnetic resonance require expensive apparatus and highly trained staff. The fluid in the cells (intracellular fluid) has mainly potassium ions, and the extracellular fluid is mainly a solution of sodium chloride.

Both also have other ions. Total body water can be estimated using different methods including dilution techniques to measure, for example, plasma volume. Body fat is estimated using different methods. Because a large portion of adipose tissue is present beneath the skin, it can be estimated by using a skinfold calliper to measure skinfold thickness in different sites. Another method is to weigh the person both in air and under water using a special apparatus and tank. This method really provides an estimate of body density. The various methods of determining body composition are described in detail in textbooks of physiology or nutrition. Body composition is much influenced by nutrition.

Body composition differs between the genders and, perhaps only slightly, among races. African Americans have been shown to have heavier skeletons than whites of the same body build in the United States. In females pregnancy and lactation influence body composition. The body composition of children is influenced by their age and growth. Disturbances of growth resulting from nutritional deficiencies influence body composition, including the eventual size of the body and of body organs. The general term for all the chemical processes carried out by the cells of the body is "metabolism". Chief among these processes is the oxidation (combustion, or burning) of food which produces energy. This process is analogous to a car engine burning petrol to produce the energy that makes it run. In most forms of combustion, be it in the car or in the human, heat is produced as well as energy. Classical physics taught that energy can be neither created nor destroyed. Although this law of nature is not completely correct, it is still true in most instances. All three macronutrients in food—carbohydrate, protein and fat provide energy.

Energy for the body comes mainly from food, and in the absence of food it can be produced only by the breakdown of body tissues. All forms of energy can be converted into heat energy. It is possible to measure the heat produced by burning a litre of petrol, for example. Food energy can also be and is expressed as heat energy. The unit of measurement used has been the large calorie (Cal) or kilocalorie (kcal) (which is 1 000 times the small calorie used in physics), but this measure is increasingly being replaced by the joule (J) or kilojoule (kJ). The kilocalorie is defined as the heat necessary to raise the temperature of 1 litre of water from 14.5° to 15.5°C. Whereas the kilocalorie is a unit of heat, the joule is truly a unit of energy. The joule is defined as the amount of energy used when 1 kg is moved 1 m by 1 newton (N) of force. In nutrition the kilojoule (1000 J) is used. The equivalent of 1 kcal is 4.184 kJ. These are units of measurement in the same way that litres and pints are measures of quantity, and metres and feet are measures of length. In many scientific journals the joule is being introduced in place of the kilocalorie, but the general public and most health workers still prefer to express food energy in kilocalories rather than joules.

The human body requires energy for all bodily functions, including work, the maintenance of body temperature and the continuous action of the heart and lungs. In children energy is essential for growth. Energy is also needed for breakdown, repair and building of tissues. These arc metabolic processes. The rate at which these functions are carried out while the body is at rest is the Basal metabolic rate (BMR). BMR for an individual person is usually defined as the amount of energy [expressed in kilocalories or megajoules expended when the person is al complete rest, both physical (i.e. lying down) and psychological. It can also be expressed as kilocalories per hour or per kilogram of weight. BMR provides the energy required by the body for maintenance of body temperature; for the work of body organs such as the beating heart and the muscles working for normal, at rest, breathing; and for the functioning of other organs such as the liver, kidneys and brain. BMR varies from individual to individual. Important general factors influencing BMR are the person's weight, gender, age and state of health.

BMR is also influenced by the person's body composition, for example the amounts of muscle and adipose tissue and therefore the amounts of protein and fat in the body. In broad terms, bigger people with more muscle and larger body organs have higher BMR than smaller people. Elderly people tend to have lower BMR than they had when they were young, and females tend to have lower BMR than males even on a per kilogram body weight basis. There are exceptions, however, to all these generalizations. BMR is important as a component of energy requirements. Of course many adult females in developing countries are smaller than 1.4 m in height and 41 kg in weight; their BMR might then be a little lower than 1 190 kcal per day. The average human burns energy at his or her BMR only when at complete rest. All ordinary movements require additional energy, and physical work, of course, requires more still.

In most in stances, when people increase their output of energy, including work, they feel more hungry and increase their consumption of their staple food, be it rice, millet, maize wheat, cassava or anything else. The energy requirements of a human being are affected by several factors. The important ones are:

— *Body size*: A small person needs less energy than a large person.

— *Basal metabolic rate*: BMR varies and can be affected by factors such as disease of the thyroid gland.

— *Activity*: The more physical work or recreation performed, the more energy is required.

— *Pregnancy*: A woman requires extra energy to develop the foetus and to carry its additional weight.

— *Lactation*: The lactating mother needs additional energy to produce energy-containing milk for the suckling baby. The relatively long duration of breastfeeding among most Asians and Africans results in a large proportion of women requiring extra energy.

— *Age*: Infants and children need more energy, for growth and activity, than adults. In older persons, the need for energy is sometimes reduced because there is a decline in activity and because their BMR is usually lower.

— *Climate*: In warm climates, i.e. in most of the tropics and subtropics, less energy is necessary to keep the body at its normal temperature than in cold climates.

The main source of energy for most Asians, Africans and Latin Americans is carbohydrates in the food they eat. Carbohydrates constitute by far the greatest portion of their diet, as much as 80 percent in some cases. In contrast, carbohydrates make up only 45 to 50 percent of the diet of many people in industrialized countries. Carbohydrates are compounds containing carbon, hydrogen and oxygen in the proportions 6:12:6. They are burned during metabolism to produce energy, liberating carbon dioxide (CO_2) and water (H_2O). The carbohydrates in the human diet are mainly in the form of starches and various sugars. The simplest carbohydrates are the monosaccharides, or simple sugars. These sugars can pass through the wall of the alimentary tract without being changed by the digestive enzymes. The three most common are glucose, fructose and galactose.

Glucose, sometimes also called dextrose, is present in fruit, sweet potatoes, onions and other plant substances. It is the substance into which many other carbohydrates, such as the disaccharides and starches, are converted by the digestive enzymes. Glucose is oxidized to produce energy, heat and carbon dioxide, which is exhaled in breathing. Because glucose is the sugar in blood, it is most often used as an energy-producing substance for persons fed intravenously. Glucose dissolved in sterile water, usually in concentrations of 5 or 10 percent, is frequently used for this purpose. Fructose is present in honey and some fruit juices.

Galactose is a monosaccharide that is formed, along with glucose, when the milk sugar lactose is broken down by the digestive enzymes. The disaccharides, composed of simple sugars, need to be converted by the body into monosaccharides before they can be absorbed from the alimentary tract. Examples of disaccharides are sucrose, lactose and maltose. Sucrose is the scientific name for table sugar (the kind that is used, for example, to sweeten tea). It is most commonly produced from sugar cane but is also produced from beets. Sucrose is also present in carrots and pineapple.

Lactose is the disaccharide present in human and animal milk. It is much less sweet than sucrose. Maltose is found in germinating seeds. The polysaccharides are chemically the most complicated carbohydrates. They tend to be insoluble in water, and only some can be used by human beings to produce energy. Examples of polysaccharides are starch, glycogen and cellulose. Starch is an important source of energy for humans. It occurs in cereal grains as well as in root foods such as potatoes and cassava. Starch is liberated during cooking when the starch granules rupture because of heating. Glycogen is made in the human body and is sometimes known as animal starch. It is formed from monosaccharides produced by the digestion of dietary starch.

Starch from rice or cassava is broken down in the intestines to form monosaccharide molecules, which pass into the bloodstream. Those surplus monosaccharides that are not used to produce energy (and carbon dioxide and water) are fused together to form a new polysaccharide, glycogen. Glycogen is usually present in muscle and in the liver, but not in large amounts. Any of the digestible carbohydrates when consumed in excess of body needs are converted by the body into fat which is laid down as adipose tissue beneath the skin and at other sites in the body. Cellulose, hemicellulose, lignin, pectin and gums are sometimes called unavailable carbohydrates because humans cannot digest them.

Cellulose and hemicellulose are plant polymers that are the main components of cell walls. They are fibrous substances. Cellulose, which is a polymer of glucose, is one of the fibres of green plants. Hemicellulose is a polymer of other sugars, usually hexose and pentose. Lignin is the main component of wood. Pectins are present in plant tissue and sap and are colloidal polysaccharides. Gums are also viscous carbohydrates extracted from plants. Pectins and gums are both used by the food industry. The human alimentary tract cannot break down these carbohydrates or utilize them to produce energy.

Some animals, such as cattle, have microorganisms in their intestines that break down cellulose and make it available as an energy-producing food. In humans, any of the unavailable carbohydrates present in food pass through the intestinal tract. They form much of the bulk and roughage evacuated in human faeces, and are often termed "dietary fibre". There is increasing interest in fibre in diets, because high-fibre diets are now considered healthful. A clear advantage of a high-fibre diet is a lower incidence of constipation than among people who consume a low-fibre diet.

The bulk in high-fibre diets may contribute a feeling of fullness or satiety which may lead to less consumption of energy, and this may help reduce the likelihood of obesity. A high-fibre diet results in more rapid transit of food through the intestinal tract and is thus believed to assist normal and healthy intestinal and bowel functioning. Dietary fibre has also been found to bind bile in the intestines. It is now recognized that the high fibre content of most traditional diets may be an important factor in the prevention of certain diseases which appear to be much more prevalent in people consuming the low-fibre diets common in industrialized countries.

Because it facilitates the rapid passage of materials through the intestine, fibre may be a factor in the control of diverticulitis, appendicitis, haemorrhoids and also possibly arteriosclerosis, which leads to coronary heart disease and some cancers. Frequent consumption of any sticky fermentable carbohydrates, either starch or sugar, can contribute to dental caries, particularly when coupled with poor oral hygiene. Adequate intake of fluoride and/ or a topical application is the best protection against caries. In many developing countries dietary fats make up a smaller part of total energy intake (often only 8 or

10 percent) than carbohydrates. In most industrialized countries the proportion of fat intake is much higher.

The term "fat" is used here to include all fats and oils that are edible and occur in human diets, ranging from those that are solid at cool room temperatures, such as butter, to those that are liquid at similar temperatures, such as groundnut or cottonseed oils. Fats in the body are divided into two groups: storage fat and structural fat. Storage fat provides a reserve storehouse of fuel for the body, while the structural fats are part of the essential structure of the cells, occurring in cell membranes, mitochondria and intracellular organelles. Cholesterol is a lipid present in all cell membranes. It has an important role in fat transport and is the precursor from which bile salts and adrenal and sex hormones are made. Dietary fats consist mainly of triglycerides, which can be split into glycerol and chains of carbon, hydrogen and oxygen called fatty acids. This action, the digestion or breakdown of fats, is achieved in the human intestine by enzymes known as lipases, which are present primarily in the pancreatic and intestinal secretions.

Bile salts from the liver emulsify the fatty acids to make them more soluble in water and hence more easily absorbed. The many fatty acids in human diets are divided into two main groups: saturated and unsaturated. The latter group includes both polyunsaturated and mono-unsaturated fatty acids.

Saturated fatty acids have the maximum number of hydrogen atoms that their chemical structure will permit. All fats and oils eaten by humans are mixtures of saturated and unsaturated fatty acids. Broadly speaking, fats from land animals (i.e. meat fat, butter and ghee) contain more saturated fatty acids than do those of vegetable origin. Fats from plant products and to some extent those from fish have more unsaturated fatty acids, particularly polyunsaturated fatty acids (PUFAs). There are exceptions, however. For example, coconut oil has a large amount of saturated fatty acids. These groupings of fats have important health implications because excess intake of saturated fats is one of the risk factors associated with arteriosclerosis and coronary heart disease.

In contrast, PUFAs are believed to be protective. PUFAs also include two unsaturated fatty acids, linoleic acid and linolenic acid, which have been termed "essential fatty acids" (EFAs) as they are necessary for good health. EFAs are important in the synthesis of many cell structures and several biologically important compounds. Recent studies have also shown the benefits of other longer-chain fatty acids in the growth and development of young children, and arachidonic acid and docosa-hexaenoic acid (DHA) should conditionally be considered essential during early development. Experiments with animals and studies in humans have shown definite skin and growth changes and abnormal vascular and neural function in the absence of these fatty acids, and there is no doubt that they are essential for the nutrition of individual cells and tissues of the body.

Fat is desirable to make the diet more palatable. It also yields about 9 kcal/g, which is more than twice the energy yielded by carbohydrates and proteins (about 4 kcal/g); fat can therefore reduce the bulk of the diet. A person doing very heavy work, especially in a cold climate, may require as many as 4 000 kcal a day. In such a case it is highly desirable that a good proportion of the energy should come from fat; otherwise the diet would be very bulky. Bulky diets can be a particularly serious problem in young children as well. A reasonable increase in the fat or oil content of the diets of young children raises the energy density of predominantly bulky carbohydrate diets and is highly desirable. Fat also functions as a vehicle that assists the absorption of fat-soluble vitamins.

Thus fats, and even specific types of fat, are essential to health. However, practically all diets provide the small amount required. Fat deposited in the human body serves as a reserve fuel. It is an economic way of storing energy, because, as mentioned above, fat yields about twice as much energy, weight for weight, as does carbohydrate or protein. Fat is present beneath the skin as an insulation against cold, and it forms a supporting tissue for many organs such as the heart and intestines. All fat in the body is not necessarily derived from fat that has been eaten. However, excess calories from the carbohydrate and protein in, for example, maize, cassava, rice or wheat can be converted into fat in the human body. Like carbohydrates and fats, proteins contain carbon, hydrogen and oxygen, but they also contain nitrogen and often sulphur. They are particularly important as nitrogenous substances, and are necessary for growth and repair of the body. Proteins are the main structural constituents of the cells and tissues of the body, and they make up the greater portion of the substance of the muscles and organs. The proteins in different body tissues are not all exactly the same.

Although proteins can yield energy, their main importance is rather as an essential constituent of all cells. All cells may need replacement from time to time, and their replacement requires protein. Any protein eaten in excess of the amount needed for growth, cell and fluid replacement and various other metabolic functions is used to provide energy, which the body obtains by changing the protein into carbohydrate. If the carbohydrate and fat in the diet do not provide adequate energy, then protein is used to provide energy; as a result less protein is available for growth, cell replacement and other metabolic needs. This point is especially important for children, who need extra protein for growth. If they get too little food for their energy requirements, then the protein will be diverted for daily energy needs and will not be used for growth. All proteins consist of large molecules which are made of amino acids.

The amino acids in any protein are linked together in chains, called peptide linkages. The various proteins are made of different amino acids linked together in different chains. Because there are many different amino acids, there are many different possible configurations, so there are many different proteins. During digestion proteins break down to form amino acids much as complex carbohydrates such as starches break down into simple monosaccharides and fats break down into fatty acids. In the stomach and intestines various proteolytic enzymes hydrolyse the protein, releasing amino acids and peptides. Plants are able to synthesize amino acids from simple inorganic chemical substances. Animals do not have this ability; they derive all the amino acids necessary for building their protein from consumption of plants or animals.

As the animals eaten by humans initially derived their protein from plants, all amino acids in human diets have originated from this source. Animals have differing abilities to convert one amino acid into another. In the human this ability is limited. Conversion occurs mainly in the liver. If the ability to convert one amino acid into another were unlimited, then the question of the protein content of diets and the prevention of protein deficiency would be simple. It would be enough merely to supply sufficient protein, irrespective of the quality or amino acid content of the protein supplied. Of the large number of amino acids, 20 are common in plants and animals. Of these, eight have been found to be essential for the adult human and have thus been termed "essential amino acids" or "indispensable amino acids", namely: phenylalanine, tryptophan, methionine, lysine, leucine, isoleucine, valine and threonine. A ninth amino acid, histidine, is required for growth and is essential for infants and children; it may also be necessary for tissue repair.

Other amino acids include glycine, alanine, serine, cystine, tyrosine, aspartic acid, glutamic acid, proline, hydroxyproline, citrulline and arginine. Each protein in a food is composed of a particular mixture of amino acids which might or might not contain all eight of the essential ones. To assess the protein value of any food it is useful to know how much total protein it contains, which amino acids it has and how many essential amino acids are present and in what proportion. Much is now known about the individual proteins present in various foods, their amino acid content and therefore their quality and quantity. Some have a better mixture of amino acids than others, and these are said to have a higher biological value.

The proteins albumin in egg and casein in milk, for example, contain all the essential amino acids in good proportions and are nutritionally superior to such proteins as zein in maize, which contains little tryptophan or lysine, and the protein in wheat, which contains only small quantities of lysine. It is not true, however, to say that the proteins in maize and wheat are not valuable. Although they contain less of certain amino acids, they do contain some amount of all the essential amino acids as well as many of the other important ones. The relative deficiency of maize and wheat proteins can be overcome by providing other foodstuffs containing more of the limited amino acids. It is therefore possible for two foods with low-value protein to complement each other to form a good protein mixture when eaten together. Humans, especially children on diets deficient in animal protein, require a variety of foods of vegetable origin, not just one staple food.

In many diets, pulses or legumes such as groundnuts, beans and cowpeas, though short of sulphur- containing amino acids, supplement the cereal proteins, which are often short of lysine. A mixture of foods of vegetable origin, especially if taken at the same meal, can serve as a substitute for animal protein. FAO has produced tables showing the content of essential amino acids in different foodstuffs, from which it can be seen which foods best complement each other. It is also necessary, of course, to ascertain the total quantity of protein and amino acids in any food. The quality of the protein depends largely on its amino acid composition and its digestibility. If a protein is deficient in one or more essential amino acids, its quality is lower.

The most deficient of the essential amino acids in a protein is called the "limiting amino acid". The limiting amino acid determines the efficiency of utilization of the protein present in a food or combination of foods. Human beings usually eat food in meals which contain many proteins; they seldom consume just one protein. Therefore nutritionists are interested in the protein quality of a person's diet or meals, rather than just one food. If one essential amino acid is in short supply in the diet, it limits the use of the other amino acids for building protein. Readers who wish to become familiar with the methods used for determining protein quality are advised to consult comprehensive textbooks on nutrition, which describe them in detail.

One method uses experiments on growth and nitrogen retention in young rats. Another involves determination of the amino acid or chemical score, usually by examining the efficiency of utilization of proteins in the foods consumed by comparing their amino acid composition with that of protein known to be of high quality, such as that in whole eggs. The chemical score may thus be defined as the efficiency of utilization of food protein in comparison with whole egg protein. Net protein utilization (NPU) is a measure of the amount or percentage of protein retained in relation to that consumed. For the professional involved in nutritional activities to help people—be it a dietitian in a health facility, an agricultural extension worker or a nutrition educator what is important is that the protein value differs among foods and that mixing foods improves the protein quality of the meal or the diet.

Proteins consumed in the diet undergo a series of chemical changes in the gastrointestinal tract. The physiology of protein digestion is complicated; pepsin and rennin from the stomach, trypsin from the pancreas and erepsin from the intestines hydrolyse proteins into their component amino acids. Most of the amino acids are absorbed into the bloodstream from the small intestine and thus travel to the liver and from there all over the body. Any surplus amino acids are stripped of the amino (NH_2) group, which goes to form urea in the urine, leaving the rest of the molecule to be transformed into glucose. There is now some evidence that a little intact protein is taken up into certain cells lining the intestines.

Some of this protein in the infant may have a role in the passive immunity conveyed from the mother to her newborn child. A little of the protein and amino acids released in the intestines is not absorbed. The unabsorbed amino acids, plus cells shed from the intestinal villi and acted upon by bacteria, together with gut organisms, contribute to the nitrogen found in faeces. Much of the protein in the human body is present in muscle. There is no true storage of protein in the body as there is with fat and to a small extent glycogen. However, there is now little doubt that a well-nourished individual has sufficient protein accumulated to be able to last several days without replenishment and to remain still in good health. Children need more protein than adults because they need to grow. Infants in the first few months of life require about 2.5 g of protein per kilogram of body weight. This requirement drops to about 1.5 g/kg at nine to 12 months of age. Unless energy intakes are adequate, however, the protein will not all be used for growth.

A pregnant woman needs an additional supply of protein to build up the foetus inside her. Similarly, a lactating woman needs extra protein, because the milk she secretes contains protein. In some societies it is common for women to breastfeed their babies for as long as two years. Thus some women need extra protein for two years and nine months for every infant they bear. Protein requirements and recommended allowances have been the subject of much research, debate and disagreement over the past 50 years.

In children inadequate energy intake also has an impact on protein. In the absence of adequate energy some protein needs to be diverted and therefore will not be used for growth. In many developing countries (though not all), the intake of protein is relatively low and of predominantly vegetable origin. The paucity of foods of animal origin in the diet is not always a matter of choice. For example, many low-income Africans and Latin Americans like animal products but find them less freely available, more difficult to produce and store and more expensive than most vegetable products. Diets low in meat, fish and dairy products are very common in countries where most people are poor. Infections lead to an increased loss of nitrogen from the body, which has to be replaced by proteins in the diet. Therefore children and others who have frequent infections will have greater protein needs than healthy persons. This fact must constantly be borne in mind, for in developing countries many children suffer an almost continual series of infectious diseases; they may frequently get diarrhoea, and they may harbour intestinal parasites.

Minerals have a number of functions in the body. Sodium, potassium and chlorine are present as salts in body fluids, where they have a physiological role in maintaining osmotic pressure. Minerals form part of the constitution of many tissues. For example, calcium and phosphorus in bones combine to give rigidity to the whole body. Minerals are present in body acids and alkalis; for example, chlorine occurs in hydrochloric acid in the stomach. They are also essential constituents of certain hormones, e.g. iodine in the thyroxine produced by the thyroid gland. The principal minerals in the human body are calcium, phosphorus, potassium, sodium, chlorine, sulphur, copper, magnesium, manganese, iron, iodine, fluorine, zinc, cobalt and selenium.

Phosphorus is so widely available in plants that a shortage of this element is unlikely in any diet. Potassium, sodium and chlorine are easily absorbed and are physiologically more important than phosphorus. Sulphur is consumed by humans mainly in the form of sulphur-containing amino acids; thus sulphur deficiency, when it occurs, is linked with protein deficiency. Copper, manganese and magnesium deficiencies are not believed to be common. The minerals that are of most importance in human nutrition are thus calcium, iron, iodine, fluorine and zinc, and only these are discussed in some detail here. Some mineral elements are required in very tiny amounts in human diets but are still vital for metabolic purposes; these are termed "essential trace elements". The body of an average-sized adult contains about 1 250 g of calcium. Over 99 percent of the calcium is in the bones and teeth, where it is combined with phosphorus as calcium phosphate, a hard substance that gives the body rigidity. However, although hard and rigid, the skeleton of the body is not the unchanging structure it appears to be.

In fact, the bones are a cellular matrix, and the calcium is continuously taken up by the bones and given back to the body. The bones, therefore, serve as a reserve supply of this mineral. Calcium is present in the serum of the blood in small but important quantities, usually about 10 mg per 100 ml of serum. There are also about 10 g of calcium in the extracellular fluids and soft tissues of the adult body. In humans and other mammals, calcium and phosphorus together have an important role as major components of the skeleton. They are also important, however, in metabolic functions such as muscular function, nervous stimuli, enzymatic and hormonal activities and transport of oxygen. These functions are described in detail in textbooks of physiology and nutrition.

The skeleton of a living person is physiologically different from the dry skeleton in a grave or museum. The bones are living tissues, consisting mainly of a mineralized protein collagen substance. In the living body there is continuous turnover of calcium. Bone is laid down and resorbed all the time, in people of all ages. Bone cells called osteoclasts take up or resorb bone, while others, termed osteoblasts, lay down or form new bone. The bone cells in the mineralized collagen are called osteocytes. Up to full growth or maturity, new bone is formed as the skeleton enlarges to its adult size. In young adults, despite bone remodelling, the skeleton generally maintains its size. However, as persons get older there is some loss of bone mass. A complex physiological system maintains proper calcium and phosphorus levels.

The control involves hormones from the parathyroid gland, calcitonin and the active form of vitamin D. Small but highly important amounts of calcium are present in extracellular fluids, particularly blood plasma, as well as in various body cells. In serum most of the calcium is in two forms, ionized and protein bound. Laboratories usually measure only total plasma calcium; the normal range is 8.5 to 10.5 mg/dl. A drop in the level of calcium to below 2.1 mmol/litre is termed hypocalcaemia and can lead to various symptoms. Tetany, characterized by spasms and sometimes fits, results from low levels of ionized calcium in the blood. All the calcium in the body, except that inherited from the mother, comes from food and water consumed. It is especially necessary to have adequate quantities of calcium during growth, for it is at this stage that the bones develop. The foetus in the mother's uterus has most of its nutritional requirements satisfied, for in terms of nutrition the unborn child is almost parasitic. If the mother's diet is poor in calcium, she draws extra supplies of this mineral from her bones. An entirely breastfed infant will obtain adequate calcium from breastmilk as long as the volume of milk is sufficient.

Contrary to popular belief, the calcium content of human milk varies rather little; 100 ml of breastmilk, even from an undernourished mother on a diet very low in calcium, provides approximately 30 mg of calcium. A lactating mother secreting 1 litre will thus lose 300 mg of calcium per day. Cows' milk is a very rich source of calcium, richer than human milk. Whereas a litre of human milk contains 300 mg of calcium, a litre of cows' milk contains 1200 ma. The difference arises because a cow has to provide for her calf, which grows much more rapidly than a human infant and needs extra calcium for the hardening of its fast-growing skeleton. Similarly, the milk of most other domestic animals has a higher calcium content than human milk. This does not mean, however, that a child would be better off drinking cows' milk rather than human milk. Cows' milk yields more calcium than a child needs.

A child (or even a baby) who drinks large quantities of cows' milk excretes any excess calcium, so it is of no benefit; it does not increase the child's growth rate beyond what is optimal. Milk products such as cheese and yoghurt are also rich sources of calcium. Although cereals and roots are relatively poor sources of calcium, they often supply the major portion of the mineral in tropical diets by virtue of the quantities consumed. The calcium content of drinking-water varies from place to place. Hard water usually contains high levels of calcium.

The absorption of calcium is variable and generally rather low. It is related to the absorption of phosphorus and the other important mineral constituents of the bones. Vitamin D is essential for the proper absorption of calcium. Thus a person seriously deficient in vitamin D absorbs too little calcium, even if the intake of calcium is more than adequate, and could have a negative calcium balance. Phytates, phosphates and oxalates in food reduce calcium absorption. Persons customarily consuming diets low in calcium appear to have better absorption of calcium than those on high-calcium diets.

Unabsorbed calcium is excreted in the faeces. Excess calcium is excreted in the urine and in sweat. It is not easy to state categorically the human requirements for calcium, because there are several factors influencing absorption and considerable variations in calcium losses among individuals. Needs for calcium are increased during pregnancy and lactation, and children require more calcium because of growth. Those on high-protein diets require more calcium in the diet. The following are recommended levels of daily calcium intake:

— adults, 400 to 500 mg;

— children, 400 to 700 mg;

— pregnant and lactating women, 800 to 1 000 mg.

Disease or malformation caused primarily by dietary deficiency of calcium is rare. There is little convincing evidence to show that the many diets of adults in developing countries supplying perhaps only 250 to 300 mg of calcium daily are harmful to health. It is assumed that adults achieve some sort of balance when intakes of calcium are low. Females who go through a series of pregnancies and long lactations may lose calcium and be at risk of osteomalacia. However, vitamin D deficiency, not calcium deficiency, is more often implicated in this condition. In children the development of rickets results from vitamin D deficiency, not from dietary lack of calcium, in spite of increased calcium requirements in childhood.

Calcium balance in childhood is generally positive, and calcium deficiency has not been shown to have an adverse influence on growth. Osteoporosis is a common disease of ageing, especially in women. The skeleton becomes demineralized, which leads to fragility of bones and commonly to fractures of the hip, vertebrae and other bones, particularly in older women. High calcium intake is often recommended but has not been proved effective in prevention or treatment. Exercise appears to reduce the loss of calcium from bones; this may explain, in part, why osteoporosis is less prevalent in many developing countries, where women work hard and are very active. There is now clear evidence that providing the female hormone oestrogen to women after menopause reduces bone loss and osteoporosis.

Additional tiny quantities are found binding protein in the blood plasma and in respiratory enzymes. The main, vital function of iron is in the transfer of oxygen at various sites in the body. Haemoglobin is the pigment in the erythrocytes that carries oxygen from the lungs to the tissues. Myoglobin in skeletal and heart muscle accepts the oxygen from the haemoglobin. Iron is also present in peroxidase, catalase and the cytochromes. Iron is an element that is neither used up nor destroyed in the properly functioning body. Unlike some minerals, it is not required for excretion, and only very small amounts appear in urine and sweat. Minute quantities are lost in desquamated cells from the skin and intestine, in shed hair and nails and in the bile and other body secretions. The body is, however, efficient, economical and conservative in the use of iron. Iron released when the erythrocytes are old and broken down is taken up and used again and again for the manufacture of new erythrocytes. This economy of iron is important. In normal circumstances, only about 1 mg of iron is lost from the body daily by excretion into the intestines, in urine, in sweat or through loss of hair or surface epithelial cells. Because iron is conserved, the nutritional needs of healthy males and postmenopausal females are very small.

Women of child-bearing age, however, must replace the iron lost during menstruation and childbirth and must meet the additional requirements of pregnancy and lactation. Children have relatively high needs because of their rapid growth, which involves increases not only in body size but also in blood volume. Iron is present in a variety of foods of both plant and animal origin. Rich food sources include meat (especially liver), fish, eggs, legumes (including a variety of beans, peas and other pulses) and green leafy vegetables. Cereal grains such as maize, rice and wheat contain moderate amounts of iron, but because these are often staple foods and eaten in large quantities, they provide most of the iron for many people in developing countries. Iron cooking pots may be a source of iron. Milk, contrary to the notion that it is the "perfect food", is a poor source of iron. Human milk contains about 2 mg of iron per litre and cows' milk only half this amount. Absorption of iron takes place mainly in the upper portion of the small intestine. Most of the iron enters the bloodstream directly and not through the lymphatic system. Evidence indicates that absorption is regulated to some extent by physiological demand.

Persons who are iron deficient tend to absorb iron more efficiently and in greater quantities than do normal subjects. Several other factors affect iron absorption.

Newborn infants are born with very high haemoglobin levels (a high red blood cell count), termed polycythaemia, which provides an extra store of iron. This iron, together with that present in breastmilk, is usually sufficient for the first four to six months of life, after which iron from other foods becomes necessary. Premature and other low-birth-weight infants may have lower iron stores and be at greater risk than other infants. An excess intake of iron over long periods can lead to the disease siderosis or haemachromatosis. Food iron is poorly absorbed. Iron is not readily excreted into the urine or the gastro-intestinal tract; thus severe iron deficiency is usually associated with an increased need for iron resulting from conditions such as pregnancy, blood loss or expansion of the total body mass during growth. Iron deficiency is most common in young children, in women of child-bearing age and in persons with chronic blood loss. Hookworm infections, which are extremely prevalent in many countries, result in loss of blood which may cause iron deficiency anaemia. In some parts of the tropics schistosomiasis is also common, and this disease also causes blood loss.

The body of an average adult contains about 20 to 50 mg of iodine, much of it in the thyroid gland. Iodine is essential for the formation of thyroid hormones secreted by this gland. In humans iodine functions as an essential component of the hormones of the thyroid gland, an endocrine gland situated in the lower neck. Thyroid hormones, of which the most important is thyroxine (T4), are important for regulating metabolism. In children they support normal growth and development, including mental development. Iodine is absorbed from the gut as iodide, and excess is excreted in the urine. The adult thyroid gland, in a person consuming adequate iodine, traps about 60 μg of iodine per day to make normal amounts of thyroid hormones. If there is insufficient iodine, the thyroid works harder to trap more; the gland enlarges in size (a condition known as goitre), and its iodine content might become markedly reduced.

Thyroid stimulating hormone (TSH) from the pituitary gland influences thyroxine secretion and iodine trapping. Iodine is widely present in rocks and soils. The quantity in different plants varies according to the soil in which they are grown. It is not meaningful to list the iodine content of foodstuffs because of the large variations in iodine content from place to place, depending on the iodine content of the soil. Iodine tends to get washed out of the soil, and throughout the ages a considerable quantity has flowed into the sea. Sea fish, seaweed and most vegetables grown near the sea are useful sources of iodine. Drinking-water provides some iodine but very seldom enough to satisfy human requirements. In many countries where goitre is prevalent the authorities have added iodine to salt, a strategy which has successfully controlled iodine deficiency disorders (IDD). Iodine has usually been added to salt in the form of potassium iodide, but another form, potassium iodate, is more stable and is better in hot, humid climates. Iodated salt is an important dietary source of iodine.

A lack of iodine in the diet results in several health problems, one of which is goitre, or enlargement of the thyroid gland. Goitre is extremely prevalent in many countries. There are other contributing causes of goitre, but iodine deficiency is by far the most common. Iodine deficiency during pregnancy may lead to cretinism, mental retardation and other problems, which may be permanent, in the child. It is now known that endemic goitre and cretinism are not the only problems caused by iodine deficiency. The decrease in mental capacity associated with iodine deficiency is of particular concern. IDD, although previously prevalent in Europe, North America and Australia, is now seen predominantly in developing countries.

Fluorine is a mineral element found mainly in the teeth and skeleton. Traces of fluorine in the teeth help to protect them against decay. Fluorides consumed during childhood become a part of the dental enamel and make it more resistant to the weak organic acids formed from foods that adhere to or get stuck between the teeth. This strengthening greatly reduces the chances of decay or caries developing in the teeth. Some studies have suggested that fluoride may also help strengthen bone, particularly later in life, and may thus inhibit the development of osteoporosis. The main source of fluorine for most human beings is the water they drink. If the water has a fluorine content of about one part per million (1 ppm), then it will supply adequate fluorine for the teeth. However, many water supplies contain much less than this amount. Fluorine is present in bone; consequently small fish that are consumed whole are a good source. Tea has a high fluorine content. Few other foods contain much fluorine. If the fluoride content of drinking-water in any locality is below 0.5 ppm, dental caries will probably be much more prevalent than where the concentration is higher. The recommended level of fluoride in water is between 0.8 and 1.2 ppm.

In some countries or localities where the content of fluorine in the water is less than 1 ppm, it has now become the practice to add fluoride to the water supply. This practice is strongly recommended, but it is only practicable for large piped-water supplies; in some developing countries where most people do not have piped water, it is not feasible. The addition of fluoride to toothpaste also helps reduce dental caries. Fluorine does not totally prevent dental caries, but it can reduce the incidence by 60 to 70 percent. An excessively high intake of fluoride causes a condition known as dental fluorosis, in which the teeth become mottled. It is usually caused by consuming excessive fluoride in water supplies that have high fluoride levels.

Zinc is an essential element in human nutrition, and its importance to human health has received much recent attention. Zinc is present in many important enzymes essential for metabolism. The body of a healthy human adult contains 2 to 3 g of zinc and requires around 15 mg of dietary zinc per day. Most of the zinc in the body is in the skeleton, but other tissues (such as the skin and hair) and some organs (particularly the prostate) have relatively high concentrations. Zinc is present in most foods both of vegetable and of animal origin, but the richest sources tend to be protein-rich foods such as meat, seafoods and eggs. In developing countries, however, where most people consume relatively small amounts of these foods, most zinc comes from cereal grains and legumes. As with iron, absorption of zinc from the diet is inhibited by food constituents such as phytates, oxalate and tannins.

No simple tests of human zinc status are known, however. Indicators used include evidence of low dietary intake, low blood serum zinc levels and low quantities of zinc in hair specimens. Much research on this mineral has been undertaken in the last two decades, and a great deal of knowledge concerning zinc metabolism and zinc deficiency in animals and humans has been gathered. Nonetheless, there is little evidence to suggest that zinc deficiency is an important public health problem for large numbers of people in any country, industrialized or developing. However, research now under way may show that poor zinc status is responsible for poor growth, reduced appetite and other conditions; in this way zinc deficiency may contribute especially to what is now called protein-energy malnutrition (PEM). Zinc deficiency is responsible for a very rare congenital disease known as acrodermatitis enteropathica. It responds to zinc therapy.

Some patients receiving all of their nutrients intravenously have developed skin lesions which also respond to zinc treatment. In the Near East, particularly in the Islamic Republic of Iran and Egypt, a condition has been described in which adolescent or near-adolescent boys are dwarfed and have poorly developed genitalia and delayed onset of puberty; this condition has been said to respond to zinc treatment. Zinc deficiency has also been reported as secondary to, or as a part of, other conditions such as PEM, various malabsorption conditions, alcoholism including cirrhosis of the liver, renal disease and metabolic disorders. Numerous minerals are present in the human body. For most of the trace elements, besides those discussed above, there is no evidence that deficiency is responsible for major public health problems anywhere. Some of these minerals are very important in metabolism or as constituents of body tissues. Many of them have been studied, and their chemistry and biochemistry have been described.

Experimental deficiencies have been produced in laboratory animals, but most human diets, even poor diets, do not appear to lead to important deficiencies.

These minerals therefore are not of public health importance. Other trace elements are present in the body but do not have any known essential role. Some minerals, for example lead and mercury, are of great interest to health workers because excess intake has commonly resulted in toxic manifestations. Cobalt, copper, magnesium, manganese and selenium deserve mention because of their important nutritional role, and lead and mercury because of their toxicity. Cobalt is of interest to nutritionists because it is an essential part of vitamin B12. When isolated as a crystalline substance, the vitamin was found to contain about 4 percent cobalt. However, cobalt deficiency does not play a part in the anaemia that results from vitamin B12 deficiency. Copper deficiency is known to cause anaemia in cattle, but no such risk is known in adult humans.

Some evidence suggests that copper deficiency leads to anaemia in premature infants, in people with severe PEM and in those maintained on parenteral nutrition. An extremely rare congenital condition known as Menkes' disease is caused by failure of copper absorption. Magnesium is an essential mineral present mainly in the bones but also in most human tissues. Most diets contain adequate dietary magnesium, but under some circumstances, such as diarrhoea, severe PEM and other conditions, excessive body losses of magnesium occur. Such losses may lead to weakness and mental changes and occasionally to convulsions.

Excess lead intake may result from consumption of lead in the household (from lead-based paint or water pipes containing lead) and from intake of atmospheric lead (from motor vehicle emissions). Mercury deficiency is not known in humans. The concern is with excessively high intakes of mercury and the risks of toxicity. Fish in waters contaminated with mercury concentrate the mineral. Vitamins are organic substances present in minute amounts in foodstuffs and necessary for metabolism. They are grouped together not because they are chemically related or have similar physiological functions, but because, as their name implies, they are vital factors in the diet and because they were all discovered in connection with the diseases resulting from their deficiency. Moreover, they do not fit into the other nutrient categories.

When vitamins were first being classified, each was named after a letter of the alphabet. Subsequently, there has been a tendency to drop the letters in favour of chemical names. The use of the chemical name is justified when the vitamin has a known chemical formula, as with the main vitamins of the B group. Nevertheless, it is advantageous to include certain vitamins under group headings, even if they are not chemically related, since they do tend to occur in the same foodstuffs. Other vitamins known to be vital to health include pantothenic acid, biotin, para-aminobenzoic acid, choline, vitamin E and vitamin K:. These vitamins are not described in detail here for one or more of the following reasons:

— deficiency is not known to occur under natural conditions in humans;

— deficiency is extremely rare even in grossly abnormal diets;

— lack of the vitamin results in disease only if it follows some other disease process that is adequately described in textbooks of general medicine;

— the role of the vitamin in human nutrition has not yet been elucidated.

Vitamin A was discovered in 1913 when research workers found that certain laboratory animals stopped growing when lard (made from pork fat) was the only form of fat present in their diet, whereas when butter was supplied instead of lard (with the diet remaining otherwise the same) the animals grew and thrived. Retinol is the main form of vitamin A in human diets. (Retinol is the chemical name of the alcohol derivative, and it is used as the reference standard.) In its pure crystalline form, retinol is a very pale yellow-green substance. It is soluble in fat but insoluble in water, and it is found only in animal products. Other forms of vitamin A exist, but they have somewhat different molecular configurations and less biological activity than retinol, and they are not important in human diets. Carotenes, which act as provitamins or precursors of vitamin A, are yellow substances that occur widely in plant substances.

In some foodstuffs their colour may be masked by the green plant pigment chlorophyll, which often occurs in close association with carotenes. There are several different carotenes. One of these, beta-carotene, is the most important source of vitamin A in the diets of most people living in non-industrialized countries. The other carotenes, or carotenoids, have little or no nutritional importance for humans. In the past, food analyses have often failed to distinguish beta-carotene from other carotenes. Vitamin A is an important component of the visual purple of the retina of the eye, and if vitamin A is deficient, the ability to see in dim light is reduced. This condition is called night blindness.

The biochemical basis for the other lesions of vitamin A deficiency has not been fully explained. The main change, in pathological terms, is a keratinizing metaplasia which is seen on various epithelial surfaces. Vitamin A appears to be necessary for the protection of surface tissue. Several studies have shown that adequate vitamin A status reduces infant and child mortality in certain populations. Vitamin A supplementation reduces case fatality rates from measles. In other illnesses such as diarrhoea and respiratory infections, however, there is not strong evidence that the prevalence or duration of morbidity is reduced by vitamin A dosing. Since pure crystalline vitamin A, which is termed retinol alcohol, is now available, the vitamin A activity in foods is now widely expressed and measured using retinol equivalents rather than the international units (IU) previously used. Humans obtain vitamin A in food either as preformed vitamin A (retinol) or as carotenes which can be converted to retinol in the body. Beta-carotene is the most important in human diets and is better converted to retinol than other carotenes.

Vitamin A itself is found only in animal products; the main sources are butter, eggs, milk, meat (especially liver) and some fish. However, most people in developing countries rely mainly on beta-carotene for their supply of vitamin A. Carotene is contained in many plant foods. Dark green leaves such as those of amaranth, spinach, sweet potato and cassava are much richer sources than paler leaves such as those of cabbage and lettuce. Various pigmented fruits and vegetables, such as mangoes, papayas and tomatoes, contain useful quantities. Carotene is also present in yellow varieties of sweet potatoes and in yellow vegetables such as pumpkins. Carrots are rich sources. Yellow maize is the only cereal that contains carotene.

However, a considerable amount of carotene is lost when green leaves and other foods are dried in the sun. Sun-drying is a traditional method of preserving wild leaves and vegetables often used in arid regions. Since serious disease from vitamin A deficiency is common in these areas, it is important that other methods of preservation be established. The conversion of beta-carotene into vitamin A takes place in the walls of the intestines. Even the most efficient intestine can absorb and convert only a portion of the beta-carotene in the diet; therefore 6 mg of beta-carotene in food is equivalent to about 1 mg of retinol. If no animal products are consumed and the body must rely entirely on carotene for its vitamin A, consumption of carotene must be great enough to achieve the required vitamin A level. Carotene is poorly utilized when the diet has a low fat content, and diets deficient in vitamin A are often deficient in fat.

Intestinal diseases such as dysentery, coeliac disease and sprue limit the absorption of vitamin A and the conversion of carotene. Malabsorption syndromes and infections with common intestinal parasites such as roundworm, which are prevalent in the tropics, may also reduce the ability of the body to convert carotene into vitamin A. Bile salts are essential for the absorption of vitamin A and carotene, so persons with obstruction of the bile duct are likely to become deficient in vitamin A. Even in ideal circumstances, infants and young children do not convert carotene to vitamin A as readily as adults do. The liver acts as the main store of vitamin A in the human and most other vertebrates, which is why fish-liver oils have a high content of this vitamin. Retinol is transported from the liver to other sites in the body by a specific carrier protein called retinol binding protein (RBP). Protein deficiency may influence vitamin A status by reducing the synthesis of RBP. The storage of vitamin A in the liver is important, for in many tropical diets foods containing vitamin A and carotene are available seasonally.

If these foods are eaten in fairly large quantities when available (usually during the wet season), a store can be built up which will help tide the person over the dry season, or at least part of it. The short mango season provides an excellent opportunity for youngsters, who may happily spend their leisure hours foraging for this fruit, to replenish the vitamin A stored in the liver. The most marked toxic effect is an irregular thickening of some long bones, usually accompanied by headache, vomiting, liver enlargement, skin changes and hair loss.

When the diet is entirely of vegetable origin, larger amounts of carotene are suggested, because the conversion from carotene to retinol is not very efficient. Deficiency results in pathological drying of the eye, leading to xerophthalmia and sometimes keratomalacia and blindness. Other epithelial tissues may be affected; in the skin, follicular keratosis may be the result. During the 1890s in Java, Indonesia, Christiaan Eijkman of the Netherlands noticed that when his chickens were fed on the same diet as that normally consumed by his beriberi patients, they developed weakness in their legs and other signs somewhat similar to those of beriberi. The diet of the beriberi patients consisted mainly of highly milled and refined rice. When Eijkman changed the diet of the chickens to whole-grain rice, they began to recover. He showed that there was a substance in the outer layers and germ of the rice grain that protected the chickens from the disease. Researchers continued to work on isolating the cause of the different effects of diets of polished and whole-grain rice, but despite many attempts it was not until 1926 that vitamin B1 was finally isolated in crystalline form.

Thiamine is one of the most unstable vitamins. It has a rather loosely bound structure and decomposes readily in an alkaline medium. Thiamine is highly soluble in water. Much research has been carried out on the physiological effects and biochemical properties of thiamine. It has been shown that thiamine has a very important role in carbohydrate metabolism in humans. It is utilized in the complicated mechanism of the breakdown, or oxidation, of carbohydrate and the metabolism of pyruvic acid. The energy used by the nervous system is derived entirely from carbohydrate, and a deficiency of thiamine blocks the final utilization of carbohydrate, leading to a shortage of energy and lesions of the nervous tissues and brain. Because thiamine is involved in carbohydrate metabolism, a person whose main supply of energy comes from carbohydrates is more likely to develop signs of thiamine deficiency if his or her food intake is decreased. For this reason, thiamine requirements are sometimes expressed in relation to intake of carbohydrate. Thiamine has been synthesized in pure form and is now measured in milligrams. Thiamine is widely distributed in foods of both vegetable and animal origin. The richest sources are cereal grains and pulses.

Green vegetables, fish, meat, fruit and milk all contain useful quantities. In seeds such as cereals, the thiamine is present mainly in the germ and in the outer coats; thus much can be lost during milling. Bran of rice, wheat and other cereals tends to be naturally rich in thiamine. Yeasts are also rich sources. Root crops are poor sources. For people on a rice diet, it is especially important to prepare rice with just the amount of water that will be absorbed in cooking, or to use water that is left over in soups or stews, for this water will contain thiamine and other nutrients.

Cereals and pulses maintain their thiamine for a year or more if they are stored well, but if they are attacked by bacteria, insects or moulds the content of thiamine gradually diminishes. Thiamine is easily absorbed from the intestinal tract, but little is stored in the body. Experimental evidence indicates that humans can store only enough for about six weeks. The liver, heart and brain have a higher concentration than the muscles and other organs. A person with a high intake of thiamine soon begins to excrete increased quantities in the urine. A daily intake of 1 mg of thiamine is sufficient for a moderately active man and 0.8 mg for a moderately active woman. Pregnant and lactating women may need more. Early work on the properties of vitamins in yeast and other foodstuffs showed that antineuritic factors were destroyed by excessive heat, but that a growth-promoting factor was not destroyed in this way. This factor, riboflavin, was later isolated from the heat-resistant portion. Riboflavin is a yellow crystalline substance. It is much less soluble in water and more heat resistant than thiamine. The vitamin is sensitive to sunlight, so milk, for example, if left exposed may lose considerable quantities of riboflavin.

Community Health

Risk management is the process of evaluating alternative actions, selecting options and implementing them in response to risk assessments. The decision making will incorporate scientific, technological, social, economic and political information. The process requires value judgements, eg. on the tolerability and reasonableness of costs. Alternative actions may be identified by the proponent or through a community consultation process. Once possible health impacts have been identified and assessed, desirable and undesirable impacts can be sorted into those of significance and those that are not. Actions to maximise potential health benefits and minimise or prevent the potential risks to health are identified. The decision making process incorporates scientific, technological, social and economic information and must take into account the community concerns identified during consultation processes.

The decision-making capacityfor an impact assessment does not lie within the health authority. This does not matter so long as the health authority is well linked in to the process and communication between health and the decision-maker is adequate. The important issue is to have health impact assessment as part of the overall impact assessment process. Negotiation may occur between the environment, planning and health agencies ii to ensure a comprehensive, coherent and workable set of changes or conditions are applied to any proposal. There are two types of monitoring and two types of evaluation that may need to be undertaken.

- monitoring of the conditions applied to a development. Routinely undertaken for many developments, both during construction and after operation of the development commences.
- monitoring of the health impacts during and/or after the development, as required.

Whilst the Inter-governmental Agreement on the Environment is aimed at environmental protection, the Rio Declaration, within the context of sustainable development and Agenda 21, makes it clear that the concept is equally applicable to human health and wellbeing. The precautionary approach is not intended to be a device to inhibit development. However, proponents may need to consider and discuss health risks that are uncertain as well as those that are well defined, including an indication of the degree of uncertainty and where the uncertainty is thought to lie. The health authority will facilitate development of the health impact statement (HIS) by the proponent through:

— discussing the Health Impact Assessment (HIA), process, methodology, specific health concerns, sources of data, resources and cost recovery (if applicable) as required - a key focus being to ensure that the overall level of effort is in proportion to the level of risk;

— providing or identifying potential sources of relevant health and demographic data, where available;

— participating in the screening and scoping processes, including visiting the site of the development if practicable;

— reviewing the health components of the draft impact assessment report;

— providing advice to the proponent when they address the concerns raised during public consultation.

In preparing a Health Impact Statement it is necessary for the proponent to consider what data need to be included. Health (or illness) data may be similarly difficult to obtain. Morbidity data collections usually cover wide areas (eg. to postcode level) and usually reflect illness rather than health. The health of the relevant population may, therefore, also require inference of health status from data available on the regional population. Very local health data, if available, may be subject to confidentiality requirements as it may be identifying. There will be ethical and confidentiality constraints on the use of any such data and it may only be accessible to the State/ Territory health authority.

Health data collected might include crude and standardised mortality data, morbidity data for diseases related to potential health impacts, eg. mosquito-borne disease notification rates, or data measuring the prevalence of chronic diseases of concern. The data collection may need to identify special populations who may be at greater risk of adverse health effects. A range of environmental factors affect health, notably food, water and air quality, and waste disposal (solid, liquid and hazardous wastes if any). It is easier, more sensitive and usually more useful to measure the hazard directly, rather than measure ill health. Indicators must be chosen that reasonably reflect both the health impacts that were identified as being of importance during the risk assessment and management steps, and the effectiveness of their amelioration. Indicators of health need to be:

— available at reasonable cost;

— valid and reliable reflections of the actual situation;

— closely linked to actual health outcome;

— timely—ie. rapidly reflect change when a health impact occurs;

— able to be acted upon directly, without further delay or further data collection; and

— readily understood by non-technical people.

Changes in indoor air quality may arise from a wide range of factors, eg. construction materials or equipment used in a building, from outdoor dust creation, from environmental tobacco smoke, or through the entrapment of other pollutants due to inadequate ventilation. Outdoor air may be affected by the handling of dusty materials, such as ores or grains, by the emission of gases such as sulfur dioxide or other smokestack emissions, including particulates or dioxins, and vehicle emissions. Whatever the source of pollution, it requires careful estimation of the area likely to be affected, the intensity and duration of the effect and the level of health impact (actual health effects) on the at risk population.

Modelling of the dispersion of airborne materials is a specialist task, as is the estimation of health effects once the dispersion model is developed. If there is the possibility of a development having an impact on the quality, quantity or the price of food this should be noted and discussed in the HIS. Impact on food production or on food producing land or water would almost certainly be addressed by an EIA but these data would be of interest to the HIA as well.

The use of local water by a proposed development and the likely impact on the surface, ground water and drinking water is a fundamental health concern. It is also an environmental concern and so will be addressed to a significant extent, if not fully, by the EIA process. However, there may be some aspects that require specific attention from a health perspective. The proponent should provide a detailed description of the local water supplies, including non-potable water, and any beneficial uses which the water is, or could be, put to. Particular attention should be paid to any impacts on the potable water supply. Impacts might be from additional consumption that depletes reserves or reduces access, chemical contaminants (nutrients, heavy metals, etc) microbial contaminants, loss of amenity of lakes or other surface water, impact on fish used for food, etc. The disposal of wastewater can have health impacts, whether or not the wastewater contains sewage. Improper disposal of stormwater can lead to loss of amenity and may be hazardous.

Disposal of sewage may be a problem in that control of nutrients and microbes can be difficult or expensive; it typically requires a considerable area of land well away from housing and most other forms of development, and improper disposal quickly becomes a health hazard. Industrial wastes pose differing hazards, depending upon their constituents. They often require further specialised treatment before discharge to sewer or to the local effluent disposal system. These details will be required for any health assessment. If wastewater is to be produced in any quantity and is not simply discharged to sewer, full information on its expected volume, content and method of disposal is likely to be required. One issue that may have significant health impact but which is not usually considered in a health context (except in relation to injury) is transport, both public and private. Improved public transport may have the effect of improving equity, improving access, reducing isolation and increasing opportunities for work and social activity. Use of public transport can even increase exercise through walking to the bus or train stop.

Cycleways provide an environmentally friendly, healthy way to travel. Improving road systems can reduce (or increase) noise, pollution, and the rate of injury to motorists and pedestrians. Areas of loading or unloading can be problematic because of noise and because of materials that may be hazardous being handled there. HIA for a development that directly or indirectly affects means of transport or traffic levels to a significant extent, needs careful consideration. It should entail description of existing services and traffic levels related to either movement of people or materials (particularly hazardous materials), the anticipated or planned changes to those services and assessment of their positive or negative effects on health and amenity.

Hazardous materials storage and handling is a good example of a health issue that is typically well addressed by current impact assessment processes and it is unlikely that further basic data would need to be provided for a HIA. The organisation of the material might need to be more focussed on human health, however, which may only require better cross referencing within the proponent's impact assessment. Social impact assessment is important to HIA in that the health and social impacts are inextricably intertwined. While these can overlap, health impact and social impact require different analytical skills and need to be assessed separately. Where social impacts are of importance to health they should be addressed by the HIA. As for social impacts, the HIA process should not become an economic assessment process. Economic impacts need only be mentioned where they are also important health impacts; their analysis should be independent from the HIA.

Recent advances in scientific techniques, such as use of novel biomarkers, in vitro toxicology, molecular modelling and computer simulations, may offer new possibilities. Furthermore, the use of such techniques should contribute to the reduction of animal use and the refinement and replacement of animal tests, a principle to which developing countries government departments and agencies are committed. The work of the Initiative is being taken forward by the Risk Assessment and Toxicology Steering Committee, which comprises participants from relevant Government departments and research councils and is co-ordinated from the Medical Research Council's Institute for Environment and Health. The Initiative aims to stimulate research so that new, improved approaches to chemicals risk assessment can be developed. It does not have its own research funds, but provides a focus, co-ordination and positive encouragement for research financed by individual Government departments or research councils.

The Steering Committee has organised a series of workshops on different aspects of risk assessment, with the aim of bringing together regulatory toxicologists, policy-makers from government and experts from academic institutions and industry to develop research specifications. The Steering Committee has also undertaken a detailed mapping of toxic risk assessment procedures across Government departments, including the issue of dealing with uncertainties. The Risk Assessment and Toxicology Steering Committee is a subgroup of the Interdepartmental Liaison Group on Risk Assessment (ILGRA). In 1995 it undertook to review the principles and practices used in Government for risk assessment with a view to identifying best practice and encouraging common approaches.

ILGRA programmes published in 1996 and 1998 discussed the use of risk assessment within Government, including issues relating to risk communication and perception. There are three important areas of Government activity in relation to chemicals and human health. These are risk assessment, risk management and risk communication:

— Risk assessment is the evaluation of the potential for adverse health effects in humans from exposure to chemicals.

— Risk management is the evaluation of alternative options and the actions taken to reduce potential risks in the light of an adverse risk assessment.

— Risk communication is the interactive exchange of information and opinions concerning risk between risk assessors, risk managers, the public and other interested parties.

In practice, however, there is often a close interface between risk assessment and risk management. Risk managers may have to set the priorities for risk assessment and frame the questions and parameters on which they need advice. Some risk assessments also implicitly incorporate decisions of a risk management nature, such as the situation envisaged as a reasonable 'worst case' for exposure. It covers effects of chemicals in air, soil, drinking water, food, the occupational environment, consumer products, human and veterinary medicines, and animal feed. It also takes into account international and European Union (EU) influences on chemical risk assessments, since a number of departments and agencies prepare risk assessments for international advisory and regulatory bodies, under the auspices of the EU, United Nations and World Health Organization (WHO). It does not address other key aspects of risk assessment, such as risks of non-chemical agents (such as radiation) and risks to the environment. Neither does it address risk management, except insofar as risk assessment and risk management are sometimes intertwined, nor does it address risk communication or risk perception. Major areas of uncertainty and weaknesses in current risk assessment procedures are identified. A basic framework for the process of chemical risk assessment for human health effects has evolved through national and international consensus and is now well accepted.

An initiative by the International Programme on Chemical Safety (IPCS) is underway, within the framework of the Intergovernmental Forum on Chemical Safety (IFCS), to examine the possibility of global harmonisation of assessment of risk from exposure to chemicals. The aim is to reach an understanding and acceptance of the various approaches used worldwide, to harmonise terminology and, in the longer-term, to achieve convergence of methodology. Risk assessments are used in different contexts within Government departments and agencies. This can influence the way in which risk assessment is approached. For example, there are clearly some constraints in the way risks can be managed when considering a chemical which is already on the market or present in the general environment compared with one that is not. Risk assessment may be required for policy advice and development, for example, to enable Ministers and Government agencies to take decisions on whether individual chemicals or classes of chemicals require closer scrutiny and/or regulation. It may be required to underpin guidance on how to assess and handle particular types of chemical risk (e.g. chemical accidents involving exposure of the general public, chemicals in the workplace). Classes of chemicals subject to these kinds of regulation include new substances, pesticides, biocides, food additives, animal feed additives and human and veterinary medicines.

In order to market or use such chemicals, permission must be sought from or a satisfactory notification must be lodged with the relevant competent authority. Risk assessments on such chemicals are then utilised at a variety of levels, to enable risk management decisions to be taken on whether a chemical or product can be freely used or whether restrictions on use are needed in order to protect human health. The setting of advisory standards, such as acceptable daily intakes (ADIs) for food additives, pesticides and veterinary residues in food, is a key component in the overall risk assessment of many chemicals subject to regulatory control. Advisory standards are also used in situations where chemicals are not directly controlled by legislative means in the medium in which they give rise to human exposure (e.g. ambient air quality standards and guidelines and drinking water guideline values); although appropriate measures may be taken if those advisory standards are exceeded.

In some cases, air and drinking water guideline values have been used in EU Directives to set enforceable standards. Legally enforceable standards are also set for certain chemicals in the workplace and for a few food contaminants. Both advisory and legally enforceable standards are usually set using the first two stages of the basic risk assessment framework described earlier, and in the case of occupational exposure limits a consideration of the third stage is also involved. Thus the majority of standards are health-based. A few, such as some water guideline values, may be based on additional, non-toxicological considerations, such as the aesthetic quality of water (e.g. taste or odour).

Risk assessment is also used to assess the health significance of situations which cross national boundaries (e.g. air pollution) and, at the other end of the scale, localised events or situations, such as accidental chemical releases, deliberate discharges from point sources, projected uses of contaminated land, and the siting of major industrial hazards. The information available for hazard identification and hazard characterisation of individual chemicals normally includes physicochemical data and toxicological data from laboratory studies on animals, animal and human cell lines, and lower organisms. Although experimental studies may be the major source of information for many chemicals, efforts continue to be made to minimise the use of experimental animals in testing. However, apart from the sector of human medicines, risk assessments frequently have to be conducted without the benefit of human data.

Occasionally, information relating biological activity to chemical structure, derived from computational or other techniques, may be available for chemicals within a related chemical group. The toxicological information needed for risk assessment of chemicals usually requires that a number of end-points be addressed in a range of tests. For the majority of chemicals subject to licensing, approval or notification, information on absorption, distribution, metabolism and excretion, general toxicity from single and repeat dose administration, reproductive and developmental toxicity, genetic toxicity and carcinogenicity may be required. For some chemicals, information on eye irritation, skin irritation and skin sensitisation may also be required, not only for the chemical itself but also for the formulation in which it will be marketed. For a few chemicals, more detailed examination of aspects of neurotoxicity, immunotoxicity, endocrine toxicity, or other special studies may be required. In some cases, knowledge of the mechanism by which the observed toxicity is induced may be required to assess whether the mechanism of action is relevant to man.

The mechanism of action may be apparent from the initial studies, or special studies may be required. However, it should be noted that many risk assessments are conducted without the benefit of mechanistic information, particularly in situations where risk assessment is used to develop a health-based standard. Risk assessments of chemicals that have been on the market for some time are needed in the areas of air and drinking water quality standards, occupational and consumer exposure, local incidents of pollution, consents for discharges, chemical accidents and the siting of major hazards. Many of these chemicals were first marketed years ago when pre-marketing notification or authorisation was not required. Risk assessments for such chemicals are generally based on whatever relevant information is available, although in some circumstances it may be possible to request additional information. Adequate physicochemical data are usually available but the extent and quality of the biological information can be very variable. Sometimes, because of experience of human exposure over time, there may be more human toxicological and epidemiological data available than is the case for newer chemicals. In contrast, a comprehensive range of in vitro and in vivo toxicological data may be absent.

To date, it is only in the area of human medicines that there has been wider international agreement on requirements for toxicological testing, under the auspices of the International Conference on Harmonisation of Technical Requirements for Registration of Pharmaceuticals for Human Use (ICH). A key aspect of harmonisation is that standard protocols for the most widely used toxicity tests have been developed and agreed within the OECD. Members of OECD, which includes all the major industrialised nations, are obliged under the Mutual Acceptance of Data agreement to accept data on chemicals for evaluation if they have been generated from studies conducted according to OECD protocols and according to the OECD principles of Good Laboratory Practice.

Harmonisation of test protocols and data requirements within chemical sectors across the EU or more globally has been beneficial in ensuring that risk assessments on new chemicals are made from an acceptable database. There is now less tolerance of gaps in databases than previously was the case. Given the global nature of trade in and use of chemicals, sectors such as pesticides, biocides, food additives and animal feed additives would benefit from global harmonisation of toxicological testing requirements. The emphasis should be on harmonisation of the minimum data needed for meaningful risk assessment.

In some chemical sectors, progression to full approval for requested uses proceeds in stages. For example, with human medicines, clinical trial certificates or exemptions are granted after scrutiny of a limited pharmaco-toxicological database that is tailored to the needs of the risk assessment required to proceed to human clinical trials. As development of the compound proceeds, further animal and/or human studies, addressing toxicological issues, are conducted, tailored to intended clinical uses, before marketing authorisation is considered. A similar, staged approval process applies to veterinary medicines during their development stage through clinical trials to full marketing. Approval of agricultural pesticides also proceeds via initial experimental permits for crop trials, which are granted on a limited toxicological database. At these early stages, risk assessment of agricultural pesticides focuses on occupational exposure; human exposure via food is not permitted unless residues are non-detectable or unless repeat-dose and teratogenicity studies are available and indicate limited exposure to residues is acceptable.

This tiered supply-based approach to toxicity testing for new substances also recognises that the cost of testing has to relate to the ability of the product to stand such costs. Furthermore, the amount of testing is also linked to the careful control of the supply and the ability to monitor the situation and take remedial action if necessary. Similarly, approval of the use of substances in food contact materials follows a tiered approach, depending on the amounts shown to be migrating into food; at very low projected human exposures only genetic toxicity studies are required, at higher projected exposures additional studies are required, and at the highest exposure levels a comprehensive set of toxicity studies is required.

Staged approaches of this nature imply acceptance of the concept that below certain levels of production/exposure only certain toxic effects are likely to occur. Such a concept is based on both scientific considerations about thresholds for toxic effects and societal considerations about acceptance of low-level risks. Other chemicals can be approved for marketing on the basis of a comprehensive set of toxicological and other studies submitted at the time approval is first sought. This situation applies to food additives, novel foods and processes, animal feed additives and certain cosmetic ingredients. When a chemical or product is subject to prior regulatory notification, approval or authorisation before it can be used or marketed, it is the responsibility of the company or consortium (the applicant) that wishes to use or market it to generate, assemble and submit the required information. This situation applies in the case of human and veterinary medicines, agricultural and non-agricultural pesticides, new substance notifications, novel foods and processes, food additives, animal feed additives, substances used in certain categories of packaging materials (plastics, cellulose film), and cosmetic ingredients in categories requiring positive approval.

At this stage there is usually little or no published information available and data generated by the applicant are often submitted 'in confidence' to the competent authorities. The authority can, where necessary, request that the applicant submit additional data. If additional studies or other information are necessary, this 'request' is, in effect, a requirement since, if not submitted, approval may be denied or a temporary approval suspended. Some competent authorities can themselves commission additional studies, though this is rarely done in the case of new chemicals. In the case of chemicals or products that are regulated or voluntarily controlled by means other than prior notification or approval, a different situation applies, since the competent authorities generally lack powers to compel chemical producers to provide information. This situation applies in the case of pollutants present in ambient air, chemicals present in drinking water, chemical contaminants in food (other than certain food packaging substances and a few other regulated contaminants) and chemicals in consumer products.

The chemical under consideration may not be synthesised commercially (e.g. dioxins or naturally occurring toxicants in food), or it may no longer be produced commercially (e.g. polychlorinated biphenyls), or it may be produced commercially but human exposure is not attributable to any one industry (e.g. pollutants and contaminants in air, water and food such as benzene, polycyclic aromatic hydrocarbons, and heavy metals). Risk assessment of occupational exposure to existing chemicals and risk assessment of major hazards and land use planning are hybrid situations. Lack of good exposure data is frequently a problematic area in risk assessment.

The type of exposure information required depends on the purpose for which it is needed. Some risk assessments require that human exposure, via ingestion, inhalation or dermal absorption, be assessed as directly as possible, in order that it may be compared with some health-based standard for human exposure, or compared with information about exposures associated with adverse effects. For many chemicals, exposure will be variable over time; the range of intakes or concentrations to which individuals are exposed may be needed, or at least an estimated 'worst case scenario'. In the case of risk assessments for which human exposure data are required, measurement of actual exposure of individuals is rarely carried out. It may be undertaken in special cases such as measurement of chemical concentrations in inspired air via personal samplers in occupational settings, or measurement of intake biomarkers in biological fluids. It is only in the special case of human medicines that the applied dose is known routinely with some certainty; exposure to the chemical at pre-specified doses is intentional and systemic exposure of the individual to the chemical is evaluated during clinical trials.

More often, population exposures are estimated indirectly, using data on measured or predicted concentrations of the chemical in air, food or water coupled with estimates or assumptions about the human body, to predict external or internal (systemic) exposures. Lack of suitable analytical methods for different media and with appropriate limits of detection may also be a factor that limits the availability of good exposure data. In certain chemical sectors where information may initially be sparse, such as new substance notifications, human exposure may have to be modelled entirely from surrogate parameters such as physicochemical properties and knowledge of the way the chemical will be manufactured and used, coupled with default assumptions about the human body.

In the case of risk assessments requiring knowledge of inputs into ambient media, the source of pollution may be a point source or a diffuse source. Concentrations at point sources and subsequent dispersion in ambient media may be measured or modelled. This type of exposure assessment requires a considerable knowledge of factors affecting the nature of releases, the ways in which the material will disperse in air, water and soil and whether dispersions from point sources overlap and need to be aggregated. It can be used to explore management options for achieving particular discharge/ emission standards. Various techniques are available for modelling each aspect of the exposure assessment and, depending on the model used, may incorporate differing degrees of conservatism. It is recommended that experience with modelling intake and exposure from point and diffuse sources is shared across Government departments and agencies undertaking such tasks, with a view to assessing the validity and utility of different exposure models.

Harmonisation of approaches both nationally and internationally would be a desirable goal. As an alternative to modelling of dispersion, actual measurements of chemical concentrations may be taken in the relevant ambient media, but this may require extensive monitoring over time and place, which presents its own difficulties. Surveillance for sporadic contaminants in large consignments of crops or food products also presents similar difficulties concerning the selection of when and where to sample. The application of statistical techniques to the design of such monitoring programmes can aid reliability and comprehensive coverage of results.

When measurements of chemical concentrations in air, water or food, or estimates of intake are used for risk assessment, 'best estimates', 'worst case' estimates, or both may be needed for the exposure assessment. 'Best estimates' are usually averages, based on mean or median concentrations or intakes. Worst case estimates, in contrast, are usually based on extreme values, though not necessarily the highest values, obtained for concentrations or intakes. Similarly, for food chemicals, provided worst case estimates do not exceed the relevant ADIs or tolerable daily intakes (TDIs), then no further action need be taken. In these situations the value of a 'worst case' estimation is that it is quickly and easily done and may enable reassuring conclusions to be drawn from the risk assessment process. Under these circumstances, the in-built conservatism of 'worst case' estimates is not a problem.

However, when considering exposure of the general public to the same chemical, 'worst case' scenarios may be used. Similarly, in the case of chemicals present in consumer products or pesticides in products for amateur home and garden use, exposure scenarios involving reasonably foreseeable misuse are considered, though deliberate ingestion with the intent to poison is excluded from consideration. For chemicals present in food, be they deliberately added, naturally present or present as contaminants, a comprehensive knowledge of food consumption patterns, coupled with knowledge of which foods contain the chemical and at what concentrations, is the key to obtaining good exposure estimates.

Information about concentrations of chemicals present in various consumer products comes largely from industry, with some from analyses commissioned by local authorities (trading standards officers/public analysts) or the Government. Measurements or estimates of exposure to chemicals present in the occupational environment may be submitted by industry and checked by the Health and Safety Executive (HSE), or HSE may make its own measurements or estimates, based on the application of models to data provided by the industry. For general pollutants present in ambient air, such as ozone, oxides of nitrogen, sulphur dioxide and benzene, both published papers and data from local measurements are utilised to assess exposure. For chemicals present in drinking water, published papers, information from the water industry and, in the case of chemical contamination, local measurements are utilised.

Exposure may be through food, water, air, skin contact, other routes (human medicines and certain consumer products), or any combination of these. For example, workers mixing and spraying pesticides may be exposed by oral, respiratory and dermal routes. Environmental pollutants, such as heavy metals or certain ubiquitous organic chemicals, may be present in food, water and air, each contributing to a greater or lesser extent to human exposure. A risk assessment may, however, be confined to the medium under detailed consideration, for example, dietary exposure to a contaminant such as benzene; this needs to be set in the context of higher exposures of the general public via ambient air and smoking. A number of Government departments and agencies emphasise the need to consider specific groups separately in risk assessments on certain substances. Failure to consider separately risks to special groups can result in misleadingly reassuring conclusions if they are based solely on risk characterisation for average adults. Relevant specific groups include those perceived as potentially vulnerable because of, for example, genetic predisposition, age, sex, pregnancy, ill-health, particular diets or high exposure.

In the case of human medicines, data from pharmacokinetic studies in special patient groups enable dose adjustments to be made prospectively. In the field of environmental air pollutants it may be the elderly and the asthmatic that are most at risk. Advice on the siting of proposed major hazard installations or on land use planning around existing installations will take into account potentially vulnerable populations such as school children or the elderly. In the case of food chemicals, infants and young children may often be at particular risk because of their smaller body weights, higher energy intakes and less varied diets. Such considerations are often a critical part of risk characterisation because they can demonstrate that only certain subgroups of the population may be at risk of adverse health effects at prevailing exposures, thus enabling more focused risk management decisions to be taken. The differing physiological conditions or requirements and differing end-organ sensitivities of subgroups of the human population are relatively under-researched areas, but they are critical to a better understanding of risks to specific groups. This also has implications for the size of uncertainty factors selected to take account of differences within human populations.

Knowledge of the range of sensitivities of subgroups of the human population and the underlying physiological or pathological mechanisms is emerging most strongly in the field of human medicine. It is recommended that, where appropriate, risk assessors maximise the use of existing knowledge about human variability and the sensitivities of subgroups of the human population to refine risk assessments and that further research in this area be encouraged. The risk assessment process, including decisions about the quality of scientific data and how they should be used, is recognised as being the proper remit of the scientific experts involved; judgements about perceived severity of effects and how to deal with or manage them are subject to wider policy considerations.

In the case of chemicals to which humans would be deliberately exposed, a chemical demonstrated to be an in vivo mutagen or genotoxic carcinogen would not normally be approved or licensed for use. This approach is applied in the regulation of pesticides, veterinary products, additives in animal feed, food additives, cosmetic ingredients, and water treatment chemicals. In the case of certain human medicines that are known or suspected genotoxic carcinogens, use may be permitted if the risk/benefit ratio to the individual patient is considered favourable. In cases where humans are inadvertently but unavoidably exposed to chemicals, such as certain contaminants in food, water and air, probabilistic risk assessment methods may be used to derive an exposure level below which the risk is regarded as very low.

Recently some other exposures (i.e. not mutagens or genotoxic carcinogens) have come to be regarded as having no threshold for toxicity, for example air pollution, based on recent time-series studies, and lead. Exposure to allergens presents a slightly different situation. Following initial sensitisation, subsequent exposure to extremely low levels of the chemical can trigger severe, life-threatening reactions. Most allergens are identified from human studies or experience because of a lack of good animal models.

Many chemicals are capable of causing allergic reactions but generally do so in only a very small proportion of the population (exceptions are allergies to certain foods and sensitisation to some industrial chemicals). Because it would be impractical to ban all chemicals which ever caused an allergic reaction, it is generally recommended that such chemicals or foods be declared on labels, so that people who are sensitive may avoid exposure. It was assumed that humans could be susceptible to the same toxic effects as those seen in the animal studies but that, dose for dose, humans in general might be more sensitive than laboratory animals, or exhibit effects which passed unnoticed in animals, and that within the human population there might be individuals who were more sensitive than the average person.

Most human exposure estimates require the use of default assumptions about the human body. They include, for example, notional figures for body weight and surface area, amounts of food and water consumed daily, respiratory rates and tidal volumes, amounts of exposed skin, amounts deposited onto exposed skin, and systemic absorption of chemicals via different routes. Many of these assumptions need to be elaborated for various human subpopulations, such as different age groups, degrees of activity and occupation. Differing default assumptions for the same parameter may be used by Government departments and agencies and some are more conservative than others. In the occupational field, for example, various operator exposure models with differing assumptions and therefore differing degrees of conservatism can be used.

A hypothetical example might be exposure of a child to dioxins, in which it is assumed that the child lives downwind from a municipal incinerator, eats a spoonful of dirt a day, eats fish from a local pond, is a 95th percentile consumer of fish, and eats food grown in the garden. However, the nature and requirements for exposure estimates in different chemical sectors and different ambient media are so different that a divergence in approach to 'worst case' estimates is to be expected.

5

Diet, Nutrition and Chronic Diseases

The rapidly increasing burden of chronic diseases is a key determinant of global public health. Already 79% of deaths attributable to chronic diseases are occurring in developing countries, predominantly in middle-aged men. There is increasing evidence that chronic disease risks begin in fetal life and continue into old age (3—9). Adult chronic disease, therefore, reflects cumulative differential lifetime exposures to damaging physical and social environments. For these reasons a life-course approach that captures both the cumulative risk and the many opportunities to intervene that this affords, was adopted by the Expert Consultation. While accepting the imperceptible progression from one life stage to the next, five stages were identified for convenience. These are: fetal development and the maternal environment; infancy; childhood and adolescence; adulthood; and ageing and older people. The four relevant factors in fetal life are:

(i) intrauterine growth retardation (IUGR);

(ii) premature delivery of a normal growth for gestational age fetus;

(iii) overnutrition in utero; and

(iv) intergenerational factors. There is considerable evidence, mostly from developed countries, that IUGR is associated with an increased risk of coronary heart disease, stroke, diabetes and raised blood pressure.

On the other hand, large size at birth (macrosomia) is also associated with an increased risk of diabetes and cardiovascular disease. Among the adult population in India, an association was found between impaired glucose tolerance and high ponderal index at birth. Higher birth weight has also been related to an increased risk of breast and other cancers. In sum, the evidence suggests that optimal birth weight and length distribution should be considered, not only in terms of immediate morbidity and mortality but also in regard to long-term outcomes such as susceptibility to diet-related chronic disease later in life. Retarded growth in infancy can be a reflected in a failure to gain weight and a failure to gain height. Both retarded growth and excessive weight or height gain can be factors in later incidence of chronic disease. An association between low growth in early infancy (low weight at 1 year) and an increased risk of coronary heart disease (CHD) has been described, irrespective of size at birth. Blood pressure has been found to be highest in those with retarded fetal growth and greater weight gain in infancy.

Short stature, a reflection of socioeconomic deprivation in childhood, is also associated with an increased risk of CHD and stroke, and to some extent, diabetes. The risk of stroke, and also of cancer mortality at several sites, including breast, uterus and colon, is increased if shorter children display an accelerated growth in height. There is increasing evidence that among term and pre-term infants, breast-feeding is associated with significantly lower blood pressure levels in childhood. Consumption of formula instead of breast milk in infancy has also been shown to increase diastolic and mean arterial blood pressure in later life.

There is increasingly strong evidence suggesting that a lower risk of developing obesity may be directly related to length of exclusive breast-feeding although it may not become evident until later in childhood. Some of the discrepancy may be explained by socioeconomic and maternal education factors confounding the findings. The risk for several chronic diseases of childhood and adolescence have also been associated with infant feeding on breast-milk substitutes and short-term breast-feeding. There has been great interest in the possible effect of high-cholesterol feeding in early life. Nevertheless, the observation of modified responses of adult cholesterol production rates, bile cholesterol saturation indices, and bile acid turnover, depending on whether the baboons were fed breast milk or formula, served to attract further interest. It was noted that increased atherosclerotic lesions associated with increased levels of plasma total cholesterol were related to increased dietary cholesterol in early life. No long-term human morbidity and mortality data supporting this notion have been reported. Short-term human studies have been in part confounded by diversity in solid food weaning regimens, as well as by the varied composition of fatty acid components of the early diet.

The ratio of low-density lipoprotein (LDL) cholesterol plus very low-density lipoprotein (VLDL) cholesterol to HDL cholesterol was lowest for infants receiving the formula in which oleic acid was predominant. Most of those infants then received an uncontrolled mixed diet and cow's milk, with no evident differences in plasma cholesterol levels by 12 months, independent of the type of early feeding they had received. A more recent controlled study suggests that the specific fatty acid intake plays a predominant role in determining total and LDL cholesterol. The significance of high dietary cholesterol associated with exclusive human milk feeding during the first 4 months of life has no demonstrated adverse effect. Measurements of serum lipoprotein concentrations and LD Lreceptor activity in infants suggests that it is the fatty acid content rather than the cholesterol in the diet which regulates cholesterol homeostasis. The regulation of endogenous cholesterol synthesis in infants appears to be regulated in a similar manner to that of adults. An association between low growth in childhood and an increased risk of CHD has been described, irrespective of size at birth. Although based only on developed country research at this point, this finding gives credence to the importance that is currently attached to the role of immediate postnatal factors in shaping disease risk.

Low birth weight Indian babies have been described as having a characteristic poor muscle but high fat preservation, so-called "thin-fat "babies. This phenotype persists throughout the postnatal period and is associated with an increased central adiposity in childhood that is linked to the highest risk of raised blood pressure and disease. In most studies, the association between low birth weight and high blood pressure has been found to be particularly strong if adjusted to current body size—body mass index (BMI)—suggesting the importance of weight gain after birth. Relative weight in adulthood and weight gain have been found to be associated with increased risk of cancer of the breast, colon, rectum, prostate and other sites. Whether there is an independent effect of childhood weight is difficult to determine, as childhood overweight is usually continued into adulthood. Relative weight in adolescence was significantly associated with colon cancer in one retrospective cohort study. Height serves partly as an indicator of socioeconomic and nutritional status in childhood. As has been seen, poor fetal development and poor growth during childhood have been associated with increased cardiovascular disease risk in adulthood, as have indicators of unfavourable social circumstances in childhood. Conversely, a high calorie intake in childhood may be related to an increased risk of cancer in later life.

Height is inversely associated with mortality among men and women from all causes, including coronary heart disease, stroke and respiratory disease. Height has also been used as a proxy for usual childhood energy intake, which is particularly related to body mass and the child's level of activity. However, it is clearly an imperfect proxy because when protein intake is adequate, genetics will define adult height. Protein, particularly animal protein, has been shown to have a selective effect in promoting height growth. It has been suggested that childhood obesity is related to excess protein intake and, of course, overweight or obese children tend to be in the upper percentiles for height. Height has been shown to be related to cancer mortality at several sites, including breast, uterus and colon.

The risk of stroke is increased by accelerated growth in height during childhood. As accelerated growth has been linked to development of hypertension in adult life, this may be the mechanism. There is a higher prevalence of raised blood pressure not only in adults of low socioeconomic status, but also in children from low socioeconomic backgrounds, although the latter is not always associated with higher blood pressure later in life. Blood pressure has been found to track from childhood to predict hypertension in adulthood, but with stronger tracking seen in older ages of childhood and in adolescence. Higher blood pressure in childhood causes target organ and anatomical changes that are associated with cardiovascular risk, including reduction in artery elasticity, increased ventricular size and mass, haemodynamic increase in cardiac output and peripheral resistance.

High blood pressure in children is strongly associated with obesity, in particular central obesity, and clusters and tracks with an adverse serum lipid profile and glucose intolerance. There may be some ethnic differences, although these often seem to be explained by differences in body mass index. A retrospective mortality follow-up of a survey of family diet and health in the United Kingdom identified significant associations between childhood energy intake and mortality from cancer. The presence and tracking of high blood pressure in children and adolescents occurs against a background of unhealthy lifestyles, including excessive intakes of total and saturated fats, cholesterol and salt, inadequate intakes of potassium, and reduced physical activity, often accompanied by high levels of television viewing. In adolescents, habitual alcohol and tobacco use contributes to raised blood pressure. There are three critical aspects of adolescence that have an impact on chronic diseases:

(i) the development of risk factors during this period;

(ii) the tracking of risk factors throughout life; and, in terms of prevention,

(iii) the development of healthy or unhealthy habits that tend to stay throughout life, for example physical inactivity because of television viewing.

In older children and adolescents, habitual alcohol and tobacco use contribute to raised blood pressure and the development of other risk factors in early life, most of which track into adulthood. The clustering of risk factor variables occurs as early as childhood and adolescence, and is associated with atherosclerosis in young adulthood and thus risk of later cardiovascular disease. This clustering has been described as the metabolic —or "syndrome X "—clustering of physiological disturbances associated with insulin resistance, including hyperinsulinaemia, impaired glucose tolerance, hypertension, elevated plasma triglyceride and low HDL cholesterol. Raised serum cholesterol both in middle age and in early life are known to be associated with an increased risk of disease later on. The Johns Hopkins Precursor Study showed that serum cholesterol levels in adolescents and young white males were strongly related to subsequent risk of cardiovascular disease mortality and morbidity.

Although the risk of obesity does not apparently increase in adults who were overweight at 1 and 3 years old, the risk rises steadily thereafter, regardless of parental weight. Tracking has also been reported in China, where overweight children were 2.8 times as likely to become overweight adolescents; conversely, underweight children were 3-6 times as likely to remain underweight as adolescents. The study found that parental obesity and underweight, and the child's initial body mass index, dietary fat intake and family income helped predict tracking and changes. The real concern about these early manifestations of chronic disease, besides the fact that they are occurring earlier and earlier, is that once they have developed they tend to track in that individual throughout life. On the more positive side, there is evidence that they can be corrected. Overweight and obesity are, however, notoriously difficult to correct after becoming established, and there is an established risk of overweight during childhood persisting into adolescence and adulthood.

Recent studies have shown that the later the weight gain in childhood and adolescence, the greater the persistence. More than 60% of overweight children have at least one additional risk factor for cardiovascular disease, such as raised blood pressure, hyperlipidaemia or hyperinsulinaemia, and more than 20% have two or more risk factors. Habits leading to noncommunicable disease development during adolescence. It seems increasingly likely that there are widespread effects of early diet on later body composition, physiology and cognition. Increased birth weight increases the risk of obesity later, but children with low birth weight tend to remain small into adulthood. In industrialized countries there have been only modest increases in birth weight so the increased levels of obesity described earlier must reflect environmental changes. The "obesogenic" environment appears to be largely directed at the adolescent market, making healthy choices that much more difficult. At the same time, exercise patterns have changed and considerable parts of the day are spent sitting at school, in a factory, or in front of a television or computer.

Raised blood pressure, impaired glucose tolerance and dyslipidaemia are associated in children and adolescents with unhealthy lifestyles, such as diets containing excessive intakes of fats, cholesterol and salt, an inadequate intake of fibre and potassium, a lack of exercise, and increased television viewing. Physical inactivity and smoking have been found independently to predict CHD and stroke in later life. It is increasingly recognized that unhealthy lifestyles do not just appear in adulthood but drive the early development of obesity, dyslipidaemia, high blood pressure, impaired glucose tolerance and associated disease risk. In many countries, perhaps most typified by the United States, changes in family eating patterns, including the increased consumption of fast foods, pre-prepared meals and carbonated drinks, have taken place over the past 30 years. At the same time, the amount of physical activity has been greatly reduced both at home and in school, as well as by increasing use of mechanized transport.

The most firmly established associations between cardiovascular disease or diabetes and factors in the lifespan are the ones between those diseases and the major known "adult "risk factors, such as tobacco use, obesity, physical inactivity, cholesterol, high blood pressure and alcohol consumption. The factors that have been confirmed to lead to an increased risk of CHD, stroke and diabetes are:

— high blood pressure for CHD or stroke;

— high cholesterol (diet) for CHD, and

— tobacco use for CHD.

Most of the studies are from developed countries, but supporting evidence from developing countries is beginning to emerge, for example, from India. In developed countries, low socioeconomic status is associated with higher risk of cardiovascular disease and diabetes. It is presumed that the disease will progressively shift to the more disadvantaged sectors of society. From a social sciences perspective, Losier has suggested that socioeconomic level is less important than a certain stability in the physical and social environment. In other words, an individual's sense of understanding of his or her environment, coupled with control over the course and setting of his or her own life appears to be the most important determinant of health. There are three critical aspects relating to chronic diseases in the later part of the life-cycle:

(i) most chronic diseases will be manifested in this later stage of life;

(ii) there is an absolute benefit for ageing individuals and populations in changing risk factors and adopting health-promoting behaviours such as exercise and healthy diets; and

(iii) the need to maximize health by avoiding or delaying preventable disability.

Along with the societal and disease transitions, there has been a major demographic shift. Although older people are currently defined as those aged 60 years and above, this definition of older people has a very different meaning from the middle of the last century, when 60 years of age and above often exceeded the average life expectancy, especially in industrialized countries. It is worth remembering, however, that the majority of elderly people will, in fact, be living in the developing world. Most chronic diseases are present at this period of life—the result of interactions between multiple disease processes as well as more general losses in physiological functions.

The main burden of chronic diseases is observed at this stage of life and, therefore, needs to be addressed. In the 1970s, it was thought that risks were not significantly increased after certain late ages and that there would be no benefit in changing habits, such as dietary habits, after 80 years old as there was no epidemiological evidence that changing habits would affect mortality or even health conditions among older people. There was also a feeling that people "earned "some unhealthy behaviours simply because of reaching "old age ". Then there was a more active intervention phase, when older people were encouraged to change their diets in ways that were probably overly rigorous for the expected benefit. Morerecently, older people have been encouraged to eat a healthy diet—as large and as varied as possible while maintaining their weight—and particularly to continue exercise. Interventions aimed at supporting the individual and promoting healthier environments will often lead to increased independence in older age.

Risk of impaired glucose tolerance has been found to be highest in those who had low birth weight, but who subsequently became obese as adults. Conversely, there is also fairly consistent evidence of higher risk of CHD, stroke, and probably adult onset diabetes with shorter stature. Impaired glucose tolerance and an adverse lipid profile are seen as early as childhood and adolescence, where they typically appear clustered together with higher blood pressure and relate strongly to obesity, in particular central obesity. Raised blood pressure, impaired glucose tolerance and dyslipidaemia also tend to be clustered in children and adolescents with unhealthy lifestyles and diets, such as those with excessive intakes of saturated fats, cholesterol and salt, and inadequate intake of fibre. Lack of exercise and increased television viewing add to the risk. In older children and adolescents, habitual alcohol and tobacco use also contribute to raised blood pressure and to the development of other risk factors in early adulthood.

Many of the same factors continue to act throughout the life course. Such clustering represents an opportunity to address more than one risk at a time. The clustering of health-related behaviours is also a well described phenomenon. Young girls who grow poorly become stunted women and are more likely to give birth to low-birth-weight babies who are then likely to continue the cycle by being stunted in adulthood, and so on. Maternal birth size is a significant predictor of a child's birth size after controlling for gestational age, sex of the child, socioeconomic status, and maternal age, height and pre-pregnant weight. There are clear indications of intergenerational factors in obesity, such as parental obesity, maternal gestational diabetes and maternal birth weight.

Low maternal birth weight is associated with higher blood pressure levels in the offspring, independent of the relation between the offspring's own birth weight and blood pressure. Unhealthy lifestyles can also have a direct effect on the health of the next generation, for example, smoking during pregnancy. There is good evidence that nutrients and physical activity influence gene expression and have shaped the genome over several million years of human evolution. Genes define opportunities for health and susceptibility to disease, while environmental factors determine which susceptible individuals will develop illness. In view of changing socio-economic conditions in developing countries, such added stress may result in exposure of underlying genetic predisposition to chronic diseases. Gene-nutrient interactions also involve the environment.

The dynamics of the relationships are becoming better understood but there is still a long way to go in this area, and also in other aspects, such as disease prevention and control. Studies continue on the role of nutrients in gene expression; for example, researchers are currently trying to understand why omega-3 fatty acids suppress or decrease the mRNA of interleukin, which is elevated in atherosclerosis, arthritis and other autoimmune diseases, whereas the omega-6 fatty acids do not. Studies on genetic variability to dietary response indicate that specific genotypes raise cholesterol levels more than others.

The need for targeted diets for individuals and subgroups to prevent chronic diseases was acknowledged as being part of an overall approach to prevention at the population level. However, the practical implications of this issue for public health policy have only begun to be addressed. For example, a recent study of the relationship between folate and cardiovascular disease revealed that a commonsingle gene mutation that reduces the activity of an enzyme involved in folate metabolism (MTHFR) is associated with a moderate increase in serum homocysteine and higher risk of both ischaemic heart disease and deep vein thrombosis. Although humans have evolved being able to feed on a variety of foods and to adapt to them, certain genetic adaptations and limitations have occurred in relation to diet. Understanding the evolutionary aspects of diet and its composition might suggest a diet that would be consistent with the diet to which our genes were programmed to respond.

However, the early diet was presumably one which gave evolutionary advantage to reproduction in the early part of life, and so may be less indicative of guidance for healthy eating, in terms of lifelong health and prevention of chronic disease after reproduction has been achieved. Because there are genetic variations among individuals, changes in dietary patterns have a differential impact on a genetically heterogeneous population, although populations with a similar evolutionary background have more similar genotypes. Most are polygenic in nature and rapidly escalating rates suggest the importance of environmental change rather than change in genetic susceptibility. There is a vast volume of scientific evidence highlighting the importance of applying a life-course approach to the prevention and control of chronic disease. The intention of primary prevention interventions is to move the profile of the whole population in a healthier direction. Small changes in risk factors in the majority who are at moderate risk can have an enormous impact in terms of population-attributable risk of death and disability.

By preventing disease in large populations, small reductions in blood pressure, blood cholesterol and so on can dramatically reduce health costs. For example, it has been demonstrated that improved lifestyles can reduce the risk of progression to diabetes by a striking 58% over 4 years. For interventions to have a lasting effect on the risk factor prevalence and the health of societies, it is also essential to change or modify the environment in which these diseases develop. Changes in dietary patterns, the influence of advertising and the globalization of diets, and widespread reduction in physical activity have generally had negative impacts in terms of risk factors, and presumably also in terms of subsequent disease.

Reversing current trends will require a multifaceted public health policy approach. While it is important to avoid inappropriately applying nutritional guidelines to populations that may differ genetically from those for whom the dietary and risk data were originally determined, to date the information regarding genes or gene combinations is insufficient to define specific dietary recommendations based on a population distribution of specific genetic polymorphisms.

An abundant stable food supply is a recent phenomenon; it was not a factor until the advent of the industrial revolution. A combination of physical activity, food variety and extensive social interaction is the most likely lifestyle profile to optimize health, as reflected in increased longevity and healthy ageing. Some evidence suggests that, within the time frame of a week, at least 20 and probably as many as 30 biologically distinct types of foods,with the emphasis on plant foods, are required for healthy diets. The current move towards increasing animal protein in diets in countries in economic transition is unlikely to be reversed in those countries where there are increased consumer resources, but is unlikely to be conducive to adult health, at least in terms of preventing chronic diseases. There is an increasing need, recognized at all levels, for the wider implications to be specifically addressed; these include the implications for agriculture and fisheries, the role of international trade in a globalized world, the impact on countries dependent on primary produce, the effect of macroeconomic policies, and the need for sustainability. The greatest burden of disease will be in the developing world and, in the transitional and industrialized world, amongst the most disadvantaged socioeconomically. In short, it may be necessary to have three mutually reinforcing strategies that will have different magnitudes of impact over differing time frames.

— With the greatest and most immediate impact, there is the need to address risk factors in adulthood and, increasingly, among older people. Risk-factor behaviours can be modified in these groups and benefits seen within 3—5 years. With all populations ageing, the sheer numbers and potential cost savings are enormous and realizable.

— Societal changes towards health-promoting environments need to be greatly expanded as an integral part of any intervention. Ways to reduce the intake of sugars-sweetened drinks and of high-energy density foods that are micronutrient poor, as well as efforts to curb cigarette smoking and to increase physical activity will have an impact throughout society. Such changes need the active participation of communities, politicians, health systems, town planners and municipalities, as well as the food and leisure industries.

— The health environment, in which those who are most at risk grow up, needs to change. This is a more targeted and potentially costly approach, but one that has the potential for cost-effective returns even though they are longer term.

Instead, consistent with the concept of a safe range of nutrient intakes for individuals, there is often a range of population averages that would be consistent with the maintenance of health. If existing population averages fall outside this range, or trends in intake suggest that the population average will move outside the range, health concerns are likely to arise. Sometimes there is no lower limit; this implies that there is no evidence that the nutrient is required in the diet and hence low intakes should not give rise to concern. It would be of concern if a large proportion of values were outside the defined goals. Ideally the definition of an increased or a decreased risk should be based on a relationship that has been established by multiple randomized controlled trials of interventions on populations that are representative of the target of a recommendation, but this type of evidence is often not available.

The recommended dietary/nutrition practice should modify the attributable risk of the undesirable exposure in that population. Consistent evidence on community and environmental factors which lead to behaviour changes and thereby modify risks has been taken into account in categorizing risks. This applies particularly to the complex interaction between environmental factors that affect excess weight gain, a risk factor which the Consultation recognized as contributing to many of the problems being considered. Evidence based on epidemiological studies showing consistent associations between exposure and disease, with little or no evidence to the contrary.

The available evidence is based on a substantial number of studies including prospective observational studies and where relevant, randomized controlled trials of sufficient size, duration and quality showing consistent effects. Evidence based on epidemiological studies showing fairly consistent associations between exposure and disease, but where there are perceived shortcomings in the available evidence or some evidence to the contrary, which precludes a more definite judgement. Shortcomings in the evidence may be any of the following: insufficient duration of trials (or studies); insufficient trials (or studies) available; inadequate sample sizes; incomplete follow-up. Evidence based mainly on findings from case-control and cross-sectional studies. Insufficient randomized controlled trials, observational studies or non-randomized controlled trials are available.

For countries where the usual fat intake is between 15% and 20% of energy, there is no direct evidence for men that raising fat intake to 20% will be beneficial. It is recognized that higher intakes of free sugars threaten the nutrient quality of diets by providing significant energy without specific nutrients. The Consultation considered that restriction of free sugars was also likely to contribute to reducing the risk of unhealthy weight gain.

Children with a high consumption of soft drinks rich in free sugars are more likely to be overweight and to gain excess weight. The Consultation recognized that a population goal for free sugars of less than 10% of total energy is controversial. However, the Consultation considered that the studies showing no effect of free sugars on excess weight have limitations.

A greater weight reduction was observed with the high complex carbohydrate diet relative to the simple carbohydrate one; the difference, however was not statistically significant. Nevertheless, an analysis of weight change and metabolic indices for those with metabolic syndrome revealed a clear benefit of replacing simple by complex carbohydrates. The Consultation also examined the results of studies that found an inverse relationship between free sugars intakes and total fat intake. Many of these studies are methodologically inappropriate for determining the causes of excess weight gain, since the percentage of calories from fat will decrease as the percentage of calories from carbohydrates increases and vice versa. Wholegrain cereals, fruits and vegetables are the preferred sources of non-starch polysaccharides (NSP). The best definition of dietary fibre remains to be established, given the potential health benefits of resistant starch. The benefit of fruits and vegetables cannot be ascribed to a single or mix of nutrients and bioactive substances. Therefore, this food category was included rather than the nutrients themselves. The category of tubers (i.e. potatoes, cassava) should not be included in fruits and vegetables.

The goal for physical activity focuses on maintaining healthy body weight. The recommendation is for a total of one hour per day on most days of the week of moderate-intensity activity, such as walking. This level of physical activity is needed to maintain a healthy body weight, particularly for people with sedentary occupations. Obviously, this quantitative goal cannot be considered as a single "best value" by analogy with the nutrient intake goals. Most countries in Africa, Asia and Latin America, the interaction or synergism of malnutrition and infection is the leading cause of morbidity and mortality in children. Viral, bacterial and parasitic infections tend to be prevalent, and all can have a negative impact on the nutritional status of children and adults. The situation was similar in North America and Europe from about 1900 to 1925; common infectious diseases had an impact on nutrition and produced high case fatality rates. The synergistic relationship between malnutrition and infectious diseases is now well accepted and has been conclusively demonstrated in animal experiments.

The simultaneous presence of both malnutrition and infection results in an interaction that has more serious consequences for the host than the additive effect would be if the two worked independently. Infections make malnutrition worse and poor nutrition increases the severity of infectious diseases. The human body has the ability to resist almost all types of organisms or toxins that tend to damage the tissues and organs. This capacity is called immunity. Much of the immunity is caused by a special immune system that forms antibodies and sensitized lymphocytes which attack and destroy the specific organisms or toxins. This type of immunity is called acquired immunity. There are two basic but closely allied types of acquired immunity. In one of these the body develops circulating antibodies, which are globulin molecules that are capable of attacking the invading agents and destroying them. This type of immunity is called humoral immunity. Antibodies circulate in the blood and may remain there for a long time, so that a second infection with the same organism is immediately controlled. This is the basis for some forms of immunization, which are designed to stimulate antibody production.

Another type of acquired immunity is achieved through the formation of large numbers of highly specialized lymphocytes which are specifically sensitized against the invading foreign agents. These sensitized lymphocytes have the ability to attach to the foreign agents and to destroy them. This type of immunity is called cellular immunity. It is a highly complex system involving many different body organs (such as the spleen, thymus, lymph system and bone marrow) and also body fluids, particularly blood and its constituents and lymph. Some of the normal defence mechanisms of the body are impaired and do not function properly in the malnourished subject. For example, children with kwashiorkor were shown to be unable to form antibodies to either typhoid vaccine or diphtheria toxoid; their capacity to do so was restored after protein therapy.

Similarly, children with protein malnutrition have an impaired antibody response to inoculation with yellow fever vaccine. An inhibition of the agglutinating response to cholera antigen has been reported in children with kwashiorkor and nutritional marasmus. Another defence mechanism that has been studied in relation to nutrition is that of leucocytosis (increased production of white blood cells) and phagocytic activity (destruction of bacteria by white corpuscles). Although malnourished children frequently have increased immunoglobulin levels (presumably related to concurrent infections), they also may have depressed cell-mediated immunity. In a recent study, the extent of this depression was directly related to the severity of the protein-energy malnutrition (PEM). Serum transferrin levels are also low in those with severe PEM, and they often take considerable time to return to normal even after proper dietary treatment. A quite different kind of interaction of nutrition and infection is seen in the effect of some deficiency diseases on the integrity of the tissues. Reduction in the integrity of certain epithelial surfaces, notably the skin and mucous membranes, decreases resistance to invasion and makes an easy avenue of entry for pathogenic organisms.

Examples of this effect are cheilosis and angular stomatitis in riboflavin deficiency, bleeding gums and capillary fragility in vitamin C deficiency, flaky-paint dermatosis and atrophic intestinal changes in severe protein deficiency and serious eye lesions in vitamin A deficiency. Infection affects nutritional status in several ways. Perhaps the most important of these is that bacterial and some other infections lead to an increased loss of nitrogen from the body. This repercussion was first demonstrated in serious infections such as typhoid fever, but it has subsequently been shown in much milder infections such as otitis media, tonsillitis, chicken pox and abscesses. Nitrogen is lost by several mechanisms. The principal one is probably increased breakdown of tissue protein and mobilization of amino acids, especially from the muscles. The nitrogen is excreted in the urine and is evidence of a depletion of body protein from muscles. Full recovery is dependent upon the restoration of these amino acids to the tissues once the infection is overcome. This requires increased intake of protein, above maintenance levels, in the post-infection period. In children whose diet is marginal in protein content, or those who are already protein depleted, growth will be retarded during and after infections. In developing countries, children from poor families suffer from many infections in quick succession during the post-weaning period, and they often have multiple infections. Anorexia or loss of appetite is another factor in the relationship between infection and nutrition. Infections, especially if accompanied by a fever, often lead to loss of appetite and therefore to reduced food intake. Some infectious diseases commonly cause vomiting, with the same result.

In many societies mothers and often medical attendants as well consider it desirable to withhold food or to place the child with an infection on a liquid diet. Such a diet may consist of rice water, very dilute soups, water alone or some other fluid with a low calorie density and usually deficient in protein and other essential nutrients. The old adage of "starve a fever" is of doubtful validity, and this practice may have serious consequences for the child whose nutritional status is already precarious. The traditional treatment of diarrhoea in some communities is to prescribe a purgative or enema. The gastro-enteritis may already have resulted in reduced absorption of nutrients from food, and the treatment may further aggravate this situation. These are all examples of how illnesses such as measles, upper respiratory infections and gastro-intestinal infections may contribute to the development of malnutrition.

Parasitic infections, particularly intestinal helminthic infections, are extremely prevalent and are increasingly being shown to have an adverse effect on nutritional status, especially in those heavily infected. Hookworms (Ancylostoma duodenale and Necator americanus) infect over µ00 million people, mainly the poor in tropical and subtropical countries. They used to cause a prevalent debilitating disease in the southern United States. Hookworms cause intestinal blood loss, and although it appears that most of the protein in the lost blood is absorbed lower down in the intestinal tract, there is considerable loss of iron. Hookworm disease is a major cause of iron deficiency anaemia in many countries. Infection densities much higher than this are not uncommon. In Venezuela, where much of this work was done, iron losses greater than 3 mg per day often resulted in anaemia in adult males, and losses of half this amount frequently produced anaemia in women of child-bearing age and in young children. Worldwide, roundworm (Ascaris lumbricoides) is among the most prevalent of intestinal parasites. It is estimated that 1 200 million people in the world (one-quarter of the world's population) harbour roundworms.

The roundworm is large, so its own metabolic needs must be considerable. High parasite densities, particularly in children, are common in environments where sanitation is poor. Complications of ascariasis can develop, including intestinal obstruction or the presence of worms in aberrant sites such as the common bile duct. In some countries ascarids are a cause of surgical emergencies in children, and many with obstruction die. In the majority of children, however, when malnutrition is prevalent, deworming improves child growth. Trichuris trichiura or whipworm inhabits the large intestine and infects about 600 million people worldwide. The worms are small and, in heavily infected children, may cause diarrhoea and abdominal pain. Many children living in poor sanitary conditions are infected with several parasitic infections at the same time. In areas where infection with these three parasites is common and where malnutrition is prevalent, deworming of children leads to an improvement in growth, a reduction in the extent of malnutrition and an increase in appetite. It also positively influences physical fitness and perhaps psychological development.

Bilharzia or schistosomiasis infections are prevalent in some countries. They also contribute to poor nutrition, poor appetite and poor growth. The three organisms that cause schistosomiasis (Schistosoma haematobium, Schistosoma mansoni and Schistosoma japonicum) are flukes, rather than ordinary worms. The fish tapeworm (Diphyllobothrium latum) has an avidity for vitamin B12 and can deprive its host of this vitamin, with megaloblastic anaemia resulting. The fish tapeworm is common in people in only limited geographic areas, mainly in temperate areas and where undercooked fish is frequently consumed. In many northern industrialized countries, farm animals and domestic pets such as dogs and cats are dewormed routinely.

Much evidence suggests that pigs grow better when they regularly receive anthelmintics. Now that highly effective, relatively inexpensive and safe broad-spectrum anthelmintics such as albendazole and mebendazole are available, routine mass deworming should be introduced where parasitic infections are prevalent in humans and where PEM and anaemia are common. Similarly, routine efforts to treat children with schistosomiasis using metrifonate or praziquantel seem highly desirable both to rid children of potential serious pathology and to improve their nutritional status. Many studies have indicated that gastrointestinal infections, and especially diarrhoea, are very important in precipitating serious PEM. Diarrhoea is common in, and often lethal to, the young child. In breastfed infants there is often some protection during the first months of life, so diarrhoea is often a feature of the weaning process. Weanling diarrhoea is extraordinarily prevalent in poor communities throughout the world, both in tropical and temperate zones. The organism responsible varies and often cannot be identified.

Diarrhoea was a major cause of mortality in children in industrialized countries up to the beginning of the twentieth century. Several studies have shown that admissions of cases of malnutrition are greatly increased during the season when diarrhoea is most common. For example, in a report from the Islamic Republic of Iran, more than twice as many cases of PEM were admitted in the warm summer than in the cold winter. Hospital and community studies indicate that cases of xerophthalmia and keratomalacia are frequently precipitated by gastro-enteritis, as well as by other infectious diseases such as measles and chicken pox. Xerophthalmia is the major cause of blindness in several Asian countries; it is also prevalent in certain parts of Africa, Latin America and the Near East. Intestinal parasites may contribute to diarrhoea and to poor vitamin A status. The exact mechanism of this relationship has not been proved, but it is likely that many infections reduce vitamin A absorption and that some result in decreased consumption of foods containing vitamin A and carotene.

Diarrhoea can be fatal, usually because it can lead to severe dehydration. Diarrhoea, and the complication of dehydration, may be said to be a form of malnutrition. Dehydration is a "deficiency" in the body of water and mineral electrolytes, and providing adequate quantities of these cures the deficiency. The term "fluid electrolyte malnutrition" (FEM) has been coined for this condition. Provision of water and adequate minerals in home-prepared food, breastfeeding or administration of oral rehydration fluids is now the accepted treatment. Although these are forms of therapy or treatment, they are really refeeding and replenishment. However, prevention requires measures and interventions to reduce infections, poverty and malnutrition. These are essential if countries are to reduce the incidence of diarrhoea. A dramatic illustration of the effect of malnutrition on infection is seen in the fatality rates for common childhood diseases such as measles. Measles is a severe disease with a case fatality rate of about 15 percent in many poor countries because the young children who develop it have poor nutritional status, lowered resistance and poor health.

Immunization against measles is proving very effective, and in many countries measles incidence has been markedly reduced. Other common infectious diseases such as whooping cough, diarrhoea and upper respiratory infections also have much more serious consequences in malnourished children than in those who are well nourished. Mortality statistics from most developing countries show that such communicable diseases are the major causes of death. It was observed in several African countries at the end of the Sahel famine that very few children were dying of starvation or malnutrition, but that deaths from measles, respiratory infections and other infectious diseases were still very much above pre-famine levels. It is clear that many, perhaps the majority, of these deaths were due to malnutrition.

The problems of infection and malnutrition are closely interrelated, yet programmes to control communicable diseases and to improve nutrition tend to be introduced quite independently. It would be much more efficient and effective if the twin problems were attacked together. Success in improving the health and reducing the mortality of children is dependent both on control of infectious diseases and on improvements in the children's food intake and care. There is increasing evidence to suggest that parents are more willing to control their family size when the chances are good that most children born will survive into adulthood. Consideration also needs to be given to providing a stimulating environment for the growing child.

All people have their likes and dislikes and their beliefs about food, and many people are conservative in their food habits. They tend to like what their mothers cooked for them when they were young, the foods that are served on festive occasions or those eaten with friends and family away from home during their childhood. The foods that adults ate without a second thought in childhood are seldom totally disagreeable to them in later life. What one society regards as normal or even highly desirable, however, another society may consider revolting or totally inedible. Animal milk is commonly consumed and liked by many people in Asia, Africa, Europe and the Americas, but in China it is rarely taken. Lobsters, crabs and shrimps are considered delicacies and prized foods by many people in Europe and North America, but are revolting to many people in Africa and Asia, especially those who live far from the sea.

On the other hand, those who overconsume animal flesh, some seafoods, eggs and other foods of animal origin will have undesirable amounts of saturated fat and cholesterol in the diet. Relatively few people or societies have strong negative feelings about consuming cereals, roots, legumes, vegetables or fruit. They may have strong preferences and likes, but most maize-eating people are also willing to eat rice, and most rice-eating people will eat wheat products. It is often stated that food habits seldom or never change and are difficult to change. This is not true; in many countries the current staple foods are not the same as those eaten even a century ago. Food habits and customs do change, and they are influenced in many different ways.

Many cultures have strong views about the consumption of milk or milk products. The customs that prohibit consumption of certain nutritionally valuable foods may not have an important overall nutritional impact, particularly if only one or two food items are affected. Some societies, however, forbid such a wide range of foods to women during pregnancy that it is difficult for them to obtain a balanced diet. Many of the nutritionally undesirable taboos that existed a quarter of a century ago have weakened or disappeared as a result of education, mixing of people from different societies and travel. Of those that remain, some food habits may seem illogical and their origins obscure, but it is not advisable for outsiders to try to alter ancient food habits without looking very closely into their origins. Moreover, it makes no sense to attempt to alter a habit that does not negatively affect nutritional status.

Nutritionally bad habits, like all other habits, are best changed by the people who have them. In this regard, influential local people, with the welfare of their fellows at heart, may join nutritionists and become part of an important alliance pledged to eradicating malnutrition. In some parts of the world the staple foods are changing or have changed. Maize, cassava and potatoes, now grown in large amounts in Africa, originated outside the continent. Since none of these foods were eaten in Africa a few hundred years ago, it is clear that the food habits of millions of people have changed. Vast numbers of people in Africa have abandoned yams and millet for maize and cassava, just as many in Europe abandoned oats, barley and rye for wheat and potatoes. Food habits are still changing rapidly. The difficulty, of course, lies in trying to guide and foster desirable changes and to slow down undesirable ones. It is often difficult to fathom what factors have been most important in stimulating or influencing changes in food habits.

The rapid increase in bread consumption in many African, Latin American and Asian countries where wheat is not the staple food is understandable. It is at least in part a labour-saving phenomenon; bread is one of the first "convenience" foods to have become available. Before leaving home to go to work one can eat some slices of bread instead of the traditional breakfast of porridge, which requires preparation time and is unpleasant cold. Bread can be carried in the pocket and eaten during a break in the working day, or when travelling. In most of the world the traditional main staple food has remained constant, irrespective of urbanization, modernization or even westernization. Thus in much of Asia rice remains the preferred staple food in rural and urban areas. Changes in food habits are not just accidental, of course; they can be deliberately initiated. At community and family level, school-age children can be important agents for change. They are still forming their tastes and developing their preferences. If they are introduced to a new food they will often readily accept it and like it. School meals may usefully introduce new foods to children and thus influence food habits. This widening of food experience in childhood is extremely important.

Children may influence the immediate family and later their own children to eat new, highly nutritious foods. Not all change is desirable, of course, and not all new food habits are good. This is an undesirable, relatively new food trend. Less attention has been given to the question of other baby foods that have been marketed and much promoted and advertised in developing countries. Locally available complementary or weaning foods, home-produced and traditionally fed, are often as or more nutritious than the manufactured baby foods, and then are always much cheaper. They are usually introduced gradually while breastfeeding continues well into the second year and beyond. Manufactured baby foods should only be promoted to those who are unable or unwilling to continue breastfeeding. They are safe and nutritionally adequate when prepared hygienically and in the right dilution. They are convenient for those who can afford to purchase them. However, such manufactured foods are expensive compared with local foods, and for most families in developing countries, other than the very affluent, they may be a waste of money.

For families who already have too little money to spend on food and other essentials, these foods are a very expensive way of buying the nutrients that they are advertised to contain. Another particularly misleading type of advertising relates to the glucose products said to provide "instant energy". Energy is present in large amounts in nearly all the cheapest foods. Similarly, drinks advertised as "rich in vitamin C" are usually unnecessary, since few children suffer from vitamin C deficiency. Vitamin C can be obtained just as well from fruits such as guavas, mangoes and citrus, or from a range of vegetables. The so-called protein-rich weaning foods are also much advertised. These are nutritionally good products, but they cost much more shall protein-rich foods available in the market such as beaus, groundnuts or dried fish, meat, eggs or milk. It usually costs much more to provide 100 g of protein from these commercially advertised products than, for example, from beans bought in the local market.

Many of the more prosperous countries, particularly in Europe, have reached the stage of zero population growth, excluding growth from immigration. This means that the number of births per year nearly equals the number of deaths. In contrast, many developing countries have far more births than deaths and, consequently, rapidly increasing populations. However, several poor countries have reduced their rate of population increase, mainly through family planning methods. Overall population growth is not the only demographic concern of many developing countries. The rapid increase in the percentage of people living in large cities is also a growing worry. Population in urban areas has increased in part because of increased fertility rates, but migration from the rural areas to the cities is also a major cause. City dwellers in general are consumers, not producers, of food; as they become more numerous relative to the rural residents, the food production burden on the few becomes greater. In 1900 there were only four cities in the world with over 2 million residents; now there are over 100 such cities, as well as a number of megalopoli with over 10 million inhabitants. The nutritional outcome of urbanization is on the whole positive.

Urbanization, together with population growth and increasing incomes, contributes to tremendous increases in food demand and thus in the volume of food required, but also to varied and dynamic changes in dietary structure. The most significant dietary change caused by the urban migration has been the substitution of staple foods such as roots, tubers and coarse grains by other sources of energy such as highly milled cereals, sugar, soft drinks and other processed foods. In the urban environment, time constraints, availability of cheap, often subsidized processed foods and convenience of preparation are important considerations in influencing food consumption patterns. The urban diet is generally more varied than the rural diet, mainly because of changes in non-staple foods. Fish, fresh vegetables, meat, poultry, milk and dairy products are consumed more often by urban people. Urban populations generally have lower energy intake than rural populations, but their physical activity may also be comparatively low. Consumption of animal protein, fat and vitamin A is higher in urban areas, and the iron consumed is better utilized. On the whole the diets of urban populations are more balanced than those of rural people.

A typical effect of urbanization is an increase in the amount of food eaten outside the home. Commercially prepared meals and other ready-to-eat foods are consumed from street vendors and food stalls. In many developing countries an informal sector for the sale of food has developed as a typically indigenous response to some of the food needs of the cities; this sector provides a cheap source of food and a significant source of income, particularly for women. Urban nutrition is also affected by the fact that in most low-income urban households women work outside the home; as a consequence there has been an almost universal decline in breastfeeding in urban areas in all regions of the developing world, with a concomitant increase in the use of more costly breastmilk substitutes and commercial weaning foods. On average, urban dwellers enjoy better nutritional status than their rural counterparts because of better health coverage and greater diversity in the diet.

A more varied urban diet with minimal seasonal fluctuations confers important nutritional benefits. FAO data show that the incidence of child malnutrition, especially chronic malnutrition, is lower in urban areas. In Ghana, the weights of the adult urban population were found to be higher than those of the rural population. In general, urban areas also have lower morbidity and mortality rates, increased life expectancy, fewer children of low birth weight and fewer growth problems. Despite rapid population growth, the world produced enough food in 1995 to feed adequately all the people on the globe—if the food were equitably distributed. Even if the population of the world doubles from the current 5 500 million to 11 000 million by the year 2030, the world's production will be capable of feeding all those people. Beyond that level, unless population growth stabilizes, serious shortages of food could result. Unlimited population increase on a planet of finite size is impossible; before too long the world would have standing room only, and each inhabitant one square metre of space. It is a credit to agricultural advances and the skills of farmers that food supplies have increased to meet population needs.

Many countries have achieved increased production levels not by expanding the land under cultivation, but by increasing the yields of cereals and other important crops per hectare farmed. This trend will have to continue. In addition, processing and marketing of foods must be improved. In most developing countries the mean age of first menstruation is 12 to 24 months later than in industrialized countries. Menarche usually occurs about 12 months after the year with the greatest growth spurt. The onset of menses signals the beginning of a female's ability to become pregnant. It is almost certain that undernutrition delays the onset of menses. In this way poor nutrition influences human fertility. Starvation and severe undernourishment, as in food shortages or famines resulting from drought, war or other factors, will usually result in cessation of menstruation in women of child-bearing age. Women who have ceased to menstruate in this way are infertile until their food intake improves. This is nature's way of preventing conception in undernourished individuals.

Psychological consequences also result. Numerous pregnancies and lactations, especially at short intervals, are likely to deplete the mother of nutrients unless she has an exceptionally good diet. Therefore, women with many children narrowly spaced are more likely to have poor nutritional status. A woman whose diet is deficient during pregnancy, especially in terms of total food and energy, is likely to give birth to a baby that is smaller than it would have been if she were adequately nourished. Since mortality is more likely in underweight babies, a poor maternal diet is seen to increase the chances of death in the baby. Pregnancies that are too numerous and too narrowly spaced may be harmful to both the mother and the child. A mother practising family planning simply to space her children more widely benefits also in nutrition and health. Family planning is intimately related to health and nutritional status.

Small family size, long intervals between pregnancies and gradual termination of breastfeeding are all associated with good health, positive nutritional status and even decreased mortality rates in the mother and family. The right to choose Family planning is a concern of the family rather than the nation. People outside the family should become involved not in trying to limit the total number of children a couple should bear, but in giving the couple the means of determining themselves how many children they will have and at what intervals. Family planning is also a right. Families, but women in particular, should be able to choose whether and when to have children. This choice used to be a luxury enjoyed only by those who had the knowledge to practice contraception and the funds to purchase contraceptive devices.

Now education and services for family planning are available to more couples, providing them with the knowledge and means to prevent unwanted pregnancies. It has been said that every child born should be a wanted child; this is indeed a goal worthy of being pursued. For many years the idea that lactation prevented pregnancy was considered an old wives' tale. Now it is known as a scientific fact that women who are intensively breastfeeding their babies do experience a longer interval before menstruation begins again, and they are therefore less likely to have an early successive pregnancy than those who do not breastfeed. Breastfeeding is likely to lengthen birth intervals by an average of five to eight months. In this way the prolongation of full breastfeeding in developing countries is having a major effect in reducing fertility, in population control and in child spacing. Breastfeeding is nature's way of helping to space children. If bottle-feeding were to replace breastfeeding without the availability of contraceptives, the result would be major increases in the number of children born. Contraceptive pills, especially high-oestrogen pills, may reduce a woman's ability to produce breastmilk. Therefore care must be taken in advising women to take contraceptive pills soon after childbirth.

In contrast, it has been suggested that the intrauterine device (IUD) may enhance or improve lactation. Some contraceptives may have an effect on nutritional status. Certain contraceptive pills are believed to cause anaemia because they affect folate utilization. The IUD may cause increased bleeding, which can lead to iron deficiency anaemia. It seems likely that a decrease in infant and child mortality is a prerequisite to the wide acceptance of family planning in those societies in which childhood deaths are common. Parents need to have confidence that their children will survive before they will risk limiting their family size. As malnutrition is one of the leading causes or contributory causes of death in children, it follows that improved nutrition will expedite the acceptance of family planning. Improved nutrition is part and parcel of a better quality of life. Having fewer children in a family means more food, more room and less poverty; these also contribute to an improved quality of life.

Wider spacing of children results in improvements in the health and nutritional status of children and their mothers. There is thus a circular effect. There is much sense in linking nutrition and family planning activities, and even in integrating them into one programme. Both are related to maternal and child health and to total family health care. It may be advantageous for the same health personnel to deal with nutrition, family planning and maternal and child health. Some countries, such as Indonesia, where family planning is having a significant impact in reducing the rate of population increase and where families are smaller shall they were 20 years ago, have combined family planning activities with nutrition and health programmes; it appears to have worked well.

Nutritionists may be concerned about the alarming rate of increase of the world's population. Kenya, for example, had a population of 26 million in 1994 and will have over 50 million people in 2020; nutritionists may be alarmed by all the implications of this population growth in terms of land shortage and mushrooming urban slums. In their work, however, nutritionists usually deal with problems of families or communities. It is important then to help people, especially women and their partners, understand the benefits of smaller families and the fact that more children require more resources: more food, more care, more time, more school fees, more money and so on. The appropriate strategy may be to persuade them that children today have a better chance of surviving than children had in 1955, and that quality of life is more important than numbers of children. It is of particular importance in many developing countries first to empower women to control their own fertility and to be in a position to have the numbers of children they desire, and second to influence men to respect these rights of their female partners. The onus of having more children falls on the whole family, but in most countries by far the greatest additional burden of work falls on the mother.

The education of girls and the empowerment of women to earn money, control resources and have more independence are all achievements that generally lead women to control their own fertility and have fewer babies. Women's support groups, sex education in schools, involvement of men in discussions, later marriage and more intensive breastfeeding are all likely to reduce the mean number of babies produced per mother. Nutrition workers, be they in the field of health, agriculture, education or social services, should make themselves conversant with modern methods of family planning. They should be able to discuss these methods with people either individually or in groups, and they should know how to advise people to use local family planning services. If these services are inadequate or cause problems for women or families, nutrition workers should be advocates for improved family planning services.

The more the choices available to women and men, the more likely it is that the babies born will be wanted babies, Of course workers must respect national laws and cultural norms. If abortion is illegal, the law will need to be respected. Communities have been most successful in limiting unwanted births where several family planning methods are available: contraceptive pills, condoms, IUDs, male and female surgical sterilization and, if legal, well-conducted abortions. In some countries newer methods such as hormone-releasing implants (Norplant) or the so-called abortion pill may be expected to help in family planning in the next five years. Nutrient requirements differ to some extent at different periods in the life cycle. Females of reproductive age have extra needs because of menstruation and, of course, during pregnancy and lactation.

Infants and children have greater requirements on a unit weight basis than adults, mainly because they are growing. Older people are also a vulnerable group; they are at greater risk of malnutrition than younger adults. Certain deficiency diseases are more prevalent in particular groups of the population. Humans get energy from the foods and liquids they consume. The nutrient requirements of women of reproductive age, of young children and adolescents and of older people are different from those of men between the ages of 15 and 60; therefore all people do not need the same amounts of food.

Women of child-bearing age have certain nutritional needs above those of adult males. One reason is that the loss of blood during menstruation leads to a regular loss of iron and other nutrients and makes women more prone than men to anaemia. In addition, however, in many developing countries women work much harder than men. In rural areas they are often heavily involved in agriculture, and in urban areas they may work long hours in factories and elsewhere; yet when they return home from the field or the factory they still have much work to do in the household, including food preparation and child care.

Frequently the heavy burden of collecting water and fuel falls on women. All of this labour increases women's needs for nutritional energy and other nutrients. The nutritional status of women before, during and after pregnancy contributes a good deal to their own general well-being, but also to that of their children and other members of the family. The field of maternal nutrition focuses attention on females as mothers. It has often concentrated on their nutritional status mainly as it is related to the well-being of the infants that they produce and their ability to breastfeed, nurture and raise their children.

The health and well-being of the mother herself has been relatively neglected. Similarly, the field of maternal and child health has put major emphasis on the child and on providing services and help to women mainly so that they can have successful pregnancies and lactations; this is also in the interests of the infant, without much concern for the mother. The dual role of women as mothers and productive workers is compromised by poor diets and ill health; not only their own well-being but that of the whole family is affected. A heavy work load may push a woman with marginal food intake over the brink and into a state of malnutrition.

A poor diet, frequent acute and some chronic infections, repeated pregnancies, prolonged lactation and a heavy burden of work may all contribute to serious physiological depletion and sometimes to overt malnutrition. The term "maternal depletion syndrome" has been suggested. In many countries young women in their late teens appear hearty, happy, healthy and attractive, but only ten or 15 years later, as young women in their late thirties, they are prematurely old, tired, down-trodden and unhealthy. Too often, the young female does not even live out her teens before her first pregnancy. During pregnancy a woman's nutritional needs become greater shall at other times in her life. Her diet needs to provide all the elements needed for the growth of a fertilized ovum or egg into a viable foetus and baby. As the woman nourishes herself she also nourishes the growing foetus as well as the placenta to which the foetus in her uterus is attached by its umbilical cord.

At the same time her breast tissue prepares for lactation. During the first half of pregnancy extra food is needed for the mother's uterus, breasts and blood—all of which increase in size or amount—as well as for the growth of the placenta. The increased need for food continues in the last half of the pregnancy, but during the last trimester the extra nutrients are required mainly for the rapidly growing foetus, which also needs to develop nutrient stores, particularly of vitamin A, iron and other micronutrients, and energy stores of fat. An adequate diet during pregnancy assists the mother to gain the extra weight that is physiologically desirable and helps ensure that the baby's birth weight is normal. Healthy women gain weight during pregnancy if they are not overworked. Just as a heavy person needs more energy to perform the same amount of physical work as a lighter person, a pregnant woman also needs more energy. In industrialized countries many women have an easy life during pregnancy; they rest frequently, thus reducing their energy needs. However, in much of Africa and some other regions, pregnant women remain active, even during their last few months of pregnancy.

The Basal metabolic rate (BMR) usually increases during pregnancy, which also raises energy requirements. Thus most women need more energy when they are pregnant, even if they are not overworked. For the overburdened woman of the developing world, who gets little rest and not much food, weight loss is a real and dangerous prospect. There is little doubt that abortions, miscarriages and stillbirths are more common in women who are poorly nourished than in those who are adequately nourished. Dietary deficiencies probably also increase the risk of producing a malformed foetus. Severe malnutrition reduces fertility and therefore the likelihood of conception. A severely malnourished woman ceases to menstruate. This is clearly a natural device to stop the loss of nutrients in the menstrual flow and to protect the woman from the rigours of pregnancy and childbirth.

The weight of the infant at birth is influenced by maternal nutrition. Low birth weights can be expected of infants born to malnourished mothers. Even a modest increase in energy intake during pregnancy tends to increase the birth weight of the infant. In many developing countries 50 to 75 percent of pregnant women have anaemia. Anaemia often contributes to high maternal mortality rates. All pregnant women should attend a clinic at regular intervals for antenatal examination which should include checking of haemoglobin levels. Practical advice should be given regarding diet, taking into account what foods are locally available and what the mother can afford. It is accepted policy in many countries that pregnant women be advised to take medicinal supplements of iron, or sometimes iron-folate. In areas where vitamin A deficiency is known to be a public health problem, infants of mothers who have poor vitamin A status are born with low vitamin A stores.

In some cultures there is a fear that extra food given during pregnancy will make the baby too large and thus cause a more difficult or complicated delivery. This is not true for healthy women of normal size. Women of short stature or with a contracted pelvis may have difficulty in delivering babies and may require special care before and during delivery. At the time of birth the mother loses blood, not infrequently 500 to 1000 ml, and she needs nutrients to regenerate that blood. In most developing countries the majority of women breastfeed their newborn infants for a period of weeks or months after delivery. The nutritional stores of a lactating woman may already be more or less depleted as a result of the pregnancy and the loss of blood during childbirth. Lactation raises nutrient needs, mainly because of the loss of nutrients first through colostrum and then through breastmilk.

Breastmilk volume varies widely, but for fully breastfed babies around four months of age, it is often 700 to 800 ml per day. It may rise later to as much as 1 000 ml or more. The nutrients present in this milk come from the diet of the mother or from her nutrient reserves. It is recommended that mothers exclusively breastfeed their infants for six months and then begin to introduce other food while continuing to breastfeed for as long as they wish, often into the second year or beyond. During the period of exclusive or full breastfeeding the woman usually will not menstruate.

The duration of amenorrhoea varies from as little as four months to as long as 18 months or more. During that time the lactating woman will not be losing the iron normally lost with each menstrual period. The conversion of nutrients in food to nutrients in breastmilk is not entire. There is a widely held belief that the composition of breastmilk varies enormously. This is not so. Human breastmilk has a fairly constant composition, and is only selectively affected by the diet of the mother. The fat content of breastmilk varies somewhat. The carbohydrate, protein, fat, calcium and iron contents do not change much even if the mother is short of these in her diet. A mother whose diet is deficient in thiamine and vitamins A and C, however, produces less of these in her milk.

Thiamine deficiency in the lactating mother can lead to infantile beriberi in the baby. In general the effect of very poor nutrition on a lactating woman is to reduce the quantity rather than the quality of breastmilk. Lactating mothers should be encouraged to attend a clinic with their babies during the months after delivery. At the clinic both mother and baby should be examined. The mother should have her haemoglobin level checked and also her weight. Medicinal iron in the same quantities as recommended during pregnancy should be given. The mother should be given advice on consuming a mixed diet. This is also a good time to discuss the mother's desire for further pregnancies and her view of the ideal spacing between pregnancies and to provide information and help regarding family planning. Relatively wide spacing between births is usually to the nutritional advantage of the mother the infant and even the next foetus. Narrow spacing between births prevents the mother from restoring her nutrient reserves before the next pregnancy, provides her with more work and a shorter time to care for her infant exclusively, and may influence her to breastfeed for a shorter period than is desirable. At each postnatal visit both the mother and the baby should be examined, and advice on the diets of both mother and infant should be provided.

Provided that the mother has adequate breastmilk, breastfeeding alone with no added food or medicinal supplementation is all that is needed for the normal infant during the first six months of life. Exclusive breastfeeding means that not even water, juice or other fluids are provided; none of these are needed. The infant should be examined regularly at the clinic, where weight gain is seen to indicate adequate nutrition. At the clinic a schedule for immunization will be set up, and this needs to be followed. Infants born with low weight (because of prematurity, for example) or twins may need special attention, and possibly iron or other supplements should be given. Up to six months of age many breastfed infants have considerable natural immunity to many infections. As the children get older they gain weight and length.

The increased energy requirements are based more on the weight of the child than on the age. Because healthy, well-nourished children follow a growth pattern, however, there is a close correlation between recommendations based on age and those based on weight. Breastmilk is relatively deficient in iron, and the infant's store of iron is sufficient only until about six months of age. From six to 12 months, the normal infant may be expected to gain between 2 and 3 kg. The infant, while continuing to receive breastmilk, will now need foods to provide extra energy, protein, iron, vitamin C and other nutrients for growth. The needed energy can usually be obtained from a gruel of whatever is the local staple food. The quantity and bulk can profitably be reduced if some edible oil or fat-containing food is also eaten. If the staple is a cereal such as maize, wheat, millet or rice, it will also provide a useful quantity of protein, but if it is plantain or a root such as cassava or yam, it will supply very little protein. In the 1950s and 1960s it was thought to be very important that complementary foods and then foods given after termination of breastfeeding should include animal protein in large amounts. This has been shown to be unnecessary.

In developing countries these foods are often too expensive for poor families or are unavailable. More important is the need to feed the young child frequently, with foods that are not too bulky and are both nutrititious and of high energy density. Ripe papayas and mangoes are excellent sources and are usually most acceptable to young children. Vitamin C can alternatively be provided by citrus fruits (e.g. Oranges) or other fruits. Gradually, as more teeth erupt, the child can be put on a more solid diet. By the age of two years, the child may have stopped breastfeeding and may be completely weaned. The term "weaning" has been used to describe the introduction of foods and fluids other than breastmilk and the transition to a solid diet without breastmilk. However, people in Northern countries also talk of "weaning from the bottle". The word is therefore often misunderstood, and it may be better not to use it because of the confusion it causes. Adult foods can be chopped up and forced through a strainer into a cup or on to a plateful of gruel for the child.

A strainer can readily be made if none is available. Otherwise, various foods can be crushed before cooking using a pestle and mortar, which are found in most households. In some societies gruel or porridge made from the local staple is made sour or partially fermented. This is a good practice. Small amounts of germinated cereal seeds, often millet or sorghum, are crushed and added to maize or other porridge. The amylase present breaks down some of the starch, causing the porridge to become thinner, so it is easier for the young child to consume, and making it more energy dense. The child can now obtain adequate nutrients in three meals per day, but until the child reaches the age of five years, parents should make certain that the child is eating adequately and getting his or her fair share of the most desirable foods, which may well be those that are most tasty and in shortest supply. Special attention may need to be given when children have a poor appetite or when they are ill and their appetite is reduced. For the whole family, but especially for children, care must be taken that food, water and other fluids are safe and not contaminated. Good personal and household hygiene are of the greatest importance. Washing hands with soap and water before meals or food handling is a good family rule.

The vast majority of schoolchildren in developing countries attend primary schools. Most are at day schools, few of which provide a midday meal. In rural areas the school is often some kilometres from the parents' home. The child frequently has to leave home early and walk a considerable distance to school. Often the child has little or no breakfast at home before he or she sets out; there is no meal at school; and the first, and sometimes only, meal of the day is late in the afternoon. The nutritional needs of a schoolchild are high. The adolescent child has proportionately higher requirements for most nutrients than the average adult. It is practically impossible for an adolescent to obtain adequate quantities of the right foods from one or even two meals a day.

It is highly desirable that school-age children cat some food before going to school and some food at school, or during the middle of the day outside the school grounds, as well as the food eaten at home. It is not practical for many mothers to rise before dawn to spend the considerable time necessary to light a fire and prepare a hot meal for children before school-time. Therefore, if no hot breakfast is available, some fruit, cold cooked potatoes, rice, cassava or even cold porridge should be left over from the previous day for the schoolchild to eat before leaving home in the morning. In some areas cold chapattis, tortillas or wheat products such as bread may be available. A midday school meal is the ideal. It should provide reasonable amounts of the nutrients most likely to be missing or short in the home diet. A whole-grain cereal as the basis and a side dish of legumes with vegetables or green leaves make an excellent school meal. There are many possibilities, depending on what foods are locally available.

The meal might include some protein-rich food and some food containing vitamins A and C. School meals are beneficial because they often supply much-needed nutrients; they can form the basis for nutrition education; they are a good way of introducing new foods; and they prevent hunger and malnutrition. School meals, in addition to improving nutritional status, may increase enrolment, especially for girls, and may reduce absenteeism. However, in many developing countries, for many reasons, school meals are unavailable. Parents' organizations can sometimes work with teachers to organize community school feeding or food supplementation or nutritious snacks. School meals can provide a good environment for nutrition education.

Further nutrition education can be carried out as an extracurricular project. A school vegetable garden or orchard can provide foods with valuable extra nutrients for the midday meal. Poultry keeping, small animal production (rabbits, guinea-pigs, pigeons, etc.) and fish pond construction, in areas where they are suitable, are educative projects and can provide food for a school meal A midday school meal might be provided by the government or local authority as part of the education system and could be paid for from the normal school fees Alternatively, a midday meal system might be started and paid for from special fees collected from the pupils daily, weekly or per term.

Local organizations might provide certain food items free or at low prices for school feeding, thus reducing the overall cost. The cost of school feeding can be reduced by local self-help efforts on the part of villagers, parents' committees and pupils These efforts may fit in well with self-help community projects For example, a small kitchen shelter can be built on a self-help basis Instead of a paid cook, a rota of parents can take turns doing the cooking. Pupils can collect fuelwood at weekends However, it must be stressed that the provision of a midday school meal must not detract from the parents' responsibilities to provide a good diet for schoolchildren at home. In the absence of a school lunch, parents should send their children to school with some food to be eaten at midday.

However, they may have real difficulty in finding suitable foods. The various foods suggested for a cold breakfast can equally provide the solution for a midday snack. The sort of food taken will vary according to what is available locally. Possibilities include a few bananas, cooked whole cassava, sweet or ordinary potatoes roasted in their skins, fruit, tomatoes, roasted maize on the cob, roasted groundnuts, coconuts, cold grilled fish, smoked cooked meat, hard-boiled eggs, a calabash of sour milk or some bread, a chapatti or tortillas. Some schools above primary level are boarding schools. These usually provide three meals a day, and the menu should be based on recommendations made to the school by someone with dietetics training. Occasionally schools plead lack of money as an excuse for an inadequate diet.

School meals need not be luxurious, but they should be balanced and should provide all the nutrients necessary for growth and health. The child with an inadequate diet will not only fail to grow properly, but may also develop anaemia and other signs of malnutrition and will not be able to concentrate on or benefit fully from the education provided. Increasingly in urban areas, and even to some extent in more heavily populated rural districts, entrepreneurs set up stalls and the like near schools so they can prepare and sell foods to schoolchildren. These "street foods" often have the advantage of providing access to cooked foods at relatively low cost, but the disadvantages include poor hygiene, poor-quality food and high prices. Where the main source of a midday snack or meal for primary or secondary schoolchildren is a vendor, the food is available only to children who have money to purchase it. Often the wealthier children participate and the children from the poorest families, or those whose parents will not provide money, do not. The health of schoolchildren also needs consideration.

In many countries school health services are non-existent or very poor. Examination for sight and hearing defects is important. Routine deworming might be initiated. Attention to micronutrient deficiencies may be needed in areas where children are at risk of iron, vitamin A or iodine deficiency. Iodine is especially important when girls reach puberty and before they have their first pregnancy. Unfortunately, in some countries a large percentage of school-age children do not attend school. In some countries far more boys than girls attend school. Out-of-school children have the same nutritional and health needs as children attending school, but they do not benefit from school meals and other services. They are an often forgotten and relatively neglected group of the population, including children from the poorest families as well as children with disabilities, either physical or psychological. Many older people, especially if unfit, take less exercise and so may need less energy. They may, therefore, eat less food and as a result get fewer micronutrients, but their needs for micronutrients are unchanged.

Consequently, conditions such as anaemia are common. Older people who have lost many or all of their teeth or who have gingivitis or other gum problems may find it difficult to chew many ordinary foods and may need softer foods. Fed on a normal family diet, they may eat too little and become malnourished. They may also suffer from illnesses which reduce their appetite or desire for food, which may also lead to malnutrition. In many rural traditional societies old people are cared for at home by relatives and others in the community.

6

Child Nutrition in India

The term 'nutrition' refers to the availability of energy and nutrients to the body's cells in relation to body requirements, while the term 'malnutrition' refers to any imbalance in satisfying nutrition requirements. Malnutrition among children is often caused by the synergistic effects of inadequate or improper food intake, repeated episodes of parasitic or other childhood diseases such as diarrhoea, and improper care during illness. Malnutrition is often cited as an important factor contributing to high morbidity and mortality among children in developing countries. The relationship between nutritional status and child mortality is not conclusive, however.

Malnutrition during childhood can also affect growth potential and risk of morbidity and mortality in later years of life. Malnourished children are more likely to grow into malnourished adults who face heightened risks of disease and death. Poor nutritional status of women has been associated with a higher age at menarche and a lower age at secondary sterility. A number of factors affect child nutrition, either directly or indirectly. The most commonly cited factors are food availability and dietary intake, breastfeeding, prevalence of infectious and parasitic diseases, access to health care, immunization against major childhood diseases, vitamin A supplementation, maternal care during pregnancy, water supply and sanitation, socioeconomic status, and health-seeking behaviour. Demographic characteristics such as the child's age and sex, birth intervals (both preceding and following), and mother's age at childbirth are also associated with child nutrition. Several studies indicate that inadequate or improper food intake and repeated episodes of infectious diseases adversely affect children's nutritional status. Proper treatment of acute infectious diseases, especially diarrhoea, has beneficial effects for children's growth and nutritional status.

Discrimination against girls in feeding and health care are often cited as reasons for poorer nutrition and higher mortality among girls than boys in many developing countries. However, most studies based on anthropometric data do not find a higher prevalence of malnutrition among girls. Many of the factors associated with child nutrition are also associated with each other. Consequently, any apparent effect of one factor on child nutrition may be due to the confounding effects of one or more of these other factors. Therefore, when assessing the effects of any one factor on malnutrition, a multivariate analysis is necessary to control for the effects of other potentially confounding factors. Using data from India's 1992-93 National Family Health Survey (NFHS), this chapter analyzes the effects of selected demographic and socioeconomic factors on various dimensions of malnutrition among children below age four, as indicated by anthropometric measurements, after statistically controlling for a number of potentially confounding variables. The chapter complements results presented in the original NFHS national report, which, however, provides only simple cross-tabulations of the prevalence of child malnutrition by selected demographic and socioeconomic characteristics without controls.

The analysis is based on data from India's 1992-93 National Family Health Survey (NFHS). Data were collected from a probability sample of 89,777 ever-married women age 13-49 residing in 88,562 households. The NFHS covered 24 states and the National Capital Territory of Delhi, which has since attained statehood. The sample represents 99 percent of India's population.

Children are the units of analysis. The NFHS collected a complete birth history, including sex and date of birth of each child, from each ever-married woman age 13- 49 in the sample. It also collected information on the height and weight of children born since a cutoff date (approximately four years before the survey), as well as a number of maternal variables relating to the care of each child. From the birth histories and information linked to them, we created a child data file, into which we also merged selected household characteristics from the household data file. Thus, the supplementation has been shown to reduce morbidity and mortality. The evidence of beneficial effects of vitamin A supplementation on morbidity and mortality in children is not conclusive, however. In as much as vitamin A supplementation reduces morbidly in children, it may also improve their nutritional status.

The three indices of child malnutrition are expressed in terms of standard deviation units from the median in the international reference population. Children who fall more than two standard deviations below the reference median are considered to be malnourished, and those who fall more than three standard deviations below the reference median are considered to be severely malnourished. Thus, children who are more than two standard deviations below the median of the international reference population in terms of their height-for-age are defined as stunted, and those more than three standard deviations below the reference median are defined as severely stunted. The categories underweight, severely underweight (based on weight-for-age), wasted, and severely wasted (based on weight-for-height) are similarly defined. Wasting is usually associated with the failure to receive adequate nutrition in the period immediately before the survey and may be the result of seasonal variations in food supply or recent episodes of illness, especially diarrhoea.

Several factors affect the validity of these measures, including coverage of the population of children and accuracy of the anthropometric measurements. In the NFHS, about 16 percent of living children below age four were not weighed and measured, usually because the child was not at home or because the mother refused to allow the measurements to be taken. These children are excluded from the analysis. Also excluded from the analysis are children whose month and year of birth were not reported by the mother and children with grossly improbable weight or height measurements. Two of the three measures of child nutrition (height-for-age and weight-for-age) are sensitive to accurate reporting of children's ages. Weight-for-height is the only measure that does not depend on accuracy of age reporting.

The weight-for-height measure is, however, sensitive to errors in the individual component measures of weight and height, especially if the errors are in opposite directions. The analysis of the effects of demographic and socioeconomic variables on the three indices of child malnutrition is multivariate and employs logistic regression models. The response (or dependent) variable in each model is a dummy (two-category) variable that simply indicates whether a child is stunted, underweight, or wasted (i.e., whether the child is more than two standard deviations below the median of the international reference population in terms of height-for-age, weight-for-age, or weight-for-height). Thirteen predictor variables are used in the analysis. All predictor variables are categorical.

The predictor variables are: child's age in months (<12, 12-23, 24-47); sex of child (male, female); birth order of child (one, two or three, four or five, six or higher); mother's age at childbirth (13-24, 25-34, 35-49); residence (urban, rural); mother's education (illiterate, literate but less than middle school complete, middle school complete or higher); religion 2 (Hindu, Muslim, other); caste/tribe 3 (SC/ST, other); exposure to electronic mass media 4 (regularly exposed, not regularly exposed); household standard of living 5 (low, medium, high); mother received iron and folic acid tablets during pregnancy (yes, no); mother received two or more tetanus injections during pregnancy (yes, no); and geographic region 6 (North, Central, East, Northeast, West, South). These variables are selected for analysis because they are known to be associated with child nutrition and because they are readily available from the NFHS.

Two additional predictor variables considered were 'received any vaccination' (yes, no) and 'received vitamin A' (yes, no). The analysis incorporating these two variables excluded children below 12 months of age because vaccinations and vitamin A supplementation are usually received during the first year of life. Neither of these variables had a significant effect on any of the three indices of child malnutrition, and their inclusion or exclusion from the regression models did not alter the effects of any of the other 13 predictor variables.

We estimate both unadjusted and adjusted effects of each of the 13 predictor variables on stunting, underweight, and wasting. In this context, 'adjusted' means that other selected demographic and socioeconomic variables are statistically controlled by holding them constant at their mean values. Present effects in the form of unadjusted and adjusted percentages malnourished for categories of each predictor variable of interest. The unadjusted percentages for categories of a given predictor variable are estimated from a separate logistic regression in which that predictor variable is the only one considered. Because each underlying regression contains just one predictor variable, the unadjusted percentages do not incorporate controls for any other, potentially confounding, predictor variables. Whereas the unadjusted percentages are based on many logistic regressions, one for each predictor variable, the adjusted percentages (for a particular response variable) are based on a single logistic regression that includes all 13 predictor variables. In calculating adjusted percentages for categories of any given predictor variable, the set of control variables consists of all the other 12 predictor variables, which are controlled by setting them at their mean values. This method of presenting results when controlling for potentially confounding variables is called Multiple Classification Analysis, or MCA.

In the logistic regression analyses, the estimation of significance levels takes into account design effects due to clustering at the level of the primary sampling unit. The regressions were estimated using the STATA statistical software package. Constant terms in the regressions are reset so that predicted percentages agree with observed percentages when all predictor variables in the regressions are set to their mean values. Because urban and rural environments in India are quite different, the factors affecting child malnutrition may have different effects in urban and rural areas. And because there is considerable discrimination against girls, especially in the northern states of India, the factors affecting child malnutrition may have different effects for boys and girls. For these reasons, the analyses of factors affecting child malnutrition are also carried out separately for urban and rural areas and for boys and girls. In some states the NFHS sample design is self-weighting, but in other states certain sectors of the population, such as urban areas, are over-sampled, necessitating the use of weights to restore the correct proportions. Some states are over-represented and others are under-represented in the sample, necessitating an additional set of weights when aggregating to the national level. All results presented in this report are based the on the weighted sample. The NFHS sample design is discussed in more detail in the original survey report.

The percentage of children below age four who are malnourished according to height-for-age, weight-for age, or weight-for-height for India as a whole and for individual states. Fifty-two percent are stunted, 54 percent are underweight, and 17 percent are wasted. The percentages who are severely malnourished according to these two measures are also substantial. Twenty-nine percent are severely stunted, 22 percent are severely underweight, and 3 percent are severely wasted.

The lower prevalence of wasting than stunting or underweight indicates that chronic malnutrition is more prevalent in India than acute malnutrition. Even so, levels of wasting and severe wasting in India are many times higher than those in the stunted. Twenty-five percent of infants and 64 percent of children age 24-47 months are stunted. A somewhat more detailed breakdown by age in Figure 3 shows that stunting is considerably less common in the first six months of life, when most babies are fully breast-fed, than at older ages. The prevalence of stunting increases rapidly up to 12-23 months of age, after which it increases more slowly. Interestingly, the prevalence of stunting is the same for boys and girls. This finding is somewhat surprising, inasmuch as there is widespread discrimination against girls in India. A separate analysis for Bihar and Kerala, the states with the highest and lowest prevalence of malnutrition, indicates that even in Bihar, in which the status of women is arguably the lowest of any state in India, there is no significant difference in the prevalence of stunting between boys and girls (results not shown).

Some other studies have also observed the absence of the expected gender differential in nutrition in India, as well as in other developing countries with widespread discrimination against girls, but no concrete reasons for this unexpected finding are suggested. Data from the NFHS are not sufficiently detailed to permit a more in-depth investigation of possible reasons for the unexpected absence of a gender differential in child nutrition favouring boys. Because competition for nutrition increases as the number of children increases within a family, one might expect that children of higher birth order would have a greater risk of stunting than would children of lower birth order. Adjusting for the other 12 predictor variables makes little difference to the effect of birth order on the risk of stunting. The prevalence of stunting also does not vary much by mother's age at childbirth. When the effects of the other predictor variables (including birth order) are statistically controlled, however, children born to younger mothers have a higher prevalence of stunting. Possibly this reflects improved expertise in childcare as parents get older.

The unadjusted prevalence of stunting is considerably lower in urban areas than in rural areas. However, once the other predictor variables are controlled, the relationship between residence and stunting slightly reverses and almost disappears. This suggests that the effects of urban/rural residence are mostly indirect, through the other predictor variables. Even after the other predictor variables are controlled, 56 percent of children of illiterate mothers are stunted, compared with 41 percent of mothers who have completed middle school or higher. Thus mother's education has large direct effects on stunting as well as some indirect effects through some of the other predictor variables. Hindus and Muslims have about the same prevalence of stunting, but children belonging to other religions have a considerably lower prevalence of stunting. Controlling for the other predictor variables, however, explains away most of the effect of religion, suggesting that the effects of religion stem mainly from the relatively high socioeconomic status of families belonging to other religions.

Similarly, children belonging to scheduled castes or scheduled tribes have a significantly higher prevalence of stunting than do other children. Again, when the other predictor variables are statistically controlled, the effect of caste/tribe on prevalence of stunting largely disappears, suggesting that the unadjusted differences by caste/tribe stem mainly from the relatively low socioeconomic status of families who belong to a scheduled caste or scheduled tribe. Children of mothers who are regularly exposed to the electronic mass media have a lower prevalence of stunting than do children whose mothers are not regularly exposed. Controlling for the other predictor variables largely eliminates the effect of mother's media exposure, suggesting that media exposure has no independent effect on stunting. The unadjusted prevalence of stunting among children in households with a low standard of living is 59 percent, compared with 37 percent for children in households with a high standard of living. This differential is reduced to 56 and 44 percent when the other predictor variables are controlled, indicating a strong direct effect of standard of living on prevalence of stunting.

Children of mothers who received iron and folic acid tablets when they were pregnant have a lower prevalence of stunting than do children whose mothers did not receive iron and folic acid tablets during pregnancy. Controlling for the selected demographic and socioeconomic variables, however, virtually eliminates this effect, and it becomes statistically nonsignificant. Children of mothers who received two or more tetanus injections when they were pregnant have a significantly lower prevalence of stunting than do children whose mothers did not receive tetanus injections during pregnancy. Controlling for the other predictor variables substantially reduces this effect, but it remains statistically significant. This finding is consistent with earlier evidence from the NFHS that a mother having two or more tetanus injections during pregnancy is a good proxy for that mother's health-seeking behaviour for her children. Controlling for the other predictor variables does not make much difference in these geographic differentials, indicating that geographic region exerts a substantial independent effect on the prevalence of stunting.

The reason for this geographic effect is unclear. It may have something to do with variations among the states in the availability and quality of health services, which are, for the most part, offered through state-level departments of health and family welfare. Only adjusted effects are presented. In both urban and rural areas, the effects of most predictor variables are similar to the effects for India as a whole. The exception is the effect of caste/tribe. Children belonging to scheduled-caste or scheduled-tribe households in urban areas have a significantly higher prevalence of stunting than do children belonging to other castes, while in rural areas there is no difference in the prevalence of stunting by caste/tribe. Thirty-one percent of infants and more than 61 percent of children age 12-47 months are underweight. For reasons that are unclear, the proportion underweight does not increase monotonically with age as it does in the case of stunting. Instead, it peaks at age 12-23 months and then declines slightly at 24-47 months. Adjusting for the control variables makes virtually no difference to the effect of age on the proportion underweight.

There is no difference in the proportion underweight by sex of child, regardless of whether the other predictor variables are controlled. The proportion of underweight children increases with birth order, again regardless of whether demographic and socioeconomic variables are controlled. The unadjusted proportion underweight varies irregularly by mother's age at childbirth, but it declines monotonically, as in the case of stunting, when the other predictor variables are controlled. The proportion underweight is considerably lower among children living in urban areas than in rural areas. When the other predictor variables are controlled, however, the effect of urban residence on proportion underweight becomes small and statistically nonsignificant. This finding indicates that the effects of urban/rural residence are felt indirectly through the other predictor variables, as in the case of stunting.

The proportion underweight among children of illiterate mothers is 60 percent, compared with 36 percent among children of mothers who have completed middle school or higher. Adjusting for the other predictor variables reduces the effect of mother's education on the proportion of children underweight, but the effect remains large and statistically significant, indicating a substantial direct effect as in the case of stunting. This finding suggests that efforts to improve women's education may contribute directly as well as indirectly to better child nutrition. An important reason for the large direct effect may be that educated women are more knowledgeable about proper nutrition and sanitation and make better use of health services. Hindu and Muslim children differ little in the proportion underweight, but a much lower proportion of children of other religions are underweight. The adjusted proportion underweight is about the same across religions, however, indicating that the lower proportion underweight among children of other religions is primarily due to their higher socioeconomic status. The proportion underweight is higher among children belonging to a scheduled caste or scheduled tribe than among other children, but the adjusted proportion underweight is about the same. This suggests that the living have large and significant effects. The adjusted effects tend to be greater in urban areas than in rural areas. The separate analysis by sex of child shows a rather similar pattern. Effects of the various predictor variables included in the analysis are quite similar for boys and girls.

The findings on wasting differ somewhat from the findings on stunting and underweight, although the two sets of findings are broadly similar. The effects of the predictor variables on wasting tend to be smaller and, in some cases, less consistent with expectation than the effects of the same variables on stunting and underweight. Child's age has an inverted U-shaped relationship with the prevalence of wasting, with children age 12-23 months more likely to be wasted than infants or children age 24-47 months. Controlling for the other predictor variables does not reduce this effect, indicating that child's age has an independent effect on the prevalence of wasting. The lower prevalence of wasting among infants may stem mainly from the fact that most infants in India are breast-feed.

Boys are more subject to wasting than girls, unlike stunting and underweight, which affect boys and girls equally. In light of the widespread discrimination against girls in feeding and medical care in India, this finding is contrary to expectation. Controlling for the other predictor variables does not alter the effect of gender on wasting, indicating that the higher prevalence of wasting among boys cannot be explained by these other variables. In contrast to the prevalence of stunting and underweight, the prevalence of wasting does not vary much by birth order of child. Mother's age at childbirth also does not have much effect on wasting, except among children born to mothers age 35-49, who have a somewhat higher prevalence of wasting. The lack of an effect of birth order may reflect the fact that wasting is primarily a result of acute malnutrition rather than chronic malnutrition. Children living in urban areas have slightly lower prevalence of wasting than those living in rural areas. When the other predictor variables are controlled, however, the adjusted effect of urban/rural residence on wasting vanishes. This suggests that the effect of residence is indirect through the other predictor variables. Although the effects are reduced after adjusting for the effects of the other predictor variables, the adjusted effects remain statistically significant.

Children belonging to religions other than Hindu or Muslim have a somewhat lower prevalence of wasting, but religion has no effect on wasting once the other predictor variables are controlled. This suggests that the lower proportion wasted among children of other religions is primarily due to their relatively high socioeconomic status, as in the case of stunting and underweight. Children belonging to a scheduled caste or scheduled tribe have a somewhat higher prevalence of wasting than do children belonging to other households, even after adjusting for the effects of the other predictor variables. Thus, the effect of caste/tribe on wasting is only partially explained by the other predictor variables, unlike the cases of stunting and underweight, where the effect of caste/tribe is completely explained by the other variables. Children of mothers regularly exposed to the electronic mass media have a lower prevalence of wasting, as expected. But, as in the case of stunting and underweight, this effect of media exposure becomes small and statistically nonsignificant once the other demographic and socioeconomic variables are controlled.

Unlike the effects on stunting and underweight, the introduction of controls considerably reduces the effect of living standard on wasting, and the adjusted effect is no longer statistically significant. Whether mothers received iron and folic acid tablets or two or more tetanus injections during pregnancy has virtually no effect on the prevalence of wasting among children. By geographic region, the east and the west regions have the highest prevalence of wasting, and the northeast region has the lowest. Boys have considerably higher prevalence of wasting than girls in rural areas, but in urban areas the gender difference is small and statistically nonsignificant. This finding is contrary to expectation, given that discrimination against girls tends to be more severe in rural areas than in urban areas. The effects of birth order and mother's age at childbirth, as estimated separately for urban and rural areas and for boys and girls, are similar to those for the sample as a whole. The effects of mother's education, however, are not similar.

Mother's education has a statistically significant effect on wasting among children living in rural areas (but not urban areas) and among girls (but not boys). The effects of religion are similar for boys and girls, but children belonging to religions other than Hindu or Muslim have the lowest prevalence of wasting in urban areas and the highest prevalence of wasting in rural areas. The effects of caste/tribe on wasting are similar for boys and girls and for urban and rural areas, but they are not statistically significant for girls or for urban areas. Media exposure has a small significant effect in the expected direction for girls, but not for boys. Standard of living has a negative but statistically nonsignificant effect on wasting for both boys and girls. It has virtually no effect on wasting in rural areas, but a negative and statistically significant effect in urban areas. The two variables related to mother's health behaviour during pregnancy have virtually no effect on wasting, either by residence or by sex of child. The effects of geographic region by residence and by sex of child resemble the effects of geographic region for the sample as a whole.

India has disproportionately large numbers of malnourished and severely malnourished children below four years of age according to anthropometric data on stunting (height-for-age), underweight (weight-for-age), and wasting (weight-for-height) from the 1992-93 National Family Health Survey (NFHS). Fifty-two percent of all children below age four are stunted, and 29 percent are severely stunted. Fifty-four percent are underweight, and 22 percent are severely underweight. Seventeen percent are wasted, and 3 percent are severely wasted. The lower prevalence of wasting than of stunting or underweight indicates that chronic malnutrition is more prevalent in India than acute malnutrition. However, the prevalence of wasting is about 8 times and the prevalence of severe wasting is about 25 times the levels in the international reference population.

There are considerable variations in the prevalence of malnutrition among states. Bihar and Kerala are the states with the highest and lowest prevalence of malnutrition in the country. Even in Kerala, which is also the state with the lowest infant and child mortality rates, 27 percent of children below age four are stunted, 28 percent are underweight, and 12 percent are wasted. Multivariate analysis of the selected demographic and socioeconomic determinants of child nutritional status indicates that the strongest predictors of child nutrition in India, once other variables are controlled, are child's age and birth order, mother's education level, and household standard of living. Older children and children of higher birth order tend to have poorer nutritional status.

Children whose mothers are more educated and those who live in households with a relatively high standard of living have better nutrition. Boys and girls have about the same level of stunting and underweight, while wasting is somewhat higher among boys than among girls. In the face of much evidence that girls receive inferior care in India, this finding that girls fare at least as well if not better than boys in terms of nutrition is difficult to explain and warrants further investigation. The findings of this study should be interpreted cautiously because of the problem of age misreporting. Previous research indicates that some births that occurred during the period 0-4 years before the NFHS tend to be erroneously reported as having occurred during the period 5-9 years before the survey. This means that some children below age four are reported as older than they really are. To the extent that this kind of age exaggeration occurs, the estimates of stunting and underweight, which are based on height-for-age and weight-for-age, of stunting or underweight indicates that chronic malnutrition is more prevalent in India than acute malnutrition. However, the prevalence of wasting is about 8 times and the prevalence of severe wasting is about 25 times the levels in the international reference population.

There are considerable variations in the prevalence of malnutrition among states. Bihar and Kerala are the states with the highest and lowest prevalence of malnutrition in the country. Even in Kerala, which is also the state with the lowest infant and child mortality rates, 27 percent of children below age four are stunted, 28 percent are underweight, and 12 percent are wasted. Multivariate analysis of the selected demographic and socioeconomic determinates of child nutritional status indicates that the strongest predictors of child nutrition in India, once other variables are controlled, are child's age and birth order, mother's education level, and household standard of living. Older children and children of higher birth order tend to have poorer nutritional status. Children whose mothers are more educated and those who live in households with a relatively high standard of living have better nutrition. Boys and girls have about the same level of stunting and underweight, while wasting is somewhat higher among boys than among girls. In the face of much evidence that girls receive inferior care in India, this finding that girls fare at least as well if not better than boys in terms of nutrition is difficult to explain and warrants further investigation.

7

Implications of Health System

The relationship between health and poverty or health and development is complex, multi-faceted and multidirectional. Poverty in its various dimensions could be a manifestation, as well as a determinant of an individual's health. In its most basic form - as a state of food deprivation and nutritional inadequacy - poverty has a direct bearing on the morbidity and longevity of people. Starvation deaths are a stark example of this reality. Similarly, nutritional deficiencies have been observed to affect physical and mental development of children, impairing health and productivity of work. Data on 'wasting' and 'stunting' as well on other nutritional deficiencies disorders such as those related to vitamin-A deficiency (nutritional blindness), iron deficiency (anaemia), iodine deficiency (goitre) or other micro nutrient deficiencies capture some of these aspects of poverty-health linkages.

The other aspects of deprivation such as lack of access to critical amenities including safe water, sanitation, non-polluting domestic fuels, connectivity to life support services and most importantly to education and general awareness, contribute to reinforcing ill health and morbidity even leading to higher mortality levels. High child mortality levels on account of supervening infections, particularly diarrhoea and respiratory infections, are fairly widespread among people deprived of these basic amenities of life.

These commonly seen childhood infections often exacerbate malnourishment and at the same time prevalence of under nourishment in children reinforces the consequences of such infections. Adequate nutrition is thus critical for child health and survival, as well as for overcoming the potential vicious cycle of poverty and under-nutrition. well-being, reinforce the transition towards better health and longevity. Better purchasing power through a more equitable distribution of employment opportunities and resources can help bring about nutritional adequacy and food security for the poor. This, coupled with public provisioning of basic amenities including water, sanitation, shelter and access to education and life support services can ensure significant improvement in health and longevity of the population.

Historically, it has been observed that in response to socio-economic development, high birth and death rates in the early stages of development, yield ultimately to low levels of births and deaths, thereby stabilising the population growth. This has been postulated as the theory of demographic transition. The transition is, however, not simultaneous in the sense that in the early stages a more rapid decline in mortality is accompanied by a gradual decline in fertility. As a result, in the initial stages of development there is a rapid population growth. The decline in population growth comes only when the fertility rates decline appreciably.

The demographic transition is, often, growth mediated, as the outcome depends on utilisation of improved economic prosperity in expanding social services including those related to nutritional security for the population, spread of education, availability of community and public health, advancement in medical services, improvement in sanitation and availability of safe drinking water. It also depends on social factors such as those that influence average age at marriage, acceptability of family planning practices, work participation rates for women, family structures, urbanisation, religious consideration, etc.

The demographic transition is generally accompanied by an epidemiologic transition. The latter relates to the changing mortality and morbidity characteristics of the population. As a society develops and undergoes demographic transition there is a shift in distribution of major causes of death. It has been observed that population with high mortality rates suffers predominantly from infectious diseases, malnourishment and reproductive health hazards. On the other hand, populations where the mortality is low, experience health problems of affluence and urbanisation such as chronic cardio-vascular diseases, cancer and diabetes.

The outbreak of AIDS has lately broken this categorisation somewhat. It has affected the poorest in Sub-Saharan Africa, as well as the more affluent in the developed countries. In mapping these transitions to ascertain the health status of individuals and societies, at any point of time, it becomes necessary to look at the relevant health and demographic indicators. The data on mortality, hence, longevity and other demographic characteristics of the population are, by and large, free of conceptual ambiguities, relatively easily quantifiable, as well as available. The same cannot be said of the information, for example, on nutrition and morbidity indicators, particularly in the Indian context.

The data on nutritional status of the population is quite inadequate in coverage and comparability over time. Even when some data is available, one has to also reckon with the issue of nutrition adaptation and inter-individualvariability, which brings out the complexities involved in the measurement of under-nutrition. It is, in fact, even argued that a person's capacity for work and productivity is not determined by his/her intake of nutrients but by efficiency with which the food energy is converted into metabolisable energy over the person's homeostatic range of intake. Similarly, in case of morbidity data, the primary source, namely, the records maintained by medical institutions and public health agencies is practically non-existent and, if available, for limited urban pockets or for some specific public health initiatives are inadequate in coverage and quality. Most of the available information on morbidity in India is based on surveys that rely on recall factor of the sample households.

For rural backward areas and among illiterate households, it may not always be the best mechanism to collect information. Moreover, to the extent morbidity in the population gets reflected in mortality and longevity outcomes for people, from the point of a country still in the middle of its demographic transition - with mortality rates quite high vis-à-vis the prevalent rates in developed countries - the exclusion of morbidity indicators from composite indices on health attainments may at best make only a limited qualitative difference. It is possible though, and there is cross-country evidence to support, that low mortality rates and, hence, higher longevity may co-exist with higher levels of morbidity for countries and regions that have completed their demographic transition or are in the midst of it but have already attained low mortality levels. In such cases, morbidity indicators may have to be necessarily incorporated in composite indices on health attainments.

The direct relevance of morbidity indicators lies more in policy planning, programme designs, and in provisioning of public resources to support the transition towards better health indicators in the society. To that end it is imperative to track the morbidity indicators. Life expectancy is an indicator of general mortality. In using life expectancy at age one, the influence of infant mortality rates and their trends, which may often be at variance with the trends in adult mortality rates, is being separated. This is important in the Indian context, as the prevalent infant mortality rates are fairly high by international standards across most States.

More importantly, by using life expectancy at age one (which is more sensitive to adult mortality rates and reflects cumulated attainments of the population), in conjunction with the infant mortality rates (which is perhaps a better indicator of the momentary changes in the overall health attainment of any population) an index is generated that balances, some what different aspects of health attainments for a population.

Much like its educational development, India's post-independence achievement in longevity and health of the population is a story of some successes and some embarrassments - perhaps in equal measures. For an average Indian the life expectancy at birth, in the last five decades, has more than doubled to over 60 years. Yet the pace of improvement does not compare favourably with most developing countries in East Asia and Latin America, where life expectancy are approaching levels of the developed world. Moreover, morbidity due to common communicable and nutrition deficiency diseases continue to be high and morbidity due to non-communicable diseases is showing a progressive increase as a result of improving longevity and changes in life styles. The national level health attainments hide the large inter and intra-State differences, as well as persisting vulnerabilities of some segments of the population.

For some States, indicators on health attainments are comparable with the middle-income countries, and in parts of others mortality levels are as high as in poorest regions of sub-Saharan Africa. The differences across the rural -urban areas and the gender divide, as well as across population segments on caste and class lines are quite striking. There are some aspects of the development process that reflect poorly on the health of country's population. Despite mounting publicly held food stocks, food and nutritional security at the household level continues to be a distant dream for a substantial section of population. With all the resources, trained manpower and even a reasonable health infrastructure at its command, a large part of the country continues to suffer from disease burden, morbidity, as well as high mortality reflective of early stages of epidemiological transition.

Life expectancy of an individual (at any age) is the number of years the person is expected to live given the prevailing age specific mortality rates of the population to which he/she belongs. It is a general measure of mortality that captures prevailing mortality rates of a population at different age groups. The need to have a measure like life expectancy arises because often the age specific mortality rates are not well correlated. This is particularly true of the infant mortality/child mortality rates and other age specific mortality rates. Besides there is a conceptual appeal in having a summary measure that provides some indication on the longevity that a person is likely to enjoy in any society. It has an intrinsic value for people and its value also lies in its instrumental attribute of enabling the pursuit of other valued personal and social goals. Moreover, the indicator life expectancy is closely related with other aspects of health attainments namely nutrition adequacy and a relative lack of morbidity.

Moreover, with the success of immunisation programmes and rehydration therapy for diarrhoea in the developing countries, the link between child mortality and mortality at other ages may have been further weakened. In addition, the indicator persons not expected to survive beyond age 40 years, based on the life tables, has been presented to reflect the deprivation aspect of longevity for use in the HPI. Life expectancy at birth has more than doubled in the last fifty years. It increased from around 30 years at the time of independence to over 60 years in 1992-96. In the period 1970 to 1996, the life expectancy at birth, at the national level improved from 49.7 years to 60.7 years as per the estimates based on the Sample Registration System (SRS), Registrar General of India.

The increase in rural areas of 11.4 years outstripping the improvement in urban areas by 7.4 years. As a result, the rural-urban gap declined from 10.9 years to 6.9 years. During the period life expectancy at birth for males increased from 50.5 years to 60.1 years, whereas in case of females it was from 49 years to 61.4 years. Till about 1970s males, at the time of birth, were expected to live longer than the females. The trend has reversed since then. Though, the females outlived males in urban areas even in early 1970s, in rural areas this has happened only in 1990s.

On the other hand, life expectancy at birth in Assam, Bihar, Madhya Pradesh, Orissa, Rajasthan and Uttar Pradesh has been in the range of 55-60 years. Among the larger States, males are still expected to outlive the females in Bihar, Madhya Pradesh, Orissa and Uttar Pradesh. The rural-urban difference in life expectancy at birth is less than a year in Kerala whereas, in Assam, Bihar, Madhya Pradesh and Orissa this difference is around 8-10 years. For males it varies from 0.8 year and 1.7 years for Kerala and Punjab respectively, at one end, to 8-9 years for Assam and Madhya Pradesh on other. For females this difference is 1 and 4 years respectively for Kerala and Punjab, whereas it is nearly 10 years for Assam, Bihar, Madhya Pradesh and Orissa in the upper end.

Life Expectancy at age one, at the national level has improved from 60.9 years to 64.9 years over the period 1981-85 and 1992-96. The increase in case of females was marginally more than that for males. In case of rural areas this increase was from 59.6 years to 63.9 years, whereas for the urban areas it was from 66.0 years to 68.9 years. Thus, there has been a decline in the rural-urban gap in life expectancy at age one from 6.4 years to 5.0 years during this period. At the State level, Kerala and Punjab have a life expectancy at age one of over 70 years, while Assam, Madhya Pradesh, Uttar Pradesh and Orissa have less than 63 years.

There are various indicators of infant and child mortality. Among the more commonly used, infant mortality rate refers to the number of deaths per thousand live births in the first year of a child's life. It reflects the probability of a child dying before attaining the age one year. Similarly, under five mortality rate refers to the probability of child dying before the fifth birthday. Unlike the indicators on life expectancy that are relatively stable and slow moving, the infant and child mortality indicators are likely to be more sensitive to changes that have a bearing on the quality of life, particularly, to the health and longevity of people.

These could be sudden adversities or non-availability of critical public health and life support services. They are, thus, more useful from the point of policy targeting and tracking changes in health attainments of a population at more frequent intervals, particularly when the population is yet to complete its demographic transition. On other hand, a reduction in this ratio would imply higher female mortality in comparison to males, indicating discrimination against girl child in availability and access to food, nutrition, health care and, perhaps, even medical support services. Between the population Census of 1981 and 1991, juvenile sex ratio declined from 958 to 946. The decline was in age groups 0-4 years, as well as in 5-9 years.

At the national level, difference between rural and urban areas was marginal, although it widened somewhat in 1991 in comparison to 1981. The ratio was more favourable for females in age group 0-4 years than that prevailing in age group 5-9 years for both the

Census years. However, the inter-State variations were quite striking. The sex ratio was relatively more favourable for females in Southern, Northeastern and Eastern States and was particularly adverse in the States of Haryana, Punjab, Rajasthan, Uttar Pradesh and Delhi.

For a majority of States both in rural and urban areas, the sex ratio was lower in age group 5-9 years than in age group 0-4 years though the differences declined over the period. The preliminary results from Census 2001 for sex ratio in age group 0-6 years was 927 females for thousand males, with a similar pattern at State level. Among the factors that explain these patterns in the sex ratios, it turns out that while female mortality was 10.5 per cent higher than male mortality in the age group 0-4 years, it was higher by 19 per cent in the age group 5-9 years in 1981.

These differences in female and male age specific mortality were much higher for rural areas than for urban. In 1991, mortality differences narrowed down considerably, to the extent that male mortality marginally exceeded female mortality in urban areas for age group 5-9 years. There are, however, wide differences in the female-male mortality at State level. For a few States, namely, Bihar, Haryana, Madhya Pradesh, Punjab, Rajasthan and Uttar Pradesh the female mortality was higher than the male for both age groups. Another factor that has a bearing on female to male ratio in the population is the sex ratio at birth.

The world over, proportion of male children at birth is more than that of female. The sex ratio at birth varies on an average between 943 to 952 females for every thousand males. It tends to progressively become favourable for females on account of higher mortality for males. In India, however, the sex ratio at birth has generally remained in the range of 900-910 females for every thousand males in 1980s, declining to 878 in 1993-95, improving marginally thereafter to 901 in 1996-98. At sub-national level, for Southern States, it is by and large, in line with prevailing trends in the developed world, but is adverse for females in the States of Bihar, Gujarat, Haryana, Punjab, Rajasthan and Uttar Pradesh. For Haryana and Punjab, the sex ratio at birth, in urban areas was at sub-800 levels in 1996-98. This points to the possibility of widespread prevalence of pre-natal sex determination and sex selection practices. It highlights the impact of perverse social and cultural factors related to marriage practices and dowry, well as role of women in household level decision making in an essentially patriarchal social context in these States.

There are significant rural-urban disparities in various mortality, morbidity and nutrition indicators. Moreover, there is multiplicity of public programmes and interventions in health sector resulting in a thin spread of available resources, manpower and infrastructure. In States where inter-sectoral linkages that influence health attainments of people, have existed either for historical reasons, or have been consciously forged as a part of planned effort, and where the health concerns the rural population have been reasonably addressed, results on health attainments, as well as demographic transition have been quite impressive.

The National Health Policy 1983 and the draft National Health Policy 2001 recognise these concerns. The Statements have highlighted a need for time-bound programme for setting up network of comprehensive primary health care services, linked with extension and health education. It talked of intermediation through 'health volunteers' having appropriate knowledge and skill. It emphasised establishment of a referral system to prevent needless load on higher levels of health care hierarchy, at the same time creating a network of super-specialty services by also encouraging private health care facilities for patients who can afford.

While there has been noteworthy success in eradication of some communicable diseases and some are expected to be eliminated in near future, the sustainability of India's health care system, as it stands today, is uncertain. Moreover, there is far greater urgency to ensure an equitable access to health care services and attain acceptable standards of good health for the population in the country. As per the Constitutional allocation of responsibilities between the Central and State Governments, health and family welfare has been identified as a State subject. The main responsibility of infrastructure and manpower building rests with the State Governments.

However, the Central Government has over the last five decades provided supplementary funds for control of major communicable, as well as non-communicable diseases, by initiating national level programmes, in some cases, with the help of assistance from foreign agencies. At the time of independence, communicable diseases were a major cause of morbidity and mortality in India. Initial efforts in public health care were, therefore, directed to their prevention and control.

National initiatives, on some non-communicable diseases that were perceived as major public health problems, have also been taken. Among these the National Goitre Control Programme (launched in 1962), the National Blindness Control Programme (launched in

1976), the National Cancer Control Programme, National Mental Health Programme (launched in 1982) and Integrated Non-Communicable Disease Control Programme (launched on a pilot basis in the Ninth Plan) are some of the major initiatives of the Central Government. In addition, the Central Government supports bio-medical research in a number of areas.

The Indian Council for Medical Research is the nodal organisation for undertaking and supervising this work. At State level, apart from the overall responsibility of providing preventive and curative health care, the Integrated Child Development Services (ICDS) Programme, the National Mid Day Meals Programme (NMMP), various micro nutrient schemes, including those targeted for improving intake of iron-folate, vitamin A and iodised salt, as well as food for work through various anti poverty programmes are some important initiatives aimed at addressing the problem of malnutrition and women and child health.

The ICDS programme providing services like supplementary feeding, immunisation against preventable childhood diseases, health checkups, health and nutrition education to women and pre-school education for children has recorded significant success in many areas, particularly in States where the primary level health care infrastructure is relatively well developed. The States that have done well include, Kerala, Tamil Nadu, Karnataka and Andhra Pradesh in the South, Maharashtra and Gujarat in the West and West Bengal in the East. Himachal Pradesh, Haryana and Punjab have also done well but it is Rajasthan and Madhya Pradesh that have of late made significant strides in improving implementation of ICDS programme in their State.

The National Mid Meal Programme (NMMP) was initiated in 1995 to improve nutritional status and learning achievements of school-going children and, more importantly, their enrolment and attendance in schools. The programme been modelled after a similar initiative in Tamil Nadu showed considerable success in attaining the stated objectives of the programme. The availability of cooked meal in schools has been found to not only improve enrolment attendance levels of the school going children but has provided critical nutrition supplements to the children. In the States where cooked meals were substituted by dry rations as, forinstance, in Andhra Pradesh, the results have not been as encouraging.

At present, the national norms envisage a Sub-Centre for population of three to five thousand; a Primary Health Centre for population of twenty to thirty thousand; and a Community Health Centre for four Primary Health Centres. The number of Primary Health Centres doctors at the national level exceeds the requirement as per the norms. There are, however, shortages in the availability of para-medics, as well as specialists at the Community Health Centres, which undermines their functioning as referral units. The disparities across States and within States between regions for infrastructure, as well as for manpower are quite striking.

Aging: Socio-economic and Health Implications

The sharp decline in mortality since 1950 and a steady recent decline in fertility has contributed to the process of population aging in India. India currently ranks fourth among the countries of the world with a large elderly population; by the year 2000, it is likely to be second only to China. Conventionally, there are two processes considered to be involved in the aging of a population, i.e., aging at the base and aging at the apex of the population.

The former results from a decline in fertility; the latter, mortality reduction among the elderly. In India, both processes are recent phenomena. The sequence of high birth rates followed by high death rates until 1951 kept the proportion of persons aged 60 or more years of age at a low level. Since 1961, a sharp decline in death rates accompanied by an increasing expectation of life at age 60 set in motion the process of aging in India; furthermore, a steady decline in the birth rate since 1971 accelerated that process.

Table 1

Crude birth rates (CBR), crude death rates (CDR), and expectation of life at age (ZcO) in census years

Census year	*CBR*	*CDR*	*Expectation of life at 60*	
			Males	*Females*
1961*	41.7	22.8	11.8	13.0
1971*	41.2	19.0	13.6	13.8
1981 +	33.9	12.5	13.8	14.7
1991++	29.7	10.7	14.5	15.5
2001++	23.7	8.4	15.2	16.4

Notes: *= Census; + = sample registration scheme; and ++ = Expert Committee on Population Projections.

Until the middle of the present century, this portion of India's population did not receive much attention.

However, the situation is changing owing to changes in kinship and family organization in the wake of urbanization, industrialization and modernization. The joint family system, which used to provide a form of social security, is disintegrating. Even in the villages where approximately three-fourths of India's population live and where the process of change has been slow, changes have been taking place which are not favourable to the elderly.

However, despite the increased vulnerability of the aged, it is fortunate that this problem has not assumed serious proportions; nonetheless, it requires attention. Since 1951, the population aged 60 years or more has grown steadily. The projected populations for the decades 1981-1991 and 1991-2001 also show an increasing trend in the growth of the elderly sector of the population. When the percentage decadal variation of the general population is compared with the population 60 or more years of age, it is found that the elderly population has grown faster than the general population, mainly because of increases in the expectation of life.

According to the Expert Committee on Population Projections, the decadal per cent increase in the elderly population for the period 1991-2001 would be 38.5 per cent - more than double the rate of increase in the general population.

In 1961, the elderly population comprised 5.6 per cent of the total, increasing to 6.2 per cent in 1981. It is likely to increase to 7.7 per cent in 2001, according to the Expert Committee. The total increase in this portion of the population during the period 1961-1981 was around 10 per cent, i.e. about 0.5 per cent per year. The Expert Committee has estimated that during the period 1981-2001, the increase would be around 1.2 per cent per year.

Table 2: Percentage of population aged 60 +, by place of residence and old age dependency ratio

Place of residence	Years 1961	1971	1981	1991	2001
Rural	5.82	6.21	6.53	6.97	8.31
	(21.0)	(27.3)	(34.3)	(42.3)	(54.9)
Urban	4.74	4.97	5.12	5.43	6.46
	(3.7)	(5.4)	(8.2)	(12.5)	(21.1)
Total	5.63	5.96	6.20	6.55	7.70
	(24.7)	(32.7)	(42.5)	(54.8)	(75.9)
Old age dependency ratio	10.6	11.4	11.5	11.3	12.6

Although the proportion of India's elderly population is small compared as a per cent of the population 15-59 years of age with that of any developed country because of the large size of India's population base, the elderly population is very large in absolute numbers. The number of persons 60 or more years of age was 24.7 million in 1961; this number increased by 72 per cent to 42.5 million in 1981. In 2001 it is expected to increase to about 75.9 million, i.e. more than three times the size of the elderly population in 1961. In other words, it will be equal to three times Canada's entire population in 1981.

The number of elderly, both in absolute and percentage terms, is larger in the rural areas of India than in urban areas. Unlike the trend in most countries, there are more males than females in the elderly population for all the years covered in this study. The usual sex ratio pattern favouring females occurs at 70 or more years of age in the case of India.

Dependency

The relatively faster increase in the elderly population will contribute to a higher dependency ratio of the population in the non-productive age group. The old age dependency ratio, which was 10.6 in 1961, is likely to increase to 12.6 in 2001. Therefore, responsibility for caring for the elderly will fall either on young wage earners or on the Government.

The sex ratio (number of females per thousand males) of the elderly population, which was 1,000 in 1961 and decreased to 950 in 1981, is projected to be 987 in 2001. Though comparatively higher than that of the general population in each decade, the sex ratio is not weighted in favour of females, as occurs in more developed countries.

By contrast, the sex ratio of the population in the 7-years-and-over age group favours females when compared with that of the population in the age groups 60-64 years and 65-69 years. As expected, it is also higher than that of the general population in all the decades studied. This indicates that there will be more women than men aged 70 years and over in 2001. Their numbers will be higher in rural areas than in urban areas. Because most of them will be without income, they will need support either from their children or the Government.

Marital status

A fairly large proportion of the elderly population is single owing to the death of the marriage partner. The incidence of widowhood is much greater among females than among males owing partly to the comparatively higher expectation of life among the older females and partly to taboos against remarriage, particularly of females.

However, since 1961, there has been a consistent decrease in the percentage of widows and widowers which is likely to continue in the future, firstly because of a relaxation of the taboos against remarriage and secondly as a result of increases in the expectation of life at age 60 and over for males and females.

Literacy

The status of literacy in the 60 and over age group and in the general population for different decades. It shows that the percentage illiterate among the elderly was higher than that of the general population during each decade. Also, illiteracy was more prevalent among elderly females than elderly males, which parallels the pattern of illiteracy among the general population. However, there was a consistent decline in the percentage of illiterate elderly males and females in succeeding decades, i.e. 70.8 per cent compared with 65.4 per cent in the case of elderly males and 95.7 per cent compered with 92.3 per cent in the case of elderly females. It has been estimated that in 2001 approximately 52 per cent of elderly males and 83 per cent elderly females will be illiterate.

The majority of the illiterate elderly were engaged either in agricultural pursuits in the rural areas or as unskilled or semiskilled workers in urban areas, many of whom most likely were living from hand to mouth with little or no savings. Since their employment was in the unorganized sectors, they would not be covered by social insurance schemes and thus would be in need of economic support. In the absence of support from their relatives, they would have to look towards the Government for support.

Elderly workers

In India, the majority of the population, including the elderly, is poor. However, one positive feature concerning the elderly population is that most of those 60 or more years old are economically active, presumably because they are engaged in sectors for which there is no specific age of retirement.

The work participation rates for the elderly population by place of residence and sex and also the proportion of elderly workers in the total working-age population. It shows that 63.7 per cent of the elderly males and 10.2 per cent of the elderly females were workers in 1981. This means that people work until they reach a relatively advanced age because the expectation of life at birth is around 55 years in India.

The proportion of workers in the elderly population was higher in rural areas than in urban areas. Since 1961, there has been a gradual decline in the labour force participation rate among the elderly in rural and urban areas, the decline being steeper among males than females. The majority of elderly workers were engaged in agriculture. Modernization of agriculture in the future (which would require fewer workers than currently) accompanied by increases in the number of young adults seeking employment are factors likely to affect adversely future job opportunities for the elderly. Therefore, planning in respect of future employment opportunities for the elderly is needed urgently before this problem grows to unmanageable proportions.

Although the decline in labour force participation rates means fewer jobs in the future, it also means that the proportion of elderly people not working will increase in succeeding decades. About 72 per cent of the elderly population are not expected to be working in 2001; in absolute numbers, this portion of the population will total about 55 million, 69 per cent of whom will be from rural areas and 62.8 per cent of whom will be female. If the percentage retired in 1981 may be assumed to remain more or less the same as in 2001, then there will be about 4.5 million elderly males and 0.9 million elderly females retired from the organized sector. Although they may not be economically dependent, they would still likely depend to some degree on their children for proper care. The remaining 15.8 million elderly males and 33.4 million elderly females will be almost entirely dependent for their livelihood on their children, charitable institutions or the Government. This would result in increased responsibility for the productive population and diversification of limited resources to provide goods and services for this portion of the population.

Health Status

The elderly are more vulnerable to disease because of decreased physiological reserves and defence mechanisms. Data on morbidity collected in the National Sample Survey - 28th Round in 1973 revealed that 28.8 per cent of the elderly population in rural areas and 25.6 per cent of those in urban areas were ill at that time.

Also, more elderly males in rural and urban areas were ill compared with elderly females.

Table 3: Prevalence of temporary illness among the elderly, by place of residence and sex (per cent)

Place of residence	*Males*	*Females*	*All*
Rural	31.3	26.0	28.8
Urban	26.1	25.1	25.6

Table 4 : Prevalence of chronic diseases among the elderly, by place of residence and sex (per cent)

Place of residence	Males	Females	All
Rural	9.2	5.3	7.4
Urban	9.4	6.4	7.9

In addition, 7.4 per cent of the elderly population in rural areas and 7.9 per cent of those in urban areas were suffering from a chronic disease, the incidence being higher among males in rural and urban areas. With regard to the overall morbidity of the elderly population, 40.5 per cent of the males and 35.5 per cent of the females in rural areas and 31.4 per cent of the males and 3 1.5 per cent of the females in urban areas were either temporarily ill or suffering from chronic disease at the time of the Survey. If it is assumed that those rates will prevail more or less the same until the year 2000, the number of elderly people who would require medical assistance in 1991 and 2001 would be quite large.

According to this estimate, there would be around 27 million elderly people ill at any given point of time in 2001. Therefore, if the goal of "health for all by the year 2000" is to be achieved, this large section of India's population, who have health problems and requirements different from those of the general population, will have to be looked after.

Table 5 : Number of elderly (in millions) requiring medical assistance, by place of residence and sex

Place of residence	*1991*		*2001*	
	Males	*Females*	*Males*	*Females*
Rural	8.8	6.3	11.3	8.2
Urban	2.2	2.0	3.6	3.4
Total	11.0	8.3	14.9	11.6

Currently, elderly people avail themselves of general medical and health services; no concerted effort has been made to provide geriatric medical care. However, there is an urgent need for specialists catering for the elderly.

Besides an increased level of illness, the aging process leads to certain disabilities such as blindness resulting from cataracts and glaucoma, deafness resulting from nerve impairment, loss of mobility from arthritis and a general inability to care for one's self. The data collected in the National Sample Survey - 36th Round in 1981 concerning disabilities among the elderly reveal that 10.9 per cent of the elderly population suffered from physical impairments. Approximately half of those affected were visually disabled. The remaining half were suffering from disabilities related to hearing, speech or locomotor functions.

If it is assumed that this rate of physical disability in the elderly population will continue for the next 10 to 20 years, the number of aged persons in 2001 who will suffer from some type of disability, would be about 8.2 million, or twice the number in 1981. These people would be dependent either on their families or charitable institutions and in the absence of such support, they would look towards the Government for assistance.

Welfare Programmes

The problem of the elderly in India was not serious in the past because the numbers were small and the elderly were provided with social protection by the family network. But owing to relatively recent socioeconomic changes, aging of the population is emerging as a problem that requires consideration before it becomes critical. However, a few studies indicate that family and relatives still play an important role in providing economic and social security for the elderly. But most of these studies relate to the middle and higher socioeconomic classes where the elderly own the means of production and have sufficient economic resources not to be affected adversely. Those in the lower levels of the social strata, who constitute the majority, will need social and economic support.

The elderly who worked in the organized sectors during their careers have been and are covered by social insurance schemes such as pensions, gratuities, leave encashment and provident fund disbursements made upon their retirement. Such systems have been in use since 1871. They cover approximately 11 per cent the population, who are likely to be economically better off compared with those who worked in the unorganized sectors; the latter constitute around 89 per cent of the elderly population. Since most worked in the unorganized sectors, the vast majority of the elderly probably worked for low wages and thus have little or no savings to enable them to meet their old-age needs.

Old age pensions have been introduced by State Governments mostly for the destitute and infirm. For example, the Government of Uttar Pradesh in 1957 became the tirst to introduce an old age pension scheme. Since then, similar schemes have been introduced by other State Governments. Such pension schemes were in operation in 16 out of 22 major States prior to 1980; all States and Union Territories, except Arunchal Pradesh, are currently providing such pensions.

India's demographic contours suggest a steep rise in the elderly population in the coming decades as a result of declining fertility, increasing expectation of life at birth and (partly) at later ages. Although the proportion of the elderly population in 2001 may be low, India will rank second in the world in absolute numbers. There will be about 75.9 million elderly people in India at that time; one out of every twelve persons will be aged 60 years or more in 2001. This phenomenon, coupled with rapid social changes resulting in the gradual breakdown of the traditional joint family system and ever-increasing financial constraints at the national level, is likely to pose serious problems for the elderly.

Two-thirds of the elderly males and 90-95 per cent of the elderly females are illiterate and a large number of them, particularly females, are single. Thus, the level of economic dependency is quite high. It has been estimated that about 18 million elderly males and 3.5 million elderly females would need jobs in 2001. These figures are based on the proportion currently working. This means that a huge amount of resources would be needed in order to create jobs for them in the future. Moreover, finances will also be required to maintain the 55 million not working, the majority of whom probably will not have adequate savings nor family assistance.

It has also been estimated that about 27 million elderly people would be ill at any given point of time in the year 2001 and thus need specialized medical care. In the absence of such medical facilities, large expenditures on infrastructure would be required to meet their needs. The occurrence of physical disabilities is another important aspect of the aging process. There will be about 17 million disabled elderly persons in India in 2001, half of whom are likely to be visually disabled. The great majority of these would not be able to work and thus would be economically dependent. In the absence of family support, they would expect help from the Government. However, the Government has no old age pension scheme nor has any provision been made for granting aid to the State Governments for this purpose. Although State Governments and Union Territories have initiated schemes to provide some financial assistance to the handicapped or the destitute, the amount of such pensions ranges from only Rs. 30 to 60 per month. Moreover, owing to the paucity of funds available, the pensions cover only a fraction of the persons eligible.

Among the positive factors which have been sustaining the elderly in India is the strong attachment of family members to the elderly. Social pressure continues to be placed on persons who fail to discharge this responsibility to their elderly family members. Thus it is important to strengthen these values and the capacity of families to cope with the problems of caring for the elderly. The elderly should be considered as human resources and their rich experience and residual capacities should be put to optimum use for the benefit of national development. Their ability to lead healthy and fruitful lives should be ensured by the Government.

Bibliography

Antia N. H., "Voluntary organizations and health care in India", *Foundation for Research in Community Health.*

Bajaj J.S et al., "Report of the Expert Committee on Public Health System", New Delhi: Government of India, *Ministry of Health & Family Welfare*, 1996.

Baru R.V., "Private health care in India: Social characteristics and trends", New Delhi: Sage Publications,1998.

Bennett S, Muraleedharan V.R., "New Public Management and Health Care in Third World", *Economic and Political Weekly*, January 8, 59-68, 2000.

Berman P, Khan M.E, eds., "Paying for India's Health Care", New Delhi: Sage Publications, 1993.

Berman P., "Health care expenditure in India", In M Das Gupta ed. Health, Poverty and Development in India, New Delhi Oxford University Press, pp 331-58,1996.

Berman, ed., "Health Sector Reform in Developing Countries", Boston: Harvard School of Public Health,1996.

Bhat P.N., et al. "Maternal Mortality in India: Estimates from Regression Model. Studies in Family Planning", 26; 4: 217-232, 1995.

Cassels A., "Health sector reform: key issues in less developed countries", *Journal of International Health Development*, 7(3): 329-349, 1995.

Chand S.K., "The Traditional Herbal Medicine System of

Chotanagpur: A study of its present status & future prospects", Ranchi: Xavier Institute of Social Service. Mimeo, 1988.

Claeson M, Bos E.R, Pathamanathan I., "Reducing Child Mortality in India: Keeping Up the Pace", *Health, Nutrition, Population Series*, 1999.

Dreze J and Sen A., "India: Economic Development and Social Opportunity", New Delhi: Oxford University Press,1995.

Duggal R., "Health Care Budgets in a Changing Political Economy", *Economic and Political Weekly*, May 17-24, 1197-1200, 1997.

Kannan K.P, Thankappan K.R, Kutty, V.R Aravindan, K.P., "Health and Development in Rural Kerala", *Kerala Sastra Sahithya Parishad*, Trivandrum, 1991.

Mathiyazhagan K., "Willingness to Pay for Rural Health Insurance Through Community Participation in India", *International Journal of Health Planning and Management*, 13: 47-67, 1998.

Ministry of Health and Family Welfare, "Bulletin on Rural Health Statistics in India", New Delhi: Rural Health Division, *Ministry of Health and Family Welfare*, 2000.

Nandraj S, Duggal R., "Physical standards in the private health sector", *Radical Journal of Health* 2(2/3):141-84, 1996.

Index

CHANGING TRENDS IN HEALTH AND NUTRITION

CHANGING TRENDS IN HEALTH AND NUTRITION

(In 4 Volumes)

Food and Nutrition Security: Urban Challenges

(Volume 3)

SUJATA K. DASS

ISHA BOOKS
DELHI—110 033

Changing Trends in Health and Nutrition
(Health)

Rs. 3200 (Set in 4 vols.)
Rs. 800 (Each volume)

ISBN: 81-8205-040-5 (Set)
ISBN: 81-8205-043-X (Vol. 3)

Published in 2004 in India by
Isha Books, D-43, Prithviraj Road
Adarsh Nagar, Delhi-110 033

Lasertypesetting by: Varsha Graphics, Delhi
Printed at: Chawla Offset Press, Delhi

Contents

Preface

The population explosion that characterized much of the 20th century is being replaced by another dramatic demographic transformation: urban population growth of an unprecedented scale. As urban expansion continues apace, the overall cost of supplying, distributing, and accessing food is likely to increase further and, with it, the number of urban households that are food insecure.

The challenge of feeding cities lies in facilitating consumer access to food and ensuring that required investments are forthcoming for increasing food production, processing, and distribution capacities and services under hygienic, healthy, and environmentally sound conditions. Adequately meeting this challenge will promote the development of peri-urban and rural areas. To feed ever-growing cities, more food will have to be imported or produced in areas presently under cultivation or on new lands.

Urban expansion and issues of food supply and distribution to and in the cities have four major consequences for urban food security. The first is the competition between demands for land needed for housing, industry, and infrastructure and land needed for agricultural production within and around cities. The second consequence is the increasing quantities of food that must be brought into cities and distributed within the expanding urban areas. The third consequence is the modification of consumption habits and food purchasing behaviours. The final consequence for urban food security is the likelihood that low-income urban households will reside farther and farther away from food markets, often in slums that do not have water, roads, or electricity.

This book explores the urban face of food and nutrition security. It will provide policy-makers, program administrators, and development practitioners a better grasp of the most important factors to consider when designing urban food and nutrition programs and policies.

Editor

1

Dimensions of Food Security

Food security is a concept that has evolved considerably over time. There are approximately 200 definitions and 450 indicators of food security. One of the most commonly accepted definitions of food security is adequate access to food at all times, throughout the year and from year to year. Access is ensured when all households and all individuals within those households have sufficient resources to obtain appropriate foods for a nutritious diet. It is dependent on the level of household resources-capital, labour, and knowledge-and on prices. Note that adequate access can be achieved without households being self-sufficient in food production more important is the ability of households to generate sufficient income which, together with own production, can be used to meet food needs.

Moving from household to individual food security requires consideration of two factors. First, how is food allocated within the household? In households where distribution is unequal, it is possible for aggregate access to improve and for some individuals to experience no change in their food security status.

A second consideration is biological utilization; the ability of the human body to take food and translate it into either energy that is used to undertake daily activities or is stored. Utilization requires not only an adequate diet, but also a healthy physical environment (so as to avoid disease) and an understanding of proper health care, food preparation, and storage processes.

The concept of food security also has spatial and temporal dimensions.

The spatial dimension refers to the degree of aggregation at which food security is being considered. It is possible to analyze food security at the global, continental, national, sub-national, village, household, or individual level.

The temporal dimension refers to the time frame over which food security is being considered. In much of the food security literature, a distinction is drawn between chronic food insecurity—the inability to meet food needs on an ongoing basis—and transitory food insecurity when the inability to meet food needs is of a temporary nature.

Transitory food insecurity is sometimes divided into two subcategories: cyclical (where there is a regular pattern to food insecurity, for example, the lean season that occurs in the period just before harvest); and temporary (which is the result of a short-term, exogenous shock such as droughts or floods). It is worth noting that because the academic literature addresses food security and differently spatial and temporal levels, the concept of food security can become confusing at times. For the purposes of operationalizing it at the level, a helpful first step is to limit these dimensions.

The physical environment plays a large role in determining the type of activities that can be undertaken by rural households. Government policies toward the agricultural sector will have a strong effect on the design and implementation of household food security interventions. For example, a pricing policy that is hostile toward agriculture will discourage production. Interventions that proceed obliviously to this fact are unlikely to succeed.

The presence of social conflict, expressed in terms of mistrust of other social groups or even outright violence, is also an important factor in the design and implementation of interventions. In such circumstances, maximizing beneficiary participation becomes especially problematic. For example, wealthier groups may take control of their own benefit, to the exclusion of poorer members. Alternatively, social conflict may encourage groups excluded from an intervention to take active steps to subvert it. A certain degree of social cohesion is necessary if group activities, such as group-based microcredit schemes or collective work on an infrastructure, are to succeed.

The resources, or endowments, of households can be divided into two broad categories: labor and capital. Labor refers to the availability of labor for production. It incorporates not only a physical dimension of how many people are there available to work but also a 'knowledge' or human capital dimension. For an agricultural household, this knowledge includes formal schooling, formal training in agricultural production, and also the informal knowledge obtained via trial and error, past farming experiences, discussions with friends and relatives, observations made about practices on neighbors' farms, and so on. Capital refers to those resources such as land, tools for agricultural and nonagricultural production, livestock, and financial resources that, when combined with labor produce income.

Households allocate these endowments across different activities such as food production, cash crop production, and nonagricultural income-generating activities (such as wage labor, handicrafts, food processing, services, etc.) in response to the returns each activity generates. In addition, households may receive transfer income from other households or from some public body such as the State or an non-governmental organization (NGO). Together, these four sources determine household income.

Households face a set of prices that determines what level of consumption can be supported by this level of income. Consumption is divided between those goods that effect household and individual food security and all other goods. Those goods that will affect food security include food consumption, or acquisition, at the household level, referred to as food access in much of the food security literature-goods directly related to health care (e.g., medicines), and goods that affect the health environment, such as shelter, sanitation, and water. These three goods, together with knowledge and practice of good nutritional and health practices-called 'care behaviors'-and the public health environment (for example, the available of publicly provided potable water), affect illness and individual food intake, which, in turn, generates nutritional status or food utilization. Stars are placed beside the household food acquisition, food intake, and food utilization boxes to emphasize that these are food security and nutrition outcomes.

Food security is not static over time. Suppose that a development agency funds that improves the provision of agricultural extension. This can be thought of as increases the human capital of the household. In turn, this raises income. Some of this income might be used to acquire additional capital stock such as agricultural implements. In turn, this raises household income in subsequent years. Allocations of food, expenditures on education, and health will affect the level and distribution of human capital within the household. These investments will also affect the household's ability to generate income in subsequent years. In other words, a well-designed intervention has the potential to set in train a virtuous circle of development whereby increased income generates greater wealth that, in turn, generates higher levels of income, consumption, food security, and nutrition. But it is also worth noting that not all these feedback effects are benign. Increased income generation may induce an offsetting reduction in private transfers received from other households, a phenomenon known as "crowding out". It is now possible to uncover the links between development and household or individual food security.

There is a series of interventions designed to improve the broader environments that affect household food security. Examples of these include field operations such as the soil, water and forest management (environment); providing an appropriate institutional environment for private agriculture (policy); and strengthening small farmers' associations (social).

There are interventions that increase the level and returns to capital. The rehabilitation of irrigation facilities, the provision of credit, and the development of new technologies are examples of this. There are interventions that increase the stock of knowledge or human capital. Examples of programmes that incorporate these include provision of extension services, rural development, that aim to provide skills training to young rural men and women, and literacy training. There are interventions that improve rural infrastructures, most notably roads. These affect household food security in two ways: by increasing the returns to undertaking activities via reducing transport costs and by reducing the costs of obtaining food and other goods for consumption.

It is worth noting that many development interventions fall into first three interventions that improve the broad environment in which households exist, or those aimed at raising levels of human or physical capital. These do not directly affect food security outcomes. Instead, they raise incomes. The links between income and these outcomes, however, are weak, and these weaknesses stem from several factors. In the case of nutritional status or food utilization, food is not the only input.

Increased food access will not necessarily improve food utilization where other factors, such as the health environment, are not favorable. A second cause is ignorance. Households and individuals may simply not be aware of all the components of a healthy diet or of good health practices. These considerations imply a complementary approach between "traditional" development activities and complementary health and nutrition interventions. The third reason for these weak links is that households, and individuals, face many competing demands for their limited financial resources. They may want to increase the level or quality of their food consumption, but they may also want to reduce labor drudgery, be better dressed, be able to send their children to school, and so on. In those programmes where there is to be an emphasis placed on beneficiary participation, it might very well be the case that beneficiaries choose interventions that have their largest impact on an outcome other than food security or nutrition.

The means by which development interventions improve nutritional outcomes can be operationalized is still evolving. It has been recognized that many programmes are constrained in their ability to optimize their impact on nutritional by a limited knowledge base. In particular, it is not clear whether the constraining factor to improved nutrition is poor access to food, weakness in the provision of health care, poor access to child care, the general health environment, or is some combination of these.

Rapid and participatory appraisal methods (PRA) techniques are "a family of approaches and methods to enable rural people to share, enhance, and analyze their knowledge of life and conditions, to plan and to act". These include mapping activities, transect walks, seasonal calendars, wealth ranking, and analytical "diagramming." Unlike traditional, more extractive data gathering methods, PRA techniques are premised on the notion that local people have an enormous amount of local knowledge. Rather than merely appropriating this information, in PRA local people dominate the agenda, decide how to express and analyze information, to plan and to evaluate. Outsiders are facilitators. They help establish rapport, and help in the use of methods.

Advantages are that these techniques are low cost, provide information quickly, require little equipment, and by deliberately seeking local opinions, provide insights that might be missed by more conventional methods. Disadvantages are that they require highly skilled personnel and are not suitable for targeting purposes. Six PRA methods are outlined: concept definition, community mapping, household food security ratings, seasonal time lines, conceptual mapping of threats to food security, and the evaluation of interventions.

Measurement is necessary to characterize the severity of the food security problem and to provide a basis for measuring the impact of development interventions at the household and individual levels.

Nutritional Dimensions of Food Security

Nutritional assessments are measurements of body size, body composition, or body function, intended to diagnose single or multiple nutrient deficiencies. Sometimes nutritional assessments consist of highly controlled technical measurements, while in other circumstances, they may be conducted in a participatory manner, fostering the processes of community involvement and ownership as a whole. Findings may be interpreted at the level of the individual, but are commonly aggregated over a community, district, or subnational region. It is clear that the link between Household Food Security and Nutrition Security is a complex one, making the naive use of nutritional measures by those seeking to draw inferences about food availability dangerous.

On the other hand, it is unquestionably the case that all nutritional measures are sensitive to changes in dietary intake. Furthermore, the supposed weakness of these measures-their multicausality-is also their strength, since those agricultural projects working together with outside institutions to incorporate health and education components into their activities find themselves armed with a uniquely direct means of assessing the gains in human welfare arising from the synergistic effects of different interventions.

There are numerous different measures of nutritional status, varying with respect to their ease of measurement, relation to dietary intake, and velocity of change following shocks or improvements in the individual's environment. Three major classes of measures may be distinguished. The first class uses clinical examinations to detect signs and symptoms of advanced nutritional depletion. Examples are surveys of goitre to detect iodine deficiency, or eye examinations to detect vitamin A deficiency. With appropriate training, lay enquirers can be used to determine levels of these conditions in the community. In contrast, laboratory methods are usually invasive (involve taking samples from sites of the body that are not immediately accessible) and therefore poorly suited to routine use in a program situation. These methods are used to detect decreased levels of nutrients in body tissues or fluids, or decreased activity of an enzyme that is nutrient-dependent. One example of a 'laboratory' method with potential for more general use is the detection of anemia by hemoglobinometry.

The third class of measurements, which will focus on in this document, is anthropometry, the measurement of body size and gross body composition. The basic principle of anthropometry is that prolonged or severe nutrient depletion eventually leads to retardation of linear (skeletal) growth in children, and to loss of, or failure to accumulate, muscle mass and fat in both children and adults. These problems can be detected by measuring body dimensions, such as standing height or upper-arm circumference, or total body mass (weight). All of these measures are expected to vary by the age of the person measured and by their sex, so that there is a need for the measurements to be standardized for age and sex before they can be interpreted. Easy-to-use computer applications are available to perform this transformation.

In particular, when children do not receive the nutrients they need, their growth is rapidly compromised, with long-term implications for their future productivity. On the other hand, although adults also lose weight in response to severe energy deficit, this effect can be very difficult to distinguish from their genetic potential. Anthropometric measurements are subject to a number of sources of error, including instrument error, investigator error, and recall error (for measures based on age). These sources of error need to be controlled, since they can easily lead to overestimates of the frequency of malnutrition, or underestimates of the effectiveness of interventions. Special standardization procedures have been developed to minimize measurement error.

Nutritional Assessment

How nutritional assessment methods may be used to improve project formulation, beneficiary targeting, monitoring, and evaluation. Many of the approaches proposed take advantage of the increase in the availability of nutritional data that has occurred since 1990.

Extant data on nutritional status may be especially valuable at the country strategy and project inception stages, both for targeting subnational regions and for needs assessment. Where nutrition security is a priority, the identification of areas of the country most at need of rural development interventions is facilitated by reference to existing sources of nutrition data. The principal nutritional indicator for targeting subnational regions is proportion (absolute numbers) of children under, or of school age (6-10 years), with low height-for-age (stunted). This indicator, more than any other, is recommended for identifying areas of greatest need for targeting economic and health interventions. Weight-based measures are, in general, too sensitive to illness and specific child-care practices, and are subject to seasonal variations. Data on stunting are available at the subnational level for virtually all poor countries, from surveys and/or from school height censuses.

The usefulness of the measure programme for targeting can be enhanced by expressing the numbers on a per kilometer squared basis. Regions/communities with large numbers of children characterized by low height-for-age are found in each of Asia, Africa, and Latin America and the Caribbean, though the condition is most common in South Asia. In Latin America and the Caribbean, the prevalence of low weight-for-age (underweight) can be used as a proxy measure for low height-for-age (stunting), since the two indicators are highly correlated in this region where low weight-for-height (wasting) is not seen. Another measure that may be of use in contexts of extreme poverty is proportion (absolute numbers) of adults and adolescents with low body mass index. This indicator identifies areas of severe food insecurity. Data are sometimes available at the subnational level from surveys. The usefulness of the measure for project targeting can be enhanced by expressing the numbers on a per kilometer squared basis. Caution should be exercised when using this measure in areas where advanced HIV disease is prevalent, since individuals with HIV disease are thin, but not as a result of food insecurity. Regions/communities with large numbers of adults/adolescents characterised by low body mass index are found in Asia and Africa. Small mid-upper arm circumference is sometimes used as a proxy measure for low body mass. It should be noted that the presence of significant numbers of adults with very low body mass index normally indicates a need for emergency relief, rather than rehabilitation or development.

Nutritional measures can be reviewed to assess the needs of beneficiaries. Normally this process is carried out for the area as a whole, but where possible, it is informative to disaggregate by variables known a priori to be linked to nutrition security, such as land ownership, gender of household head, sanitary/health care resources, etc.

The needs assessment process should start by collating nutritional data from as many different population-based sources as possible. The information should be arranged by indicator, age group studied, and year of collection.Conflicting evidence from different sources should be carefully reviewed with the help of local experts to identify the source of the discrepancy. Subsequently, it may be helpful to rank the different problems identified according to their frequency in the population. It is useful to compare the same indicator across different age/sex groups. For example, stunting in children where adults are also short may be more suggestive of intergenerational deprivation effects than of current food access or health problems; similarly, while wasting in children may indicate poor feeding practices or health problems, the combination of wasting in children and low body mass in adults indicates a crisis in entitlements to food.

Specific nutrient deficiencies are not uncommon in children due to poor feeding practices; however, when they are also found in adults, a problem of food access should be suspected. It is also important to contrast different indicators: substantial childhood wasting in the absence of stunting, for example, indicates a nutritional crisis of very recent advent; stunting in the absence of wasting, on the other hand, indicates a complex and deep-rooted nutritional problem, sometimes not directly related to food availability at the household level. Similarly, specific nutrient deficiencies in the absence of stunting or wasting may indicate either poor feeding practices or a general problem of dietary quality, while combined with stunting and/or wasting, they are more likely to indicate profound poverty of resources at many levels.

Table 1
Nutritional indicators for needs assessment exercises

Indicator	*Interpretation*
Prevalence of low height-for-age (stunting) in preschool or school-age children	Children's skeletal *(linear)* growth compromised due to constraints to one or more of nutrition, health, or mother-infant interactions. In some populations, these constraints are already apparent in utero.

Prevalence of low weight-for-height (wasting) in preschool or school-age children	Quality of diet a more frequent limitation than inadequate quantity.
Prevalence of low weight-for-age (underweight) in preschool or school-age children	Children suffer *thinness* resulting from energy deficit and/or disease-induced poor appetite, mala-bsorption, or loss of nutrients. Energy deficit may be due to lack of food in household or feeding of low energy density foods that satiate before the child meets its energy require-ments.
Prevalence of low body mass index in adults or adolescents	This indicator confuses the two processes described above and is therefore not a good indicator for needs assessment purposes.
Prevalence of low mid-upper arm circumference in adults/ adolescents	Adults suffer *thinness* as a result of inadequate energy intake, an uncompensated increase in physical activity, or (severe) illness.
Prevalence of low serum retinol in preschool children.	As above. Restricting analysis to the arm has the advantage of reflecting the mass of just three tissues—bone, muscle, and fat—the last two of which are particularly sensitive to body weight gain/loss.
Prevalence of low hemoglobin (anemia) in preschool or school-age children	Children suffer vitamin A deficiency, either as a result of low intake of vitamin A in the diet, or because there is a high frequency of infection, leading to sequestering of vitamin A from the blood.

Prevalence of low hemoglobin (anemia) in nonlactating, nonpregnant women	Children suffer from anemia, either as a result of low iron intakes or poor absorption, or as a result of illness. Severe protein-energy malnutrition and vitamin B12/folate deficiency can also lead to anemia.
Prevalence of low hemoglobin (anemia) in men	Women suffer from anemia as a result of low iron intakes, poor absorption, illness, or excessive losses of blood. Severe protein-energy malnutrition and vitamin B12/folate deficiency can also lead to anemia.

Just as nutrition data can assist with targeting and needs assessment at the project formulation stage, so they can also be of assistance for small-area targeting and sequencing of interventions in the implementation phase.

The potential of small-area targeting has been discussed elsewhere. This procedure is greatly facilitated when nutritional data are available at a fine level of disaggregation, permitting the identification of priority-need small areas (usually districts or municipalities) within the overall area of influence of the project. School height censuses are an obvious source of such data, but detailed nutritional surveys are also occasionally available.

Where these data are not available, conducting a large-scale nutritional survey for the purpose of small-area targeting is likely to be very cost-ineffective; other indicators should therefore be used. Only in exceptional circumstances are nutritional data available at a level of disaggregation sufficiently fine to permit community-level targeting. Often, however, socioeconomic data can be collected that permit the estimation of the expected rate of malnutrition in the community.

For a number of reasons, it is unwise to use nutritional measures for household-level targeting in rural development programmes. These reasons include the following:

— Most nutritional measures are age-sensitive, so that a two-year-old child is much more likely to be stunted than a one-year-old, even though the conditions of the household are identical.

— Some measures of nutritional status change in a relatively short time, so that a child who has just been ill can easily be wasted even where the household's conditions are generally good.

— Many other measures reflect past conditions, or even inter-generational effects, more strongly than current conditions.

— The cut-offs used to determine the presence or absence of malnutrition are arbitrary, so that a child with a height-for-age Z-score of -2.1 is classified as stunted while one with a Z-score of -2.0 is not, even though there is little reason to include the first family in a development program and not the second.

— Finally, there have been instances where families in areas with programmes using individual targeting-based nutritional status have actually withheld food from children so that their nutritional status will deteriorate and the family will be entitled to participate in the programmes.

The search for interventions should be guided by an analysis of the constraints to nutrition security in each of its contributing areas: household food security, health, and mother-infant interaction. As nutritional indicators represent the joint outcome of all of these factors, there is only a limited amount of information that they can provide on the causes of, and solutions to, nutrition insecurity.

Monitoring and Evaluation

Nutritional assessment can be an extremely valuable element of the monitoring and evaluation process in rural development programmes for a number of different reasons:

— Nutritional measurements provide a measure of human welfare that is sensitive to changes in food supply, as well as to other community development processes.

— Nutritional measurements provide a nonsubjective, quantitative assessment of progress towards a fixed goal (the elimination of malnutrition).

— Nutritional measurements cannot easily be falsified by individuals with vested interests in the outcome of the interventions (including the subjects themselves).

— Nutritional measurements are relatively easy to obtain, either in sentinel sites for the purpose of ongoing monitoring, or in a sample of the entire study area for the purpose of evaluation.

In order to assess whether programme interventions have improved nutrition security among beneficiaries, it is first necessary to identify which nutritional indicators could plausibly have been altered by project interventions, and which subgroups of the population are most likely to have benefitted. For example, its sole aim the promotion of home gardening should not be expected to produce an impact on adult BMI, since vegetables are, in general, rich in micronutrients but not in energy. Similarly, a programme aimed at increasing basic grain production in rural Africa is unlikely to affect the nutritional status of infants less than six months of age, since these infants usually consume only breast milk and are therefore unaffected by changes in the family diet.

The length of time that an intervention has been in place is also an important variable to take into account when selecting nutrition indicators and study populations, since different indicators reflect events in the recent and distant past with different intensities, and take different amounts of time to respond to such changes. There any many different ways of using nutritional assessment to determine whether project interventions are improving, or have improved, the nutrition security of the beneficiary population.

The most important element of a successful monitoring system is a mechanism for ensuring that the data are promptly collated and analyzed so that they can feed into decisionmaking processes without delay. Nutritional indicators should be selected on the basis of the simplicity of measurement: weight-for-age would be the indicator of choice in many communities, although mid-upper arm circumference may be as good or better in communities where acute or seasonal food shortages are known to occur and to result in fluctuations in body mass.

The analysis of the data should focus on obtaining moving averages that reflect important changes in nutritional status without being excessively dominated by short-term 'blips'. It is likely to be necessary to control for the effect of the aging of the study cohort over time, as this leads to apparent improvements in nutritional status that are-sadly-illusory. Samples of approximately 100 individuals are likely to be sufficient for the monitoring of trends over time, with measurements perhaps every two or three months.

One popular way of determining the impact of project activities on nutrition security is to conduct one survey prior to implementation and another at the end of the evaluation period, examining changes in the nutritional profile of the population over the two points in time. This type of evaluation is credible if it can be demonstrated that the population surveyed is the same at each period in time (e.g., a representative sample of all adult women in the project zone of influence). It is not necessary for the individuals in the survey to be the same; indeed, often it is unavoidable that the individuals are different, such as when the nutritional status of children under five is measured before and after a five-year development.

The comparison may be strongly influenced by factors specific to the timing of the two surveys. This is particularly the case when nutritional measures are used that are sensitive to short- or medium-term fluctuations in intake (e.g., serum vitamin A). It is less of a problem when using measures such as height-for-age Z-scores, which reflect cumulative influences over a substantial period of time. When the beneficiary population alone is studied, the evaluation can determine whether the observed changes in nutritional status are of the expected direction and magnitude, but is unable to causally link program activities to observed changes. When a 'control' group is also measured at the same time points as the intervention group, it is possible to infer whether changes in nutritional status appear to be more beneficial in the intervention group than in the control group.

The before-after comparison is usually expressed as the change in mean values of the nutritional indicator, but can also be expressed as the relative (or absolute) change in the proportion of the population with values below some critical measure. The latter comparison may be more relevant from a human welfare perspective, but requires larger sample sizes than the comparison of means approach. One factor specific to studies with nutritional status as outcomes is that the interpretation of the results will be strongly influenced by the age composition of the study population. If the age composition has changed between initial and final surveys, or if the intervention group has a different age structure to the control group, be it ever so slight, this MUST be taken into account in the analysis. Since adjusting for age effects requires some knowledge of statistical methods, the utmost care should be taken to ensure comparability of the initial and final samples.

In some situations, it is possible to track individuals over time and to examine associations between programme activities and changes in nutritional status at the individual level. This approach to measuring project impact is expected to be far more sensitive than the approach outlined above. An individual's final height minus initial height is referred to as gain in height, while their final weight minus initial weight is referred to as weight gain. Since the amount of gain in height and/or weight is dependent on the time elapsed between the two measures, it may be appropriate to express these measures as gain per unit time, usually referred to as height or weight velocity. It is very important to realize that height and weight velocity are both sex- (and especially) age-dependent, so that analysis must take account of different age structures of intervention and control groups.

One other complication that should also be borne in mind is that many individuals will not be able to be traced at the time of the second survey. Since these individuals are always different from those who remain traceable, the picture of project impact obtained may be unrepresentative. It is not a good idea to calculate an individual's change in Z-score from one time period to another, since, for example, a half Z-score deterioration in nutritional status in an infant can have very different physiological implications from a half Z-score deterioration in an older child.

In the absence of data on nutritional status prior to intervention, it is possible to directly compare the attained nutritional status of children of project beneficiaries with the attained nutritional status of children of nonbeneficiaries. In order to be able to interpret the results of such a comparison, it is necessary either to assume that beneficiaries and nonbeneficiaries were comparable prior to the project intervention, or else to adjust statistically for variables known to affect beneficiary status. If all concerns about using these methods are satisfied, beneficiaries may be compared to nonbeneficiaries either with respect to average (mean) nutritional status, or with respect to the proportions falling below a critical cut-off point. If this method is used, it is particularly important to select an indicator that can reasonably be expected to be sensitive to dietary intake and changes in the household environment over the period of evaluation.

Some degree of internal control may be obtained by comparing the experience of a subgroup of the population who can be expected to have been responsive to the project interventions to that of a subgroup who would not be expected to have responded to the particular kind of interventions implemented, or within the time frame under consideration.

2

Household Food and Nutrition Security

Households are considered food secure when they have year-round access to the amount and variety of safe foods their members need to lead active and healthy lives. Thus, household food security has three key dimensions, the availability of food, access to food, and utilization of food. Household food security should be recognised as a dynamic and relative state for many households and assessed accordingly. For example, food insecure households may either lack access to nutritionally adequate food supplies or be at risk of losing such access. Vulnerability increases when households have to cope with recurrent shocks, forcing them to sell their assets, thus reducing their coping capacity and progressively leading them to destitution.

Good nutrition is an outcome of household food security, appropriate caring practices, including infant and child feeding practices, and access to health care and proper environmental health. Food insecurity and poor nutritional status are highly correlated with poverty and social inequity. Efforts to secure adequate food are central to the livelihood strategies of poor households. Household food security is a complex phenomenon attributable to a range of factors that vary in importance across regions, countries and social groups, as well as over time. These factors include among other things are given below:

— annual and seasonal food availability (including own production) and prices; household income (levels and flows); household expenditures at different times of the year; consumer preferences, perceptions and behaviours; household size, labour demands, social discrimination, and gender and age bias

— access to resources such as land, water, employment opportunities; access to improved technologies to enhance productivity; existence of institutional and physical infrastructure as well as overall macro economic environment and good governance

— adequate utilization of food requires ingesting enough of the right kinds of foods to meet nutritional requirements, including those requirements that are elevated by physical growth, parasitic infections, illness, high workload, pregnancy and lactation.

Secure access to food is an essential condition for nutritional well-being, but is not sufficient in itself. Households without enough food (in terms of both quantity and variety) cannot be well nourished. However, households that can access the food they need, can still present cases of malnutrition due to inappropriate allocation of resources, inadequate care and feeding practices (in particular for small children) or poor health. Poor nutrition is both a symptom and a cause of poverty. It reduces the ability of the poor to maximise the benefit of their main assets, their mental capacity and their potential for physical labour. When their members suffer from poor nutrition, food insecure households have limited access to development opportunities, and little time or energy to invest in acquiring skills which could improve their long-term prospects.

The prevalence of food insecure households is usually higher in marginalised areas where a variety of constraints contributes to vulnerability: environmentally fragile ecosystems, low productivity, geographical isolation, and limited access to health or education services. Hardship and lack of economic opportunities increasingly lead individuals and families to migrate on a temporary or permanent basis, altering existing social and family structures and often decreasing the capacity of families and communities to care for themselves. Crisis situations (due to natural disasters, conflicts, severe economic crisis or major epidemics such as HIV/AIDS) usually exacerbate the vulnerability of food insecure households and/or plunge vulnerable households into food insecurity and destitution.

Food insecure households can, however, be found in all areas. Households or population groups can be marginalised from the local socio-economic development process due to insufficient access to assets (e.g. land, income) or information, social services and low social status (linked to ethnicity, caste, religious or political reasons, immigrant status, disease).

Urban food insecurity has become an increasing problem in many countries as the purchasing power of poor or impoverished households does not allow them to cover their basic needs. The vulnerability of food insecure households in urban areas is closely linked to access to employment opportunities and food prices. Household food security is necessary to ensure that all members of a household have an appropriate dietary intake. It is particularly important that women of childbearing age and small children cover their nutritional needs. To a large extent, feeding practices are determined by indigenous knowledge and the allocation of tasks, responsibilities and resources within the household, in which gender often plays a major role.

In many cases people lack the required information, do not give sufficient priority to this matter or face constraints-especially in terms of time—resulting in chronic malnutrition. Poor households must make difficult decisions regarding competing needs (food, housing, clothing, education, health care, transportation, investments, agricultural inputs, etc) in the short and mid-term, and achieving household food security is only one (even if it is often the main one) of their objectives.

In certain circumstances, they may actually choose to cut down on their food expenses or even go hungry to preserve their assets and protect future livelihoods. In many cases, poor households are compelled to sell their assets, jeopardising long term food security in order to ensure immediate food consumption needs.

The rural poor tend to be risk averse (e.g. reluctant or unable to adopt new production techniques) and avoid activities that bring no immediate benefit (e.g. soil conservation measures). This is particularly true of situations where people have no reliable access to land (e.g. for land tenure or security seasons). While household food security must remain central to poverty alleviation strategies, it should be considered within a sustainable livelihood approach.

Mechanisms that minimize risk or strengthen coping strategies are important aspects of improving food security in vulnerable settings. Nutrition and food security indicators provide comprehensive and accurate measures of human well-being at both individual and community levels.

Particular attention should be paid to indicators of the nutritional status of young children and women of reproductive age, as poor nutrition at these times of life have lasting effects. Indicators of childhood malnutrition (underweight and stunting) should be regularly used in poverty alleviation programmes, both as tools for targeting the most vulnerable and as measures of impact. Other locally appropriate indicators, such as micronutrient deficiencies and adult Body Mass Index (BMI), should be included where necessary.

Natural disasters and conflicts are increasingly common impediments to household food security and often cause widespread under-nutrition and micronutrient deficiencies. Emergencies manifest their effects through a number of different mechanisms, including problems with food production, storage, transport, and marketing; household food preparation and feeding practices; income generation, and various social networks. Existing livelihood systems and development activities are disrupted and most population groups in the areas concerned are affected directly or indirectly.

Household Food Insecurity and Poor Nutrition

The poor and food insecure may suffer more than other groups from macro-economic disequilibria such as high inflation or unrealistic exchange rates that discriminate against local labour and production. This is particularly true in rural areas as many such policies also specifically discriminate against the rural and agricultural sectors. High rates of food insecurity and under-nutrition are commonly found in low-income food deficit countries with limited or stagnant economic growth, inadequate food supplies, and an inability to import.

People who have little or no involvement or input in the development of local and national policies and resource allocation are often at great risk of poverty, food insecurity, and under-nutrition. Accordingly, the meaningful participation of local organisations and food insecure communities and households in the identification and implementation of food security strategies and coping mechanisms is essential if the primary causes of poverty, food insecurity and poor nutrition are to be addressed in a sustainable manner. Even more important is the creation of conditions in which such population groups can effectively participate in, guide and benefit equitably from social and economic development processes. Education, information, communication and access to opportunities are important for timely and informed decision-making.

Household food security and nutrition are also good entry points for community participation. Food insecure people are usually marginalised from development activities, as they often do not have the time, resources or interest to participate. Since access to food, care and health are daily problems, these topics are of immediate concern to poor communities and households. With the appropriate assistance, they may, therefore, be more likely to participate actively in finding appropriate solutions. Achieving the objectives of HFS and nutrition requires co-ordination among local institutions that can or should support food insecure groups.

Throughout much of the world, women play a central role in ensuring household food security. Women are the majority of the world's agricultural producers, with decisive roles in the management of fisheries, forestry and farming resources. In many places, women are responsible for providing most of the food required by their families, either by producing it, or by earning the income for its purchase. They are also almost universally responsible for household food processing, storage and preparation, and for feeding and caring for the family. Women's roles in household food security can vary significantly across social groups and cultures, even within relatively close geographic areas.

The low social status of women in many societies, as well as their multiple and time-consuming responsibilities, works against their full participation in the development process. Their status varies, however, according to their age and social position. Many women and certain age groups face constraints and attitudes that increase their daily workload and hinder their participation in decision-making and development activities. They may be constrained culturally or even legally from having equitable access to various resources and services, sometimes even to household food resources.

Despite their significant contributions to household food security, women tend to be invisible actors in development and often their work is not recorded in statistics or mentioned in official reports. As a result, their contribution is poorly understood and often underestimated. It is important to recognise that in most food insecure households, all members contribute in some way to productive and reproductive activities related to food and nutrition. Their roles vary by cultural norms, gender, age and livelihood systems. Children may not be able to attend school in order to fulfill tasks that are regarded as essential, undermining long-term prospects for improved food security. Efforts should be made to adapt training and education activities to fit with household and community requirements.

Improving Household Food Security

The International Conference on Nutrition in 1992 endorsed a three-tiered model for addressing problems of household food insecurity and under-nutrition. Broad-based action is required within three overlapping domains. At the national level, it is recognised that macro-economic, social and trade policies, as well as appropriate investments in infrastructure, social services and rural development, can have pronounced effects on the ability of poor households to acquire and utilise food effectively. Ensuring that policies, legislation and investments promote sustainable economic growth, equity and social justice is crucial for creating the conditions in which all population groups can meet their nutritional needs.

Understanding and monitoring the impact of macro-economic policy and development investments on poor and food insecure households is important for developing and implementing more effective policies and programmes. Such monitoring is also important for mitigating any unintended or unavoidable negative effects on specific population sub-groups. The second domain entails sector-specific policies and programmes. Given the multifaceted causes of household food insecurity and malnutrition, action in various sectors can have a pronounced impact on food and nutrition. Planners and policy-makers in Ministries of agriculture, health, education, water development, social welfare, and women's affairs can significantly affect household food security and nutrition by including nutrition objectives and considerations in their policies and programmes.

The key element is to ensure that the poor and malnourished benefit directly from the various sectoral programmes. The third domain consists of strong community-based action, as it is at this level that many of the above-mentioned sectoral interventions come together. To be effective much of the work needed must take place at the community level. Targeted and co-ordinated efforts focussing on improving household food security, fostering people's participation and empowering women and marginal groups are needed to address local food and nutrition problems.

Such community-based programmes may involve participatory appraisal and planning methods; expanding and diversifying food production and ensuring availability at the local market; improving food preservation and storage; improving water supplies; expanding and diversifying income generating activities; providing nutrition education and training; ensuring access to basic health care and care systems; supporting small animal husbandry; and strengthening local institutions.

A key dimension of community-based action is enabling households to maximize food security and nutrition with existing household resources while also striving to increase such resources. Experience has shown that some households can significantly improve child nutrition through improved feeding practices, hygiene, household budgeting and women's education.

In order to achieve this objective, it is important:

— to ensure peace, security and good governance

— to stabilise the economy, control inflation and reduce economic distortions

— to promote investment in food and agricultural development

— to promote rural and urban employment opportunities

— to promote efficient and equitable markets

— to facilitate expanded opportunities for regional co-operation and trade

— to analyse and monitor the impact of socio-economic policies, programmes and interventions on poverty, HFS and nutritional well-being

— to ensure that safety nets such as direct transfers are developed and targeted to the poorest and most vulnerable households

— to develop pro-poor legal and regulatory frameworks

Major policies should be systematically screened in terms of expected impact on the ability of poor households to acquire and utilise nutritionally adequate and safe foods. Accompanying interventions may have to be set up as and where needed to mitigate negative impacts that may not be avoidable.

It is important to promote actions that will strengthen the functioning of food markets, and stabilise food supplies at accessible prices. In general, it is agreed that poverty can best be attacked through market-based strategies that provide opportunities to trade goods and services competitively, and provide income and employment opportunities for the poor. Strategies that encourage the expansion and diversification of food systems, and that promote employment, small-scale industries and trade can be particularly effective.

In order to ensure that poor and food insecure households can take advantage of such opportunities and be able to purchase or produce nutritionally adequate foods, they must have or develop access to the following:

— literacy training, in particular for women

— basic health care and sanitation

— health and nutrition education

— resources such as land, water, agricultural inputs and income, improved technologies to enhance productivity

— appropriate training opportunities

— market infrastructure (transportation, storage and processing),market information and advice

— effective rural financial systems

— safety nets for marginalised and dependent people

Household food security and good nutrition are recognised as both outcomes of development and as important investments in equitable development. Healthy, well-nourished people are essential contributors to social and economic development. Realising the commitment to improve household food security and nutrition has wide-ranging benefits: children can grow and develop normally, cognitive abilities improve, and productivity increases.

Policies and programmes in various sectors or Ministries (agriculture, health, water development, social welfare, women's affairs, education, transportation, HIV/AIDS prevention, and migration) can have a significant impact on HFS and nutrition. This impact, which can be direct or indirect, can vary for different population groups and is usually a combination of positive and negative effects. Understanding what these effects are, or may be, in order for planners to strengthen the positive ones and mitigate the negative ones, is essential.

The development of sectoral interventions to address specific nutrition problems is also needed (e.g. promoting home gardens through the Ministry of Agriculture to combat micronutrient deficiencies, incorporating nutrition education into school curricula, promoting female education, etc.)

Community based programs that focus on household food security and nutrition practices are key. Specific attention should be given to improving conditions among food insecure groups and poor households in both rural and urban areas. Ensuring that women benefit equitably from policy and programme initiatives is particularly important.

Special attention should be paid to addressing the nutritional problems of pregnant and lactating women, and children as nutritional deficiencies in these groups can have profound and long-lasting effects. Improving food consumption of the poor and the nutritional status of women and children are key, objectively verifiable outcome measures that should be used to gauge the success of food security programmes.

At the policy level, action may be required to address negative social discrimination and gender bias. Women's education, which has proven to be a key element for reducing child malnutrition, is particularly important to any long-term strategy to promote good nutrition and food security.

The agriculture sector should play a key role in assisting poor people in rural areas. It is important that policies and programmes focus on diversifying and improving local food production and access (while exploring the feasibility of commercial crops), address issues of land tenure and access to common property resources, and promote the integration of women farmers and small-hold producers into commercial agriculture.

In most contexts, raising household incomes and advancing market-based approaches will provide a major contribution to the promotion of household food security. However, an over-emphasis on the promotion of cash crops can be detrimental to household food security if such promotion is undertaken without understanding the likely impact on household incomes and expenditures.

In some cases, the income generated through the sale of cash crops may either not be adequate or not be allocated towards purchasing the foods needed. Reallocation of time within the household may also lead to decreased caring capacity. It should be recognised that a large and growing part of the incomes of the poor are derived from off-farm income. Efforts to increase income-earning opportunities are essential to ensuring household food security and good nutrition.

To achieve maximum impact on household food security and nutrition, research needs to target food insecure communities, focusing on small resource-poor farmers and landless agricultural workers. Research should be directed at all stages of the food chain (e.g. diversification in agricultural production, improvement of post-harvest technologies with a view to facilitate consumption and marketing of safe foods).

Priority should be given to operational research, and communities should participate in the research and extension programmes, in order to build upon local strengths (including indigenous knowledge). Farmer-researcher-extension linkages are essential. Involvement of the private sector should be encouraged as long as the outcomes of the research contribute to improved food security for poor households.

Food resources that have often received limited attention in the past (such as root crops, tubers, millet, and sorghum) should be given higher priority, wherever they can provide a sustainable contribution to household food security or the resilience of livelihood systems. Crops traditionally grown by women are particularly important as they are usually intended for home-consumption.

Biotechnology could provide a useful contribution if geared towards the needs and constraints of poor farmers. Particular attention should be given to labour-saving technologies for women in production, processing, marketing and income generation. At the Community Level: developing participatory interventions to improve the livelihoods of food insecure households

While macro and sectoral approaches are essential to establish a coherent framework for sustainable development, there is a simultaneous need to provide direct assistance to food insecure communities and groups to enable them to benefit from the development process. Food insecure households should be the primary focus of community-based projects. Projects should ensure that poorer households are systematically involved in problem identification, action planning, implementation, monitoring and evaluation.

Community members and local organisations need to be involved in understanding the causes of food insecurity and nutrition problems, and why certain households are able to cope better than others within the same environment. On this basis, they will be able to develop appropriate activities and strategies to increase the self-reliance of vulnerable households. Projects should specifically address vulnerability issues to prevent marginal groups from slipping deeper into food insecurity. Minor deficits in rainfall, crop yields, pasture, land, access to natural resources or employment can cause shocks to vulnerable households, resulting in severe food insecurity. The poorest households can become increasingly sensitive to shocks and less able to return to pre-shock levels.

Women play a key role in household food security, care and health, therefore household food security and nutrition projects work primarily with women. Such projects are conducive to women's empowerment and welfare through the provision of information, education, training, organisation and resources.

Dimensions of HFS and nutrition

These different approaches should not be seen as mutually exclusive, but as a necessary combination in order to achieve a reduction in household food insecurity and poverty. Local strategies cannot be implemented in a sustainable way in isolation. They require an enabling context in terms of policies, institutions, infrastructure, and economic and social organisation. In order to support these different approaches, the following issues are particularly important:

— strengthening capacity of local organizations in assessment, planning and implementing household food security and nutrition activities where relevant

— facilitating feedback from local planning to the policy making level and back

— developing integrated Food Insecurity and Vulnerability Information and Mapping Systems (FIVIMS) to support planning, monitoring and evaluation

— developing and synchronising famine early warning systems and mitigation strategies

— strengthening national and regional capacities for programme/project development and backstopping

— enabling the poor and socially disadvantaged to participate in local decision making and governance

— creating appropriate financing mechanisms for local development initiatives

It should also be recognised that more affordable consumer prices and increased household incomes alone do not automatically translate into either household food security or better nutrition. Several factors need to be in place to ensure that increased household income contributes to household food security and nutrition. Local food supplies must be adequate to meet household/community demand, and households must have the time, knowledge and motivation to make best use of their limited resources to achieve the nutritional well-being of all household members. Nutrition education, delivered through appropriate mix of communication channels, can effectively empower households to improve nutrition.

Achieving household food security and nutritional well-being is at the heart of efforts to alleviate poverty and promote sustainable livelihoods. As such, household food security and nutritional well-being can serve as primary objectives of development, as a targeting device, as a guiding principle, as an integrating concept, and as a measure of impact. Accordingly, programmes and relevant components aimed at achieving household food security and better nutrition can provide real substance to poverty alleviation and sustainable livelihood initiatives.

The most fundamental issue is to make improvements in household food security and nutrition specific objectives of development and to work to mainstream these into virtually all aspects of development assistance where relevant.

— *Targeting:* Food insecurity and under-nutrition are highly correlated to poverty. Participatory poverty assessments can play a major role in the identification of suitable location-specific goals and indicators. Food consumption and anthropometric indicators constitute good proxies for food insecurity and human well-being. Global, national and local food and nutrition information systems (such as FIVIMS, Vulnerability Analysis and Mapping systems, and nutrition surveillance systems) must be supported by UN and bilateral donors to enable informed decision making. These should track changes in vulnerability to food insecurity, particularly in zones prone to recurrent natural disasters or conflict.

—*Designing strategies:* Ensuring household food security is at the core of poor households' livelihood strategies and the poorest people often have the most complex strategies. Understanding how poor households gain access to and utilise their food is important for designing effective and sustainable strategies and approaches to achieving food security and for determining how best to help them cope with their problems. Understanding how poor households ensure resilience against shocks is key to strengthening their livelihood strategies. Food insecure households must be systematically involved in identifying and testing solutions to their problems. Community participation is necessary in all stages of poverty alleviation programmes (problem identification, planning, implementation, monitoring and evaluation).

In order to design and implement effective poverty alleviation and sustainable livelihood initiatives, it is important to know which households are food insecure and assess how their constraints, opportunities and coping mechanisms vary over space and time. Adequate attention must be given to changes in individual food requirements at different points in the life cycle. Young children and women of reproductive age are often most at risk of food insecurity and malnutrition. Adolescents and the elderly can also represent vulnerable groups.

—*Monitoring and Evaluation Using appropriate indicators:* Anthropometric, food consumption, and income indicators should regularly be used as a measure of impact on poverty. Gender-disaggregated indicators should systematically be used. It is particularly important to monitor the nutritional status of young children and women of reproductive age, as poor nutrition at these times of life can have lasting effects on the individual, and also on the next generation.

Further work and inter-agency collaboration for the identification and management of appropriate indicators and information systems is ongoing and should be encouraged.

The factors influencing HFS and nutritional well-being are beyond the capacity or mandate of any one organisation. There is therefore a need - and an opportunity - for intensified inter-agency co-ordination of policies and actions, at local and community level (micro and sectoral project design, implementation, monitoring and evaluation), at national level (policy and strategic planning) and at global level (inter-agency policy).

Working towards a common understanding of problems and possible solutions:

— There is a need for more information on experiences in joint planning and implementation of specific projects and collaborative efforts at the programme level. Specific areas could be selected by the different UN agencies in order to develop and test collaboration mechanisms with a view to disseminate lessons learned and best practices.

— Formulation of better co-ordinated policies, programmes and strategies in the areas of HFS, health and nutrition, with a particular focus on marginal areas and population groups.

— A systematic search for complementarity and clearer distribution of responsibilities among the various actors.

— Long-term investment in HFS and nutrition assessment and in training capacity.

— *Developing operational tools:* There is a need for common efforts to develop and test more user-friendly, practical and cost-effective tools and guidelines for:

— Assessing and evaluating the impact of policies, programmes and projects on household food security and nutrition.

— Ensuring the incorporation of household food security and nutrition into development policies and programmes.

— Formulating, implementing, monitoring and evaluating HFS and nutrition projects or project components for replication on a wider scale.

The FIVIMS initiative (along with the Vulnerability Analysis and Mapping system, and nutrition surveillance systems) could provide a collaborative mechanism to address some of these needs.

—Strengthening institutions: Priority should be given to strengthening the capacity of institutions to develop, implement and monitor the multi-sectoral approaches needed to promote household food security and good nutrition. Increasing the capacity of district level staff from government to work in collaboration with NGOs and the private sector to provide better support and services will contribute to the present efforts to ensure good governance alleviate poverty and promote sustainable livelihoods.

Improving inter-agency collaboration: The ACC Subcommittee on Nutrition (SCN) has identified three main areas for action in its Strategic Plan to improve nutrition globally: (i) to promote harmonized approaches among the UN agencies, and between the UN agencies and governmental and non-governmental partners, (ii) to review the UN system response to malnutrition, monitor resource allocation, and collate information on trends and achievements reported to specific UN bodies, and (iii) to advocate and raise awareness of nutrition issues at global, regional and country levels.

For the Strategic Plan to lead to sustainable improvements in nutrition, it is essential that the importance of household food security and its interactions with nutrition be recognised and addressed accordingly. The SCN should develop relevant areas of the Strategic Plan into time bound actions, with targets and administrative arrangements.

— *Collaborating at country policy and strategy level:* The World Food Summit goal can only be achieved if household food security and nutritional well-being are adopted as central strategic goals within the framework of the United Nations Development Assistance Framework (UNDAF) at the country level.

Yearly Common Country Assessments (CCA) should systematically review the food and nutrition situation in country and monitor food insecurity. It is expected that national Food Insecurity and Vulnerability Information and Mapping Systems (FIVIMS) will provide a significant contribution to that effect. Improving household food security and nutrition should be a standard strategic issue in CCAs.

The ACC Network on Rural Development and Food Security should assist thematic groups in country and encourage greater collaboration and synergy among UN agencies. Establishing administrative, technical and funding modalities to encourage inter-agency co-operation in the area of household food security and nutrition: Both the international Conference on Nutrition and the World Food Summit called for greater action and collaboration among UN agencies to address the widespread problems of food insecurity and malnutrition around the world. Within this process, the concept of household food security needs to be emphasised, and agency actions should specifically aim, inter alia, to strengthen the capacity of households to serve as viable social and economic units able to meet the food and nutritional needs of all members.

3

Urbanisation: Challenges to Food and Nutrition Security

The population explosion that characterized much of the 20th century is being replaced by another dramatic demographic transformation: urban population growth of an unprecedented scale. The urban population in the developing world is expected to double to 4 billion by 2025, accounting for about 90 percent of global population growth. In contrast, rural population will grow slowly and stop when it reaches 3 billion. China and India epitomize the huge shifts underway.

China, now two-thirds rural, will become predominantly urban in the next 25 years, and the 600 million people to live in urban India by 2025 will approximate the combined total population of the United States, Russia, and Japan. By 2015 the number of cities in developing countries with 1 million or more residents is expected to reach 400, more than quadruple the number of such cities in 1975. While forecasts of city sizes are subject to error, some large cities, such as Dhaka, are grow by 1 million or more persons per year for the foreseeable future.

Experts in a number of disciplines are concerned about these projections of rapid urban growth. Many demographers warn that cities will be unable to accommodate large population increases—a fear similar to the one voiced a generation ago about global population growth. For these Malthusians, world population growth must be managed by reducing unwanted fertility in urban areas of developing countries and among potential migrants living in rural areas. Unwanted fertility can be reduced most directly by improving access to modern methods of contraception.

Reducing fertility is essential because urban populations are particularly skewed toward peak reproductive ages between 15 and 40. Most migrants move to the city between the ages of 12 and 29. Some public health specialists raise different concerns. They see the poor health conditions suffered by now-developed countries in Europe and North America during 1875–1900, the period of most rapid urban growth, as a possible fate of developing countries. Despite comparatively modest population growth and great economic progress, industrializing cities in the late 19th century experienced higher mortality levels than did rural areas.

Urban health services and sanitary infrastructure could not keep up with the demand generated by in-migration. Given such a precedent, these specialists believe, it behooves developing-country governments to increase budgetary allocations to the health sector, direct public health resources toward urban centres in accordance with exceedingly rapid growth rates, and maintain adequate urban water and sewage systems. Environmentalists too worry about large, modernizing cities in poor countries because these cities contribute to the destruction of the world's ozone layer.

Modern urban systems require a great deal of energy, and the consequent emissions of carbon monoxide, carbon dioxide, and nitrogen oxide from fossil fuel combinations blanket the earth, trapping excess heat and leading to global warming, climate change, rising sea levels, change in vegetation. To limit such damage, environmentalists call for innovations in urban planning that would reduce the dependency on motor vehicles—the primary polluting agent in cities—and on air-conditioning. Also of growing concern to environmental scientists is the heavy toll on human life taken by floods and other natural disasters in ecologically fragile zones.

Colonialists established large cities of the developing world along routes most suitable for trading, usually coastal areas. They did not choose these locales for their environmental safety standards, nor for their ability to accommodate millions of new residents. Nor has a sensitivity to the possibility of disaster guided the development of these cities. Political scientists commonly view rapid city growth with some alarm because they believe that unmanageable city sizes can lead to civil violence,. a weakening of the state, growing radical religious fundamentalism, revolution, and a general deterioration in the quality of urban life.

The World Bank predicted in 1990 that urban poverty would become the most significant and politically explosive problem in the next century. Current estimates of urban poverty in developing countries lend credence to such claims. The United Nations (UN) concluded in 1996 that more than 500 million urban residents in less-developed countries, or almost 30 percent of the world's urban population, were living without adequate shelter.

Future urban population change in the developing world is likely to pose different challenges in different regions. Latin America, for instance, has already reached the urbanization level of the developed world, with three-quarters of the population living in cities and towns. Despite this urban sprawl, virtually all cities in the region that currently contain 2 million residents or more likely will have to absorb at least an additional million residents by 2025.

In most large cities of Africa, the population is increasingly moving to unplanned settlements on the periphery where land is cheapest. In contrast to Latin America, however, this horizontal expansion does not involve job relocation, and it reduces the efficacy of major urban infrastructure such as piped water, electricity, sewerage, and roads. The projected average annual growth rate of the urban population in Africa during 2000–20, 3.9 percent, portends that settlements will only deteriorate, particularly in the absence of sustained economic growth. Of equal concern to some commentators is the proliferation of 'urban villages' of 200,000 to 400,000 residents, large towns and small cities that typically lack the most basic amenities for a decent standard of living. The UN anticipates that in 2020 60 percent of urbanites in Africa will reside in cities with fewer than 500,000 residents, making urban development planning for small locales a continued priority. The challenge facing China and India is one of magnitude:

> the rapid urbanization that will occur in these two countries during the next quarter century is unprecedented in terms of numbers. Moreover, in South Asia—as in Sub-Saharan Africa—urban growth has been fueled less by economic dynamism than by rural poverty and continuing high fertility, a pattern likely to continue in the immediate future. In contrast, urban population change in more prosperous Southeast Asia has been distinguished by dynamism, resulting in the blurring of rural-urban boundaries as major expressways and railroad lines radiate out from urban cores, giving rise to new towns, industrial estates, and other urban forms in areas hitherto agricultural.

For governments that wish to manage urban population growth in the future, three policy options have received priority attention.

Contrary to conventional wisdom, urban growth in developing regions has stemmed more from natural increase (an excess of births over deaths) than from rural out-migration. This pattern is likely to continue in the near future. To control population, therefore, particular emphasis should be given to measures that provide women in urban areas and potential migrants in rural areas with the means to regulate fertility. This strategy has been implemented effectively, for instance, by Profamila, the national family planning agency of Colombia. By contrast, efforts to reduce city sizes by restricting migration have largely failed, even under the most coercive regimes (with the exception of South Africa under apartheid).

Many scholars accept that rapid urban growth in the developing world is inevitable but do not accept dire predictions of its consequences. These optimists maintain that city governments with good management capabilities can absorb large population increases without diminishing human welfare or the quality of the environment. The key is a commitment to undertake and sustain policies that, among other things, maintain infrastructure, increase productivity of the labor force, and alleviate poverty. A frequently cited example of success is Curitiba, a city in Brazil that has avoided the degradations experienced in most other developing-country cities of comparable size by implementing low-cost public transport as an alternative to cars, preserving green spaces, promoting multisectoral planning, and introducing other sound urban management measures.

Effective urban governance is an additional mechanism by which cities can overcome population pressures. Though good governance practices for cities have been articulated only recently and not yet been implemented fully anywhere, they include engaging nongovernmental actors—communities, civic groups, private contractors—in meeting basic needs; decentralizing decisionmaking authority and control of municipal resources to local indigenous groups; and making city governments more responsive to local needs, more accountable for actions, and more transparent with respect to financing.

Urban growth rates rise when developing countries favour urban manufacturing over rural agriculture. Rural-to-urban migration is heavier when well-paying jobs are plentiful in urban industry but scarce in village farming and when rural laborers cannot obtain desirable prices for their goods. An unexpected outcome of the structural adjustment programs of the 1980s, which raised the price of food for urban consumers, has been slower urban growth in many countries than was anticipated 20 years ago. In the future, governments themselves conceivably can manage the pace of urban growth by promoting equitable economic policies between urban and rural areas.

Countries, and avoiding the bleak vision of the pessimists, is possible only if governments act energetically on a number of different fronts: reducing urban poverty and inequity, helping women achieve their fertility preferences, improving urban infrastructure, removing bias against rural-based agriculture, and building good governance.

Conditions for Nutrition Security

Large increases in urban poverty and malnutrition as growth in urban areas outstrips the capacity of the city to provide jobs, or to build the necessary infrastructure for urban agriculture, effective markets, health, and good water and sanitation. Generally, policymakers, donors, and other development practitioners believe that rural conditions are much worse than urban ones; so does this mean that resources should not be directed to the urban poor and malnourished? The prevalence of urban poverty in each country is highly dependent on country-specific experiences and policies. Higher prevalence could result from civil wars that drive people into the cities, as in Somalia, or from implementation of an industrial strategy that builds on unequal income distribution, as in Brazil, even when average levels of economic development are similar.

Furthermore, levels of urban and rural poverty are linked, underscoring the profound positive impact that broad-based economic growth can have on overall poverty reduction. However, that the sectors with the highest rates of growth do not necessarily have the highest rates of poverty alleviation, because they attract more (often poor) people than they can absorb. This could be one explanation for the fact that in many countries, rural poverty rates are decreasing much more rapidly than urban poverty rates (which may even be increasing). While urban-based employment is growing and helping to decrease rural poverty, it cannot absorb all the additional supply of labor coming from the countryside. Moreover, poverty alleviation within particular sectors can be offset by large income inequalities. In fact, such inequalities, as well as the type of growth pursued in the urban sector, may be much more important to the location of poverty than the aggregate growth and distribution effects.

Availability of food, access to food, and risks related to either availability or access are the essential determinants of food security. National food security implies that within a country the amount of food available, if evenly distributed, is enough to meet people's food needs. At the household level, "a household is food secure when it has access to the food needed for a healthy life for all its members (adequate in terms of quality, quantity, safety, and culturally acceptable), and when it is not at undue risk of losing such access". The broad area of food security may be usefully disaggregated into questions relating to adequacy of food availability and stability of both food availability and access. This approach focuses on conditions necessary to achieve food security and highlights the need to consider both the nature of the food itself and the range of factors determining security of food availability and access.

Adequacy of food availability means that the overall supply should potentially cover overall nutritional needs in terms of quantity (energy) and quality (providing all essential nutrients); furthermore, it should be safe (free of toxic factors and contaminants) and of good food quality (taste, texture, and so on). Last but not least, the types of foodstuffs commonly available (nationally, in local markets, and eventually at the household level) should be culturally acceptable. Stability of the food supply and of access to food presupposes environmental sustainability, implying that there is a judicious public and community management of the natural resources that have a bearing on the food supply; and also presupposes economic and social sustainability in terms of conditions and mechanisms securing food access.

This implies just income distribution and effective markets, together with various formal (public-sector) and informal safety nets. These could be public social security schemes, programmatic interventions, income-generating programs, and numerous forms ofcommunity transactions, and self-help and solidarity networks, the latter taking on particular importance when people have to cope with shocks and crisis situations of various kinds.

In urban areas, the main determinants of food availability at the household level are prices and income, access to home production (urban agriculture), and access to formal and informal transfers. Household behaviors, influenced by cultural factors and knowledge, also affect patterns of food demand and distribution within the household.

The second condition for nutrition security is adequate care. Care is the provision in the household and the community of time, attention, and support to meet the physical, mental, and social needs of the growing child and other household members. Care encompasses a number of critical factors in the development of nutritional well-being among individuals-especially the most vulnerable groups in society: young children and pregnant and lactating women.

The third condition for nutrition security is health, which is largely a consequence of adequate prevention and control of diseases. The issue of chronic diseases will not be addressed, although it is recognized as an increasingly important health concern in urban areas.Health is determined by a series of factors that act at three levels. At the community level, factors such as the quality of the overall environment (biological pathogens and chemical pollutants in air, food, and water), and the availability, cost, and quality of services such as water, electricity, sewage, refuse disposal, and health services are important health determinants. At the household level, the most important factors include the general conditions of the household, including the type of housing, the availability and cost of water and hygienic facilities, and the number of rooms per household member (an indicator of crowding); the availability of food; and household caring behaviors related to the use of preventive and curative health services, the use of water and hygienic facilities to provide a healthy, hygienic, and safe environment, and food-related behaviors such as the acquisition of food, the intrahousehold allocation of resources, feeding practices (including breast-feeding), and food preparation methods. At the individual level, the determinants of health relate to the interactive mechanisms among an individual's food and nutrient intake, nutritional status, and health status.

Young children are more susceptible to infectious diseases, malnutrition, and poor growth, and are likely to suffer long-term negativeconsequences of these insults on their physical, cognitive, and reproductive performance in adulthood. Mothers are also more biologically vulnerable to ill-health because of their reproductive role. Maternal health is of special concern because of the excessive demands on their body, and the particular health risks associated with pregnancy and child birth.

In addition, maternal health and nutritional status are important for maintaining a safe pregnancy, ensuring adequate growth of the fetus, and experiencing satisfactory lactation. In urban areas, the health of women is also crucial for their role as income earners and ability to provide adequate care for their children and family.

Urban Food Sources

Historically, the most significant difference between food access in urban and rural areas has been that rural people can often produce their own food, whereas urban people are more dependent on food purchases. A recent study in Accra found that households purchase 90 percent of their food. This dependence on markets is further increased because, unlike their rural counterparts, urban dwellers cannot exploit natural resources to provide for housing, energy, and water. Food expenditures can make up as much as 60 to 80 percent of total income among low-income urban households. People can get their food from three sources: the market, their own production, and transfers from public assistance programs or other households.

The efficiency of the food marketing and distribution system, household purchasing patterns, the household's ability to produce its ownfood, as well as the household's access to public transfers, such as food subsidies or food aid programs, or private transfers, such as exchange relationships with rural relatives, are among the most important factors affecting the cost of food for the urban household.

Urban Agriculture

Urban agriculture, defined as production in the home or plots in urban or peri-urban areas, is more widespread and important than generally thought. Some believe that it is not only a potentially significant source of income, food, energy, and micronutrients for family members, but that it can also benefit the environment by providing a way to reuse solid wastes and water. A number of studies now exist on the topic.

Most of the studies on Africa note that the importance of urban farming increased in the 1970s and 1980s as urban populations in much of the region grew at record levels and urban economies began to crumble. Virtually all of the empirical studies carried out in Africa characterize urban agriculture as a means of obtaining some amount of food for household consumption through nonmarket or subsistence means. In Latin America and Asia, commercial urban farming is more highly developed, especially with regard to vegetable and perishable-food production, but much of this production is also for home consumption.

As with any farm household, a household involved in urban agriculture is both producer and consumer.

Urban agriculture also improves access to food by raising incomes if production is sold. The significance of urban agriculture can be measured in several ways: in terms of the proportion of the urban population engaged in the practice, in terms of income and employment, in terms of total production, and in terms of the impact on access to food and nutrition. Farming is practiced by a surprisingly large proportion of urban populations, up to as much as 40 percent within African cities and 50 percent in Latin America. Urban farming is not simply a marginal activity of recent migrants from the countryside: migrants may stay in cities for 5-10 years before acquiring land for cultivation.

Several studies note that while many socioeconomic groups in the city may farm, farming constitutes a crucial form of food access for the lower income groups. Yet, because farming requires access to land, those who practice urban agriculture may not be among the poorest of the poor. Reliable data about the proportion of the total urban food supply coming from urban production are scarce. For some commodities, especially vegetables or poultry, the proportion of total urban consumption coming from urban agriculture can be quite high.

UNDP cites figures as high as 70 percent of poultry products (meat and eggs) and 90 percent of vegetables consumed in some cities in Asia and Africa coming from producers within urban areas. Maxwell and Zziwa (1992) estimate that 15-20 percent of the total consumption of staple foods in Kampala comes from urban agriculture. Some estimate the monetary value of urban agriculture in Kenya in 1985 at $4 million. But studies are scattered, often location-specific, and use varying definitions of 'urban agriculture,' so the estimates remain rough. In any case, the importance of urban agriculture varies with the city. Availability of land and agricultural inputs and municipal policies toward farming determine the extent of urban agriculture in most cases.

The green spaces available in Kampala, Uganda, for example, are not so prevalent in Accra, Ghana, and very few urban households in Accra farm. As a secondary or complementary economic strategy, even when households farm, only a limited number of urban households are entirely dependent on farming for their livelihood. In Dar es Salaam, for instance, about 55 percent of peri-urban households in selected wards farmed, but, on average, they depended on agricultural production for food only 2 to 3 months of the year. The majority of urban farmers in Africa are women-figures range from slightly over 50 percent in surveys where the household head was asked who farmed, to about 85 percent in time allocation studies. Only a few studies have explicitly explored intrahousehold division of labor and responsibilities related to urban agriculture.

Most studies describe urban agriculture as a 'household survival strategy,' and to the extent that urban agriculture is characterized in theoretical terms, it is most often placed as a special subcategory of the urban informal economy.

Urban agriculture uses resources, products, and services found in and around the urban area and, in turn, often supplies resources, products, and services to that area. Urban agricultural systems include horticulture, floriculture, forestry, aquaculture, and livestock production.

The United Nations Development Programme estimates that 800 million people are engaged in urban agriculture worldwide, with the majority in Asian cities.

Of these, 200 million are considered to be market producers, employing 150 million people full time. Urban agriculture is thus an important supply source in developing-country urban food systems, a critical food-security valve for poor urban households. It affords a cheap, simple, and flexible tool for productively using open urban spaces, treating and recovering urban solid and liquid wastes, generating employment and income, adding value to products, managing freshwater resources more sparingly, and resolving otherwise incompatible urban land use issues.

Urban agriculture's nature and magnitude vary, of course, depending on agroecological conditions; national, regional, and local policies; market conditions; and household characteristics, but it has become an important part of the urban scene.

Urban agriculture complements, rather than supplants, rural supplies and imports of food and will continue to do so. Cities will continue to depend largely on rural agriculture for bulkier, less perishable foodstuffs. But urban agriculture can provide significant amounts of food at small scales and for specific items. It can generate goods valued at tens of millions of dollars in any given major city. By growing their own food, cities lower their food deficits and obtain an important source of fruits and vegetables and livestock products, including dairy. Urban agriculture provides an estimated 15 percent of all food consumed in urban areas and is likely to double that share in the next couple of decades. Cities with more advanced urban agriculture sectors, particularly in Asia, have become largely self-sufficient in higher-valued, nutritious perishables. Some cities even export surpluses abroad.

Urban agriculture is also integral to city life, a vibrant part of urban economic and ecological systems. Urban farmers use urban land, public services, inputs, and even urban wastes in production. They then sell to local markets and often reinvest profits into goods produced or sold at city outlets. Urban agriculture can be an important supplement to household income. In Cairo, the rearing of small livestock, practiced by over a quarter of households, provides more than 60 percent of household income. In Dar es Salaam urban agriculture is the second largest employer. High-valued specialty foods and nonfood crops (such as ornamental flowers) that require little space for production are especially good for providing needed cash.

Still, the great majority of urban farmers are poor and grow food mainly for their own subsistence, with little support or protection, on small plots that they do not own. These households can secure food from urban agriculture that they could not afford otherwise. Studies in Harare, Kampala, and Nairobi found that urban agriculture can improve nutritional status of household members, as measured by caloric and protein intake, meal quality, or children's growth rates.

Many discussion indicate that women predominate in urban agriculture, which conveniently enables women to earn income, improve household diets, perform household chores, and exert greater control over household resources, budgets, and decisionmaking.

The poor can be constrained from doing well with urban farming for many reasons, including lack of access to land, credit, water, and other inputs or legal obstacles arising from concerns about public health. Urban farmers often use public spaces, and if they lack title to the land they use, they cannot be assured they will actually reap the benefits of their investment. Without title, the majority of low-income urban producers cannot get formal loans that require assets as a guarantee nor can they get support from national farmers' unions, whose members' activities must be legally sanctioned. Women may be constrained by extension or credit services that disregard the knowledge women farmers have of crops, input combinations, and cultivation methods. Aridity, unreliable supplies of piped water, and violent rainfalls can all critically constrain many production systems.

If improperly managed, urban agriculture can even exacerbate environmental degradation, including soil erosion, loss of vegetation, siltation, and depletion of water resources. Public health concerns stem from misuse or mishandling of agrochemicals; the application of untreated or improperly treated wastes to food crops; the exposure of crops to air, water, or land pollution, including possible contamination from heavy metals; and unsafe disposal of vegetable and animal wastes.

Some threats, such as those from agrochemicals, are less prevalent than commonly believed because the poor usually cannot afford inorganic inputs. Consequently they grow crops or raise livestock organically. However, the poor often have no option other than to grow their crops in hazardous conditions, and threats from authorities may only deter them from investing in safer production methods.

To improve urban agriculture and make it more sustainable, farmers must use better practices and governments must promote or better manage it through more informed policies. Nongovernmental organizations (NGOs) can support these efforts. Legitimizing urban agriculture can help its low-income practitioners gain access to land, needed services, and credit. Policymakers can legitimize and promote urban agriculture through public appeals, as in Uganda.

Governments can provide land for urban agriculture in city master plans, support greenbelt projects, and set up a network of input and service centers. They can engage directly in urban agricultural production by leasing out public land; assigning undeveloped, public land to farmer organizations; partnering with producers; or becoming producers themselves. Urban laws and regulations can be revised to be compatible with people's survival options, as in Kampala, where bylaws now allow for certain kinds of farm production in certain zones. Governments can also tolerate urban agriculture as interim land use in public housing schemes or incorporate it as a way to productively manage open urban spaces.

Some development banks in South Africa and Tanzania have also provided credit by supporting revolving funds for cooperatives of urban farmers. Farmers' organizations can also help to legitimize the sector and organize access to credit, inputs, and markets. There is enormous potential for reducing risks to public health by educating and empowering urban producers, as opposed to ignoring or harassing them. Farmers can reduce environmental risks and gain financially by making appropriate choices about what crops to grow. For example, increasing the use of short-cycle crops boosts productivity and decreases the use of potentially contaminated water. Because many safe practices are knowledge-based, they are also affordable and easily adopted by farmers.

Producers can be taught to avoid the use of polluted organic or chemical fertilizers on specific crops or to draw water from wells instead of rivers. Urban farmers can have mutually beneficial contracts with municipal waste-disposal services, and nonfood urban agriculture can be used to rehabilitate contaminated water bodies and soils, generating income in the process. NGOs can help determine the scale of composting that would be both cost-effective and environmentally suitable. Cities can treat and recirculate wastewater. When cities introduce treatment of water for irrigation, they should also devise creative cost-recovery mechanisms (for example, bartering agreements) instead of penalizing wastewater-using farmers.

Challenges to urban agriculture remain to be addressed from the community up to the national level. Governments must apply the wealth of local experiences to creating institutional structures for implementing urban agriculture policies. Overall, experience shows that prohibition of urban agriculture has been ineffective. Governments now should move beyond accommodation and into issue resolution: multiple-stakeholder governance so far seems to be the best approach to creating a sustainable urban agriculture that is friendly to small farmers. NGOs can help create and mediate among the various organizations. Experience also has shown that urban agriculture is most viable where it is mainstreamed into robust strategies for land use, poverty alleviation, economic development, and sound environmental management. Outside Asia, few national food policies seek synergies between rural and urban production or guide integrated urban agricultural programs. Land-use and regulatory systems must be designed and enforced for fairer access to land, water, and markets.

Agricultural extension must be adapted to the needs of urban producers. Agricultural research stations and urban planning departments must collaborate. Model health and land-use codes need to be developed. Regional and global networks are developing, but national and local networks must also be created and supported. Public policy should also acknowledge women's knowledge, constraints, and opportunities and act upon them to enhance women's citizenship. Governments throughout the developing world must recognize the place of urban agriculture in the city's development and in securing food and nutrition security of its residents, a place it has long held without recognition and, moreover, a place that is now expanding.

It is widely agreed that urban agriculture increases food access and availability, but the actual impact on food security and nutrition has rarely been empirically measured. The environmental and health impacts of urban farming are potentially both positive and negative. Previous research highlights the potential of urban agriculture to recyclewastewater and organic materials, and thus help resolve both solid and liquid waste disposal problems in rapidly growing cities. But these suggestions add to concerns about food safety, particularly contamination from the use of untreated wastewater for irrigation.

The intensive use of agricultural chemicals in a densely populated environment and urban livestock production also pose potential dangers to health and nutrition. On balance, researchers seem to agree that urban agriculture could have a beneficial impact on the urban environment through recycling wastes, stabilizing drainage and run-off, and making productive use of green spaces, but serious research and assessment is needed to ensure that urban farming employs techniques and technologies that will also safeguard human health.

Urban agriculture in most cities is a precarious enterprise. Reluctance to change the legal status of urban agriculture stems partly from biases against urban agriculture on the part of urban authorities, and partly from concerns about food safety and the health and environmental impact of urban agriculture discussed above. In many cities, agriculture remains technically illegal despite the potential benefits. In Nairobi after World War II, the government passed a law ordering all crops within the city to be cut down. Livestock and horticulture remain illegal today. In Kampala, more than one-fourth of farmers face harassment and eviction from the city council or landowners.

The most critical institutional constraint to urban agriculture, particularly crop cultivation, is access to land. The institutional conundrum of urban farming is that the practice is dependent on access to land, but the group to whom farming is most important is the least able to gain secure access to land. While some forms of urban agriculture are so intensive that they can actually compete with other land uses on an economic basis, much of the subsistence production by the urban poor relies on informal access to underutilized or unutilized urban land. Frequently, farmers do not own the land but use publicspace or use vacant lots owned by private owners, with or without their permission.

Landowners and farmers may enter into informal agreements but, because of the lack of an adequate legal framework governing tenancy, lease, and appropriate use, private landowners will not formally lease their land or not lease their land at all. With low tenure security and questionable legality, the farmer is not motivated either to be efficient or to care for the land. Insecurity of tenure and other institutional constraints to land access effectively prevent technological improvements. The uncertain legal status of urban agriculture is such that official projects or programs aimed at improving urban agriculture have been relatively rare. Typically, urban agriculture is not taken into account in the urban planning process.

In India, agriculture is not part of the master plan of any city. In combination with a weak legal framework, the lack of awareness and government recognition means planners often do not think about how to provide water and drainage infrastructure to handle urban farming, and governments make little provision for research on and extension for urban farming techniques. For instance, Tanzania's National Urban Water Agency strongly opposed the use of water for urban farming, and imposed a fine for use of water for agriculture in the city. Property rights could be designed to give landowners and farmers the security of tenancy they need to be more productive and to farm in an environmentally friendly way, but negative planning and cultural attitudes toward urban agriculture mean there is little movement to remove existing policy, administrative, and legal hurdles for urban agriculture.

These constraints are often exacerbated by the fact that in many cities, it is mostly women who are involved in urban agriculture. Legal and cultural biases against women owning or even leasing land make their attempts at urban farming even more difficult. Success with urban agriculture does exist, however. For decades, city authorities in Lusaka, Zambia, enforced laws against crop production in the city as a health hazard. Farming of vacant land was illegal. Legal action was rarely taken but authorities often cleared land of crops. Faced with economic decline in the 1970s, however, the presidenturged urban dwellers in 1977 to grow their own food. In response, the Lusaka City Council stopped enforcing the antiurban agriculture laws. Government stores even made subsidized seeds for fruits and vegetables available. In 1977, 43 percent of Chawama, one of the largest slums in Lusaka, had home gardens. A decade later, 40 percent of households still had home plots. In a few cases in Accra, land in peri-urban areas has been deliberately protected for agricultural use. The fate of any given community in the process of urbanization depends on local leadership and the commitment of the leadership to the development of the local community.

In addition to a general lack of studies, the lack of a common definition of urban agriculture and the precise definition of an 'urban area' has hampered efforts to draw on available findings to state conclusively what the impact of urban agriculture is on poverty, health, food security, nutrition, and the environment. Urban agriculture appears to have greater significance for these issues, however, than most policymakers and researchers have suspected. At this stage, it seems clear that the importance of urban farming varies with the conditions found in the cities. In some areas, urban farming is clearly an important coping strategy for households and in others, it has the potential to be. For lower-income groups, whose monetary incomes are insufficient to purchase adequate food, farming can constitute a crucial form of land access, although because farming requires access to land, those who farm tend not to be among the poorest of the poor. Because women often have responsibility for food procurement for the household, women are frequently involved in urban agricultural production and sales.

The practice of agriculture in the city, however, presents a number of challenges, from competition for scarce available land to use of techniques and technologies that degrade the soils, pollution, and increase of poisoning and infectious diseases. At the same time, urban agriculture offers new potential for recycling urban wastes, saving onmarketing transport costs, and providing poor segments of the population with employment possibilities.

Urban food and nutrition security depends on strong links between urban and rural areas. But policymakers and urban planners often ignore this interdependence. There are two broad, often overlapping, categories of rural-urban linkages. 'Spatial' links refer to the movement of people, goods, money, and information between urban and rural areas. 'Sectoral' links describe the interdependence between agriculture on the one hand and industry and services on the other. In the next two decades, three main issues related to rural-urban interdependence are likely to emerge:

— Changes in land use around urban centers, from farmland to residential or industrial use;

— Greater diversification of income sources in rural and urban areas, often involving people migrating or commuting between the countryside and urban centers; and

— Changes in the direction and composition of internal migration.

The areas surrounding urban centers play an important part in the provision of food to urban consumers, and the proximity of these areas to urban markets lowers food transport and storage costs. At the same time, urbanization is at its most intense in these peri-urban areas. The process of urbanization transforms land-use and farming systems, patterns of labor-force participation, infrastructure requirements, and natural resource systems. Peri-urban areas show wide regional variations. Southeast Asia's extended metropolitan regions involve a mix of agriculture, cottage industry, industrial estates, suburban development, and other residential settlement over a wide radius. But in Sub-Saharan Africa, where the industrial base is usually weaker, agriculture prevails around cities, although with important transformations in land ownership and use.

Uncontrolled urban growth can pose a major threat to agricultural land and in many cases benefits mainly middle- and upper-income groups. Speculative purchases can also withdraw agricultural land from food production. In Manila's extended metropolitan region, for example, large areas of rice land have been converted to industrial, residential, and recreational uses or have lain idle while owners awaited either development permits or more propitious market conditions. Such changes eliminate highly fertile agricultural land from production that urban households would otherwise rely on for affordable food. Although small-scale peri-urban farmers contribute significantly to food production, in the process devising ways of using degraded land and large volumes of waste, proximity to urban markets does not guarantee them access to urban consumers.

Around Paraguay's capital, for example, limited access to credit severely constrains the capacity of small farmers to grow produce, which is in high demand among urban consumers. On the outskirts of Bamako, Mali, the lack of transport makes it difficult for many small-scale fruit and vegetable producers to reach the city's markets. Social networks among traders and middlemen can also exclude small producers from access to local markets. These constraints affect not only the income of small producers but also the food and nutrition security of urban consumers. The transformation of peri-urban agricultural land, likely to intensify in the next few decades, raises two important issues for policymaking. First, to avoid increases in poverty, better working conditions and alternative employment opportunities are required for workers in these areas. Increased mechanization of production will reduce the number of agricultural workers. Those that remain will be mainly wage workers, often hired on a seasonal basis. These workers will need to supplement their incomes with other urban-based activities. Second, sound management of natural resources will become increasingly necessary as commercial agricultural production competes even more intensively with urban industry and households for essential resources such as water.

A large number of households in both rural and urban areas rely on different income sources for their livelihoods, which span the rural-urban divide. In Colombia much of the temporary work-force employed during the coffee harvest comes from urban areas. These workers usually stay on the farm over the week and return home for the weekend. In Zimbabwe low-income urban residents make ends meet by working seasonally on farms. Rural residents, on the other hand, increasingly make their living from sources outside agriculture. Low-income rural people, for example, supplement their income with petty trading, which can involve commuting or circular migration to urban centers.

In many cases those who migrate semipermanently remain closely in touch with their relatives back home. Parents working long hours in the urban informal sector tend to send their children to live with relatives in their home villages. This is because living conditions, including access to health services, are sometimes better in rural areas than in the cities, especially when nongovernmental organizations (NGOs) are active there. Even long-term migrants maintain close rural ties because keeping a rural base provides a safety net to cope with times of economic hardship or political violence. In Botswana as many as half of the low-income urban residents keep either land or cattle in their home village. In addition, in exchange for help from relatives, relatively settled migrants in urban areas support newly arrived migrants and secondary school students from their extended families. These obligations make additional demands on the already insufficient housing situation of low-income urban households. Policies often ignore the extent to which low-income groups rely on both urban and rural resources to make a secure living. By overlooking these complexities, policies can undermine the survival strategies of the poor.

The government housing program in South Africa, for example, provides grants that can be spent only in rural or urban areas but not both. This makes it difficult for households to maintain links with home areas. In Brazil, many housing programmes allow residents to take in only members of their nuclear household. This rule prevents residents from fulfilling their social obligations, thereby weakening social networks and safety nets.

Policies must not create additional burdens for the poor by assuming that low-income people live their lives only in one location. Rural development initiatives need to take into account nonagricultural activities and encourage and support them. At the same time, urban policies must be flexible about housing needs and recognize the importance of rural social networks and social relations even in urban dwellers' lives.

Internal migration is another key facet of rural-urban interdependence. It cannot be measured easily, however, partly because censuses do not register short-term movements. Not all migration is rural-to-urban: in Latin America most movement occurs between urban centers, while in Sub-Saharan Africa rural-to-rural movement is important. Anecdotal evidence on return migration links it to worker retrenchments in the formal sector, especially during the implementation of structural adjustment programs in the 1980s. These different kinds of migratory patterns point to the varied influence of regional and national economies. For instance, the relocation of Mexican industries to secondary cities because of government incentives has precipitated the movement of skilled, middle-class workers out of Mexico City.

Economic imbalance between locations is not the only cause of migration. Changing social relations, especially between gender and generational groups, and improved access to information are also important. As young men and women migrate to seek greater financial and social independence, they often tend to remit less than their predecessors, generally because of the increased cost of living in the cities. Another major cause of migration is the higher demand for women workers in the service industry and in light manufacturing linked to export processing. This trend is likely to continue in the next few decades and will have a major impact on labor markets. Policymakers need to identify and support the positive aspects of this urban influx and minimize the negative ones, such as the lack of child care for mothers who work.

Migration will play an increasingly central role in economic and social change over the next decades. But it will be a complex affair, involving different directions for different groups. Children may be looked after by older generations in home villages while their young parents move to urban centers for specific periods of time. After accumulating capital during that first period of urban employment, the parents are likely to move on to invest the capital. Policymakers need to carefully consider the relationships between migrant parent, child, and home village, all of which are bound up by the economic web of remittances.

Policymakers have usually ignored the importance of rural-urban interdependence, or attempted to curb it, as in the case of migration. Inevitably the living conditions of lower- and middle-income groups have worsened. As a first step, policy-makers need to identify and soften or eliminate policies that have a negative impact on rural-urban linkages. The next step is trickier because rural-urban linkages are highly context-dependent. Policies based on generalizations about the scale and nature of linkages have usually failed.

Local government can play an important role in addressing local needs and priorities, but action at the local level generally must be supported at the regional and national levels. This support includes managing natural resources while responding to both urban and rural demands; assisting local economies by providing physical and social (health and education) infrastructure; and facilitating the efforts of low-income households to make a living by drawing on a variety of resources, including migration. Given the difficulty of making specific policy recommendations, what is more important initially is for various government, NGO, and other groups and actors to recognize the centrality of urban-rural interdependence to both urban and rural livelihoods, to understand the local and national problems associated with it, and to conduct a democratic dialogue to arrive at a negotiated set of strategies for nurturing and benefiting from this interdependence. Understanding the importance of rural linkages to urban livelihood, food, and nutrition security is critical if policies are to improve the lives of the urban poor, rather than making them even more difficult than they already are.

Urban Food Marketing Systems

Clearly, food prices and the ability to earn cash income are crucial to the achievement of food security in urban areas. Food prices are dependent on a number of factors, including the efficiency of the food marketing system and availability and access to food subsidies or other food programs. Inefficient food marketing systems linking rural and urban areas can increase the costs of food for the urban poor. For example, bad roads and inadequate storage facilities can lead to high losses that increase costs as goods are transported to towns from agricultural production areas. Within the city, urban food distribution systems are highly diverse. Food for the cities can come from areas of agricultural production either at home or abroad, rural or urban, or from international trade or aid.

Traders, distributors, processors, and retailers are major participants in the marketing chain that gets food from producer to consumer, with each actor potentially performing multiple functions or overlapping with others. Almost 20 years ago, the problems that continue to affect urban food supply and increase urban food costs today. Wholesale markets that connect producers and traders with retailers are often run-down and obsolete, with ineffective management. Generally built decades ago, they do not have sufficient space or storage facilities to handle the large volumes of food currently processed. Frequently located in highly urbanized areas, traffic congestion around the markets is immense.

Urban retail markets are often small and scattered. This means that, although they are able to create employment and effectively meet the demand of poor urban consumers who need easy access to markets and make purchases in small quantities, gains from economies of scale are difficult. Macroeconomic policies also have a significant impact on the price of urban food. For many years, and in many countries, "cheap food" policies deliberately kept the price of urban food low, but structural adjustment programs in the 1980s and 1990s have reversed many of these policies. Virtually all single-city case studies and review articles of urban food security note that the price of food has risen faster than the general cost of living since the mid-1980s, and much faster than increases in income.

The impact of structural adjustment on prices has been felt mainly through the deregulation of domestic food markets, but also through the devaluation of currencies and the price of imported foods. On the other hand, prices for urban food could fall in some countries if deregulation were broadened to include the food-processing sector.

Tight time constraints, coupled with an income pattern where wages are earned and spent daily, often compel the urban poor to buy their food in small quantities from neighborhood shops rather than central markets. These latter facilities usually offer bulk food at lower prices, but do not provide the option to buy in small quantities. Development-associated increases in income and the opportunity cost of time, especially women's time, as well as exposure to advertising, also have tended to favor a shift to processed foods more widely provided by supermarkets and street vendors than by traditional markets. Furthermore, with increasing development and the burgeoning size of cities, producers, retailers, and wholesalers have tended to become more specialized and distinct.

The structure of food retailing has also been affected by the introduction of new technologies such as refrigeration, which has prolonged the storage, transport, and shelf-life of perishables. However, despite the rising importance of supermarkets, has insisted on the continued vital role of the traditional, 'petty commodity' sector. The tiny quantities in which food is often sold in this sector make food more accessible to the poor, who may have very little to spend and cannot afford the cheaper bulk purchases possible from supermarkets. Street foods can also be a significant source of food for many urban dwellers, both in terms of energy intake and food expenditure. In Indonesia and the Philippines, urban households spend up to 25 percent of their food budgets on street foods, a proportion that remains constant across income groups. In Ibadan, Nigeria, 98 percent of schoolchildren bought their breakfast in the streets.

In many cases, street foods are cheaper than home-prepared meals, especially when time spent shopping and cooking and the cost of transport and fuel are factored in. Smaller and poorer families tend to spend more on street foods than other households. Households in the poorest expenditure quintile spent an average of 39 percent of their total food budget on foods purchased away from home, compared to 26 percent of the top quintile, a finding confirmed in cities of Bangladesh and the Philippines. Also, small families in urban areas of Thailand spent 58 percent of their food expenditures on street foods, compared to 36 percent of families with eight members or more.

Street foods may also be, in some cases, the lowest-cost foods available. Vendors may be able to acquire raw materials through family or ethnic networks, or purchase discounted quantities at reduced prices. They may also rely on unpaid (in wages) labor from family members. Even if more expensive per unit than raw foods, purchase of prepared street foods can free-up time for the worker to engage in income-generating activities that have a greater benefit to the household than food preparation, especially in cases where traditional foods require long preparation times.

Urban residents may gain access to some amount of food through their own production. This may be from urban agriculture, farming operations outside the city, or the peri-urban areas. Even if the proportion of the total household food supply coming from own production is small, it is important in the sensethat the household can access this food at critical times, such as when income is insufficient for food purchases.

Private food transfers often take the form of reciprocal exchanges between urban and rural households. Rural kin provide urban families with food, and urban family members may remit some of their cash income to rural households, or provide some other service in return, such as assisting family members in obtaining employment or schooling in the city. The literature on urban-rural linkages makes numerous references to this type of exchange, but exchanges involving food are rarely quantified. The strength and persistence of such rural-urban ties is also the subject of debate, particularly in Africa, where the level of urbanization is the lowest but the rate of urbanization highest.

Interviews with poor households that dependence on rural areas for food or support was not widespread. Only about 35 percent of households received any food from rural areas in the year previous to the interview, and only about a quarter of them visited their home village. Private transfers can also come from companies that, through company cafeterias, use food as part of 'wages.' In this case, food compensates for low cash wages and can help to reduce absenteeism.

Public Transfers Governments and NGOs also have social assistance programs that provide food to targeted households. School feeding programs for children or food baskets given at health clinics are two such examples. Although programmatic food transfers are not by any means unique to cities, by virtue of their population density and infrastructure, a larger variety of food assistance programs is often available in cities. Emergency relief programs to prevent famine are also usually logistically easier to mount in cities than in rural areas. Indeed, in the late 20th century, outright famine is largely a rural, not urban, phenomenon.

Urban food systems that the poor rely on are fragmented, and this leads to inefficient marketing and an increase in the unit cost of food. The fragmentation of the food distribution system is partially linked to the level of economic development. Increased efficiency and integration are difficult without adequate transportation and storage facilities and without good information systems and access to credit. Improved integration of the food distribution system is also hard when a large proportion of the population is poor and can only afford to buy small amounts of food at a time. This demand pattern logically leads to a large number of sellers who sell small quantities of food, which are generally higher in price per unit than bulk purchases. With economic development, a shift occurs in how and where people obtain their food. Supermarkets replace traditional street sellers and central markets. This leads to increased consumption of processed products.

Urban living also increases the amount of food prepared and eaten away from home. Processed foods may be more expensive than nonprocessed ones, butsave preparation time, but street foods may actually cost less on a per-nutrient basis. Urban agriculture and private and public transfers may be particularly important for urban dwellers who have few other alternatives than purchasing their food.

In urban areas, households buy most of their food, so lack of income is the main challenge to food security. The importance of being able to earn cash income also means that the ability to stay healthy, to get a good job (and therefore the ability to acquire good education and training), and to have access credit to smooth consumption or expand or start up businesses are critical to urban food and nutrition security. With enough income, prices can rise and families can still buy enough to eat. Millions of urban poor, however, are vulnerable to prices rises or sharp declines in income, say due to illness or loss of job by the principal income-earner. Unfortunately, governments and NGOs simply do not have the resources to support programs to meet the needs of all those who are poor and food insecure. Unable to turn to social assistance, these households must work to earn a living as best they can. Consequently, outright unemployment in developing countries is relatively low. In large cities in Latin America and Asia, unemployment is generally less than 10 percent. Yet, the majority of the urban labor force works in sectors like petty trade and services where wages are low and job tenure uncertain. In urban Sub-Saharan Africa, employment in sectors that pay regular wages, such as manufacturing and industry, accounts for less than 10 percent of total employment. Urban poverty thus is not primarily the result of lack of work but the lack of well-paying, steady jobs.

Labor Market Issues

The quality of work opportunities—low wages, precarious working conditions, and insecure job tenure—is a crucial constraint to improving the livelihoods of the urban poor, especially since labor is poor people's greatest asset. As urbanization proceeds in the coming decades and continues to provide opportunities for residents of as well as migrants to urban areas, the labor market increasingly becomes a key determinant of wealth and poverty. If policymakers do not address labor market issues, urbanization may intensify poverty in cities and shift the primary location of destitution from rural to urban areas.

Urbanization implies a transition from agricultural to industrial employment and, particularly, to service-sector jobs. According to International Labour Organization (ILO) estimates, the share of industrial employment in developing countries rose only from 11 to 14 percent between 1965 and 1990 (and only from 8 to 9 percent in Sub-Saharan Africa), while service-sector employment increased from 17 to 25 percent (13 to 24 percent in Sub-Saharan Africa). With urbanization, cities also account for an increasing share of national income. Urban areas now generate 55 percent of gross national product in low-income countries—although the urban population share is much lower—and 85 percent in high-income countries.

Dynamic cities represent engines of economic growth. They bring benefits through economies of scale and the higher productivity of many urban economic activities. Urban incidences of poverty tend to be lower than rural ones precisely because expanding urban economies offer significant employment opportunities. However, the contribution of urbanization to improving the livelihoods of poor people in urban and rural areas is more modest than these positive outcomes may suggest, for the following reasons:

— Urban growth is often supported by government bias against rural and in favour of urban areas when allocating investment funds.

— A nation's overall poverty level may be reduced much more by rural development than by urban growth, especially in highly rural regions such as Asia and Africa.

— Often the poorest people from rural areas are not able to migrate to cities because of the financial investment and networks that migration usually requires.

— Many urban workers are badly paid, have insecure employment, or are overworked.

During the 1950s and 1960s, many experts expected that urbanization in developing countries would be accompanied by growth of a modern industrial sector that would provide permanent, protected employment. Instead, large numbers of urban inhabitants ended up working in the informal sector. In developing-country cities most people, particularly women, worked outside large, modern enterprises. Many of these jobs were insecure and did not pay well. With economic crises and adjustments during the 1980s and 1990s, the percentage of people working in this urban informal sector increased.

Jobs in urban areas show great diversity—from regular, secure government jobs; to well-paid independent jobs; to skilled, manual jobs in large-scale industries; to visible kinds of "informal" jobs. The last category is extremely heterogeneous, including relatively better-offtaxi drivers and market vendors as well as rickshaw pullers, beggars, prostitutes, and others. Many urban occupations are also marked by seasonal variations in availability of work. Moreover, job characteristics are linked to social differentiation. People of particular groups, ethnicity, castes, gender, or age often find employment only in particular segments of the labor market. Although women's role in the labor market is changing with urbanization, women's work is concentrated in a limited number of sectors.

During the last three to four decades the global female labor force expanded nearly twice as much as men's, but women still tend to be over represented in less-secure and irregular jobs. Even when they work in the same types of jobs or sectors as men, they get paid less than men. When countries experience economic crises, the burden tends to fall heaviest on urban women, who must continue to work and devise innovative coping strategies to care for other members of the household. The complexity of urban labor markets is augmented by the fact that people usually derive incomes from various sectors.

Members of a household often work in different occupations and sectors. People in secure jobs whose pay has eroded with inflation may take up extra jobs, such as vending or driving a taxi. In many cases, urban households cross rural–urban boundaries, with their rural base continuing to function as a social and economic safety net. Urban workers often return to their villages when they lose their jobs during crises.

Some urban dwellers maintain ties to the land in another way, through urban agricultural production that provides income and improves nutrition for as much as 40 to 50 percent of the African and Latin American urban population. This extra food and income is important for lower-income groups, particularly women, and often serves as a means of coping with increases in urban poverty, higher food prices, or food shortages.

The general tendency globally is toward more flexible labor markets, with less employment security and more differentiation among types of jobs. In Africa, Asia, and Latin America, flexibility in employment has been reinforced by economic stagnation since the 1980s and continuing policies of liberalization. The fall of communism also has led to more diverse forms of employment, away from state-guaranteed work.

— China state enterprises have been dismantled, employment security has declined, and a huge urban "floating population" of migrants has rapidly emerged.

— The East Asian miracle itself was based on flexible labor markets, with large companies employing a core group of workers and using subcontractors to employ large numbers of additional workers, with little employment protection.

— In India growth of modern employment stagnated even in the 1980s, and large numbers of laborers worked for subcontractor.

— In Africa, with the lowest levels of urbanization and continued economic crisis, flexible forms of labor have remained the norm.

— Latin America urbanized and industrialized early, and here flexible employment perhaps has been most prominent. Trends in wages have also been diverse. For example, positive trends in employment in Chile and Indonesia were accompanied by declines in real manufacturing wages.

The poor work in a variety of jobs, but working long hours in often precarious conditions for low wages is a constant. Jobs tend to be irregular and tenure is insecure. The urban poor may work in garment factories or at home for piece-rate work, operate small shops, sell food or cigarettes in the street, scavenge in garbage dumps, sweep streets and clean latrines, drive rickshaws, or seek day-work in construction. In the smaller cities, service jobs in the informal sector dominate because there is little manufacturing. Perhaps because of their concentration in these unskilled, irregular jobs, seasonality affects the earnings of the urban poor just as surely as it does those of the rural poor. CARE Bangladesh reports on the decrease in income and job availability among casual laborers such as rickshaw drivers and construction workers in Dhaka in the rainy season. This is primarily due to the outdoor nature of their work and the increased likelihood of illness.

The informal sector, where many of the poor work, is so large that it can no longer be seen as a marginal sector. In most countries it plays a central role in the economy. On average, 40 to 60 percent of urban workers in Asia are in small-scale enterprises, the Asian Development Bank's (ADB) preferred term for the informal sector. Fifty-two percent of urban workers in Sri Lanka and 30 percent in Thailand work in such small businesses. Thirty percent of all employment in Latin America is in the informal sector, rising to 50 percent if wage laborers in small-scale enterprises are included. About 1.7 million people work in the informal sector in the urban areas of Central America. The informal sector is at or near three-fourths of the labor force in Guatemala, El Salvador, and Honduras. Of course, this means that one-fourth of the labor force is in the formal sector.

The numbers of workers in the informal sector are significant, but can fluctuate widely over time. For example, in Nicaragua in 1985, the informal sector was substantially larger than formal but substantially smaller in 1993. Around 40 percent of the urban work force finds employment, including self-employment, in the informal sector in Kenya, and as much as 90 percent of the urban work force is in the informal sector in Freetown, Sierra Leone. Wage workers seem to be relatively rare in Africa, amounting to only about 25 percent of informal labor. It is generally assumed that family labor composes the bulk of the informal-sector labor, but apprentices may be one-half to four-fifths of the informal labor force in some countries in Africa, although significantly less in east Africa.

Whether a person finds a job in the formal or informal sector is to a large extent determined by education and training. But factors such as an economic sector where employment can be found, skills, neighborhood, caste, and gender can be even more important than human capital. In Central America, those employed in the informal sector tend to be the least educated; the youngest and the oldest; and female.

Informal-sector work is less assured than formal-sector work, but it can also possess a dynamic, entrepreneurial character that contrasts with the traditional view that it provides employment to those who cannot find formal-sector jobs. Average incomes from formal- and informal-sector work are often similar. Yet the "informal" label disguises the existence of at least two distinct strata: employers, including the self-employed, and intermediary traders in one group, and family laborers, employees, and apprentices in another. Even then, 'self-employed' covers a wide range of activities, where small owner-operators have wages roughlyequivalent to informal-sector wage labor, and may include those who work on commission. Differentiation among these groups is more apparent in Latin American cities but is also present in Africa.

Some interpret these statistics as evidence that, instead of being marginalized, informal-sector workers can earn and invest enough to climb out of poverty. Yet only a few really earn enough to do so. For example, in Africa, only informal urban workers with incomes in the highest 20 percent could be classified as genuine entrepreneurs, as owners of enterprises in more skill- and capital-intensive subsectors such as manufacturing and trade. Because a certain minimum of skills and capital is necessary to undertake these activities, successful workers are not drawn from the ranks of the unemployed but from those who are already employed and so have access to the necessary social, physical, and financial resources. Even for these workers, backward linkages to other informal activities that provide inputs are more prevalent than forward linkages to formal-sector businesses, especially in Africa.

While acknowledging the potential for dynamism, weaknesses inherent in the informal sector inhibit it from generating escapes from poverty for everyone. Lack of capital is one obstacle. Urban livelihood assessments in Bangladesh and Tanzania have pointed out the great need for additional credit facilities for both men and women. These assessments showed that many of the urban poor did participate in savings groups of some sort, including funeral funds or rotating funds, but the amounts of credit available for, say, business expansion were limited. In Tanzania, for example, most poor urban households relied on friends, relatives, or shopkeepers for credit when needed, and less than 10 percent had access to microcredit finance schemes or formal banks.

In developing countries where mechanization is still limited, human labor provides much of the power for productive economic work. For the poor, labor is their most important asset. Work capacity, performance, and productivity of workers are therefore generally important for income. This can lead to a situation where poor, malnourished workers perform poorly because of decreased working capacity, and therefore do not get access to better-paying jobs. Various studies support this assumption, showing positive associations between wage achievement and nutritional status as proxied by either body weight, body-mass index, stature, or caloric and protein intake.

In urban Brazil, this was true for both men and women and associations of wages with body-mass index in men were stronger among the less-educated. It is interesting to see that not only current short-term nutrition (reflected by body weight, body-mass index, and nutrient intake) is important for income, but also past chronic malnutrition (reflected in attained adult height), thus emphasizing the importance of nutrition during early life for human capital formation. An urban area of Bangladesh, illness-induced loss of employment was highly prevalent, particularly among the poorest households, and that it resulted in substantial losses of income. Households with a chronically incapacitated principal income earner were also two-and-a-half times more at risk of having a severely malnourished preschooler and at high risk of having other undernourished household members. Thus, poor adult health and nutritional status may be a serious constraint to the household's ability to generate income and protect its members from food insecurity and malnutrition.

Underemployment, rather than outright unemployment, is an important constraint to adequate income in many urban areas. The urban poor often have low-paying and unstable jobs in the informal sector.

Although the informal sector often pays low wages, many analysts also see the sector as a promising source of economic growth fueled by small entrepreneurs. Because labor is often the poor's only productive resource, their dependence on highly variable wages and employment puts them at high risk of poverty and food insecurity. The ability of the poor to cope with the vagaries of the labor market, but ultimately to take advantage of it to overcome their poverty, depends critically on their own skills, their access to functioning labor markets, and their health and nutritional status. Women often fare worse than men in the labor market because they often have less access to well-paying jobs in the formal sector and frequently work as unpaid family workers or in the informal sector.

Female labor-force participation has been steadily increasing throughout the developing world, particularly in Southeast Asia and Latin America. More than 60 percent of total female employment in the majority of West African cities is in the informal sector. In West Africa, women are 60-80 percent of the urban work force in trading; in Asia and Latin America, women dominate trading and manufacturing in the urban economy. Distinctions among informal- and formal-sector work blur for women, as it does with men. Women in Sub-Saharan Africa may leave formal-sector jobs like teachers or nurses to work in more lucrative informal-sector activities. Also, as do the men, women may hold multiple jobs, which they combine with their household and child care activities. These household responsibilities may force women to take part-time informal sector jobs or work at on flexible hours at home. Indeed, women have less access to better-paying jobs in the formal sector and are disproportionately represented among unpaid family workers and in the informal sector. Such gender distinctions are apparent in the study in Ghana, where 60 percent of the men are in wage labor while 75 percent of the women are self-employed.

Consequently, women's wages overall are usually lower than men's, and differences may be higher in the informal than in the formal sector. In India, women's wages are only 17 percent of men's; in Kenya, women's wages are 18 percent lower than men's. In Latin America, on average, females receive 51 percent of the average male's wages. The gap is due in part to women's generally lower level of education and their unavailability for night or overtime work because of legal barriers or family responsibilities. The lack of access to assets, such as education, training, and credit, continues to inhibit women's ability to acquire higher-paying jobs. Still, even after taking into account differences due to level of education, skill, and experience, a significant gap between the wages received by women and those received by men remains.

Challenges of Globalisation

Urbanization is increasingly accompanied by globalization through trade and financial liberalization, both of which reinforce the importance of cities and economies of scale. Urban labor markets in 2020 are likely to become even more competitive and flexible. To take advantage of open, expanded, but highly competitive markets, governments need to react rapidly to demands imposed by a global labor market and now rely less on inward-oriented development policies.

Highly diverse urban labor markets are here to stay. Rewards from these markets will differ dramatically, depending on each economy's ability to respond to and take advantage of global markets. Inequality is already quite pronounced in urban areas—and between urban and rural areas—and may become even more pronounced. Therefore, public policies that support urban labor will be needed to reduce the tensions that may arise from globalization and to ensure equitable access to rewarding labor markets, especially for the poor.

Many policymakers have indicated a desire to reduce rates of urbanization, but this is not a reasonable strategy. Continued economic growth under open markets will remain the most likely development scenario, one that probably will not lead to de-urbanization. Policies should focus on improving the effects of inevitable urbanization and migration, for example, by providing support to migrants rather than discriminating against them. Certainly in many countries rural development will remain crucial to reducing poverty and improving food security and nutrition, but this should not bar urban policies from supporting the livelihood strategies of both urban migrants and urban residents. Macroeconomic policies have tended to assume that liberalization and deregulation would lead to economic growth and creation of employment.

However, such policies by themselves may have only limited impact on poverty and may even have specific negative consequences for the urban poor. Macroeconomic policies need to be context-specific and sensitive to their effects on urban labor markets, especially on the conditions that need to be fulfilled to enable the urban poor to participate in the benefits of economic growth on an equitable basis. Policymakers must also create targeted programs for the urban poor and food insecure. Up to now, urban policies, particularly those of donors, have tended to focus on issues of service delivery, shelter, and infrastructure. More thought needs to be given to employment-guarantee schemes in urban areas.

Macroeconomic policies and safety-net programs, however, are only part of the urban employment agenda. Policies need to pay more attention to enhancing productive employment for the urban poor—that is, ensuring employability of and equal opportunities for the urban poor in an increasingly competitive urban labor market. Policies should promote access of the poor to financial capital through microfinance schemes; build the capabilities of the urban poor through formal education and training so that they can secure high-quality employment; and take into account the heterogeneity of labor markets and fluctuating nature of labor supply and demand. Governments may also need to pursue special policies to reduce gender disparities and to break through the labor market segmentation that inhibits certain groups from taking up jobs in more rewarding activities.

Urban expansion and issues of food supply and distribution to and in the cities have four major consequences for urban food security. The first is the competition between demands for land needed for housing, industry, and infrastructure and land needed for agricultural production within and around cities. Agriculturally productive lands are likely to be lost in this competition.

The second consequence is the increasing quantities of food that must be brought into cities and distributed within the expanding urban areas. This means more trucks coming into cities, contributing to traffic congestion and air pollution. It also means additional stress on existing food distribution infrastructure and facilities, most of which are already inefficient, unhygienic, and environmentally unfriendly. The third consequence is the modification of consumption habits and food purchasing behaviours. Consumers in urban areas—who generally pay up to 30 percent more for their food compared with their rural counterparts—have less time to spend preparing food. Therefore, the demand for more convenience and processed meals increases, raising issues of food quality and safety in terms of the use of appropriate inputs, particularly safe water, in food processing.

The final consequence for urban food security is the likelihood that low-income urban households will reside farther and farther away from food markets, often in slums that do not have water, roads, or electricity. Since these households are also less likely to have refrigerators, they face additional time and transport costs in accessing food daily.

As urban expansion continues apace, the overall cost of supplying, distributing, and accessing food is likely to increase further and, with it, the number of urban households that are food insecure. The challenge of feeding cities therefore lies in facilitating consumer access to food and ensuring that required investments are forthcoming for increasing food production, processing, and distribution capacities and services under hygienic, healthy, and environmentally sound conditions. Adequately meeting this challenge will promote the development of peri-urban and rural areas.

To feed ever-growing cities, more food will have to be imported or produced in areas presently under cultivation or on new lands (which are likely to be more distant and less productive).

Urban and peri-urban agriculture can be an important source of food for some cities, especially when the national rural food production, marketing, and transportation systems are not well developed. However, urban and peri-urban agriculture pose a number of problems that stem from their close proximity to densely populated areas, with animals and humans sharing the same air, water, and soil resources. Inappropriate use of chemicals and solid and liquid wastes in farming can contaminate food, soil, and water resources used for drinking and food processing. Raising livestock in and close to urban areas may also increase health risks for residents. While many of the problems could be solved by information and extension assistance, local city authorities have often responded instead by destroying food crops and evicting food producers from public lands.

Much of the expected higher cost of feeding cities is likely to be accounted for by transportation costs as well as by posthar-vest food losses from inappropriate food handling and packaging, the need to collect food from a large number of small farmers, and frequent delays from road check points and (often illegal) taxation. These food losses can be as high as 35 percent for perishable food products, while transportation costs can reach as high as 90 percent of the overall food marketing margin.

In developing countries, a large share of food passes through wholesale markets and is then redistributed within the urban area through retail markets, shops, street sellers, and supermarkets, all of which have problems. Many wholesale markets are old, have not adapted to the increase in food quantities, are not properly managed and maintained, and are in areas that urban expansion has transformed into central, high-density spots. The latter factor increases traffic congestion and eliminates space for market expansion. Storage facilities, particularly cold storage, are insufficient or badly managed or both. These difficulties create additional costs and losses for traders and lead to increased food contamination.

At the retail level, supermarkets and hypermarkets (combined supermarkets and department stores) play only a minor role in urban food distribution in developing economies. Even in Latin American cities this sector accounts for only 30 percent of food retail sales, even though it has developed rapidly since the 1970s. Such markets usually cater to the needs of high-income families, are located in middle- to high-income urban areas, and distribute mainly manufactured food products and imports. Staples produced locally are only a small part of these markets' food sales. They usually rely instead on direct contracts with distant food producers for their supplies.

The traditional retail food sector dominates developing-country markets, making it central to improving food distribution in cities. But public retail markets, which tend to be concentrated in city centers, are usually congested, unhealthy, and insecure. Spontaneous markets are often seen by local city authorities as a cause of traffic, health, and safety problems, and the sellers are consequently harassed by municipal police. In recent times many cities have experienced a steep rise in informal-sector retailing, which fills an important gap in the distribution chain because it is a convenient source of cheap food for low-income urban consumers. It also serves as an important source of revenue for low-income households engaged in these activities.

Most city and local authorities believe that food supply and distribution issues are not their responsibility and instead concentrate on public health, education, housing, sanitation, and transport. However, these authorities affect food supply and distribution systems directly or indirectly through, for example, health and housing regulations and construction and management of processing and market infrastructure. Fortunately, awareness is growing of the need for city and local authorities to play a proactive and coordinating role in actions to improve urban food security.

City authorities need to adopt policies that support those involved in food supply and distribution activities by promoting private investment, getting involved in food supply and distribution themselves (by facilitating urban and peri-urban agriculture and by providing the necessary planning, infrastructure, facilities, services, information, and regulations), coordinating public and private development initiatives, and mediating between the central government and the private food sector. When formulating food supply and distribution policies and strategies, city and local authorities should rely on four strategic principles:

1) adopt an approach that is consultative, participatory, open-minded, alliance-seeking, and technically sound and involves the private sector;

2) promote competition and reduce the influence of large intermediaries;

3) leave to the private sector facilities and services that can best be run as businesses; and

4) encourage effective development that lowers the cost of living and stimulates employment growth in the city.

City and local authorities can also play a crucial role in national food-security policies by complementing efforts by farmers' associations and local rural authorities to lobby governments on programs that will reduce food production and marketing constraints. City and local authorities also need to support urban and peri-urban agriculture with information campaigns to minimize adverse health and environmental consequences and with appropriately enforced regulations that allow and facilitate urban and peri-urban agricultural activities. City and local authorities can play a fundamental role in ensuring that food distribution issues are appropriately considered when new infrastructure, facilities, and services are being planned. These considerations include location, type, and standards of the services and structures, as well as the financial capacity of the users, in order to enable them to pay usage fees and keep up market facilities. Other key issues are the management of markets and the criteria for allocating space for building markets.

While much of the food production and distribution is out of the control of city and local authorities, these authorities must coordinate with other organizations that are major stakeholders in the food production and distribution system, and they should promote and support policies that ensure urban food security and stimulate private investment as well as private participation in planning decisions. Only if low-income urban households have access to affordable, good-quality food through the programs and policies noted here can they achieve food security.

Role of Women in Urbal Food Security

As the urban population in all developing regions grows over the next 20 years, governments and families will face unique challenges in their efforts to ensure the well-being of millions of children. They will have to take into account changes in women's roles, in strategies for childcare, and in the means of obtaining food security. All these changes will have major implications for the livelihoods of people residing in the new urban megacities.

Many studies in developing countries show that women contribute as much or more than men do to family food security and children's nutritional status when unpaid work is included in the estimation. Nowadays more women also work for income than ever before. Globally women's rates of participation in the labor force were 54 percent in 1950 and 66 percent in 1990 and are projected to reach almost 70 percent in 2010. Urban women now are more likely to work for income when their children are very young and to stay in the labor force longer than they were previously. Worldwide they enter the labor market at high rates in their 20s, increase labor force participation through their 30s and 40s, and leave work only after age 50. The percent of households that rely on women's financial contribution for food security is also increasing.

Women provide the main source of income in more than 20 percent of households in Latin America, Sub-Saharan Africa, and most of Asia. Even in dual-parent families, women are contributing a higher percentage of income than before. The forces that have increased women's labor force participation—urbanization and globalization—have pulled women into jobs that are of lower quality (low-skilled jobs with no security or protection), part-time, home-based, or all of these.

More than 80 percent of women work in largely gender-segregated occupations, and women on average still earn less than 70 percent of what men earn. Since women are in lower-skilled and temporary jobs, they are more likely to lose jobs than are men during financial crises. Women also still lag far behind men in having the skills to handle new technologies, making them less likely to get higher-paying jobs that require these skills.

Urban residence can have mixed consequences for women and children. On the one hand, women workers in an urban economy can potentially earn a higher percentage of the family income. Since percentage of income earned has been shown to relate to decisionmaking in the family, these women might be less tied to traditional restrictions, such as food taboos during pregnancy. According to a recent United Nations study, urban women also have fewer children, and they and their children are much more likely to be literate than rural women and theirs.

Services such as family planning may be more available in urban areas, and women's increased independence may lead to higher self-esteem and recognition of rights. On the other hand, urban women who work may be more vulnerable to violence and harassment at the workplace than rural women and may be forced into informal work such as street vending that offers few protections.

Many women with little income must raise their children surrounded by the inadequate infrastructure of urban slums. For new migrants to urban squatter settlements, support systems may be weak, leading to stress and family dysfunction. Poor or sporadic job opportunities for men, as well as the need to obtain food with cash, may result in a decline in male support for families and less food security.

Women are now much more likely to work when their children are under 12 months old, a period of time when children have the greatest need of intensive care for good growth and development. Workers in the formal sector, for example, are limited to 12 weeks of maternity leave in most countries, even though about 6 months of exclusive breastfeeding is recommended. For women working in the informal sector, any leave at all is taken at the risk of losing income and job opportunities. Although in some countries working mothers breastfeed less, work itself does not necessarily limit breastfeeding, nor does mothers' work seem to affect children's nutritional status in some developing countries.

In two studies in urban Latin America, income earned by the mother when the child was at least 12 months of age was positively associated with the child's nutritional status when income levels were controlled for. Women's income had a stronger positive association with children's nutrition than men's income. However, when women did not have the power to decide how to spend their income on children, wage work led to negative effects on children's nutritional status.

Adequate childcare is essential for working mothers. In urban Ghana, women's strategies for providing childcare were more important for children's nutritional status than family income.

In urban Guatemala, maternal employment did not increase children's chances of malnutrition unless they were cared for by a preteen. Work at home, however, often considered to be a positive option, has been associated with poorer nutritional status for children if demands of the work are intense and time-bound (for example, piecework). In sum, when mothers are poor—with time-intensive, low-paid, and inflexible work; no control over earnings; and no good alternative caregivers—infants are at risk of poor growth.

Some women who work during their child's first year of life have no other sources of support. For these women, work is a survival strategy; the alternative is starvation for mother and child.

Day care in the urban slums of developing countries, particularly for children under three, is usually woefully inadequate in coverage and quality. The most common day-care centers are run by governments or private voluntary organizations. These centers are likely to be attended only by children over three and have extremely limited coverage because of the large investment needed in buildings and equipment. Yet childcare is clearly necessary. United Nations data from 23 countries in Africa, Asia, and Latin America show that a majority of working women with children under five work away from home.

Some innovative approaches to childcare include family day-care homes, in which one mother watches five or six neighbour children in her home; or mobile crèches, which involve childcare facilities set up near the employment site of working mothers. In lieu of day-care options, families use older female siblings (much more than male siblings), thus keeping girls out of school; other family members; and neighbours. There are cases of families resorting to drastic strategies, such as giving children a dose of opium so that they will sleep during the day.

More women will work for earnings in the next 20 years, particularly when their children are young. Although the smaller family sizes associated with urbanization should decrease the time needed for childcare, this may turn out not to be the case. Many urban parents will want their children to be schooled in order to attain the best opportunities for a successful life. The consequent focus on developing children's language and social skills may increase rather than decrease time commitments for care.

Three factors have been shown to reduce the negative effects of maternal work on young children: helping mothers not to work when their children are very young, providing an adequate wage rate and flexible working hours, and providing reasonable alternative childcare. Ensuring these will be necessary for the health and well-being of an urbanizing society. Policies are also needed that provide women protection against returning to work too soon after giving birth.

Maternity protection legislation is woefully inadequate. Whereas 192 countries have ratified the Convention on the Rights of the Child, only 38 have ratified the International Labour Organization's 1952 Maternity Protection Convention. Even if signed, the latter's provisions apply to only a small proportion of the population.

Cultural and social attitudes also need to reflect women's equality in the work force. For example, although girls are attending school at much higher rates and are performing as well as or better than boys in many countries, these gains have not been translated into correspondingly equal employment and training opportunities, according to the International Labour Organization's 1999 World Employment Report.

Policies can go a long way toward improving women's income by, for example, implementing gender-blind minimum wage rates, organizing informal or self-employed labor, and supporting urban development programmes.

To improve outcomes for children, governments can legalize squatter settlements after a period of time to allow people living in them access to services, and they can invest in health, day care, and infrastructure. Training women for skilled jobs is also a key component for raising incomes and thereby improving child health. Outside pressures, such as the Beijing Conference on Women, and efforts of United Nations and bilateral agencies, can help, but sustained efforts are needed within countries to implement and monitor good policies.

Caring adequately for urban children will be essential for their nutritional status and the health of urban society. Providing alternative childcare means that women's work in childcare, which was traditionally unpaid, must now be paid for. Model urban programs, such as Child Friendly Cities Programs, do invest in childcare for working women, but these efforts are not enough. Innovative approaches are needed to provide good child-care, especially for the youngest age group. These approaches must rely on partnerships between employers, workers, and government to provide adequate care. Innovative strategies could include support for parental childcare cooperatives, social insurance to enable mothers or fathers to stay home after the birth of a child, childcare linked to schools, and even the involvement of elders in childcare. Good childcare is not cheap, but the investments made at this age are perhaps the most important for the next generation and for working women themselves.

4

Food Security and Health Systems

A number of factors will affect the future shape of urban food insecurity and malnutrition. Because urban dwellers must buy most of their food, urban food security depends mostly on whether the household can afford to buy food, given prices and incomes. High per-unit costs of food result from inefficient urban food-marketing systems and the fact that the poor usually can buy only small quantities of food at a time rather than in bulk. Macroeconomic policies are also important. Inflation, depreciation in the exchange rate, and the removal of key consumer or producer subsidies can all push prices up.

Policies to improve urban food security must therefore seek to improve market efficiency and maintain stable prices. Logically, income security is also crucial to food security for urban dwellers. Yet with little human or financial capital, the poor are forced to take casual, insecure jobs. These jobs often experience seasonal ups and downs, just as in rural areas. For example, demand for construction workers can decline drastically during the rainy season. Garment workers may be laid off when the holiday rush dies down. With their abundance of labor, but often little else, the poor find competition for jobs is fierce. To lift the poor from poverty, programs and policies should concentrate on creating jobs and on increasing the capacity of the poor to find and hold more-secure, higher-paying jobs or to expand their own businesses and generate new jobs.

Governments, communities, and the private sector should cooperate to provide the elements for private sector success, much of which depends on a capable, if not extensive, government. At the same time, targeted income or food programs and more general social security and unemployment programs will continue to be necessary to provide for those who are left behind or who cannot work, including the elderly and the sick. Programs may also need to address issues of land and housing security, as secure tenure helps ensure that the poor do not lose their investments in tangible assets or in social networks. However, efforts to improve urban livelihoods must go beyond a focus on urban jobs.

Urban and rural lives are intertwined through goods, services, and people. In many cities, a majority of urban dwellers depend indirectly on agriculture for their livelihoods, through employment in food transport, retailing, and processing. Survival strategies may involve maintaining links with a home community in rural areas, through a plot of land or continued connections with family. Policies for improving urban livelihoods, then, must take into account the complexity of urban–rural links and recognize that rural conditions affect urban livelihoods as well.

Urban food security may also have a more direct link with agriculture. Even in large, congested cities, the urban poor may have a home garden or raise small animals as part of a coping strategy. This urban production, often done by women, can complement household incomes and improve the quality of urban diets. Urban planners and local governments should consider how to incorporate environmentally sound urban agriculture in their plans. Of course, food security is not enough for good nutrition. A healthy household environment and good care and feeding practices are essential as well. The threats to good nutrition for both adults and children in urban areas differ from those in rural areas. The most substantial threats to health of the poor in the cities come from flimsy and overcrowded housing amid filthy conditions—uncollected garbage unsafe water, overflowing sewers—and from the inability of the poor to get good health care. Even when health facilities are available, the poor often have no access to these services because of an inability to pay.

According to UNICEF and the World Health Organization, for example, globally less than 20 percent of the urban poor have access to safe water, compared with 80 percent of the rich. Poverty and inequality are clearly major determinants of health and nutrition outcomes in the city. Potentially harmful changes in diets also accompany urbanization. Because urban dwellers often face time constraints and have greater exposure to advertising and easier access to supermarkets and fast-food vendors, they often consume more processed and prepared foods. The typical urban diet results in higher levels of some micronutrients and animal proteins than the rural one, but it also means higher intakes of saturated and total fat and sugar and lower intakes of fiber.

Combined with a sedentary lifestyle, this diet increases the risk of chronic diseases, including obesity. The public health sector faces a significant challenge in trying to overcome the malnutrition and poor health caused by poverty at the same time it responds to diseases associated with wealth and industrialization. Challenges to child nutrition come from this unhealthy physical environment and from inadequate caring and feeding practices.

Urban women end breastfeeding two to three months earlier than rural women, perhaps depriving their children of needed nutrients and reducing immunity. Women in urban areas also often work outside the home, which may mean they have less time and more difficulty in caring for their children. Policies to promote child nutrition in urban areas should focus not only on increasing incomes, especially women's, but also on encouraging good feeding and caring practices, including provision of easily accessible quality child care for those mothers who work.

Good caring practices are possible even for the poor—as they frequently depend more on knowledge rather than income levels—and have been shown to counter the effects of low income on nutritional status. The greatest difference between solutions to food and nutrition insecurity in rural and urban areas is probably that in rural areas development can often be addressed through broad-brush interventions affecting agriculture, which drives the rural economy. While agricultural growth may also help to reduce urban food insecurity, the income sources in urban areas are more diverse, as are underlying causes and actors in the urban environment.

Effective policies and programs will require a holistically conceived response that coordinates actions across actors and levels—from the household (to raise incomes, for example), to the community (to install a water system), to far beyond (to promote labor-intensive growth by the government). In any case, the most effective, relevant policies will emerge from a system of governance that firmly connects the needs of the poor to a politically responsive local government that has the technical and institutional capacity to act. Programs should work to strengthen the poor's ability to organize, make demands, and affect local authorities and to strengthen the municipality's understanding of its responsibility to respond.

Some argue that concern about urban poverty is misplaced—that rural areas continue to hold most of the poor, food insecure, and malnourished and that they will for many years to come. Many analysts and governments seem complacent because their countries are not industrialized or highly urban. As we look to 2020, is such complacency justified? Clearly not. First, the experiences of the industrialized world clearly show that developing countries are simply not going to "urbanize" themselves out of poverty. Governments and development agencies must take seriously the shift in poverty, food insecurity, and malnutrition from rural to urban areas. Second, in highly urbanized regions such as Latin America, the geographic center of poverty has already shifted: in these countries more poor people already live in the cities than in the countryside. Finally, even in countries that are still highly rural and where rural poverty predominates, millions of poor people live in cities. These people deserve not to be forgotten.

The perception that urban poverty exists only in industrialized countries is not matched by reality. In Mozambique, for example, with a poverty rate of 69 percent, 2 million poor people live in urban areas, more than the number of urban poor in highly urbanized Colombia and more than half the number of urban poor in much more populous Indonesia. Even in highly rural countries, then, urban poverty, food insecurity, and malnutrition are problems of today, not tomorrow. For the sake of the millions of hungry and undernourished people living in cities today, as well as for the sake of those millions who may be forced to live there tomorrow, governments, development agencies, and communities must act now.

They must work forcefully, confidently, and reasonably to promote policies, including those that promote rural development, to confront the rising specter of urban poverty, hunger, and malnutrition and so achieve the 2020 vision of sustainable food and nutrition security for all.

Urban Diets

There is ample evidence that urban diets are quantitatively and qualitatively different from rural diets in all regions of the developing world. In general, rural dwellers tend to eat more cereals, especially coarse grains, while urban dwellers tend to eat more varied diets with higher levels of animal protein and fats.

Meat, poultry, fish, and milk products were all consumed more frequently by small-town and, especially, large-city dwellers. In Burkina Faso, rice accounted for 35 to 46 percent of the cereal expenditures of residents of the capital city (all income groups) compared to insignificant amounts in three different rural areas of the country; and in Kenya, 'quasi-urban' groups devoted a proportion of their total cereal expenditures to bread (as opposed to maize) that was threefold greater than agricultural households of similar incomes. Finally, in a weighed intake study in Bangladesh, urban slum dwellers consumed more oils, leafy vegetables, pulses, and potatoes than a predominantly landless group of rural peasants, but consumed less cereals and other vegetables. Similar findings have been reported from Brazil, Turkey, and Pakistan.

The different composition of urban diets relative to rural diets has important implications for the nutrient adequacy of urban dwellers. This may relate to different age/sex compositions of urban households, different activity levels, and, therefore, different energy requirements, or perhaps inadequacies of the data collection methods in capturing the more diverse food sources in urban areas, particularly snacks and street foods. The digestibility of the rural diet was lower than that of the urbandiet, with an apparent absorption of energy of 89 percent (rural) versus 95 percent (urban). Even bigger discrepancies were seen for protein, with apparent digestibilities of 67 percent and 90 percent for rural and urban, respectively. The studies noted above all suggest that the micronutrient intake of the urban poor is likely to be higher than that of their rural counterparts, particularly for vitamin A, vitamin C, folate, and some minerals. These differences may affect even the nutritional status of breast-fed infants, since multicountry studies of the nutrient content of human breast milk have indicated that protein, nitrogen, vitamin A, and iron levels tend to be lower in rural than in poor urban samples.

The controlled trial of urban and rural Mexican diets that both iron and calcium intakes were higher for the rural diet, while zinc intakes were similar. The particular interest of this study lies in the fact that the authors were able to investigate the relative bioavailability of zinc, iron, and calcium in the two diets. All three minerals were markedly better-absorbed from the urban-type diet than from the rural-type diet, presumably because of the lower concentration of inhibitors such as phytates, the greater concentration of promoters such as ascorbic acid, and the contribution of animal food sources, which contain more available forms of iron (heme-iron) and promote absorption of calcium. There are various reasons why urban diets tend to be more diverse than rural diets-namely higher income, changing values and norms, and cultural diversity.

The towns of Africa, working women have less time for food preparation and have a tendency toward higher-priced, 'convenience' source of calories; the higher price is counterbalanced by savings in time and transport. In an urban area of Sri Lanka provides strong evidence that the opportunity cost of women's time can be an important determinant of food consumption patterns. The value of time of the primary woman had a positive effect on bread consumption and a negative impact on rice consumption, which requires preparation and cooking time. Furthermore, because of the greater availability of different foodstuffs in the urban market, urban consumers (especially those at low-income levels) tend to be more price sensitive than rural consumers, and to switch between substitute foods more easily. In times of crises, poor urban households in Guayaquil substituted potatoes with plantains and fresh fruit juices with powdered fruit-flavored drinks. Some of the substitutions are likely to have a negative nutritional impact, especially when they involve replacing nutrient-dense foods with 'empty calories' as is the case with the fruit juice example above.

The poor sanitary conditions of many developing-country cities are notorious. Combined with poor hygiene practices, these conditions create a situation in which food safety is severely compromised. Street foods make up a large proportion of the foods eaten in developing-country cities, especially for certain age groups. In a food frequency survey of secondary school students in Port-au-Prince, Haiti, it was found that, on average, 25 percent of the students' daily energy and 15 percent of their daily protein were obtained from street foods. Similar results were obtained in a study of Nigerian adolescents, who also obtained 25 percent of their daily energy from street foods, as well as more than half their total intakes of protein, iron, calcium, vitamins A and C, and thiamin. Other studies have shown that in Kuala Lumpur, Malaysia, and Iloilo, the Philippines, almost 25 percent and 30 percent of household expenditure, respectively, are spent on street foods. In Accra, households spend one-third of their food budget on street foods. The importance of street foods in the diets of vulnerable groups in developing countries (especially preschool children and pregnant and lactating women) has not been adequately documented. Thee high levels of sugar, salt, and fat in many street foods, a factor that should be taken into account when assessing the overall impact of street food consumption on dietary intakes.

With respect to the safety of street foods, both the Expert Consultation of the Food and Agriculture Organization of the United Nations in 1988 and the results of a multicountry the types of pathogens found in street foods were similar to those found in foods prepared and served indoors, and that food hygiene practices of street vendors were similar to those of indoor restaurant workers. A study carried out in Colombia suggested that foods of animal origin, those with a high protein or moisture content, a relatively high pH, or a relatively large number of ingredients tended to present the highest risk of contamination.

Constraints to better practices identified were the lack of potable water for cooking, drinking, washing utensils, and hygiene; improper handling and storage of ingredients and cooked foods; lack of facilities for waste disposal; use of unlawfuladditives, and poor personal hygiene by street vendors. One study in India analyzed water and food samples from both ambulant vendors and restaurants in the city of Pune, and found that the restaurants were no more hygienic than the ambulant vendors. There are no available data comparing the levels of microbial contamination in street foods and the foods poor city dwellers commonly prepare and eat at home. The determinants of reliance on street foods have not been well documented, although several possible determinants are mentioned in the FAO Expert Consultation report. These include reduced transportation costs and time needed to obtain meals; high opportunity costs of cooking at home for working women; lack of appropriate cooking facilities in many urban dwellings, and the fact that street foods are often cheaper because vendors can take advantage of economies of scale in their preparation.

Major qualitative differences are seen between rural and urban diets. These differences persist even when analyses are restricted to groups with broadly similar incomes and result in significant rural-urban differentials in intakes of many nutrients. Even those nutrients such as iron, which do not appear to be consumed at consistently higher levels in urban diets, may be better absorbed because they are obtained from animal rather than vegetable sources. The relatively high cost of traditional staples in urban areas, the greater range of potential 'substitute' foods, and the opportunity costs of women's preparation time have all been suggested as possible determinants of the greater diversity of urban diets. Street foods are a major feature of urban eating, but the health and nutritional consequences of this pattern-especially for young children and women-have not been investigated. The trade-off between greater convenience and perhaps lower cost on the one hand, and poor nutritional quality and higher risks of contamination on the other, remains to be fully explored.

Nutrition Transition

Increasing urbanization in the developing world has brought a remarkably rapid shift toward a high incidence of obesity and noncommunicable diseases such as diabetes and coronary problems, at a time when large segments of the population still face undernutrition and poverty-related diseases. Obesity and its related diseases, for example, affect 25–50 percent of the population in countries as disparate as Kuwait, Mexico, Thailand, and Tunisia. This "nutrition transition"—a term used to describe shifts in diet, physical activity, health, and nutrition—can be traced to higher incomes, the influence of mass media and food marketing, and a range of changes in the nature of work and leisure. Where a person stands in the nutrition transition depends on how far that person has moved away from a traditional diet and toward a diet common in the West, with all the accompanying changes in physical activity and body composition.

According to this qualitative measure of transition, urban areas throughout the developing world are much further along in the process than rural areas. On a regional basis, most Latin American and Caribbean countries and selected countries in North Africa, the Middle East, and East Asia have shifted the most in nutritional status and dietary and activity patterns. The most promising policy option for remedying the ill effects of this transition appears to be a combination of price policies, education, and specific program actions at the school level.

Urban residents have vastly different lifestyles than rural residents. These lifestyles create their own patterns of food demand and time allocation. The consequences for diets, physical activity, and health have been enormous. The urban diet. Urban residents obtain a much higher proportion of energy from fats and sweeteners than do rural residents, even in the poorest areas of very low-income countries. Most urban dwellers also eat greater amounts of animal products than their rural counterparts.

Urbanites consume a more diversified diet and more micronutrients and animal proteins than rural residents but with considerably higher intakes of refined carbohydrates, processed foods, and saturated and total fat and lower intakes of fiber. Countries that have an urban population share of 75 percent consume about 4 percentage points more energy from vegetable and animal fat and 12 percentage points more energy from sweeteners than countries with an urban population share of 25 percent. This holds true even at low levels of gross national product (GNP). Related research has shown that lower-income countries are able now to afford far more energy from fat than they could in the past at the same level of GNP. Thus, not only are urban diets changing, but they are changing at an earlier stage of economic development.

Increasing incomes partially explain this turn toward fattier foods and sweeteners, but there also seems to be an upward shift in consumer demand for sweeteners and higher-fat products at any given income level. Greater penetration of mass media and modern marketing approaches into the lives of urban residents may account for this shift in food choices. Little is understood, though, about the impact of media and marketing on the nutrition transition. Economic work that relies on income and price changes cannot account for these shifts in behaviour. The ability to produce lower-cost foods that contain oils and sweeteners has facilitated the transition as well. In the last half century, new technologies and new oilseed varieties, for example, have made it much easier to create high-quality, low-cost edible oils as alternatives to much more expensive animal fats. Urban physical activity patterns.

New technologies in work and leisure, along with shifting diets, have increased obesity levels in the urban areas of developing countries. Body composition has changed in tandem with the transformation of the preindustrial agrarian economy into an industrial, urban one. As this transformation has accelerated, the service sector has grown rapidly, capital-intensive processes have come to dominate industrial production, and time-allocation patterns have changed dramatically. Urban work now requires less physical exertion and allows more leisure. Leisure activity has been transformed, particularly by changes in food preparation, production, and processing and by the revolutionary penetration of the mass media into the developing world. Almost all Chinese households, for example, owned at least one working television set by 1997.

Changes in diet and physical activity have accelerated the rate of increase in obesity in the developing world. Trends in obesity are not limited to one region, country, or racial or ethnic group. In many cases, such as with women in Egypt and South Africa and across ages and sexes in Mexico, the lower- and middle-income countries have overweight levels that match those of the United States and exceed those of most European countries. Obesity levels are much higher in urban areas: in China and Indonesia adult obesity is twice as prevalent in urban areas as it is in rural areas; in the Congo it is almost six times as prevalent. The Middle East, the Western Pacific, and Latin America have far higher levels of obesity than other developing regions.

Higher-income populations in the developing world also have much higher levels of obesity. This relationship also held a century ago among European and North American populations, but the reverse is now true: the poor in Europe and North America experience far higher levels of obesity and diet-related chronic diseases than their rich counterparts. This reversal has occurred recently among urban Brazilian women and in Chile. A range of changes in health have accompanied this nurition transition. Most immediate among these seems to be the emerging epidemic of diabetes, stroke, and hypertension, all diet-related chronic diseases. The evidence from some Asian and Latin American countries is particularly worrying. The economic costs of diet-related noncommunicable diseases in fact have surpassed the cost of malnutrition in China. A unique issue emerging from this transition is the increasingly frequent double burden of undernutrition and obesity in the same household. The prevalence of households with both overweight and underweight members in Brazil, for example, is 11 percent.

How can the food policy and public health communities, already burdened by the challenges of poverty, undernutrition, and underdevelopment, deal with the seemingly contradictory goal of promoting both greater and lesser food intake? How can they address the prevention of obesity when they focus on undernutrition and poverty?

The solutions common to both undernutrition and overnutrition and promoting them through education and more direct interventions. Promulgating nutrient-dense fruits and vegetables, for example, would reduce caloric intake and improve micronutrient status. Another such solution is breast-feeding, which offers food rich in nutrients and reduces obesity and coronary heart disease. Policymakers must also take direct action to reduce obesity at all age levels. Few large-scale efforts have done this successfully, though Scandinavian countries did change their diets and reduce coronary heart disease between 1976 and the 1980s. To do so, the Scandinavians focused on price and other policies, such as fish subsidies, to encourage healthier diets.

During the 1990s Singapore reduced child obesity through a combination of changes in school diet and increased fitness and physical activity programming. A major first step toward a healthier population is awareness of the problems related to the nutrition transition. Many developing countries are realizing the importance of this issue. They must continue their efforts and develop programs and policies for agricultural production, nutrition, food marketing, and education that will help them to successfully confront the nutrition transition and achieve sustainable food and nutrition security.

Threats to Urban Health

The future looks more urban than ever. As urban demographer Ellen Brennan has observed, "In a few years, roughly around 2006, a crossroads will be reached in human history, when half of the world's population will be residing in urban areas." By 2030, three-fifths of the world's population will live in urban areas. Evidence indicates, though, that this future may be more unequal than ever.

The majority of urban people will live in Asia, Africa, and Latin America—in countries that are getting relatively poorer, not richer. The latest World Bank data show the ratio of income per capita in the richest countries over that in the poorest countries has increased from 11 to 1 in 1870, to 38 to 1 in 1960, and to 52 to 1 in 1985. And poverty in the poorest countries appears to have become more urbanized. An urban world with growing inequality bodes ill for the health of urban dwellers. In addition, globalization—the rapid global movement of capital, ideas, skills, and employment connected to the concentration of power in the private sector—is changing the urban physical and social environment. Consequent changes in diet and physical activity are affecting the health of all urban people.

Accompanying these changes is the fact that the poor rely increasingly on the wealthy.

The United Nations Environment Programme (UNEP) reports that private foreign investment controlled by corporations was worth US$250 billion in 1996, in contrast with less than US$50 billion in official development assistance. In the same year, foreign exchange trading by big investors amounted to US$350 trillion—more than 10 times the world's gross domestic product. The wealth of the world is now in the hands of a tiny minority of people. The ratio of the average income of the world's wealthiest 5 percent to the world's poorest 5 percent increased from 78 to 1 in 1988 to 123 to 1 in 1993. This shift of financial and political power influences development opportunities for urban areas. Cities compete against each other for foreign and private investment on the basis of their population and resources.

Urban development relies on low-cost urban labor in one city or country competing with low-cost urban labor in another. As a result the well-being and health of the world's urban people can become precarious.

Urban areas could be healthy places for people to grow, live, and work. Health depends on equitable availability of a simple set of good physical conditions, such as clean and plentiful water, clean air, uncontaminated and adequate food, access to sanitary home and work environments, protective shelter, safe and remunerative employment, and safe environments in which to move around. At first, the urban health picture looks quite simple. Urban development, based on industrial or manufacturing processes, provides employment, which leads to a wealthier society.

A richer society, in turn, can pay for better delivery of water, sanitation, health services, and education. Ultimately this translates into better health. Witness the mortality rate of children under five of 5 per 1,000 in highly urbanized industrialised countries, as opposed to about 170 per 1,000 in 30 percent urbanized Sub-Saharan Africa and about 120 per 1,000 in 27 percent urbanized South Asia. But this simple view conceals the impact on health of inequalities between and within urban centers.

Urbanization in developing countries has not taken place in a context that enables good physical conditions for health to be easily realized. Historically, the industrialized countries of the northern hemisphere built their economies by transforming and trading the natural-resource bases of Asia, Latin America, and Africa. These northern countries went on to control the trade system, limiting the ability of the so-called "developing" countries to follow the same route toward urbanization and development.

Developing countries have three significant urban health agendas, each linked to the issue of inequity between and within cities: the resolution of health problems stemming from (1) urban poverty, such as infectious diseases and poor nutrition, (2) the current "dirty" industrialization process, and (3) the social and political environment within cities.

An estimated 600 million or more people live in low-income settlements in African, Asian, and Latin American cities and towns. This urban poverty is generally accompanied by limited and poor-quality water, food, and housing, as well as limited education and low-paid hazardous work. Urban poverty is the most direct result of constricted urban development opportunities, which are driven by inequalities between countries and cities. Undernutrition, malnutrition, and infectious diseases are widespread in African and Asian urban centers because of poverty. Malnutrition increases the risk of infectious disease. Death rates for infectious diseases—such as diarrhea, measles, and tuberculosis—and for infant mortality among urban poor children in developing countries can be up to 100 times higher than those for urban children in industrialized countries. The World Bank calculated that in 1998 acute respiratory diseases (about 111 million years of life lost) and diarrheal diseases (about 94 million years of life lost) were the world's major health problems, and they were concentrated in urban areas of developing countries. In one poor part of Calcutta that contains 4 million people, about one out of every fifth child under 5 and adult over 65 dies due to diarrheal and respiratory diseases. Malaria and dengue fever represent significant health problems in urban areas of Africa and Asia. Thus the first challenge is to provide a solution to the disease-causing environments propagated by poverty.

Pollution from dirty industrial development adds to health risks. Metropolitan areas in developing countries often rely on attracting investment for rapid, environmentally dirty industrial development. Transportation also contributes significantly to local air pollution and global warming. UNEP says that 1 billion urban residents are exposed to health-threatening levels of air pollution, creating the double health burden city dwellers face of poverty and environmental degradation. This type of double health burden is linked to the dilemma of developing-country cities being forced to compete against each other in dirty development: attracting investment on the basis of extremely low environmental standards and extremely poor labor conditions. This kind of development is hazardous for the current generation but also toxic for the future. It raises the challenge of providing a form of urban development that eliminates urban poverty without introducing the effects of dirty, unsustainable industrialization.

Good urban health also depends on the urban social and political environment. The shift toward inequality within countries is evident in almost every city and town internationally, regardless of its wealth, and has been linked to social and health impacts such as increases in violence and poor mental health. Evidence shows that urban violence stems from political disempowerment, unequal access of some people to opportunity and justice, frustrated aspirations, and perpetual confrontation with lack of change. Death rates from urban violence in the low-income areas of cities are high. More than twice as many poor in São Paulo, for example, die a violent death compared with the rich. Poor urban children, particularly boys, are greatly affected by the trauma of urban violence. All these issues raise the third challenge for urban health: developing urban areas in a way that provides equal opportunity and benefits to all.

Malnutrition and Ill-health

Urban/rural comparisons regarding food consumption, nutritional status, mortality, and prevalence of disease are often used as evidence of urban bias and the rationale for a focus on rural, not urban poverty. Indeed, most simple comparisons of energy intake and prevalence of childhood malnutrition or infant mortality indicate that, on average, urban populations are better-off than rural populations. The literature on urban/rural comparisons in selected health and nutrition indicators is presented below, followed by a compilation of data from the demographic health surveys conducted in 35 countries between 1985 and 1996.

Urban/rural differences in infant and child mortality have been analyzed for 64 countries (including both developing and developed countries), and for 24 countries, using data from DHS. Overall, approximately 75 percent of the countries had lower infant and child mortality rates in urban areas. The range of infant mortality rates in less developed countries is approximately 12 times greater than in developed countries, that the overall mean is 5 to 8 times greater, and that urban/rural differences are much greater than in developed countries. Data on the prevalence of infectious diseases among preschoolers are scarce, but information from four countries suggests greater prevalence of diarrhea, fever, and other illnesses in urban areas, although the magnitude of the rural/urban differences is generally small.

Relative to childhood malnutrition, urban/rural differences using survey data from FAO in 11 countries, most of which were in Africa. Data were from the late 1970s and early 1980s. They found that chronic malnutrition (low height-for-age, or stunting) was generally greater among rural populations. The prevalence of stunting in urban areas was between 55 and 78 percent of the rates found in rural areas, except for Mauritius, where it was 32 percent. With respect to acute malnutrition (low weight-for-height, or wasting), however, differences between urban and rural samples were generally small and the overall prevalence in both areas were either equal or lower than expected in a normal population (2.3 percent).

Some argues that urban/rural differences in malnutrition using data from the 1970s and the 1980s that were compiled by the United Nations Children's Fund (UNICEF) for 33 countries in Africa, Asia, and the Americas. Stunting and low weight-for-age (underweight) were consistently higher among rural children, and were on average 1.6 and 1.5 times greater, respectively, than in urban areas. Wasting was higher in urban areas in 9 of the 33 countries studied, but the prevalence of wasting was generally low and urban/rural differences were of small magnitude.Analysis of DHS Data from 35 Countries Data from 44 DHS conducted in 35 countries between 1985 and 1994 were examined for urban/rural differences in childhood mortality, morbidity, and malnutrition patterns. Eight countries had data at two points in time, which were used to look at changes over time within urban and rural areas.

The main findings are as follows: infant, child, and under-five mortality rates were generally larger among rural populations except for five countries (on one or more indicators). When urban populations had higher mortality rates, however, the percentage difference between urban and rural samples was generally small (less than 12 percent, except for Paraguay, where the difference was 30 percent). Note that the magnitude of the urban advantage was greater for child (1-4 years) than for infant (0-1 year) mortality, suggesting that children between 1 and 4 years of age are more sensitive to the negative factors associated with life in rural areas than during their first year of life. It is likely that breast-feeding plays a major role in protecting rural infants during their first year of life.

The prevalence of stunting and low weight-for-age among preschoolers was consistently lower among urban samples, and the percentage difference between urban and rural ranged from 16.5 percent to 100 percent for weight-for-age and from 0 to 53 percent for stunting. Urban/rural differences in wasting, however, were inconsistent and of small magnitude-three countries showed no difference, and 8 had higher and 21 had lower prevalence of wasting in urban areas.

Differences in childhood morbidity from respiratory infections and diarrhea show inconsistent patterns, but overall childhood morbidity was greater in urban areas in approximately 25 percent of the countries studied. In general, however, the magnitude of the urban/rural differences in morbidity were smaller than the differences in infant and child mortality or malnutrition among preschoolers. Eight countries had data from DHS surveys at two points in time, usually four or five years apart. Differences in the percentage change over time were examined for these countries. Infant and child mortality decreased much more over time in the urban than the rural areas in Ghana, Bolivia, and Indonesia. Cities in Zimbabwe experienced an increase in infant, child, and under-five mortality over time, whereas rural populations had decreasing patterns. For other countries, the percentage change over time was comparable between urban and rural areas. Except for Ghana, the data on changes in nutritional status over time cannot be interpreted because the age groups differed from one period to the other. In Ghana, the reduction in the percentages of underweight or stunted children were much larger in urban areas than in rural areas. Wasting, on the other hand, increased between 1988 and 1993 in both rural and urban areas, with larger increases among the rural sample.

Simple comparisons between urban and rural areas, however, may be misleading. Basta in 1977 first highlighted the fact that statistics of cities as a whole mask important differences between social classes.

City health statistics usually tend to look much better than rural ones. The reason is either because the squatter or slum inhabitants do not appear in the statistics (they are not 'official' residents of the city in many cases), or else because their inclusion is obscured by the enormous difference that exists between their status and that of the middle-to-high income parts of the city. To illustrate his point, Basta gathered data on health and nutrition outcomes and compared squatter and nonsquatter urban areas, or squatter and whole city averages. He demonstrated that the overall prevalence of most diseases, such as typhoid, diphtheria, and measles, was 50 percent greater in squatter areas than for the city as a whole; average death rates from dysentery were three times larger in squatter areas; energy intake was one-half to two-thirds that of city averages; health coverage was sometimes two to ten times worse; anemia was twice as prevalent; and malnutrition was three times greater in squatter areas. In most cases for which data were available, it was also clear that intra-urban differences were of much larger magnitude than urban/rural differences.

A review of the literature the urban poor have a health profile different from other urban groups both in terms of mortality and morbidity. Similar to the findings published that infant mortality rates in squatter areas of Latin American cities are often up to three times larger than among higher income groups. They present similar data for malnutrition, morbidity from diarrheal diseases, and the prevalence of parasitic infections. Even the causes of death are strikingly different between poorer and wealthier segments of the urban population. Among the poor, 51 percent of infant deaths were caused by infectious diseases, whereas deaths among the wealthier group were largely due to problems of gestation, delivery, or the early postnatal period, as found in more developed countries.

The DHS data to compare differentials in child mortality, morbidity, and anthropometry within the urban sector of four countries. The authors found that there were major socioeconomic differentials in child health and mortality within the urban sector of all four countries, and that except for Egypt, mortality rates among the urban poor were at least as high as those of the rural population. The authors also showed that the patterns of within-urban differences vary between countries according to the overall degree of national development and the particular history of urban development. For instance, while socioeconomic differentials in child mortality within the urban sector of Ghana are moderate, they are large in Egypt and very large in Brazil.

A representative survey of Accra revealed that the prevalence of underweight children among households from the lowest income quintile (23 percent) was three times higher than that in the highest income quintile (6 percent). The difference in stunting was twofold. The proportion of children who had diarrhea in the two weeks prior to the survey was also larger among the poorest income quintile (32 percent) than among the wealthiest group (22 percent). Recent analysis of DHS data from 20 countries shows a clear relationship between childhood mortality and access to piped drinking water. In all countries studied, all four types of childhood mortality were higher among rural households, followed by urban residents without piped water, and finally urban residents with piped water. In some countries and at certain ages, mortality rates were higher among poor urban groups than among the rural group. Overall poor urban children had a 57 percent greater under-five mortality rate than wealthier urban children, and a 17 percent lower mortality rate than rural children.

The results from the earlier and more recent data sets reviewed lead to surprisingly similar conclusions, namely that childhood mortality, stunting, and underweight are generally lower in urban than rural areas, whereas wasting and morbidity from infectious diseases are often higher in urban areas. The consistency of these findings across data sets is impressive, considering that different combinations of countries were represented and that the studies covered two decades. Caution is needed when comparing urban and rural areas, however, because city averages do not capture the large heterogeneity in poverty, morbidity, mortality, and nutritional status found within urban areas. There are often enormous differences between poor and middle-to-high income parts of the city. Generally the intra-urban differences are of a much larger magnitude than urban/rural differences.

Diseases due to malnutrition

This section emphasizes the various poverty-related diseases, rather than chronic diseases such as cancers and cardiovascular diseases. Thus, diarrhea, respiratory infections, and malaria are emphasized because they play a crucial role in the etiology of malnutrition and because they are important causes of death among young children. Nutritional deficiencies such as protein-energy malnutrition, and deficiencies in vitamin A, iron, and zinc, which are associated with reduced immunity and increased vulnerability to infections, are also discussed.

Acute Respiratory Infections (ARI). Acute respiratory infections are the leading cause of death among children under five years and are also important causes of morbidity. ARI are responsible for the deaths of between 4 and 4.3 million children under five years of age each year-this represents 25 to 30 percent of all child deaths. Almost all of these deaths are due to pneumonia, and children under 3 years of age are the most affected. Little information exists on ARI morbidity and mortality in urban areas, but it is generally believed that ARI in urban areas are more severe and more prevalent than in rural areas, mainly as a result of outdoor and indoor air pollution and crowding. An analysis of infant mortality in Porto Alegre, Brazil, found that 21 percent of all deaths were due to pneumonia, with mortality from pneumonia six times higher in the shantytowns than in other areas. Pneumonia was the leading cause of infant deaths in the slum areas of the city, whereas it was third in other areas of Porto Alegre.

Diarrheal diseases : In 1985, diarrhea caused 5 million deaths in developing countries, 80 percent of which were among children under 5 years of age. Recent data reveal some improvement, but diarrheal diseases are still estimated to have caused 3.2 to 3.3 million child deaths in 1990 and 3 million in 199. About 80 percent of these deaths occurred in the first two years of life. Although no information is available on the percentage of diarrheal deaths that occurred in poor urban areas, it is generally recognized that severe diarrhea is among the most serious and prevalent health risks faced by children exposed to unsanitary and contaminated environments such as urban slums. Estimates from the early 1980s suggested that in one year alone, more than 2 million urban preschoolers died as a consequence of diarrhea-related dehydration.

Global estimates derived from surveys coordinated by WHO in 60 developing countries indicate that, on average, children suffer 3.5 episodes of diarrhea per year, with higher incidences found in Latin America and Sub-Saharan Africa. Highest incidence rates are found among 6-to-11-month-old children, who experience a median of five episodes per year. Poor urban slums, however, may have diarrhea incidence rates as high as 8 to 13 episodes per year. Each episode of diarrhea has the potential to contribute to malnutrition, and the longer the episode, the larger the negative impact on growth.

Malaria: Recent estimates suggest that malaria is probably responsible for between 1 and 2 million deaths in developing countries each year, 75 percent of which are among children under five. Data on childhood mortality from malaria in urban areas were not found, but it is widely recognized that malaria is an urban problem, mainly because the breeding of the Anopheles mosquito, the carrier of malaria, is facilitated by the pools of stagnant water commonly found in slums. Similarly, dengue and dengue hemorrhagic fever, which are also associated with poor sanitation, overcrowding, and inadequate water storage, are highly concentrated in urban areas of the developing world. Dengue, which affects millions of people yearly and is responsible for thousands of deaths, tends to affect disproportionately young children and the elderly.

Parasitic infections: Parasitic infections are rarely fatal in themselves, but they are responsible for a large burden of morbidity. Data on parasitic infections are not usually disaggregated by age group, but a high prevalence of a variety of parasites is documented in the urban studies. The authors highlight the magnitude of intra-city differences between poorer and wealthier groups.

The malnutrition-infection-malnutrition deprivation cycle, describes the synergistic effect of malnutrition and infectious disease. The cycle is particularly acute in its effects on young children living in poor environments. The phenomenon can be summarized as inadequate nutrient intake leads to malnutrition, which results in increased vulnerability to infectious diseases as a result of a depressed immune system; infections, in turn, further exacerbate poor nutritional status as a result of reduced appetite and food intake, increased intestinal losses of nutrients, and increased nutrient requirements. This phenomenon is true both for rural and urban populations, and for areas with different levels of diarrhea and malnutrition.

Micronutrient deficiencies: No data were found on global estimates of micronutrient deficiencies among urban children from the developing world. Various urban case studies from countries in Asia, Africa, and Latin America, however, report high prevalences of iron-deficiency anemia and vitamin A deficiency. In Sao Paolo, Brazil, the prevalence of severe anemia in 1984 was 22 percent among children living in slum areas compared to 13 percent among those who lived in residential areas. In Guatemala, no significant differences were found in mean hematocrit (packed red cell volume) or low hematocrit values (< 38 percent, corrected for altitude) between rural and urban samples of both preschool and school-age children. Only a small predominance of low ferritin levels (an indicator of iron reserves) was found among preschoolers from rural areas, compared to children from the city.

Every year, approximately half a million women die from causes related to pregnancy and the birth process. Maternal mortality rates in developing countries are, on average, 450/100,000 live births, in sharp contrast to the 30/100,000 found in developed countries. Although less emphasized, maternal morbidity is also highly prevalent in developing countries and includes problems such as anemia, hypertension, eclampsia, hemorrhage, sepsis, abortion-related infections, reproductive tract infections, and acquired immune deficiency syndrome (AIDS). No data were found on maternal morbidity and mortality in urban areas.

Iron-deficiency anemia is the most widespread nutritional problem among women. Estimates from UN ACC/SCN indicate that the highest prevalences of anemia among adult women of reproductive age (15-49 years old) are found in South Asia (64 percent), followed by Southeast Asia (48 percent), Sub-Saharan Africa (42 percent), Near East/North Africa (33 percent), Middle America/Carribean (28 percent), China (26 percent), and South America (23 percent). Overall, half of all pregnant women and 41 percent of nonpregnant women in the developing world are anemic. Prevalences of anemia are generally at least 20 percent higher among pregnant than among nonpregnant women, except for South Asia, where both groups have equally high prevalences. No data were found on global estimates of maternal anemia in urban areas. At the microlevel, a study in Guatemala in 1984 showed lower prevalences of low hemoglobin values among urban women (7.6 percent), compared to two rural samples (12.5 percent and 45.4 percent, from the southern coast and the poor highlands, respectively). Differences in ferritin levels showed similar patterns (15 percent among urban women, compared to 26 percent and 47 percent for the two rural samples). Recent estimates among lactating women (between 3 and 10 months postpartum) from poor urban areas of Guatemala city revealed prevalences of low hemoglobin values as high as 35 percent (< 12.8 g/dL, corrected for altitude).

Nutritional status of mothers

Data on the nutritional status of women of reproductive age (assessed by anthropometry) are also available from the data sets compiled by UN ACC/SCN. Maternal stunting (height < 145 cm), which is associated with high reproductive risks and low birth weight, is particularly prevalent in Asia and Central America (> 15 percent). Women in Africa are significantly taller (averaging 154 to 158 centimeters) compared to the Middle and South Americas (152 to 154 cm) and Asia (150-151 cm). The prevalence of underweight follows the same regional patterns, but is much higher: 60 percent in Southeast Asia, 45 percent in South Asia, and 20 percent in Sub-Saharan Africa and Middle America. Body-mass index, used to measure adult wasting, is highest in South and Southeast Asia (around 40 percent), followed by Africa (20 percent). No data were found on maternal anthropometry for urban areas.

Mothers with poor health or nutritional status may have decreased energy levels and a reduced capacity to perform certain caregiving activities. Studies show that maternal deficiencies in iron and certain vitamins result in less active caring behaviors. Results from Egypt indicate that anemic women spent substantially less time caring for their children than non-anemic women, and that mothers with low vitamin B-6 status were less responsive to their infant's vocalization and distress, and were more likely to request help from older siblings for caregiving duties. Severe maternal malnutrition is also known to be associated with reduced lactational performance, potentially reducing both milk quantity and quality. Thus, maternal malnutrition can negatively affect breast-feeding, which is one of the most important caring behaviors for protecting the health and nutrition of children in the developing world.

Unfortunately, data on the health and nutritional status of women in urban areas are scarce, let alone data on the effect of this status on maternal caring behaviors. Mental Health of the Caregiver Studies have reported high levels of stress and depression among women in developing countries. Urbanization has also been shown to be associated with mental disorders, probably as a result of changes in social support and life events. The physical and mental health of family members both before the onset of rapid urbanization and after the peak of the urbanization trend (1965 and 1980, respectively), 40 percent of mothers reported being anxious or depressed after urbanization. A study in urban slums in Bangladesh reported anecdotally that some women were extremely socially isolated, and were often so depressed that they were unable to care for their children properly.

Environmental determinants of health

Recent reviews of the environmental determinants of health in cities have emphasized the importance of assessing both the physical environment (such as the quality of air, water, food, and housing), and the social environment (such as alienation, unemployment, ethnic tensions, violence, and stress). It is likely that the health of young children will be affected more directly by characteristics of their physical environment, whereas the social environment will affect them indirectly, mainly through the impact on the mental health, physical health, and caring ability of their main caregiver.

Urban health problems, their determinants, the risk groups most affected, and the actions that should be undertaken by each sector to alleviate the problems. As indicated by the authors poverty and the lack of formal education are determinants of all the illnesses listed and, therefore, are not repeated for each illness separately. The following discussion is based on this table.

Few relevant population-based studies are available to evaluate the causal factors of ARI, but a number of risk factors have been suggested, with overcrowding and urban pollution (both indoor and outdoor) being the most frequently mentioned. High levels of outdoor pollution, especially suspended respirable particles like sulphur dioxide, nitrogen dioxide, and ozone, are possible factors causing ARI. Exposure to indoor air pollution from coal and biomass combustion for cooking and/or heating has also been associated with pneumonia in children. Studies in Nepal have also shown an association between time spent in proximity to wood stoves and symptoms of chronic bronchitis and impaired lung function in women.

Overcrowding, inadequate ventilation, and dampness are also thought to be associated with the incidence and severity of respiratory infections. High population density and the concentration and proximity of infective and susceptible people in urban areas promote the transmission of infectious agents. Crowding is a potentially important risk factor for ARI mortality, measles, and tuberculosis. Attendance at day-care centers, an increasingly common phenomenon in many urban areas of the developing world, has also been linked to increased respiratory morbidity in young children.

The most important factor in the etiology of diarrheal diseases and helminth (worm) infections in urban areas is water (access and availability, quality, and quantity used). The predominant infectious agents responsible for diarrhea are transmitted by fecal contamination. Human feces remain one of the world's most hazardous pollutants, and related water and sanitation inadequacies still constitute one of the world's most serious health problems. The ingestion of contaminated water, the use of insufficient amounts of water for personal and domestic hygiene, and the inadequate disposal of feces, all characteristics of urban environments, are the most effective routes of transmission of diarrheal pathogens. Waterborne diarrheal diseases are estimated to be highly prevalent in urban areas, mainly as a result of contaminated water and food, crowding, limited access to water, and poor food and household hygiene.

It is important to note, however, that on average, households in urban areas have better access to potable water and appropriate sanitation facilities than households in rural areas. A number of urban studies have shown a strong association between morbidity and mortality from diarrheal diseases, on the one hand, and the quality of the water consumed and the quantity available for personal and domestic needs on the other. Similarly, evidence of reductions in morbidity and mortality from diarrheal and parasitic infections following water and sanitation interventions is widely documented, although mainly in rural areas. A review of the impact of water and sanitation interventions indicates a median reduction in diarrheal morbidity and mortality of 27 and 30 percent, respectively. More recent reviews have confirmed these findings.

The determinants of nutritional deficiencies are those identified previously as playing a key role in the malnutrition-infection deprivation cycle, including inadequate nutrient intake and poor utilization of nutrients due to ill-health. It is generally believed that malnutrition and micronutrient deficiencies are less prevalent among children in urban areas because of increased incomes, food access, and household food availability.

However, very little is known about how these various factors interact in urban areas and how they affect the nutritional status of the vulnerable groups. Child feeding practices, including breast-feeding, during the first two years of life are particularly important for the growth and development of the child.

The concentration of iron in breast milk is not sufficient to prevent anemia beyond 6 months of age, but the contribution of bioavailable iron from breast milk may be important. Breast-feeding also protects the child against vitamin A deficiency, even in areas where vitamin A deficiency is a public health problem. Thus, continued breast-feeding beyond the period of exclusive breast-feeding is important for the child, but may be difficult for working urban mothers to practice.

The high rates of diarrhea and other infectious diseases documented in urban areas are another factor that may predispose children to malnutrition and micronutrient deficiencies. It may be that even though children's diets in urban areas are better overall than rural diets, the high rates of infections do not allow children to maintain optimal nutritional status. The burden of parasitic infections in urban areas may also exacerbate malnutrition.

The four main causes of maternal mortality related to child bearing in developing countries are hemorrhage, infections, obstructed labor, and eclampsia. The first three are caused or exacerbated by poor maternal nutrition. The severity of postpartum hemorrhage, for instance, is aggravated by maternal iron-deficiency anemia. Poor iron status reduces immunocompetence, which, in turn, increases maternal susceptibility to infections. And short maternal stature (a reflection of past, childhood malnutrition) is associated with obstructed labor. Teenage pregnancies are also associated with higher risks of maternal mortality, mainly because of the competition for nutrients for growth between mother and fetus. Thus, nutritional stress plays an important role in causing or aggravating maternal mortality in developing countries. There are a number of reasons for supposing that maternal health may be better in urban than in rural areas. Diets in urban areas may be higher in energy relative to requirements and may be higher in bioavailable iron than in rural areas. Prenatal care is also usually more widely available and mothers are more likely to deliver in health facilities as opposed to at home with the assistance of midwives. At the very least, health care facilities are easier to reach in situations of emergencies, and this may reduce the risks of maternal mortality related to complications of pregnancy or childbirth. Urban areas, however, expose women to different types of health hazards.

Environmental pollution combined with indoor exposure to smoke from cooking stoves makes women more vulnerable to chronic respiratory infections. Pregnancy may also make women more vulnerable to some chemical toxins that they may be exposed to at work, and to certain diseases such as malaria. Prostitution, which is more common in urban areas, is associated with increased risk of sexually transmitted diseases including AIDS. Teenage pregnancies are also thought to be more prevalent in urban areas. Finally, violence against women may be exacerbated in urban areas by poor living conditions, unemployment, and stress.

Poor urban communities suffer an alarming lack of access to basic water, sewage, and rubbish disposal services, which make it virtually impossible for them to reduce contamination of water and food, maintain adequate levels of hygiene, or control insect-vectors of disease. While infant and child mortality are generally lower in urban than in rural areas, the incidence of a number of common childhood diseases such as diarrhea and respiratory illness may actually be higher. However, nationally or regionally representative data on the distributions of these diseases are scarce. As in rural areas, infections may lead to malnutrition, which, in turn, may result in increased vulnerability to further infections.

The precise levels of childhood malnutrition (and especially micronutrient malnutrition) in urban areas remain unknown. Similarly, the magnitude of maternal mortality, morbidity, and malnutrition in urban areas is undocumented, as are the specifically urban hazards that may predispose women to these outcomes.

Education of caregivers

Maternal education has been consistently associated with positive child health and nutrition outcomes. The mechanisms by which maternal education is beneficial for the child, however, are not well understood. It is not clear whether maternal education influences health through an improvement in child care practices directly (such as with the development or enhancement of caring skills and better use of health care facilities), or whether the influence is more a result of increased maternal income resulting from better employment opportunities, or both. There is evidence that in some cases, maternal education and socioeconomic status interact so that maternal education is more important among poor households that have access to a minimum level of resources. In Accra, maternal education was the single most important determinant of good care practices, whereas household income, assets, and food availability were not associated with good care practices.

The impact of maternal education on the nutritional status of children was mediated through improved care practices. Maternal education also appears to have a greater effect on children's nutritional status at certain ages. Where maternal education was significantly associated with height-for-age Z-scores only among children less than two years of age. Income, on the other hand, was important only for older children. Results from Ecuador, Mexico, Paraguay, Peru, and the Dominican Republic showed that maternal schooling was associated with increased use of health services. In the Philippines, maternal schooling had a positive effect on children's energy intake, maternal practices related to hygiene, and the use of health services for preventive purposes (immunization). These positive behaviors, in turn, reduced the incidence of diarrhea among young children.

The characteristics of employment in urban areas may make the provision of adequate caring for children more difficult. Many women in cities are more active in the informal sector, where wages are generally low and hours often uncertain and long. The conditions of many urban occupations may be less compatible with child care in that they make it more difficult for a mother to take a child with her if the work is on the street or in an office, as opposed to out in the field as in a rural area.

A comparative analysis of demographic health survey (DHS) data from 15 countries estimated the proportion of breast-milk-substitute use attributable to employment away from the baby during the first 6 months of life. The results showed that, contrary to general beliefs, maternal employment was not a main determinant of breast-milk-substitute use in developing countries. The proportion of breast-milk-substitute use attributable to maternal employment ranged from 0.7 to 22 percent and was less or equal to 5 percent in 10 of the 15 countries studied. Similar findings were reported in studies undertaken in Nairobi, Bogota, Bangkok, and Semarang (Java), where maternal employment per se was not found to be a consistent predictor of breast-feeding duration and use of infant formula.

Overall, the impact of maternal employment on child health and nutritional status appears to be linked not only to income, but to other related factors such as type of work (for example, wage labor and self-employment), place of work, length of working day, the availability and quality of substitute child care, and the child's age. In times of recession, maternal employment had a negative impact on child caregiving time and on children's nutritional status, not only because more women started to work and tended to work longer hours, but also because women returned to work when their children were younger.

An important source of support for a caregiver is the family, regardless of the environment. Changes in family structure related to the transition from rural to urban areas, and their impact on caring behaviors and the health and nutritional status of family members, are not well researched or understood. Fathers are a potentially important source of support to the caregiver, both physically and emotionally, and the opinions of fathers may have significant consequences on the initiation of certain caring behaviors, such as breast-feeding. The community structure is clearly different in urban and rural areas. As a result, the opportunities and resources available for caring are different as well. Residents in urban areas, however, may develop new networks, or may recreate networks based on the rural ones in an attempt to adapt to the new urban situation.

A common pattern of child care, especially in developing countries, is for the mother to provide the primary care during a child's first year, and then share the caring responsibilities with the child's older siblings or other adult family members, once the mother takes on employment responsibilities outside the home. There is no consistent relationship between who provides childcare and the health or nutritional status of the child, but adult caregiving was generally positively associated with children's health and nutrition, whereas sibling caregiving was detrimental to the child. Other studies suggest that care by a preteen caregiver is associated with lower nutritional status of a child under 2 years old, controlling for maternal education and socioeconomic status.

Little data exist on the availability of older siblings as caregivers in an urban setting. However, with increased school attendance in urban areas, their availability is likely to be limited. The number of children left without any form of child care is difficult to ascertain. Anecdotal stories of children left alone, locked in the house, are frequently heard in large cities of the developing world, but systematic data on this phenomenon are not available. Institutional day care could be a good alternative for child care in urban areas. Traditional institutional care, however, is usually too expensive for poor urban households, which results in low coverage underutilization of these services. Many governments in Latin America and some countries of Africa and Asia have started to implement community day care centers to support working parents living in poor urban slums. These programs have enormous potential to relieve some of the time pressures on working mothers and may be particularly indispensable for the large number of women head of households living in urban areas.

Breast-feeding is the best example of a caring behavior that provides unequivocal nutritional, health, and emotional benefits to the child, as well as potential positive effects to the mother. Breast-feeding also provides immunity to the child and protection against infectious diseases. The beneficial effect of breast-feeding is thus particularly important for children living in contaminated environments such as urban slums. In these settings, where it is almost impossible to prepare complementary liquids or breast-milk substitutes hygienically, infants exclusively breast-fed have significantly lower diarrheal morbidity and mortality, compared to those who receive mixed feeding. Thus, exclusive breast-feeding for the first 4 to 6 months may be particularly important in urban areas.

There is a general belief that urban mothers are less likely to initiate breast-feeding and more likely to wean earlier if they do breast feed. This is supported by studies carried out in Thailand, Egypt, and Ghana. Although the percentage of children ever breast-fed and the median duration of breast-feeding tend to be lower in urban areas, the pattern is not fully consistent and differences are often of small magnitude. Urban mothers were found to initiate breast-feeding at a surprisingly high rate (greater than 90 percent, except in the Philippines, where the percentage was 82 percent). The median duration of breast-feeding, on the other hand, was consistently shorter in urban areas, with maximum urban/rural differences of 4-6 months. Exclusive and full breast-feeding duration was much shorter than the recommended 4-6 months for both urban and rural populations in all countries reviewed.

Some studies suggest that, in relation to breast-feeding and child care practices, the work-related variables, such as flexibility, number of hours, types of environment, and levels of stress, are more important than work per se or urban versus rural location. Intrahousehold Allocation of Resources and Maternal Control over Resources Several studies suggest that income earned by mothers and the autonomy that they have over this resource are among the most important factors that determine the health and nutritional status of their children. These studies suggest that mothers are more likely than fathers to allocate resources under their domain to children. It is not surprising, therefore, that the children of female-headed households often do well in this regard. A study conducted in Jordan found that the degree of autonomy of mothers within households was the most significant factor associated with child nutritional status, after controlling for women's age, education, and household size. In another study in Malawi, the author found that the most malnourished children were those of mothers with low status in the household.

Residing in an urban area may influence a mother's autonomy and control over the resources available to her because of the increased probability that she will be an income-earner, which often goes hand in hand with an increase in her authority in the home. On the other hand, it may also be the case that the more traditional domains under a mother's control in the rural areas, such as child rearing and food provision through agricultural production, are weakened in the urban environment.

Health-seeking behaviors include those practiced in the home, such as providing rehydration solution for a child with diarrhea, as well as those practiced outside of the home, such as taking a child to a health clinic for treatment of an illness. A great deal of care that falls under this heading occurs in the home by the household's primary caregiver. When attempts to reduce the symptoms of a child's illness or injury fail, the caregiver will often seek help outside the home and get assistance from traditional healers, local pharmacies and dispensaries, and hospitals. The options available in urban settings are generally different, and formal health care facilities are usually more accessible. The decision to use the facilities, however, will depend on a variety of factors such as the cost of transportation to and use of the clinic; the opportunity cost of time for traveling, waiting, and being treated; and the quality of attention and the perceptions about the benefits of using the facilities. In Sierra Leone, distance was a common reason given by rural women for not attending immunization clinics, whereas urban women were more likely to report that they did not attend for lack of time.

In peri-urban areas of South Africa, a marked drop in immunization coverage between the second and third doses of DPT/oral poliomyelitis vaccine was associated with mothers' return to work when their children were between 5 and 8 months of age. Because of these time constraints, the so-called "supermarket" organization of health services, which consists of offering immunization coverage at all times instead of on special days, has proven particularly successful in urban areas. The availability of health care facilities is generally greater in urban rather than rural areas, and most immunization data indicate higher coverage in urban areas.

Families in urban areas also tend to use health services more frequently than in rural areas for curative purposes-when children have acute respiratory infections (ARI), fever, or diarrhea. There is a consistently greater percentage of urban children taken to health services for diarrhea and ARI compared to rural children.These data, however, are city averages and pockets of undercovered population are known to exist in poor shantytowns, which also experience the greatest risk of infectious diseases. Lower education levels and greater time constraints, combined with poorer knowledge and awareness of the availability and potential benefits of health services, make the urban poor less likely to use the facilities.Additionally, the lack of supplies, the unfriendly attitude of some health workers, the unsanitary conditions, and the overcrowding that plague many of the health services in urban slums may discourage any human being from using them.

The issue of autonomy and control over resources is also important with respect to the discussion of health-seeking behaviors. Income in the hands of women is associated with increases in the share of the household budget spent on health, education and housing as well as improvements in child health. A study in South India showed that children were more likely to receive medical attention if the mother had more assets. It is unclear, however, whether differentials in resource allocation between men and women hold true across income groups and cultural boundaries.

Household hygiene and maternal hygiene behaviors are strong determinants of childhood infectious diseases, including diarrhea, and malnutrition. Maternal hand-washing behavior, and the use of soap in particular, is also recognized as an important factor in the incidence of diarrhea and nutritional status of children. The median reduction in diarrheal rates achieved with hygiene education interventions is 26 percent, while hand-washing interventions alone reduced diarrheal morbidity by 35 percent (median value). It is clear that hygiene and sanitation are pervasive problems in much of the developing world's urban areas. What is less clear, however, is the degree to which the specific actions of a caregiver can reduce the exposure to certain pathogens and, hence, protect the health and nutritional status of young children, given the fundamentally unhygienic environments in which they live. The literature on water and sanitation interventions, although largely from rural areas, suggests that maternal behavior related to the use, maintenance, or enhancement of the new technologies for improving water and sanitation conditions is likely to be the key determinant of whether an intervention is successful.

An intervention in rural Bangladesh that combined the introduction of hand pumps and hygiene education showed a larger decrease in diarrhea incidence among children of mothers who used at least three of the four hygienic practices taught, compared to those who received the hand pumps but did not change their hygiene practices. Reductions in diarrheal morbidity and mortality following water and sanitation interventions are on the order of 27 to 30 percent. It is estimated that combining these interventions with hygiene education could achieve reductions in diarrheal morbidity of 35 to 50 percent.

This category of caring behaviors relates to the emotional support provided by caregivers to the child. It is well-known how important positive interactions are, both emotionally and physically, to the overall development of children, especially with respect to the child's mother or primary caregiver. Some of the specific caring behaviors that have been found to influence children's nutrition include frequent physical contact, a consistent responsive reaction to the child's needs, and showing affection to the child. Changes in the sources of support for and interaction with children, such as transformations in family structure due to migration from rural to urban areas, are important to consider for their potential health and nutritional consequences.

The community structure and the opportunities and resources available for care are different in urban and rural areas. In particular, maternal employment outside the home is more common in urban areas, and this may result in lower breast-feeding rates and inadequate complementary feeding practices. At this point, one cannot conclude whether, overall, the potential costs to a child's health and nutritional status of reduced maternal time for care (and for breast-feeding in particular) are outweighed by the additional income generated by the working mother. Maternal malnutrition and poor health may reduce mothers' capacity to perform caregiving activities, respond to children's demands for attention and care, and interact with other family members to seek assistance. Finally, the general lack of public services such as water, sanitation, and refuse disposal in urban areas is likely to represent an important physical barrier to good caring behaviors.

Strategies for Urban Well-being

Many now believe that the three urban health challenges outlined above could be met if urban policymakers focused more on environmental and social sustainability. Sustainability could help reverse trends in inequality because it emphasizes equity in consumption and resource distribution. If equitable, sustainable development is to be achieved, a first step may be to emphasize the use of health as a means of identifying priorities in urban policy. This would enable the urban development agenda to be guided by the long-term goal of human well-being rather than the short-term goal of economic well-being.

Governmental, nongovernmental, and international organizations are developing urban initiatives—such as the highly participatory Local Agenda 21 plans, Healthy Cities, and Sustainable City Networks—that emphasize healthy and sustainable development. These initiatives incorporate intersectoral collaboration; the participation, particularly of the poor, in setting priorities; equity in distribution of services; and sustainability in decisions about investment. The forces of globalization must also be turned toward environmental and social justice, and thus to the advantage of the urban majority and the urban future.

Against the attempts to shift toward equity and intersectoral collaboration, urban services have become part of the globalized economy, with large-scale privatization of urban services, including education, water, waste disposal, energy, housing, sanitation, and health. Privatization policies were intended to improve efficiency and extend delivery, but urban services appear to be moving into the hands of major multinational corporations, who then control many aspects of urban policy that were formerly in the hands of local government. The result often has been a narrowing of delivery.

Macropolitical and macroeconomic processes influence the ability of decisionmakers to improve the conditions that affect the health and well-being of urban citizens. Many specialists argue that only when local governments gain control of the destiny of their cities will sustainable urban development become a reality and will we be able to achieve health security for all.

Governments, development agencies, and communities are attempting to improve urban livelihoods and reduce urban poverty and food and nutrition insecurity. However, much of their understanding builds on a rural and agrarian knowledge base or focuses on providing urban public services and infrastructure.

Developing more effective urban programs requires considering some key characteristics that affect the livelihoods of the urban poor:

— Greater dependency on cash income and less reliance on agriculture and natural resources

— Low wages from work at insecure jobs

— A large number of women working outside the home

— Legal obstacles, including insecure land and housing tenure

— Inadequate access to safe water, sanitation, and health services

— Frequently weak social networks, which often transcend the geographic boundaries of communities.

In urban settings diagnostic tools must be able to grapple with livelihood systems that are complex and constantly changing, often span economic sectors, and often involve linkages with rural areas. Standard approaches may be stymied because the poor may not readily disclose coping strategies, which are frequently illegal, and because safety considerations may constrain data collection, with interviews having to be carried out before dark. Targeting programs may also be difficult. Community-based targeting may not work well in urban areas because poverty and malnutrition are widely dispersed in pockets across the city and because people move frequently and often work outside of the areas where they live. Local, municipal, and national governments, along with community organizations and nongovernmental organizations, combine with political interests from inside and outside a community to exert influence over local activities.

Lack of skills, poor health, and inadequate access to capital often limit the poor to jobs that are insecure, temporary, and casual. Incomes, too, are often subject to significant seasonal swings, just as in rural areas. For example, in the rainy season, the government may shut down foodsellers because it fears an outbreak of cholera. Insecure access to affordable, decent housing also consigns the poor to livelihoods that are unlikely to improve. This is because a house in an urban area serves not only as a base for household enterprise but also as the center of social relations useful for finding jobs, getting credit, or acquiring food. Eviction can be a tragic disruption of these strategic networks.

Lack of secure tenure can also inhibit community development. Donors or governments may hesitate to invest in infrastructure without being assured that people have a stake in maintaining the investment or that they will still be there when construction is completed. Slum improvements may even negatively affect the poor if the poor do not have secure tenure because with improvements, landlords may raise rents, forcing out the very group the improvements were intended to benefit.

Creating successful employment is also difficult. Income-generation and credit schemes tend to be small in scale. While perhaps helping some individuals to cope with deprivation, they often fail to provide permanent escape from poverty. Business-training programs often have difficulty identifying those individuals who are true entrepreneurs and who can generate a significant number of higher-quality jobs. Still, experience suggests that effective programs must ensure that the poor receive training in job and life skills and have access to sufficient credit. Income-support programs need to keep the seasonal dimension in mind as well. Communities must work with the private sector and government to ensure that available labor is matched up with available opportunities and to provide an economic and regulatory environment that promotes business expansion.

Existing services in urban areas are often overwhelmed by crowded conditions and poor infrastructure maintenance. Dangerous environments are made more so by inadequate health facilities, erratic water supplies, poor drainage, and infrequent refuse collection. Government agencies may not have the capacity or resources to adequately support these services. Privatization may hold out hope for more efficient service, but private companies are likely not to be concerned with distributive justice. They may raise prices beyond the ability of the poor to pay, increasing inequity in access to basic services. In pursuit of profit, private companies may also worsen environmental conditions and raise risks to the health of the poor. Proposed solutions for improving service delivery must include input from, and meet the needs of, those the system will serve.

Community water systems, for example, must be financially viable for the supplier but also must not exclude the poor who may not be able to pay full recovery-cost prices. Poor peoples rights to access basic services must be ensured, even in a competitive, free-market world, and government agencies, civic groups, and the private sector should work together to design and implement effective, sustainable systems. Experiences even in such countries as Haiti have shown that communities can work with the private sector to devise creative, low-cost, often low-tech solutions that accomplish that goal.

Nongovernmental organizations can play an especially important role as facilitators among these groups, providing technical capacity, or knowledge of other experiences, when needed.

People rely on social networks to create opportunities or manage risk. In an urban setting, increased mobility leads to weak social cohesion and fewer opportunities for establishing a sense of community. In addition, networks that are differentiated and decentralized replace the family- and geographic-community-based networks of rural areas. Individual-level social capital based primarily on an ability to reciprocate becomes the back-bone of these new urban networks. With so little to give, the destitute may soon be left out of these networks.

Negative forms of social capital can arise, with organized crime providing a system of protection and assistance for many. The resulting crime and violence can seriously restrict mobility for social interaction, eroding the space for developing trust and cooperation in the community even further. Programs should be careful not to displace beneficial social networks where they exist. They should be sure to take into account the resources, current social networks, and coping strategies of the poor. Where community cohesion is weak, initial efforts might concentrate on focused—such as water and sanitation infrastructure—that will help the community establish trust and mechanisms for further cooperation. Building community infrastructure using community labor is one way to provide employment and contribute to community cohesion. Special efforts should be made to involve those whose social ties may be weak and have few resources, other than their labor, to offer.

Unemployed youth may be a particularly vulnerable group. Providing this group with job and life skills, improving their connections to employers, and augmenting their sense of self-worth may help to address problems of crime, violence, and sexually transmitted diseases, especially HIV/AIDS.

Conflicts in rural areas causing flight to urban areas or in cities themselves put immense strains on often-impoverished governments—disrupting services, distorting markets, and eliminating employment opportunities. Conflict may erase any sense of governmental authority and scatter populations in and around the city, complicating service provision. Even in the midst of conflict, organizations must strive to promote a functional, nondiscriminatory authority to protect the population's access to services, food, and other goods.

Relief programs may provide goods directly to needy areas, although sometimes providing cash directly to the poor may be best. At the same time, efforts must be carried out on a continuing basis, with all parties drawn into negotiations, to guarantee a minimal set of interventions for providing basic services.

In addition to the factors mentioned here that complicate urban programming, a number of trends will also affect the design of future programs. Past urban interventions focused on supplying infrastructure and related services or were sectorally focused. Donors now place greater emphasis on designing strategies that emerge from an integrated understanding of the lives of the urban poor.

Donors and development organizations are also placing greater emphasis on the community's participation in and control of the development process. Instead of providing services or managing interventions directly, they facilitate development processes led by communities, linking communities with local governments and other key players. Donors must acknowledge that this process will take more time than is traditionally allotted, and must incorporate a flexible workplan, because they must consult with, and often improve the capacity of, all stakeholders, including municipal governments.

Safety nets programmes

Safety net programs are usually designed to protect people who fall into two broad categories of poverty-those who suffer from "chronic poverty" and those who suffer from "transient poverty." Countries have experimented with a wide range of interventions, from cash and in-kind transfers, price subsidies, and food stamps to income-generation programs. Formal safety nets, however, are not the only mechanism available for crisis management. Families and individuals often adopt their own coping and adaptive strategies, which are referred to as informal safety nets. The following sections briefly discusses formal and informal safety nets as they relate to the urban context.strategies, which are referred to as informal safety nets. The following sections briefly discusses formal and informal safety nets as they relate to the urban context.

Although many formal safety net programs have been implemented in urban areas of the developing world, the literature on specific issues related to the effectiveness and impact of these programs on the urban poor is extremely scant. Overall, however, governments and donors alike are renewing their interest in safety net programs as a way of protecting incomes and living standards, particularly when declines result from structural adjustment and macroeconomic stabilization measures. There is also increasing pressure to ensure that social assistance programs are effective in reaching the needy and in reducing poverty, food insecurity, and malnutrition, while, at the same time, pressure exists to reduce overall costs of the programs. Often, the response of governments is to examine how targeting of the programs can be redirected from urban to rural areas. In many developing countries, however, conventional programs of social insurance and unemployment compensation are not fiscally feasible, or are unable to respond adequately to economies with large informal sectors and widespread open unemployment in urban areas.

In the late 1980s, structural adjustment programs began to incorporate specific measures to mitigate the impoverishment of vulnerable groups. The most prevalent interventions in Latin America and Africa have been social action programs, social funds, or social investment funds. These funds generally provide money for activities geared toward employment creation and social service delivery, including infrastructure development and support for microenterprises. In South Asia, food subsidies and public employment programs have been the most notable forms of intervention.

Although the urban poor may have better access to formal support networks, households often also use family support systems and private income transfers to cope with temporary economic distress or protect those who are permanently unable to help themselves. In some cases, urban dwellers may rely on families in rural areas to supply them with food or income as they cope with the stress caused by rising food prices or loss of employment. Vulnerability to food insecurity in cities is, first and foremost, vulnerability to fluctuations in the price of food and income. As a result, urban residents have developed strategies for reducing vulnerability that are markedly different from those of rural areas.

Adaptive strategies of low-income urban residents deal with longer-term changes in the economy and are generally attempts to diversify sources of either income or food to minimize the probability that at some point the household will have no food. Agricultural production by an urban household within or outside the city is one such strategy. Increased female participation in wage labor and informal trade is another. A recent World Bank study that examined household responses to poverty and vulnerability in four poor urban communities in different regions of the world found that a frequent response to declining real incomes was for poor households to mobilize additional labor, usually women's labor, and, in the poorest households, children's labor as well. An increase in women's labor-force participation occurred in the areas of petty trading and services within the informal sector. Poor families have their children work because of the need for extra income. As parents' incomes rise, they are able to send their children to school rather than to work.

In Egypt, a 10 percent increase in mothers' wages was found to result in a 15 percent decline in labor among children ages 12 to 14, and a 27 percent decline among 6-to-11-year-olds. The growth of the "petty commodity" food market is another adaptive strategy, as is reliance on nonmarket exchanges between the city and the countryside. In Sub-Saharan Africa, urban residents often receive transfers of food from family members still living on the farm. Other long-term adaptations to food insecurity may involve changes in family or household composition, including fostering of children outside urban areas.

Coping strategies, on the other hand, are short-term mechanisms for dealing with immediate insufficiencies of food or income. Strategies may include substitution of cheaper food, borrowing food or purchasing on credit, cutting nonfood expenditures or selling assets, sending household members elsewhere to eat, maternal buffering, and cutting back on the number of meals or rationing the amount of food apportioned. In other instances the urban poor may attempt to pool resources to make food available less expensively through community meals or communal kitchens. In some cases, community kitchens may be supported programmatically with food aid or other inputs; in other cases, these kitchens may be self-help efforts. In Peru, the number of community kitchens grew from 100 in 1978 in the whole country to about 5,000 by 1991 in greater Lima alone.The community kitchen experience illustrates potential problems with programs that draw on community resources, especially women's participation. The costs of the program in terms of foregone income, reduced time for child care, and less interaction with the family are not well understood.

The importance of urban ties to rural areas as an element of either adaptive or coping strategies of the poor is subject to some debate. Substantial literature exists on urban-rural links, and recent case studies provide good illustrations of different perspectives and city experiences. About 90 percent of these households, drawn from central as well as peri-urban areas, had been Dar es Salaam for more than five years, which may have allowed them to form their own urban networks and reduce the strength of ties to rural areas, a point also made. Generally, these households stated that they were too busy to go home to rural areas for short periods. "Going home" to rural villages seemed to be a strategy that served as an "ultimate safety net" or part of a way to deal with long-term crises or periods of unemployment. Reliance on rural ties for food or assistance was not part of a short-term or day-to-day coping strategy.

In Durban, South Africa, he found that some households continue to regard their rural homestead as their real home (48 percent of his sample), while others, over time, lose all links with rural areas (19 percent). The importance of urban ties to rural areas thus probably varies with conditions in the specific city and country, as well as with the assets and ability of the household to form new support networks in urban areas.

Social assistance programs must also be careful not to inhibit private responses to crises. Several examples of situations where public programs negatively affected private coping strategies. With a school feeding program, for example, households may reduce the food given to a child at home and increase the allocation to other household members, thus defeating the purpose of the additional meal at school. A situation in Sri Lanka where a food stamp scheme resulted in a two-to-three-day reduction in labor market participation per month, approximately one-third of the value of the original food stamp subsidy. In one urban community in Zambia, 90 percent of the women stopped other income-generating activities to work on a self-help project. Although it was their choice to work on the programme, women supplanted their long-run coping strategies with the need to provide for their families in the short-run by taking the food-for-work job. A critical issue, then, is how to ensure that public safety nets complement informal coping strategies rather than inhibit them. This question is relevant for both the urban and the rural contexts.

The ability to measure poverty and identify the poor is often a crucial aspect of program design. There are three main types of targeting mechanisms: individual assessment; group or geographical targeting; and self-targeting. Two-stage screening is also used at times, whereby a geographical location is selected first (say, urban areas), and individual targeting (of poor households, for example) is done at a second stage. The more common criteria used for individual assessment include means testing (based on income) and the use of gender of household head or nutritional status. Group or geographical measures target beneficiaries who live in a particular area known to be poor or schools located in a particular region known to have high malnutrition rates. Self-targeting programs are usually designed in a manner to discourage participation of nonpoor individuals.

Informal and formal safety nets are important elements of a comprehensive social strategy. The design of effective formal safety nets depends on external government, donor, or NGO assistance and must take into account the nature and determinants of poverty and food and nutrition insecurity in urban areas. Formal safety nets must also ensure that they do not undermine the household's own private logic and response as it deals with falls in income or threats to food and nutrition security.

A number of safety net programs exist, ranging from general price subsidies to cash transfers to specific nutrition interventions. Some general principles about what kinds of programs work best under what conditions do exist, but they are few and in most cases have not been adequately studied. Information on how programs work together to form a complete antipoverty or food and nutrition strategy is lacking. In any case, programs will have to be adapted to local conditions, so situation-specific information is critical to the process of program choice and design. Community involvement in such identification of priorities and appropriate design and implementation is critical to sustainability and success. External support of a process through which the poor can redefine the relationships among themselves and with local authorities may be just as important as support of a specific project intervention.

5

Food and Nutrition Security in India

At the time of independence, India was faced with two major nutritional problems. One was the threat of famine and the resultant acute starvation due to low agricultural production and the lack of an appropriate food distribution system. The other was chronic energy deficiency due to:

— low dietary intake because of poverty and low purchasing power;

— high prevalence of infection because of poor access to safe-drinking water, sanitation and health care;

— poor utilisation of available facilities due to low literacy and lack of awareness.

The major public health problems were chronic energy deficiency (CED), kwashiorkor, marasmus and micronutrient deficiencies such as goitre, beriberi, blindness due to Vitamin-A deficiency and anaemia.

The country adopted multi-sectoral, multi-pronged strategy to combat these problems and to improve the nutritional status of the population. Article 47 of the Constitution of India states that "the State shall regard raising the level of nutrition and standard of living of its people and improvement in public health among its primary duties". Successive Five-Year Plans laid down the policies and strategies for achieving these goals.

The Green Revolution ensured that the increase in food production stayed ahead of the increase in population. The country has moved from chronic shortages to an era of surplus and export in most food items. The country is self sufficient in food grain production and currently there is a buffer stock of over 60 million tonnes. Along with the steps to achieve adequate production, initiatives were taken to reach foodstuffs of the right quality and quantity to the right places and persons at the right time and at an affordable cost.

Initiatives to improve nutritional status of the population during the last five decades include:

— Increasing food production- building buffer stocks

— Improving food distribution- building up the Public Distribution System (PDS)

— Improving household food security through

— Improving purchasing power

— Food for work programme

— Direct or indirect food subsidy

— Food supplementation to address special needs of the vulnerable groups-Integrated Child Development Services (ICDS), Mid-Day Meals

— Nutrition education especially through Food and Nutrition Board (FNB) and ICDS

— Efforts of the health sector to tackle

— Adverse health consequences of undernutrition

— Adverse effects of infection and unwanted fertility on the nutritional status

— Micronutrient deficiencies and their health consequences

Over the years, there has been improvement in access to food through the PDS; the food for work programme has addressed the needs of the vulnerable out-of-work persons. The ICDS programme aimed at providing food supplementation for pre-school children, pregnant and lactating women, nearly covers all blocks in the country.

The Mid-day-meal programme aimed at improving the dietary intake of primary school children and reduction in the school drop out rates has been operationalised. There has been substantial improvement in access to health care.

National programmes for tackling anaemia, iodine deficiency disorders and Vitamin-A deficiency are being implemented. As a result of all these interventions, there has been a substantial reduction in severe grades of under-nutrition in children and some improvement in the nutritional status of all the segments of population. Kwashiorkor, marasmus, pellagra, lathyrism, beriberi and blindness due to severe Vitamin-A deficiency have become rare.

However, several challenges remain. To meet all the nutritional needs of the growing population, the country will have to produce an extra five million tonnes of food grains annually and increase the production of livestock, fish and horticultural products. This has to be achieved in the face of shrinking arable land and farm size, low productivity, growing regional disparities in productivity and depletion of the natural resource base.

Appropriate steps have to be taken to minimise the potential adverse consequences of globalisation on domestic production, employment and price stability of food commodities. In spite of huge buffer stocks, 8 per cent of Indians do not get two square meals a day and there are pockets where severe under-nutrition takes its toll even today.

Every third child born is under weight. Low birth weight is associated not only with higher infant mortality but also long-term health consequences including increased risk of non-communicable diseases. In the last five decades, the mortality rate has come down by 50 percent and the fertility rate by 40 percent but the reduction in under nutrition is only 20 percent. Around half of the pre-school children suffer from under-nutrition.

Micronutrient deficiencies are widespread; more than half the women and children are anaemic; reduction in Vitamin-A deficiency and iodine deficiency disorders (IDD) is sub-optimal. Under-nutrition associated with HIV/AIDS will soon emerge as a public health problem. Alterations in lifestyles and dietary intake have led to the increasing prevalence of obesity and associated non-communicable diseases.

The country will have to gear itself up to prevent and combat the dual burden of under-nutrition and over-nutrition and associated health problems.

Major nutrition-related public health problems inlude:

— Chronic energy deficiency and undernutrition

— Micro-nutrient deficiencies

— Anaemia due to iron and folate deficiency

— Vitamin A deficiency

— Iodine Deficiency Disorders

— Chronic energy excess and obesity

During the Tenth Plan there will be focused and comprehensive interventions aimed at improving the nutritional and health status of the individuals.

There will be a paradigm shift from:

— household food security and freedom from hunger to nutrition security for the family and the individual;

— untargeted food supplementation to screening of all the persons from vulnerable groups, identification of those with various grades of under-nutrition and appropriate management;

— lack of focused interventions on the prevention of over-nutrition to the promotion of appropriate lifestyles and dietary intakes for the prevention and management of over-nutrition and obesity.

Interventions will be initiated to achieve:

Adequate availability of foodstuffs by:

— ensuring production of cereals, pulses and seasonal vegetables to meet the nutritional needs;

— making them available throughout the year at affordable cost through reduction in post harvest losses and appropriate processing;

— more cost-effective and efficient targeting of the PDS to address macro and micronutrient deficiencies. This may include providing coarse grains, pulses and iodised/ double fortified salt to below poverty line (BPL) families through the targeted PDS (TPDS);

— improving people's purchasing power through appropriate programmes including food for work schemes.

Prevention of under-nutrition through nutrition education aimed at:

— ensuring appropriate infant feeding practices (universal colostrum feeding, exclusive breast feeding up to six months, introduction of semisolids at six months);

— promoting appropriate intra-family distribution of food based on requirements;

— dietary diversification to meet the nutritional needs of the family.

Operationalising universal screening of all pregnant women, infants, preschool and school children for under-nutrition. Operationalisation of nutrition interventions for the management of under-nutrition through:

— targeted food supplementation and health care for those with under-nutrition;

— effective monitoring of these individuals and their families;

— utilisation of the panchayati raj institutions (PRIs) for effective inter-sectoral coordination and convergence of services and improving community participation in planning and monitoring of the ongoing interventions.

Prevention, early detection and appropriate management of micronutrient deficiencies and associated health hazards through:

— nutrition education to promote dietary diversification to achieve a balanced intake of all micronutrients;

— universal access to iodised/double fortified salt;

— early detection of micronutrient deficiencies through screening of all children with severe under-nutrition, pregnant women and school children;

— timely treatment of micronutrient deficiencies.

Promotion of appropriate dietary intake and lifestyles for the prevention and management of obesity and diet-related chronic diseases Nutrition monitoring and surveillance to enable the country to track changes in the nutritional and health status of the population to ensure that:

— the existing opportunities for improving nutritional status are fully utilized; and

— emerging problems are identified early and corrected expeditiously.

Research efforts will be directed towards:

— review of the recommended dietary intake of Indians;

— building up of epidemiological data on:

 — relationship between birth weight, survival, growth and development in childhood and adolescence;

 — body mass index norms of Indians and health consequences of deviation from these norms.

In view of the massive inter-state variations in the access to nutrition related services and nutritional status, state specific goals to be achieved by 2007 have been worked out taking the current status into account. National goals have been drawn taking into account the state specific goals.

Sustainable Food Production

One of the major achievements in the last 50 years has been the green revolution and self-sufficiency in food production. Food grain production has increased four-fold.

Food Production

Progress achieved:

— the country has achieved self-sufficiency in food grains to meet the needs of the growing population;

— there are ample food grain stocks.

Current Problems:

— 'Green Revolution Fatigue' in some areas;

— productivity remains low;

— improved food grain availability has not resulted in eradication of hunger or reduction in under-nutrition especially in vulnerable groups.

— very little attention is being paid to achieve integrated farming systems that will ensure sustainable evergreen revolution essential for appropriate dietary diversification to achieve nutrition security.

Paradigm shift needed:

— from self sufficiency in food grains to meet energy needs to providing food items needed for meeting all the nutritional needs;

— from production alone to reduction in post harvest losses and value addition through appropriate processing;

— from food security at the state level to nutrition security at the individual level.

Challenges:

— continue to improve food grain production to meet the needs of the growing population;

— increase production of coarse grains to meet the energy requirements of the BPL families at a lower cost;

— increase production of pulses and make them affordable to increase consumption;

— improve the availability of vegetables at an affordable cost throughout the year in urban and rural areas.

Opportunities:

— achieve substantial improvement in nutrition security;

— achieve decline in macro and micronutrient under-nutrition.

Interventions to Improve Food Production

Food grain production

Inputs needed to achieve a sustainable increase in food grain production to meet the needs of the growing population have to be provided. Locally produced and procured coarse grains made available through the TPDS at a subsidised rate may substantially bring down the subsidy cost without any reduction in calories provided. This will also improve targeting as only the most needy are likely to buy these coarse grains. Millets are rich in minerals and micronutrients and hence increased consumption will improve the intake of these vital nutrients by the poor.

Pulse production

In the last two decades, there has been a progressive decline in pulse consumption, especially among the poorer segments of the population. This is due to stagnant production and the rising cost of pulses. This trend has to be reversed. Measures to improve pulse production may include reactivation of the pulse component of the Oil Seed and Pulse Mission, a major thrust on research and development and innovative community-based efforts similar to the M.S. Swaminathan Research Foundation's efforts in Tamil Nadu to improve pulse production.

Horticultural production

Available data on the current production of fruits and vegetables and the projected demand for 2006 are shown in Table 1. Per capita consumption of these in the country is very low. Consumption of adequate quantities of vegetables, especially green leafy ones, is essential for meeting the dietary requirement of vital micronutrients. Besides, vegetables also provide several phytochemicals and fibre.

Table 1: Fruits and vegetables (in million tons)

	Demand 2006	Production 1997/98
Fruit	50	40.05
Vegetables	130	72.83

At present, there is insufficient focus on the cultivation and marketing of low-cost, locally-acceptable green leafy vegetables, yellow vegetables and fruits. As a result, these vegetables are not available at affordable cost throughout the year.

Health and nutrition education emphasising the importance of consuming these inexpensive but rich sources of micronutrients will not result in any change in food habits unless the horticultural resources in the country are harnessed and managed effectively to meet the growing needs of the people at an affordable cost. Horticultural products provide higher yields per hectare and sell at higher prices. The processing, storage and transportation of horticultural products in a manner so that there is no glut and distress sales will make their production economically attractive to farmers and improve availability to the consumers.

Homestead production for dietary diversification

Homestead production is another method of increasing consumption of vegetables, milk and animal products and reduces the gap in consumption. Strategies can be worked out for using degraded lands for vegetable production. Farm wastes as well as food grains unfit for human consumption can be used to feed backyard poultry in order to increase homestead production of eggs and chicken and also increase consumption of these at home.

Table 2: Per capita availability and deficit

Food items	Per capita availability	ICMR dietary guidelines for Indians	Per capita deficit
Milk	216 g**/day	300 ml*/day	34 g/day
Egg	30 eggs/annum	180 eggs/annum	150 eggs/annum
Meat	3.24 kg/annum	10.95 kg/annum	7.71 kg/annum

* milli litre ** grams

Food Processing and Preservation

Post harvest losses especially in vegetables and fruits are presently in the range of 20 to 30 percent and contribute directly to higher costs and reduce availability of these commodities. Precision farming and food processing based on science and technology are both intellectually stimulating and economically rewarding, they can increase farmers' income and rural employment considerably. This will not only help in retaining educated youth in the farm sector but would also enable the micro-nutrient needs of the population to be met through a sustainable food-based approach.

Equitable Distribution of Foodstuffs

Achievement of food adequacy at the national level is a necessary, though not sufficient, precondition to ensure the achievement of household nutrition security. Buffer stocks do help to combat acute transient food scarcity, caused by natural disasters like floods and droughts. Early warning systems are in place and food can be rushed to areas of threatened distress fairly rapidly. What is proving more difficult is the task of combating chronic mild / moderate under-nutrition in a large number of poor households. Inequitable distribution of available food among different segments of the population and even within the family is one of the major factors responsible for under-nutrition / over-nutrition. Good governance and health and nutrition education hold the key to improving equitable distribution of food based on need.

The TPDS was introduced in June 1997 in an attempt to limit the mounting cost of subsidy, and at the same time, ensure that the BPL population does get subsidised food grains. Under this system subsidised foodgrains are provided only to people below the poverty line. Taking the average household size as 5.51 (1991 Census), the monthly requirement of food grain for a household is 73 kg. TPDS meets only a part of the total requirement of food grains for the family.

Apart from TPDS, other initiatives to improve food security of families include:

— Allocation of food grains to institutions where indigent people live at rates similar to that for BPL population;

— Annapoorna Scheme to provide foodgrains to indigent old persons;

— Antyodaya Anna Yojana to provide food grains to the poorest of the poor families among the BPL population at the rate of Rs.2 per kg for wheat and Rs.3 per kg for rice;

— Sampoorna Grameen Rozgar Yojana for rural poor in need of wage employment; preference is given to scheduled castes, scheduled tribes and parents of children withdrawn from hazardous jobs.

Role of the Community

Innovative local efforts can go a long way in improving nutrition security especially for the poorer segments of the population living in vulnerable areas. Formation of local food grain banks under the supervision of the PRIs to help in achieving nutrition security for all and insulating the economically and socially deprived sections of the community from seasonal food insecurity has been suggested.

During the Tenth Plan period every effort will be made to:

— identify vulnerable groups/families, undernourished individuals and provide them with well-targeted subsidised food items through TPDS. In addition to the supply of rice and wheat, locally procured coarse grains, pulses and iodised salt may be provided;

— test and evaluate various modalities of improving the efficiency of the systems currently in operation to improve household nutrition security;

— choose appropriate modalities for making optimal use of available subsidies to meet the needs of the vulnerable segments of the population; and

— ensure that there is no duplication of schemes for improving nutrition security to vulnerable groups.

Community Food bank

Main features of the proposed food bank are:

- one bank for every village or cluster of villages with population ranging from 2000 to 5000;
- supervised by a society or council chosen by the gram sabha;
- managed by a stakeholder council, with different operations assigned to different self-help groups;
- to be implemented with honesty, political neutrality, fairness, absence of discrimination based on religion, caste, class, gender and political belief.

Managment of Transient Food Scarcity

Though the country has averted large-scale severe under-nutrition or famine in the past five decades, droughts do pose a major threat to food security. Over the years, the country has developed a system for the early recognition and management of transient food scarcity in times of drought. During the Ninth Plan period, Rajasthan, Andhra Pradesh and Gujarat were affected by drought. Of the various relief measures, Andhra Pradesh benefited only from additional ration through PDS. In the other two states, additional measures such as food for work, supply of drinking water, essential medicines and cattle feed were also in operation.

The National Institute of Nutrition (NIN), Hyderabad conducted a survey in the drought-affected districts in these three states to assess the impact of drought and the ongoing intervention programmes on the diet and nutritional status of the population. In

Rajasthan, there was no increase prevalence of CED in adults as compared to the non-drought period. However, there was an increase in the prevalence under-nutrition in pre-school children (64.8 per cent) as compared to non-drought period (46.7 per cent). In Gujarat and Andhra Pradesh, prevalence CED in children and adults was not more in the drought-affected districts. These data suggest that except in the case of children in Rajasthan, the adverse consequences of drought on the nutritional status were prevented due to intervention programmes.

During the Tenth Plan period, efforts will be made to monitor rainfall data to provide early warning of drought. Monitoring agricultural production will provide information about impending food insecurity. In drought-prone areas intensive monitoring of the nutritional status of pre-school children based on ICDS reporting system will help assess the severity of the problem at block level. Timely relief measures can be organised based on these data. Apart from other process indicators for monitoring the relief operations, monitoring the nutritional status of pre-school children through the ICDS system will be used for assessing the out reach, adequacy and impact of relief measures.

Nutritional Status of Tribal Population

The tribal population is not a homogeneous group. There are wide variations among the groups nutritional status and access to and utilisation of nutrition and health services. The tribal populations the north-eastern states have high literacy levels; they access available facilities, and hence their nutritional and health status is better than the national level. On the other hand, primitive tribes such as the Onges in the Andamans have very little awareness or access to either nutrition or health care. Differential area-specific need assessment, strategies and programmes to improve access and utilisation of nutrition services have to be developed for each of the tribal areas.

Higher prevalence of under-nutrition in tribal population is due to

— poverty and consequent under-nutrition

— lack of awareness about, access to and utilisation of the available nutrition supplementation programmes;

— social barriers preventing the utilisation of available nutrition supplementation programme and services.

— poor environmental sanitation and lack of safe drinking water, leading to increased morbidity from water-borne infections;

— environmental conditions that favour vector-borne diseases;

— lack of access to health care facilities resulting in increased severity and /or duration of illnesses.

The tribal population is recognised as socially and economically vulnerable. Their lifestyles and food habits are different from that of their rural neighbours. They depend on minor forest produce, are employed in manual labour and may not have adequate income. Their food consumption pattern is dependent on the vagaries of nature and varies from extreme deprivation to high intakes. Several focused interventions for tribal development and improvement in their health and nutritional status have been initiated in the last three decades. In order to assess the impact of these, the National Nutrition Monitoring Bureau (NNMB) carried out a repeat diet and nutrition surveys of the tribal populations living in the Integrated Tribal Development Project (ITDP) areas in 1998-99. These covered the states of Kerala, Tamil Nadu, Karnataka, Andhra Pradesh, Maharashtra, Gujarat, Orissa and West Bengal, where the NNMB had carried out an earlier survey in 1985-87. Comparison of data of the two surveys showed that there has not been any improvement in the food and nutrient intake. However, there has been some reduction in the prevalence of severe forms of under-nutrition and in nutritional deficiency signs. The tribal population is more under-nourished than their rural counterparts.

There were substantial differences in the food and nutrient intake and nutritional status between tribal populations living in different states. In some population groups, there was adequate intake of minerals and some micronutrients even though the diet was inadequate in terms of meeting energy and protein needs. The nutritional status of women and children in some of the northeastern states with a predominantly tribal population is better than the national average.

Table 3: Inter-State Differences in Nutrient Intake

	State with	
Nutrient Intake	*Lowest*	*Highest*
1-3 age-group		
Protein	10g	24.5g
Energy	466 k cal	1000 k cal
Vit. A	34 μg	264 μg
4-6 age-group		
Protein	19.8 g	36.3 g
Energy	756 k cal	1524 k cal
Vit. A	51.2 μg	502.7 μg
>18 years males		
Protein	47.0g	59.5g
Energy	1932k cal	2503k cal
Vit. A	8 μg	57 μg

Table 4: Nutritional Status in North Eastern States

State	% Tribal population as per 1991 Census	Weight-for-age % below -3SD children < 3 years	% ever married women with Height below 145 cm	BMI < 18.5 kg/m²	BMI > 25 kg/m²
Arunachal	63.7	7.8	11.9	10.7	5.1
Meghalaya	85.5	11.3	10.3	18.8	10.8
Mizoram	94.8	5.0	21.1	25.8	5.8
Nagaland	87.7	7.4	10.7	22.6	5.3
All-India	8.1	18.0	13.2	20.3	10.6

During the Tenth Plan, monitoring nutritional status of the tribal population, especially of those who have poor access to services, will be continued. Monitoring of the ICDS reporting will provide early warning of any deterioration in the nutritional status in pre-school children so that appropriate intervention can be initiated. Research studies on dietary habits that contribute to good nutritional status as well as those that make the tribal population vulnerable to diseases will be carried out. Based on the data, specific intervention programmes will be taken up to improve nutritional status and to eliminate dietary habits that are likely to cause ill health.

Energy Requirement of Indians

Energy requirement is defined as the amount that will balance the energy expenditure of the individual consistent with long-term good health. This intake will allow for the maintenance of economically necessary and socially desirable physical activity. In children and pregnant/ lactating women, the energy requirement will include energy needed for deposition of tissue and secretion of milk at the rate consistent with good health.

All estimates of requirement are based on habitual intakes and though these are expressed as daily intake, it is not implied that these amounts must be consumed on a daily basis. Estimates of requirement are derived from actual data of individuals on intake and expenditure. Actual intakes and expenditure of people of the same age, sex, similar body size and performing similar physical activity are used to compute average energy requirement for tne groups.

The recommended intake of energy of a group is equal to the average energy requirement of individuals of the group because both lower and higher energy intake are associated with health hazards. This is in contrast to other nutrients. For example, the recommended safe level of protein intake is the mean +2 SD value of the group because with this over 97 per cent of the persons in the group would get their requirements. Studies have shown that Indians have about 5 per cent lower Basal Metabolic Rate (BMR) than those predicted on the basis of WHO/ FAO/ UNU equations. The possible causes of lower BMR among Indian include:

— under-nutrition with low body weight and low BMI (weight in kg/ height in metre 2);

— under-nutrition resulting in lower protein turn-over (which accounts for 20 per cent of BMR);

— difference in proportion of muscle and viscera;

— lower oxygen supply to the muscle;

However, the energy cost of work done computed in terms of basal energy cost or physical activity ratios are similar. For computing RDA, the ICMR has taken body weight of 'reference man' as 60 kg and that of 'woman' as 50 kg. Average weight of Indian men is 52 kg and women 44 Kg. For children and adolescents, weight for age from NCHS / well-to-do Indian children have been utilised by ICMR for deriving the RDA so that energy intake enables optimum growth. However, as in adults, majority of children and adolescents weigh substantially less and hence their energy requirement is lower. In view of these, it is likely that the energy requirement of Indians is likely to be substantially lower than the current ICMR recommendations.

Over the last few decades there has been a reduction in the physical activity and hence reduction in the energy needs in all the age and weight categories. Obesity rates in all age groups are increasing mainly because of the reduction in physical activity without concomitant reduction in energy intake. In view of the known adverse health consequences of both excess and deficient energy intake, it is essential that appropriate recommendation for the RDA for Indians is evolved. This has to be done quickly as the country is entering an era of dual disease burden of CED and infections on the one hand and that of obesity and non-communicable diseases on the other.

Table 5:ICMR's RDA for Energy
(reference body weights and actual body weights)

Sex	Ref. body weight	Actual body weight	activity category	Energy for ref. body weight	RDA for actual body weight	percent difference
			Sedentary	2425	2115	13
Man	60.0	52.0	Moderate	2875	2492	13
			Heavy	3800	3293	13
			Sedentary	1875	1740	12
Woman	50.0	44.0	Moderate	2225	1958	12
			Heavy	2925	2594	11

During the Tenth Plan, review of the RDA for Indians will be taken up on a priority basis. The ICMR has reconstituted its Expert Committee on RDA which will take all the above factors into consideration and come up with an appropriate recommendation regarding the dietary intake of Indians.

One of the priority areas of research during the Tenth Plan will be studies to define the BMR and energy requirement of healthy adult Indian men and women, adolescents, children and the elderly. Simultaneously studies will be taken up to define the dietary intake needed to correct the chronic energy deficiency or obesity in each of these groups.

Assessment of Nutrional Status

Anthropometric indices (height, weight and BMI) are widely used for the assessment of the adequacy of energy intake. Body weights and heights of children reflect their nutritional and growth status; weights and heights of adults represent the cumulative effect of dietary intake over a long period. The BMI is the most widely used anthropometric index for the assessment of the nutritional status in adults as it reflects the effect of both acute and chronic energy deficiency/excess.

BMI, however, does not clearly bring out the entire extent of chronic under-nutrition. For instance those who are stunted and have low body weight may have normal BMI. An increase in energy intake will result in improvement in BMI both in adults and in children, but in adults and children with severe stunting, improvement in dietary intake will not result in an improvement in height. Continued over-consumption of energy especially in stunted individuals could lead to over-nutrition, obesity and increased risk of non-communicable diseases. It has also been reported that the body fat content for a given BMI is different not only between men and women but also among countries.

BMI has been used to assess energy deficiency as well as energy excess. The currently used norms (<18.5 - undernutrition and >25 over-weight) were evolved on the basis of data from the developed countries where adverse health consequences of under-nutrition have been shown to be associated with BMI values below 18.5 and the health hazards of over-nutrition have been reported with BMI of over 25. The mean and frequency distribution of BMI of Indians are substantially different from developed countries. It is, therefore, possible that the currently used classification may be satisfactory for developed countries but not for India.

There are wide variations in height, weight, body composition and BMI right from birth through childhood and adolescence between countries and different income groups in the same country. Birth weight and growth of Indian children from well-to- do segments of the population are similar to United States National Center of Health Statistics (NCHS) standards but adult heights and weights in India are lower.

The functional significance of inter-country variations in stature are not yet clearly understood. However, the existing gap between the stature of Indians from well-to-do families where there are no nutritional constraints and under-nourished persons from poorer segments of the population is clearly due to poor nutrition and health care. The short-term nutritional goal of the country is to identify individuals and families, who are under-nourished and provide them with adequate nutrition and health care so that they do not incur health hazard associated with under-nutrition.

As both CED and obesity are associated with adverse health consequences, it has been suggested that each country should develop its own norms for BMI and cut-off points indicative of various degrees of under-nutrition and over-nutrition based on their own data on health problems in persons with varying BMI levels. In view of the profound implications of these suggestions it is essential that research studies are taken up during the Tenth Plan period to examine the usefulness of currently used cut-off points of BMI as indicators of CED, metabolic functions, work capacity and health indices. It is also important to collect data on BMI of well-nourished Indians in different regions and the health profile of adults with different BMI. Epidemiological data on the risk of non-communicable diseases among different BMI groups in India will have to be collected to evolve appropriate cut-off points for BMI in Indians so that those at risk can be identified and appropriate interventions undertaken.

Dietary Intake and Nutritional Status of Adults

Over the last three decades, there have been substantial changes in the socio-economic status of people, some increase in the dietary intake of men and women especially of the affluent segments in rural and urban areas, ready availability of fast foods, ice creams and other energy rich food items at affordable costs have resulted in increased energy consumption.

About 48 per cent of the households consumed more than adequate amount of both proteins and calories, while 20 per cent of households consumed inadequate amounts of both the nutrients. With increasing access to cooking gas, piped water supply, labour-saving gadgets and transport, there has been a substantial reduction in the physical activity pattern and energy expenditure, especially in the middle and upper income groups.

Data from NNMB repeat surveys indicate that there has been some reduction in under-nutrition and some increase in obesity over the last two decades. Data from National Family Health Survey-2 (NFHS) confirms that currently both under-nutrition and over-nutrition are problems in women and that there are massive inter-state differences. The percentage of women with under-nutrition varies from 10.7 in Arunachal Pradesh to 48 in Orissa and those who are over-weight from 3.7 in Bihar to 33.8 in Delhi. The country will, therefore, have to gear up to prevent, detect and tackle the problems of both under-nutrition and over-nutrition in the next two decades.

Over the last two decades there have been a growing number of reports that Indians are a very high-risk group for cardiovascular diseases and diabetes. A majority of them are not obese and do not have risk factors associated with non-communicable diseases in the developed countries.

The higher prevalence of non-communicable diseases among persons whose birth weights were low has been documented. It has been hypothesised that people who have lived under nutritional constraints over millennia have 'thrifty genes' which enable them to survive and sustain themselves with lower energy intake. In such a population, any rapid increase in energy intake may result in increased risk of non-communicable diseases. This is an area where further research studies need to be done.

The amount by which the dietary intake should be increased or decreased to correct CED/ obesity in adults will depend upon the rate at which the desirable weight is to be achieved and the extent to which the deficit or excess in weight is due to lean and fat tissue. Since adults cannot grow, the appropriate weight for actual height is to be calculated and the appropriate dietary intake to correct under-nutrition or over-nutrition computed.

In adults who are seriously under-weight for their height, there will generally be a loss of both fat stores and lean body mass. Therefore, bringing their weight into the normal range requires additional amounts of both energy and protein. Clinical experiences suggested that under-weight adults who are free from disease could be rehabilitated fairly rapidly if they eat to appetite.

For correction of obesity, a low energy diet coupled with adequate exercise will be needed. If low energy diet is to be continued for a long period to achieve desired reduction in weight, it is essential to ensure adequate amounts of protein and micronutrients intake. For sedentary adults food low in energy density, rich in fibre containing lot of vegetables and adequate exercise would go a long way in terms of providing satiety and preventing obesity.

During the Tenth Plan, the major thrust would be to undertake massive health and nutrition education to encourage appropriate dietary intake and healthy life styles among all segments of the population. Epidemiological studies will be initiated to obtain data on dietary intake, nutritional and health status to define levels at which functional impairment in health status occur.

Geriatric Nutrition

With increasing longevity, the proportion and number of persons in the age group of 60 years and beyond is rapidly increasing, with women out- numbering men. The population of elderly has been projected to double from6.23 crore in 1996 to 11.29 crore in 2016. With increasing age, there are metabolic changes and also reduction in physical activity and, as a result, their energy requirement is substantially lower than younger adult.

Elderly individuals face problems in ensuring appropriate dietary intake because of alteration in taste with increasing age and loss of teeth. The reduction in physical activity with increasing age, not accompanied by a concurrent reduction in energy intake, makes the elderly prone to obesity. Due to low intake of vegetables, food rich in micronutrients and increased susceptibility to infection, anaemia and Vitamin B complex deficiency may be more common in the elderly.

Adequate dietary calcium intake from birth to 30 years is critical for the development of peak bone mass. Osteoporosis occurs more commonly in women than in men as bone loss occurs earlier and more rapidly in women as compared to men. With increasing longevity, there will be an increase in the number of persons with osteoporosis. There is very little data on the incidence of osteoporosis in India.

Lack of social support, breaking up of the joint family system, changing lifestyles all aggravate the health and nutritional problems of the elderly. Available data from nutrition surveys indicate that the dual problem of chronic energy and micronutrient deficiency on the one hand and obesity on the other are seen among the elderly. Innovative efforts to provide societal support, health care and nutrition services to the elderly are currently being taken up by several agencies. Simultaneously, there are efforts to improve family and societal support to elderly within the existing cultural ethos in different regions. Successful models for improving quality of life will have to be replicated.

In many states elderly persons who are without any financial support get old age pension. The amount as well as coverage varies between states but, on the whole, the amount provided is too low to meet the nutritional needs of the elderly person. Following reports of severe under-nutrition among the elderly and destitute persons in several states, the central and the state governments initiated steps to improve the access of these segments to food-grains. The National Policy on Older Persons announced in January 1999 provides a framework for welfare of the elderly persons including improved financial security and increased access to health and nutrition services. It is envisaged that National Plan of Action for the implementation of the policy will be drawn up. The policy also recommends research to expand the knowledge base on nutritional needs of the elderly.

During the Tenth Plan, a database on the magnitude of the nutritional problems in the elderly (under-nutrition, micronutrient deficiency and obesity) will have to be created through the ongoing diet and nutrition surveys. Based on the data appropriate area- specific intervention programmes can be drawn up. While the technical inputs will come from the nutritionists, implementation of the programme will largely rest with the families, community and the PRIs.

Nutritional Status of Adolescents

Projections made by the Technical Group on Population Projections indicate that the number of adolescents (in the 10-19 age group) will increase from 200 million in 1996 to 215.3 million in 2016. Adolescents, who are undergoing rapid growth and development, are one of the nutritionally vulnerable groups who have not received the attention they deserve.

Adolescents gain 30 per cent of their adult weight and more than 20 per cent of their adult height between 10 and 19 years. Taking into account, the desirability of achieving full potential for growth, ICMR has used NCHS/well-to-do Indian children's body weight for computing RDA for adolescents. However, children from the poorer segments of the population in India are shorter and weigh less. It is unlikely that any extra food at this stage can accelerate or extend the duration of physical growth. Additional dietary intake at this period can only lead to adolescent obesity. The ICMR Expert Committee for RDA may have to take all these into account and evolve appropriate recommendations for dietary intake in Indian adolescents. Data from NNMB also shows that over this period there has been some increase in obesity among adolescents especially for those from the affluent groups both in the urban and rural areas. The prevalence of micronutrient deficiencies are high. With the onset of menstruation, girls in this age group are vulnerable to anaemia and all its adverse consequences.

Data from NFHS-2 indicate that the median age at marriage of girls in India is 16 years and 61 per cent of all girls were married before the age of 18. There are large inter-state variations in age at marriage. The mean age at first birth is 19.2. Under-nutrition, anaemia and poor ante-natal care inevitably lead not only to increased maternal morbidity but also to higher incidence of low birth weight and peri-natal mortality. Poor childrearing practices of these girls will add to infant morbidity and under-nutrition, thus perpetuating the intergenerational cycle of under nutrition. Appropriate education, nutrition and health interventions, delay in age at marriage, optimum health and nutrition interventions during pregnancy are some of the inter-sectoral initiatives to break this vicious cycle.

With a view to minimising these adverse effects, appropriate nutritional and health interventions for adolescents are being taken up under the ICDS and Reproductive and Child Health (RCH) Programmes. The Department of Women and Child Development has launched Kishori Shakti Yojana.

Prime Minister in his Independence day address in 2001 stated that food grains will be provided to combat under-nutrition in adolescent girls and pregnant and lactating women. A pilot project is being initiated to operationalise the announcement of the Prime Minister. The project, initially for a period of two years, will be taken up in two of the backward districts in each of the major states and most populous district (excluding the capital district) in the remaining smaller states/Union Territories. The funds for 2002-03 is being given as special additional central assistance to the states so that they can provide food grains through TPDS totally free of cost to the families of identified under-nourished persons. The programme will be operationalised through the Department of Women and Child Development in the centre and in the states.

During the Tenth Plan, studies to improve the understanding of the relationship between energy requirements, body composition, endocrine changes and micronutrient status in children and adolescents will be taken up so that appropriate focused interventions can be initiated. Programmes to improve the nutrition and health status of adolescents will be effectively implemented.

Adolescent girls fall into two categories—those who are in school and those who are not. The focus of efforts to improve the health and nutritional status of those who are in school will have to be through the school health system. Efforts will be made to screen all for anaemia and under-nutrition and provide appropriate management. Screening will also enable the identification of obese adolescents and the initiation of appropriate remedial measures. Appropriate information, education, communication and motivation (IECM) to delay marriage until at least the age of 18 and postpone child-bearing till the age of 20 will be vigorously taken up.

A majority of the girls in the out-of-school category marry during their early teens and conceive soon after. The focus of any strategy will be to get these girls to the anganwadi so that the anganwadi worker, in collaboration with the auxiliary nurse midwife (ANM), can undertake the following activities:

— screening for under-/over-nutrition and micro-nutrient deficiencies;

— targeted interventions to tackle the nutritional problems of adolescents, especially girls;

— introduction of community-supported supplementary nutrition programmes using community food and food prepared by women's groups using locally-available commodities and given on a priority basis to adolescent girls who are under-nourished or pregnant;

— IEC to improve awareness;

— health and nutrition education to prevent early pregnancies and under-nutrition; and

— appropriate antenatal and intrapartum care and contraceptive care when needed.

Nutritional Status of Pregnant and Lactating Women

Traditional belief was that pregnant and lactating women require additional dietary intake as they have to meet their own nutritional requirements and also supply nutrients to the foetus and the infants. Some available data indicated that a low dietary intake, especially in already chronically undernourished women, had adverse effects on the health and nutritional status of the mother, the course and outcome of pregnancy and the birth weight of the offspring.

Both the ICMR and the WHO Expert Groups recommended additional intake for pregnant and lactating women. The WHO had recommended an additional 300 kilo calories (Kcal) throughout pregnancy and 500 additional Kcal during the first year of lactation. The ICMR has recommended an additional intake of 300 Kcal during the second and third trimester of pregnancy, 550 Kcal during the first six months of lactation and 400 Kcal during 7- 12 months of lactation.

Epidemiological data from the developed and developing countries, however, indicate that there is no increase in dietary intake during pregnancy and lactation among habitually well-nourished women who eat to appetite. This did not have any adverse effect either on their own nutritional status or on the course and outcome of pregnancy. Studies undertaken during the 1980s have shown that there are adaptive changes during pregnancy.

There is a reduction in BMR and physical activity and there might be some improvement in the as yet unmeasured efficiency of energy utilisation. The energy and nutrients saved due to these adaptive processes are sufficient to meet the increased requirements for nutrients during pregnancy. So long as there is no reduction in the habitual dietary intake, there is no deterioration in the maternal nutritional status either during pregnancy or during lactation. In well-nourished individuals, additional intake during pregnancy and lactation results in excessive weight gain and this may lead to obesity.

However, there are limits to adaptations. Studies from developing countries have shown that reduction in dietary intake below habitual levels and increased workload above the habitual levels are associated with deterioration in maternal nutritional status and reduction in birth weight. Some such readily identifiable situations are:

— reduction in habitual dietary intake during drought and the pre-harvest season;

— increase in work e.g., newly inducted manual laborers;

— combination of both the above (food for work programmes);

— adolescent pregnancy;

— pregnancy in a lactating woman; and

— pregnancy occurring within two years after last delivery.

Research studies in India and elsewhere have shown if pregnant women in whom there has been a reduction in habitual dietary intake or excess energy expenditure or whose body weight is less than 40 kg are identified and given adequate continuous food supplementation and antenatal care there is substantial improvement in outcome of pregnancy, birth weight and neonatal mortality.

Encouraged by such data, almost all developing countries embarked on food supplementation programmes for pregnant and lactating women. None of these programmes screen pregnant women or provide supplements only to those with energy gap or those with moderate/severe undernutrition. When food supplements are provided without screening, targeting supplementation and monitoring the programme, the improvement in maternal nutrition, and birth weight, if any, is very limited.

One of the major problems is to reach food supplements to the under-nourished women. Even when the logistics of reaching the food to women is meticulously worked out and efficiently carried out, food sharing patterns within the family results in the 'target' women not getting the supplements in significant quantities. Obviously this is one of the factors responsible for the demonstrated lack of beneficial effect. The lack of adequate antenatal care and continued physical work during pregnancy are two other factors responsible for the lack of impact.

Under the ICDS programme, food supplements are being provided to pregnant and lactating women who come to anganwadis. The reported coverage is between 15 and 20 per cent in most blocks. The women who receive supplements are not being chosen on the basis of their nutritional status and may not be the most needy ones. There has not been any evaluation studies on this component of the ICDS. However, data from nutrition surveys indicate that there has not been any significant decline in maternal under-nutrition over the last decade.

During the Tenth Plan efforts will be made to weigh all women as early in pregnancy as possible and to monitor their weight gain. Well-nourished women will be advised not to increase their dietary intake to prevent over nutrition and obesity. Women who weigh less than 40 kg will be identified and

— given food supplements consistently throughout pregnancy;

— given adequate antenatal care;

— monitored for weight gain during pregnancy and, if weight gain is sub-optimal, identify the causes and attempt remedial measures; and

— given appropriate antenatal, intrapartum and postpartum care.

Effective intersectoral coordination between ANMs and anganwadi workers will enable the identification of and provision of appropriate care to undernourished pregnant women. The PRIs can play an important role by ensuring that these women receive food supplement throughout pregnancy. The methods by which food supplements can be provided to identified undernourished pregnant and lactating women may vary. In some cases the food may be provided at the work site. In yet other cases, it might be possible to link antenatal care and the provision of free food-grains for pregnant and lactating women on lines similar to the Mid-day-meals scheme to increase enrolment. With the empowerment of the PRIs and nagar palikas, it might be possible to monitor these programmes at the local level and consequently achieve better coverage. If well-targeted intervention to identify undernourished women and provide them health and nutrition education and ante-natal care are implemented effectively, there can be substantial reduction severe under-nutrition in pregnant women and low birth weight. The feasibility, utilisation, cost and impact of such well-directed, innovative strategies involving close local monitoring need to be assessed.

Maternal Nutrition and Birth Weight

It is estimated that one-third of Indian neonates weigh less than 2.5 kg at birth. There are substantial differences in the maternal body weight and birth weight between income groups, which are partly due to differences in the nutritional status and partly due to differences in health care.

Table 6: Birth Weight and Socio-economic Status

	Poor Income	Middle Income	High Income
Age (years)	24.1	24.3	27.8
Parity	2.41	1.96	1.61
Height (cm)	151.5	154.2	156.3
Weight (kg)	45.7	49.9	56.2
Hb (g/dl)	10.9	11.1	12.4
Birh weight (kg)	2.70	2.90	3.13

Identification of infants weighing less than 2.2 kg and referring them to hospitals where a paediatrician is available will substantially reduce neonatal mortality. During the Tenth Plan, efforts will be made to ensure that the anganwadi workers report all births in the village, weigh all neonates delivered at home soon after birth and refer those weighing less than 2.2 kg to a hospital with a pediatrician. This will enable development of referral services, reduce neonatal mortality and generate nation-wide data on birth weight and prevalence of low birth weight.

Growth During Infancy

Energy requirements during infancy are very high because this is one of the periods of very rapid growth. The energy cost of growth in infants and children include two components: the energy value for the tissue and the energy cost of synthesising the tissue. This has to be taken into account along with the basal energy needs and energy needs for activity in infants and children. Available data suggest that energy needs are highest during the first three months and then fall over the next six months when the growth rates are lower. It rises again after nine months as the child becomes physically more active. The RDA for infants drawn up both by WHO and by ICMR takes this phenomenon into account.

Growth during infancy and childhood depend upon birth weight, adequacy of infant feeding and absence of infection. Available data clearly indicate that in India exclusively breast-fed infants thrive normally during the first six months of life and have lower morbidity episodes than those receiving supplements in addition to breast milk. In view of this, promotion of universal exclusive breast-feeding for the first six months of life has been the national policy. Breast milk alone is insufficient to meet the growing baby's needs after six months and appropriate semi-solid complementary foods have to be introduced to enable them to meet their nutrient needs. Care should be taken to reduce the chances of infection by providing freshly prepared food.

In India, steps taken for the protection and promotion of the practice of breast-feeding have been effective and breast feeding is almost universal. However, the message that exclusive breast feeding up to six months and gradual introduction of semisolids after that are critical for the prevention of under-nutrition in infancy has not been as effectively communicated. Data from NFHS-2 indicated that exclusive breast-feeding among infants in the age group of 0-3 months was only 55.2 percent. In spite of the emphasis on the need for timely introduction of complementary food only 33.5 per cent of the infants in the age group of 6-9 months received breast milk and semi- solid food.

There are substantial inter-state differences in exclusive breast feeding and timely introduction of semi-solid food. While Andhra Pradesh and Kerala fare well in terms of appropriate infant feeding practices, the too early introduction of supplements is a major problem in states like Delhi, Himachal Pradesh and Punjab and too late introduction of supplements is a big problem in Bihar, Uttar Pradesh, Madhya Pradesh, Rajasthan, and Orissa. Both these practices are associated with increased risk of under-nutrition and infection.

As a result of these faulty infant feeding habits, there is a steep increase in the prevalence of under-nutrition from 11.9 per cent at less than 6 months to 58.5

per cent in the 12- 23 months age group. Correction of these faulty infant feeding practices through nutrition education will prevent the steep increase in under-nutrition in the 6-24 months age group.

During the Tenth Plan the major focus will be on:

— promotion of exclusive breast feeding in the first six months;

— nutrition education for the introduction of appropriate low-cost, energy dense complementary food at six months of age;

— three-monthly monitoring of weight in infancy and childhood; and

— detection of infants with faltering growth and initiating appropriate steps to improve their nutritional status.

Studies carried out at the NIN had shown that if roasted, coarsely ground cereals, pulses and oil seeds mixture is provided to households free of cost, the mothers were willing and able to give this to young children three to four times a day; as a result there was improvement in timely introduction of complementary food.

In an effort to find out if this could be replicated at the national level, Additional Central Assistance is being given since 2000-01 under the nutrition component of PMGY to provide such a mixture once a week to BPL families totally free of cost. The progress and impact of this will be assessed during the Tenth Plan period. The goals for the Tenth Plan are to

— enhance early initiation of breast-feeding (colostrum feeding) from the current level of 15.8 per cent (as per NFHS 2) to 50 per cent;

— enhance the exclusive breast-feeding rate for children up to the age of six months from the current rate of 55.2 per cent (as per NFHS 2) to 80 per cent; and

— enhance the complementary feeding rate at six months from the current level of 33.5 percent (as per NFHS 2) to 75 per cent.

Growth During Childhood

The WHO/FAO/ UNU and the ICMR Expert Committee took note of the fact that Indian children are smaller at birth, infancy,childhood and adolescence but suggested that it is desirable that the growth potential of children should be fully expressed and that the estimates of energy and protein requirement should allow for this. However, as the normal Indian children are smaller and they weigh less, the actual energy requirements may be substantially lower. It is a matter of concern that even this small amount is not fully met.

Low dietary intake is associated with short and long term metabolic, biological, genetic, social and behaviourial adaptations. Reduction in physical activity could be behavioural adaptation in children to low energy intake. While this could be considered as a protective adaptation to ensure continuing growth, it may impair the child's curiosity, exploration or play and hence have adverse consequences on intellectual and social development. Research studies are needed to define adaptation to low dietary intake and its functional consequences.

Even though, Indian children have lower birth weight, dietary intake, growth trajectories and body size than their counterparts from developed countries, those with mild under-nutrition do not have any major functional or intellectual impairment. However, those with severe under-nutrition incur health hazards such as increased susceptibility to infections. The vicious self-perpetuating cycle of under-nutrition rendering them susceptible to infection and infections aggravating under-nutrition can at times result in death. Efforts are, therefore, directed towards screening all under five children for under-nutrition and initiating appropriate health and nutrition intervention to combat adverse health consequences of under-nutrition.

In order to enable children with under-nutrition to catch up' with those who are well-nourished, it is essential to provide them with additional food and excellent health care. Quantitative estimates of the dietary requirements for catch up growth in children are very difficult because the targeted body weight in a growing child is not fixed but increases with time; the longer the period of rehabilitation, the greater is the gap to be filled. Milder form of CED of short duration in a child leads to low weight (wasting) but does not affect the height. This can be easily corrected with adequate dietary intake.

More severe or prolonged CED can result in stunting and wasting. Adequate dietary intake at this stage may reverse wasting but the child may not be able to catch up with the deficit in height. The relative contributions of these two factors and their severity will vary in different communities. It is impossible to make generalisations about the amounts of additional energy and protein needed for catch up growth in children who have become under-nourished as a result of prolonged inadequate dietary intake. Clinical monitoring is critical to achieve optimal results.

Diets consumed by Indians from low-income group families are predominantly cereal-based, have low fat content and are not energy dense; young children share the food from the family pot. Infants and young children require more energy per kg weight than adults but they have a relatively small stomach capacity. As a result, unlike adults who, with their larger stomach capacity, can readily meet their energy needs through the cereal pulse diet taken as three meals, the children have problems in meeting their energy needs unless fed five to six times a day. It is, therefore, imperative that nutrition education should clearly focus on the need to ensure that children are fed more often -at least once in four hours - so that their nutritional needs are met from even this type of food.

Whereever feasible, efforts may be made to increase the energy density of the food provided to them by adding sugar/jaggery and oil seeds/ oil to their food. Because of the low stomach volume, pre-school children can consume a cereal-pulse mix providing only about 150-200 calories in one meal. This has to be kept in mind when food supplementation programmes are planned for these children. Food supplements aimed at providing adequate nutrients needed for catch up growth in undernourished children must compromise energy-dense food and these have to be fed at least once in four to five hours to the child daily. It is not possible to provide the needed amount of food for catch up growth in under-nourished children through on-the-spot feeding at anganwadis.

Health - Nutrition Interactions

Dietary intake is a critical, but not the sole, determinant of the nutritional status of the population. Low birth weight, poor infant feeding practices, infections due to poor sanitation, lack of safe drinking water and poor access to health care are other major factors responsible for under-nutrition. In spite of low dietary intake, the prevalence of severe under-nutrition and under-five mortality is lower in Kerala because of more equitable distribution of food between income groups and within families and better access to and utilisation of health care facilities.

However, in Uttar Pradesh, Madhya Pradesh and Orissa, under-nutrition and under-five mortality rates are higher, in spite of higher average dietary intake, because of the lack of equitable distribution of food and access to health care. Identification and appropriate nutrition and health interventions among 'at risk' groups and under-nourished children are essential for optimal results. Equally important are interventions from related sectors to provide safe drinking water and improve environmental sanitation so that morbidity due to infections is reduced. In spite of high per capita income, dietary intake and access to health care, both under-nutrition and infant mortality rates (IMR) are relatively high in Punjab. It is imperative that health and nutrition programmes are co-ordinated to achieve optimal synergy between the two interventions so that there is improvement in the nutritional and health status in all states.

Nutrition-Fertility Interactions

The association between low birth weight, under-nutrition during infancy and childhood and high infant mortality on the one hand and high parity and low inter birth intervals on the other have been well documented by research studies. Currently, birth order of three or more form over 50 per cent of all births in Uttar Pradesh, Madhya Pradesh and Bihar.

In Kerala and Tamil Nadu, birth order of three or more constitute less than 30 percent of all births. Efforts to meet all unmet needs for contraception in the poorly performing states in order to reduce the high order of births would indirectly have a beneficial effect on child nutritional status, especially in terms of reduction in severe grades of undernutrition. Coordination between ICDS and health functionaries to achieve optimal synergy between the interventions is critical for improving the nutritional and health status of women.

In the last two decades, there have been reports on the health status and growth performance of Indian children from the low-income group who have been adopted and grew up without nutritional constraints during childhood. Data from these studies suggest that these children have a substantially higher prevalence of obesity during childhood, adolescence and in adult life. Girls have higher body weight and body fat and, compared to their counterparts, attain menarche one or two years earlier. This, in turn, may result in their being shorter than their counterparts as skeletal growth ceases after menarche.

In view of the changing dietary habits and life styles and the increase in obesity, research studies may have to be taken up to document the growth pattern of Indian children living not only under nutritional constraints but also among affluent groups and their impact on adult stature and reproductive function.

Trends Nutritional Status of Pre-School Children

Pre-school children constitute one of the most nutritionally vulnerable segment of the population and their nutritional status is considered to be a sensitive indicator of community health and nutrition. There has not been a substantial improvement in their energy intake over the last two decades. However, there has been a reduction in moderate and severe under-nutrition.

Though there has not been any improvement in micronutrient intake over the years, there has been a substantial decline in the prevalence of nutritional deficiency signs. This is, perhaps, because of the better access to health care and effective treatment of infections. The decline in fertility and reduction in the higher order births may also have contributed to this because prevalence of severe forms of under-nutrition is higher among higher order births.

Intra-familial Distribution of Food

It is widely believed that in India, especially among the rural poor, food distribution is not based on 'need'. The breadwinner gets sufficient food, the children get the next share and the women take the remains. In times of scarcity, the dietary intake of women and children are likely to be most adversely affected. Several small studies in different states have reported that intra-familial distribution of food follows this traditional pattern even today.

Data from surveys showed that there has been reduction in the proportion of families where both adults and pre-school children were having inadequate food intake. However, it is a matter of concern that the proportion of families where the dietary intake of adults is adequate but that of pre-school children is inadequate has nearly doubled. Nutrition and health education on child-feeding and child-rearing practices are of paramount importance in improving the dietary intake and nutritional status of children through appropriate intra-familial distribution of food.

Programme for Improving Nutritional Status

The ICDS scheme was initiated in 1975 with the following objectives:

— to improve the health and nutrition status of children in the 0-6 age group by providing supplementary food and coordinating with state health departments to ensure the delivery of the required health inputs;

— to provide conditions necessary for pre-school children's psychological and social development through early stimulation and education;

— to provide pregnant and lactating women with food supplements;

— to enhance the mother's ability to provide proper child care through health and nutrition education;

— to achieve effective coordination of policy and implementation among the various departments to promote child development.

The initial geographic focus of ICDS was on drought-prone areas and blocks with a significant proportion of scheduled caste and scheduled tribe population. In 1975, 33 blocks were covered under ICDS. Over the last two decades the ICDS coverage has progressively increased. The nutrition component of the ICDS aims at providing food supplements to pre-school children between the age of six months to six years, pregnant and lactating mothers and adolescent girls. The type of food supplements in the ICDS programme varies widely, from ready-to-eat food to the supply of supplements cooked in the anganwadi.

The emphasis was initially on providing cooked food through on-the-spot feeding in the anganwadi because it was believed that

— this would ensure that the targeted child would get food supplements, which would not be shared between other members of the family; and

— the anganwadi centres would provide practical nutrition education to women on cooking and feeding young children.

However, the on-the-spot cooked food feeding programme has several disadvantages as well. They are:

— children especially those in the age group of 6-36 months cannot consume the entire amount of food provided because of a smaller stomach capacity;

— even if older children do eat the food provided in the anganwadis, this acts mainly as a substitute, and not an addition, to home food;

— the most needy segments viz., children in the critical 6- 36 month age group and women, may not be able to come to the anganwadis duty and receive the food;

— providing food supplements only to the children from BPL families or those with under-nutrition is not possible as it may be difficult to feed one child and withhold food from another in the same anganwadi;

- cooking food, feeding the children and cleaning the vessels and the anganwadi take up most of the time of the anganwadi workers and helpers, leaving them little time for other important activities such as growth monitoring, nutrition education, or pre-school education;
- in any mass cooking and feeding programme, the monotony of the food provided and relatively poor quality of the preparations is a problem;
- cooking in poor hygienic conditions and keeping left-over food may result in bacterial contamination of food;
- under-nourished children, even those in the 3- 6 year age group, if given double rations, cannot consume all the food at one sitting in the anganwadi.

Evaluation of the Nutrition Component of ICDS

The nutrition component of the programme was evaluated by the Nutrition Foundation of India (NFI), Delhi, National Institute of Public Cooperation and Child Development (NIPCCD), Delhi, and the National Council of Applied Economic Research (NCAER), Delhi. In addition, there have been several small-scale evaluations.

There were major reviews of the nutrition sector and ICDS programme by the World Bank and the Government of India in 1997 and 2001. The findings showed:

- ICDS services were much in demand but there are problems in delivery, quality and coordination;

— the programme might be improving food security at the household level, but does not effectively address the issue of prevention, detection and management of the under-nourished child/mother;

— children in the 6-36 months age group and pregnant and lactating women do not come to the anganwadi and do not get food supplements;

— available food is shared between mostly children in the 3-5 years age group irrespective of their nutritional status;

— as there was no attempt in ensuring that all children are weighed, the children with severe CED could not be identified and offered double the rations as envisaged in the ICDS guidelines. As a result, there is very little focussed attention on the correction of under-nutrition, prevention and management of health problems associated with moderate and severe under-nutrition.

— child care and nutrition education of the mother is poor or non-existent.

— there were gaps in the training and knowledge of anganwadi workers. Also, supervision of the programme, community support and inter-sectoral coordination was poor.

Nutrition Component of PMGY

Under Pradhan Mantri Gramodhaya Yojna 15% funds are earmarked for Nutrition Component. As the funding for PMGY is through the Gadgil-Mukherjee formula, the populous poor states with high under-nutrition rates do not get sufficient funds. The Department of Women and

Child Development implemented the nutrition component of the programme providing take-home food supplements to children in the 6-36 months age group in the first two years viz., 2000-01 and 2001-02. From 1st April 2002, the Planning Commission has taken over its implementation. Some of the available data indicate that in many states:

— there was difficulty in procuring locally available take-home food supplements;

— relatively expensive ready-to-eat food, and not cereal-pulse-oilseed mix was provided;

— the funds provided under the nutrition component of PMGY were not treated as an additionality but were substituted for state's own Plan funds for nutrition;

— there has not been any substantial improvement in the enrolment of children.

The guidelines laid down for the nutrition component of PMGY emphasise that all infants and children should be weighed at least once in three months to detect those who are under-nourished so that health and nutrition interventions could be undertaken. Even though growth monitoring is an essential component of ICDS, this actually has not been operationalised.

ICDS During the Tenth Plan

During the Tenth Plan, every effort will be made to strengthen India's commitment and institutional capacity to combat under-nutrition in pre-school children and pregnant and lactating women. The nutrition component of ICDS will be specifically directed to achieve reduction in both micro and macro-nutrient under-nutrition. The focus will be on:

- strengthening the nutrition and health education component so that there is appropriate intra-familial distribution of food based on needs;
- reaching children in the 6-36 months age group, pregnant and lactating women;
- weighing all vulnerable population, identify those with CED and provide integrated health and nutritional support so that they recover within the next three months;
- ensuring universal screening of all children at least once a quarter to identify those children with growth faltering;
- focusing health and nutrition intervention to ensure that children in Grades III and IV under-nutrition are in Grade II by the next quarter;
- looking for and treating health problems associated with severe under-nutrition;
- enhancing the quality and impact of ICDS substantially through training, supervision of the ICDS personnel and improved community ownership of the programme;
- concentrating on the improvement of the quality of care and inter-sectoral coordination and strengthening nutrition action by the health sector;
- creating nutrition awareness through IEC at all levels (community, women's group, village- level workers, PRIs, programme managers and policy makers at the state and central levels);

— establishing a reliable monitoring and evaluation mechanism

There is a shift in focus from providing cooked food at anganwadis to take-home food supplementation (under the PMGY and the pilot project providing food-grains to under-nourished pregnant and lactating women and adolescent girls). Undoubtedly, the take-home food supplements provided will be shared with the family, but that would add to household food security. When coupled with nutrition education, the under-nourished persons may get their due share.

Nutritional education and careful monitoring of weight of the under-nourished individual will go a long way in ensuring that the person does get her due share. This shift may free the anganwadi workers and helpers from the time-consuming task of cooking and cleaning, giving them time for their other designated tasks for child development.

During the Tenth Plan, inter-sectoral linkages between the health and the ICDS programmes will be strengthened. The Health sector will:

— invest in upgrading the nutritional knowledge and skills of all health care workers;

— focus on the management of health problems in moderately and severely under-nourished children; and

— train health and anganwadi workers so that they provide nutrition and health education on feeding of infants and young children and nutrition counseling to parents with sick children.

Simultaneously, efforts will be made to build up institution capacity for strengthening:

— advocacy for nutrition among policy makers, programme implementers, women's groups, PRIs etc;

— country's capacity for nutrition action, training and research; and

— the network of medical colleges, home science colleges, centres undertaking nutrition monitoring and nutrition education.

Priority areas for research in nutrition during the Tenth Plan will include:

— operational research to identify and eliminate constraints in the ongoing programme; and

— analysis of nutrition needs at the local level and tailoring ongoing nutritional interventions to meet these needs.

Funding of the Nutrition Component of the ICDS Programme

The ICDS programme is a centrally sponsored one in which the Centre bears the cost of maintaining the infrastructure, while the states bear the expenditure on the food component. The programme has expanded and central expenditure on the scheme has increased from Rs.1.54 crore in 1975-76 to Rs. 1,000 crore in 2000-2001. With the increase coverage, there is an increasing need for funds for the food supplements as well. Though the central expenditure has increased over the years, there has been no corresponding increase in the states' own plan expenditure on food supplements.

The World Bank computed the information on expenditure relating to nutrition in 12 major states. In addition to ICDS, some states have supplementary feeding programmes, like the Mid-day meals programme in Tamil Nadu. States' expenditure on supplementary nutrition does not have any correlation with level of under-nutrition state domestic product. States with a higher prevalence of under-nutrition are not investing higher amounts in food supplementation programmes. However, expenditure on supplementary nutrition is not the only critical determinant of the level of under-nutrition. Kerala, which is spending very little on supplementary nutrition programmes, has the lowest under-nutrition rates, perhaps due to more equitable distribution of food and effective health care.

The Planning Commission reviewed the current funding of the ICDS food supplementation programme. The funding requirements were calculated for different scenerios: on the basis of the ICDS norms (1999), for providing food supplements only to persons from BPL families, for providing food supplements to undernourished children and pregnant women or providing double the rations to children with severe under-nutrition. The total funds available for procuring food supplements i.e., state nutrition allocation under Plan and the PMGY nutrition outlays were taken into account while computing the gaps. Currently, in most states there are substantial gaps between the requirement and the actual funds provided. However there are other states where the funds provided are more than what is required. It is a matter of concern that states like Bihar with high rates of poverty, under-nutrition and birth rates have substantial gaps.

However states like Gujarat, Tamil Nadu and Delhi are spending more than the required minimum amount.

In spite of this, the nutritional status of children in these states is not better than the national average. It would, therefore, appear that while funding constraints is a problem in some states, effective implementation may be the bottleneck in other states. The critical role of the family in ensuring intra-familiar food distribution based on needs to prevent under-nutrition cannot be overestimated.

During the Tenth Plan efforts will be made to:

— persuade states to provide more funds;

— optimally utilize funds provided under PMGY;

— improve targeting by providing available food on a priority basis to those with under-nutrition;

— improve health care for under-nourished children; and

— monitor children / women with severe grades of undernutrition who are receiving food supplementation and assess improvement in their nutritional status.

Given the current financial constraints, States may find it difficult to increase the amount of funds currently being allocated to the programme. However experience in Orissa has shown that even with the existing outlay it is possible to achieve significant reduction in severe grades of undernutrition by identifying the children with severe grades of undernutrition and ensuring that they get the required health and nutrition inputs. It is essential that appropriate guidelines for screening all children and identification of those with undernutrition and utilizing the available food supplements to fully meet the requirement of these children on priority basis are drawn up and agreed to by the centre, state, PRI and the community; the PRI and the community should play a major role in ensuring the effective implementation of the programme.

The National Programme of Nutritional Support to Primary Education commonly known as Mid Day Meals Scheme was launched in August, 1995 as a 100% centrally funded Centrally Sponsored Scheme. The objective of the programme is to give a boost to universalisation of Primary Education by increasing enrolment, retention and attendance and simultaneously improving nutritional status of students in primary classes.

Micronutrient Deficiencies

Goitre due to iodine deficiency, blindness due to Vitamin A deficiency, dry and wet beriberi and pellagra were the major public health problems in pre-independent India. Sustained dietary changes resulted in the elimination of beriberi and pellagra. Kerato malacia due to severe Vitamin A deficiency is no longer a public health problem. However, there has not been any decline in the prevalence of anaemia due to iron and folic acid deficiency; the decline in Vitamin A deficiency and iodine deficiency disorders has been very slow.

The Tenth Plan envisages a paradigm shift from food security to nutrition security to meet the needs of the macro, micro and phyto nutrients through dietary diversification. There will be sustained efforts to reduce/ eliminate micronutrient deficiencies including universal salt iodisation to eliminate Iodine Deficiency Disorders (IDD) and a multi-pronged strategy to reduce the prevalence of anaemia and associated health hazards.

Anaemia

In India, the prevalence of anaemia is high because of:

— low dietary intake, poor iron and folic acid intake;

— poor bio-availability of iron in phytate fibre-rich Indian diet; and

— infection such as malaria, hook worm infestations. like copper, zinc, pyridoxine and Vitamin-B12 are rare in India. Studies conducted by the ICMR and NNMB show that the prevalence of anaemia is high among pregnant women (50-90 per cent) and children (50-70 per cent).

India was the first developing country to take up a National Nutritional Anaemia Prophylaxis Programme to prevent anaemia among pregnant women and children. Screening for anaemia and iron-folate therapy in appropriate doses and route of administration for the prevention and management of anaemia in these vulnerable groups have been incorporated as an essential component of antenatal care and paediatric practice. In spite of all these efforts anaemia continues to be a major problem affecting all segments of the population and there has not been any substantial decline in the adverse consequences of anaemia. A nation-wide survey on anaemia using the cyanmeth-haemoglobin (Hb) method is currently under way and will provide data on the prevalence of anaemia in pre-school children, pregnant women and adolescent girls.

Pregnant women with Hb less than 8 g/dl show functional decompensation and constitute a high-risk group. A single Hb estimation done around the twentieth week of pregnancy is sufficient to detect the high-risk anaemic pregnant women.

The RCH programme envisages screening all pregnant women for anaemia by Hb estimation utilising the ANM and laboratory technicians in the primary health centres so that anaemia in pregnancy could be detected and effectively treated. Unlike the situation elsewhere in the world, oral iron therapy is not effective in correction of moderate or severe anaemia in Indian pregnant women, within the short time available because of the poor bio-availability of iron in the Indian diet.

The Ninth Plan envisaged the prevention, detection and management of anaemia in pregnant women as a priority intervention but this has not yet been operationalised. Evaluation of the ongoing RCH programme by the Rapid Household Survey, Department of Family Welfare and NFHS-2 showed that a majority of pregnant women are not screened for anaemia and their iron and folic acid tablet (IFA) intake is erratic.

Poor quality and inadequate supply of IFA tablets, erratic distribution due to poor worker motivation and erratic intake by woman are some of the major problems which are responsible for anaemia among them. The recent efforts to improve packaging and availability of these IFA tablets has not yet had an impact on the regularity of intake. As a result very high rates of anaemia in pregnant women persist and the impact of severe anaemia on birth weight and maternal mortality remain unaltered.

The prevalence of anaemia in childhood is very high and contributes to poor scholastic performance and increased susceptibility to infection. In India, anaemia is caused by (a) inadequate intake of food (cereals and pulses) and vegetables rich in iron and folate; (b) poor bio-availability of iron; and (c) high incidence of hookworm infestation and incidence of malaria. Several investigators have taken up small-scale intervention studies to address each of these problems. These small research studies have proved the beneficial effect of these interventions.

However, the larger programmes had very little impact. Pre-school children have been one of the target groups to receive IFA tablets under the National Nutritional Anaemia Prophylaxis Programme. But both access to and intake of IFA tablets by children have been very poor and there has been very little impact in terms of reduction in anaemia in childhood. Neither the RCH nor the school-based programmes have operationalised the programmes for detection and treatment of anaemia in children in the country. There are inter-state and perhaps inter-district variations in the prevalence of anaemia in children and the data from the RHS Survey is expected to provide information on this.

Strategies for the Prevention

The major intervention strategies required for the prevention and management of anaemia are:

— improve dietary intake to meet RDA for all macro and micronutrients;

— dietary diversification-inclusion of iron folate rich foods as well as food items that promote iron absorption;

— food fortification, including introduction of iron and iodine-fortified salt and other iron-fortified items;

— health and nutrition education to improve over all dietary intakes and promote consumption of iron and folate-rich foodstuffs; and

— screening for early detection of anaemia among vulnerable groups such as pregnant women.

Management of anaemia depends upon its severity and chronicity and the physiological status of the individual and the time available for correction of anaemia.

Infants:

— exclusive breast feeding for six months, and introduction of green leafy vegetables along with cereal/pulse/oilseed mix in the sixth month for the prevention of anaemia;

— screening for anaemia in pre-term, low birth weight infants and those with growth faltering and repeated episodes of infection; and

— appropriate treatment for anaemic infants. Preschool children:

— advocacy with regard to dietary diversification for the prevention of anaemia;

— all growth retarded children and those with repeated infections should have Hb estimation carried out; and

— those found to be anaemic must be provided with appropriate treatment.

School children:

— Operational research needs to be done to assess the feasibility of at least once-a-year screening for detection and correction of anaemia as a part of the school health check up; and

— set up mechanism to cover out-of-school children among whom anaemia is likely to be more prevalent; efforts may have to be made to explore the mechanism for the prevention, detection and management of anaemia in this group.

- In hookworm endemic areas, it will be necessary to improve;
- sanitation and educate people not to walk barefoot;
- treat children with a history of passing worms with broad spectrum anti-helminthics; and
- screen all anaemic children for hookworm infestation and treat them.

Adolescents

Wherever possible, attempts should be made to screen adolescent girls, especially those who are undernourished or have menstrual problems, for anaemia and provide appropriate treatment. Adolescents who are pregnant should receive very high priority for screening and management of anaemia.

Pregnant women

The multi-pronged strategy for the control of anaemia in pregnancy include:

- fortification of common food items such as salt with iron to increase the dietary intake of iron and improve the haemoglobin status of the entire population, including girls and women prior to pregnancy;
- screening of all pregnant women for anaemia using a reliable method of haemoglobin estimation;
- oral iron folate prophylactic therapy for all non-anaemic pregnant women (with haemoglobin more than 11 g/dl);
- iron folate oral medication at the maximum tolerable dose throughout pregnancy for women with haemoglobin level between 8 and 11 g/dl;

— parenteral iron therapy for women with haemoglobin level between 5 and 8 g/dl if they do not have any obstetric or systemic complication;

— hospital admission and intensive personalised care for women with haemoglobin less than 5 g/dl;

— screening and effective management of obstetric and systemic problems in all anaemic pregnant women; and

— improvement in health care delivery systems and health education to the community to promote utilisation of available care. Elderly people

— research studies to assess the magnitude of the problem; and

— mount an appropriate intervention programme based on the findings. Research and Development

— evaluate the safety, efficacy, acceptability and cost effectiveness of double (iodine and iron) fortified salt so that decisions regarding universal double fortification of salt and its supply through TPDS system could be taken; and

— evaluate the safety, feasibility, efficacy and cost effectiveness of fortifying food items like atta with iron.

Monitoring and Surveillance

Initiatives for monitoring the programme for preventing and controlling anaemia will include:

— strengthening routine reporting under the RCH programme to include percentage of pregnant women in whom haemoglobin estimation has been done, percentage anaemic, percentage given IFA tablets, compliance in IFA intake and the percentage given parenteral iron therapy; and

— requesting PRIs, Women's Self Help Groups and Anganwadi Worker's to monitor intake of IFA tablets.

Evaluation of the ongoing programmes through process and impact can be done as a part of the Rapid Household Surveys by including questions regarding haemoglobin estimation, IFA coverage and intake. In addition as and when large-scale surveys are done, information can be collected on the prevalence of anaemia in pregnancy, childhood, adolescents and the elderly so that it is possible to asses the impact of ongoing interventions.

Tenth Plan goals include:

— screening of children for anaemia wherever required and appropriate treatment of those found anaemic;

— universal screening of pregnant women for anaemia and appropriate treatment; and

— reducing the prevalence of anaemia by 25 per cent and moderate and severe anaemia by 50% in children, pregnant and lactating women and adolescents;

Iodine Deficiency Disorders (IDD)

Iodine deficiency disorders have been recognised as a public health problem in India since the 1920s. Unlike other micronutrient deficiencies, iodine deficiency disorders are due to deficiency of iodine in water, soil and foodstuffs and affect all socio-economic groups living in defined geographic areas. Initially, Iodine deficiency disorders was thought to be a problem in sub-Himalayan region. However, surveys carried out subsequently showed that iodine deficiency disorders exist even in riverine and coastal areas.

No state in India is completely free from iodine deficiency disorders. It is estimated that 61 million people are suffering from endemic goitre and about 8.8 million people have mental/ motor handicap due to iodine deficiency. Universal use of iodised salt is a simple, inexpensive method of preventing iodine deficiency disorders.

Following the successful trial of iodized salt in the Kangra Valley, Himachal Pradesh, a National Goitre Control Programme (NGCP) was launched in 1962. Initially the programme aimed at providing iodised salt to the well-recognised sub-Himalayan 'goitre' belt. However, there was no substantial reduction in iodine deficiency disorders due to the erratic availability of salt, availability of cheaper non-iodised salt and the lack of awareness regarding the need to use iodised salt.

In view of the fact that no state was free of iodine deficiency disorders, a decision was taken for the universal iodisation of salt for human consumption, which was implemented in a phased manner from 1986. The progress in implementation of this programme was tardy as the production and availability of iodised salt was a fraction of what was required. In August 1992, the NGCP was renamed as the National Iodine Deficiency Disorders Control Programme (NIDDCP), taking into its ambit the control of a wide spectrum of iodine deficiency disorders with the goal of reducing the prevalence of IDD below 10 per cent in endemic districts of the country. Based on the recommendations of the Central Council of Health, the Government took a policy decision to iodise the entire edible salt in the country by 1992. There has been a steady progress in the production of iodised salt over the past few years in India.

Available data suggest that there has been substantial increase in the availability and consumption of iodised salt during the 1990s. However, the NFHS-2 showed that even in the late 1990s only 49 per cent of households use cooking salt that is iodised at the recommended level of 15 the parts per million or more, about 28 per cent of the households use salt that is not iodised at all and 22 per cent use salt containing less than 15 ppm of iodine. In coastal states like Tamil Nadu, Andhra Pradesh, Kerala, and Gujarat, the percentage of households consuming adequate iodised salt is much lower than in many of the northern states where the availability of iodised salt is more than 90 per cent. One of the reasons could be that the salt transported by road are not subject to any kind of check regarding iodisation and this loophole in the law permits transport of non-iodised salt by road to areas upto 250 km. Therefore, these areas have ready access to non-iodised salt.

A national consultation was held in April 1999, to discuss the scientific and epidemiological evidence on benefits and safety of iodised salt in the prevention and control of iodine deficiency disorders; the consensus statement from the consultation confirmed that under the existing conditions in India universal iodisation of salt for human consumption was safe and will enable the country to combat IDD. In October 2000, the central government lifted the ban on sale of non-iodised salt for human consumption. However all the states and Union territories, except Kerala and Gujarat, have issued ban notifications on the sale of non iodised salt for human consumption in their entire territories under the Prevention of Food Adulteration Act. There is a partial ban in Andhra Pradesh and Maharashtra.

Strategies for Prevention

It is essential to ensure that only iodised salt is made available for human consumption in order to enable the children of the 21st century to attain their full intellectual potential and take their rightful place in a knowledge based-society. Efforts to improve the quality of iodised salt will include:

— mandatory certification of the adequacy of iodisation as a pre-requisite for getting priority for the transportation of salt;

— ensuring that the salt is packed in half or one kg consumer poly pack at production site itself to prevent deterioration in quality during transportation and storage;

— periodic checking of the iodine content of salts available at wholesale/retail outlets; and

— quality check at the household level through anganwadi/school-based testing using salt iodine test kit.

IEC to increase the demand for good quality iodised salt will have to continue. Efforts to reduce price differentials between iodised and non-iodised salt and provide ready access to iodised salt through TPDS will have to be considered. Monitoring of the production, distribution, quality of salt at various levels, along with the studies on goitre prevalence among school children, urinary iodine excretion status, thyroid status of school children, neonatal thyroid status by appropriate screening techniques, may be used to assess the progress of reduction in iodine deficiency disorders. In areas where iodine deficiency disorders continue to be high, despite the adequate availability and extensive use of iodised salt, the possible role of goitrogens may have to be investigated.

The Tenth Plan goals are to:

— achieve universal access to iodised salt;

— generate district-wise data on iodised salt consumption; and

— reduction in the prevalence of iodine deficiency disorders in the country to less than 10 per cent by 2010.

Vitamin A Deficiency

Vitamin A is an important micronutrient for maintaining normal growth, regulating cellular proliferation and differentiation, controlling development, and maintaining visual and reproductive functions. Diet surveys have shown that the intake of Vitamin A is significantly lower than the recommended dietary allowance in young children, dietary adolescent girls and pregnant women. In these vulnerable sub-groups multiple nutritional problems coexist including inadequate intake of energy as well as of micronutrients other than Vitamin A. Inspite of the fact that there has not been any significant improvement in the dietary intake of Vitamin A and coverage under Massive Dose Vitamin A programme has been low, there is a decline in clinical Vitamin A deficiency in under-five children in the country. This could perhaps be due to increase in access in health care, consequent reduction in severity and duration of common childhood morbidity due to infections.

It is estimated that the prevalence of Vitamin A deficiency signs during pregnancy and lactation ranges between 1 and 5 per cent. Small-scale studies have reported large inter state and inter district variation. However, nation-wide comparable data is not available. There are reports of night blindness occurring during pregnancy and disappearing after delivery without any treatment. Sub-clinical Vitamin A deficiency might perhaps be more widespread. It may not be feasible to undertake large-scale studies to estimate prevalence as biochemical estimation of Vitamin A deficiency during pregnancy present several problems.

There is very little data on the prevalence of Vitamin A deficiency during lactation. In spite of continued secretion in breast milk, available limited data does not suggest increased prevalence of Vitamin A deficiency during lactation. Unlike anaemia, Vitamin A deficiency in pregnant and lactating women is not associated with any increase in morbidity and mortality. There is no ongoing programme for the prevention, detection and treatment of Vitamin A deficiency in pregnant and lactating women.

During the Tenth Plan period, the detection and management of clinical Vitamin A deficiency will be included as a component of antenatal care. Night blindness and Bitot's spot are readily identifiable clinical entities. Women with these symptoms / signs will be identified by the ANM and 10,000 IU of Vitamin A administered daily for four weeks. Efforts to promote cultivation and consumption of micro-nutrient rich vegetables will be taken up for prevention of clinical deficiency.

Vitamin A deficiency in childhood is mainly due to inadequate dietary intake of Vitamin A. Some of the earlier studies from developing countries have shown that Vitamin A administration could have beneficial effect on growth, morbidity and morality in children but more recent studies do not confirm this. The association between measles, severe protein energy malnutrition and keratomalacia and high fatality in such cases was reported by many paediatricians.

In the 1950s, prevalence of night blindness and Bitot's spot in pre-school children ranged between 5 per cent and 10 per cent in most states. Paediatricians in major hospitals in most of the states reported that blindness due to Vitamin deficiency is one of the major causes of blindness in children below five years. A five-year long field trial conducted by NIN showed that if massive dose Vitamin A (200,000 units) is administered once in six months to children between one and three years of age, the incidence of corneal xerophthalmia is reduced by about 80 per cent.

In view of the serious nature of the problem of blindness due to Vitamin A deficiency, it was felt that urgent remedial measures in the form of specific nutrient supplementation covering the entire population of susceptible children should be undertaken. In 1970, the National Prophylaxis Programme Against Nutritional Blindness was initiated as a centrally sponsored scheme. Under this scheme, all children between ages of one and three years were to be administered 200,000 IU of Vitamin A orally once in six months.

This programme had been implemented in all the states and union territories during the last thirty two years. The major bottleneck during the 1970s was lack of infrastructure at the peripheral level to ensure timely administration of the dose. In the 1980s there was considerable improvement in the infrastructure. The lack of adequate supply of Vitamin A which came in the way of improved coverage was also corrected. However coverage levels continued to be very low. Ninth Plan strategy to improve the coverage of all doses of massive dose Vitamin A administration:

— increased inter-sectoral coordination between ICDS and family welfare workers -anganwadi workers may be requested to administer second and subsequent doses;

— ensure adequate availability of Vitamin A;

— health education to improve consumption of foods rich in B-carotene to be continued and backed up by efforts to improve their availability at affordable cost.

The goal for the Ninth Plan was to control Vitamin A deficiency so that the incidence of blindness due to this becomes less than one in 10,000 not only at the national level but also in every state.

In an attempt to improve the coverage, especially of the first two dose, it was decided to link Vitamin A administration to the ongoing immunisation programme during the Eighth Plan period. Under the revised regimen a dose of 100,000 IU of Vitamin A was administered to all infants at nine months along with measles vaccine and a second dose of 200,000 IU was administered at 18 months of age along with booster dose of DPT and OPV. Subsequently, the children were to receive three doses of 200,000 IU of Vitamin A every six months until 36 months of age. The reported coverage figures under the modified regimen indicate that there has been some improvement in coverage with the first dose. However, the coverage for subsequent doses is low.

Available data suggests that during the Ninth Plan there has not been any substantial improvement in the coverage level of the second and subsequent doses of Massive Dose Vitamin A. In an attempt to improve the coverage, Orissa linked administration of Vitamin A with the pulse polio immunisation campaign. It is reported that the state took precautions to prevent overdosing by stopping Vitamin A administration in the preceding six months.

Planning Commission, the Department of Family Welfare and the Indian Academy of Paediatrics stated that this strategy is inappropriate because:

— while all children in the 0-5 age group get polio vaccine only those in the 1-3 age group receive Vitamin A. It may not be easy to give the latter only to 1-3 year children as the PPI is a massive campaign covering over 120 million children and the booths are manned by persons who are not health professionals;

— there would be difficulties in keeping adequate record of Vitamin A dosing; as a result, there will always be a possibility of toxicity or side effects due to multiple dosing within six months. Stopping Vitamin A dose six months prior to PPI will have a negative impact on Vitamin A administration through the routine services;

— the second dose of Vitamin A for the year has to be administered through an alternative strategy; and

— when the pulse polio programme ends, the re-initiation of routine Vitamin A administration would pose problems.

During the campaign mode administration of Vitamin A, along with pulse polio, in Assam in November 2001 deaths among children who were administered massive dose Vitamin A were reported. Some of these deaths could be coincidental where Vitamin A had been administered to ill children, but the possibility that some of the deaths could have been due to Vitamin A toxicity (either due to administration of higher dose or a massive dose Vitamin A administration earlier) cannot be ruled out. Since then, the Department of Family Welfare reiterated the earlier recommendation that the campaign mode -administration of Vitamin A along with pulse polio immunisation should not be taken up.

Strategies for Prevention

Clinical Vitamin A deficiency often coexists with other micro-nutrient deficiencies and, hence, there is a need for broad-based dietary diversification programmes aimed at improving the overall micro-nutrient nutritional status of the population. In addition, the ongoing Massive Dose Vitamin A supplementation programme in children in the 9-36 month age group will be continued and its implementation strengthened.

Strategies in specific groups are indicated below.

Infancy

— health and nutrition education will be taken up to encourage colostrum feeding, exclusive breast feeding for the first six months and the introduction of complimentary feeding including mashed greens and yellow/orange fruits/ vegetables at sixth month;

— 100,000 IU dose of Vitamin A will be given at nine months along with the measles vaccine; and

— every effort will be made to ensure the early detection and prompt treatment of infections.

Childhood

— ensure adequate intake of Vitamin A rich food throughout childhood;

— early detection and prompt treatment of infections; and

— massive dose Vitamin A administration at 18,24,30 and 36 months of age; in order to improve coverage without too many logistic problems, these four doses are to be administered by anganwadi worker during April and October each year (pre-summer/pre-winter period) under the supervision of the ANM.

Sick Children

— all children with xerophthalmia should be given two doses of synthetic Vitamin A as per the present schedule of the Government under the RCH programme;

— all children suffering from measles should also be given one dose of Vitamin A, if they have not received it during the previous one month;

— all cases of severe CED (based on weight for age criteria or clinical signs) should be given one additional dose of Vitamin A.

Research studies may have to be taken up to identify:

— food items, conventional as well as non-conventional, which are rich in vitamin A;

— functional decompensation associated with Vitamin A deficiency in various stages in different age and, physiological status groups;

— time trends in the prevalence of sub-clinical and clinical Vitamin A deficiency in different regions.

Goals for the Tenth Plan

— achieve universal coverage for each of the five doses of Vitamin A;

— reduce prevalence of night blindness to below 1 per cent and that of Bitot Spots to below 0.5 per cent in children between six months to six years of age;

— eliminate Vitamin A deficiency as a public health problem.

Dietary Improvement and Diversification

There are three approaches for combating micro-nutrient deficiencies: medicinal supplementation, food fortification and dietary diversification with increased intake of micro-nutrient- dense foods. The first two approaches can take care of only one or two nutrients. Dietary diversification is the most appropriate and sustainable option ensuring adequate intakes of all micronutrients and phytochemicals. Availability, affordability, access and awareness are some of the major determinants of sustained dietary diversification in families and communities.

Dietary diversification can be made possible through community effort through increased production of micronutrientdense foods and reduced wastage through appropriate processing. It can be linked to income generation, particularly for the rural women. Micronutrient intake in children and women can be improved if the community contributes locally produced millets, fruits and vegetables for supplementary feeding programmes such as ICDS, and Mid-day Meal. It is important to update and expand available data on the micro and phyto nutrient content of conventional and unconventional food items so that optimal use is made of the country rich diverse plant resources to eliminate micro nutrient deficiencies.

Research

India is one of the pioneers in nutrition research not only in the Asian region but also in the world. Several research institutions and universities are carrying out the research studies with assistance from ministries and research funding agencies such as Indian Council of Agricultural Research, Indian Council of Medical Research, Council for Scientific and Industrial Research, Department of Bio-Technology and Department of Science and Technology. Basic, clinical, applied and operational research studies have identified major nutritional problems in the country, their aetiology, appropriate remedial and preventive measures, and the modalities of effectively operationalising the intervention programme at the regional and national level.

Initially the focus of research was on deficiency diseases and chronic energy deficiency, the health hazards associated with them, methods for detection, treatment and prevention. It is noteworthy that the major interventions such as food supplementation programmes, the National Anaemia Prophylaxis Programme, massive dose Vitamin A supplementation programme have all been initiated on the basis of research work carried out in the country. Over the last two decades, responding to the changing spectrum of nutrition-related disorders, research studies have been initiated on food and drug toxins and nutritional risk factors associated with non-communicable diseases.

During the Tenth Plan period basic, clinical, applied, operational and socio - behavioral research in nutrition will continue to receive priority attention so that the country can effectively and rapidly tackle the dual disease burden due to under- and over-nutrition. Networking of the research institutions and universities carrying out research studies on nutrition will be attempted, so that there is no unnecessary duplication of efforts and the available resources are fully utilised.

Priority areas for research in nutrition include:

— nutritive value of food items - for macro, micro and phyto nutrients using newer techniques; analysis of uncommon food stuffs for their nutritive value;

— food safety including food contaminants, adulterants and genetically modified food items;

— dietary intake and nutritional requirement of Indians;

— evolving and testing better tools for assessment of nutritional status;

— evolving appropriate norms for assessing the nutritional status of Indians;

— assessing the determinants of nutritional status;

— nutritional status and health, especially epidemiological data on the health consequences of deviation from the norms;

— nutrition-fertility and nutrition-infection interactions;

— micro-nutrient deficiencies and their health consequences;

— changing dietary habits and lifestyles focusing on obesity and noncommunicable diseases;

— increasing longevity-nutritional implications;

— nutritional problems of the elderly;

— clinical nutrition, including nutritional management during illness and nutritional rehabilitation;

— emerging changes in nutritional status due to changing ecology, agriculture, life style and social policy;

— effectiveness of nutrition intervention as assessed by health and nutritional benefit and cost of different interventions; socio-behavioural research on lifestyle modifications, IEC&M to the population to alter lifestyles;

— operational research to improve the efficiency of the implementation of on-going programmes.

Nutrition Monitoring

Nutrition monitoring refers to repeated measurements of changes in the nutritional status of individuals and groups at regular intervals. In India, there are huge differences in per capita income, purchasing power, availability of food items, dietary habits, lifestyle and nutritional status between and within states, among urban, rural and tribal population.

The country is currently going through demographic, economic, social, educational, agricultural and health transition, all of which can modify nutritional status. Sound, reliable data is needed for appropriate, decentralised planning and monitoring of interventions to meet the local needs. It is important, therefore, to strengthen, streamline and effectively utilise the existing mechanisms for monitoring the nutritional status of the population.

The National Nutrition Policy, drawn up by the Department of Women and Child Development and adopted in 1993, envisaged the building up of a "regular monitoring and surveillance system and developing a reliable database in the country not only to assess the impact of ongoing nutrition and development programmes but also to serve as an early warning system for initiating prompt action."

The ICDS functionaries regularly file monthly progress report on nutritional status. However, there are lacunae and delays in the collection, reporting, collation and analysis of data. Monthly progress reports are not utilised for district level monitoring and midcourse correction of ongoing programmes. During the Ninth Plan, the NIN, at the request of the Department of Women and Child Development, conducted a study in Andhra Pradesh for improving the monthly progress reports of the ICDS workers and improving monitoring of the ICDS programme at the district level. The data from the study indicated that it was possible to train and orient the ICDS functionaries to improve the quality and timeliness of the reporting. Analysis of the data and discussions on the implications of the reports with the functionaries facilitated the implementation of mid-course corrections and led to improved performance.

When data from the Andhra Pradesh study was used for Geographical Information System (GIS) mapping, it showed that the data generated by anganwadi workers are useful for monitoring the situation at the block/district levels and for building up, over time, a database for nutritional surveillance. Orissa had utilised 'routine' reporting of the ICDS workers for block-wise GIS mapping of the severe and moderate under-nutrition in the 0-6 years age groups. The GIS maps clearly brought out trends in under-nutrition in different areas, different seasons and in different age groups. Meghalaya, Rajasthan, Maharashtra, Madhya Pradesh and Karnataka have initiated projects to improve nutrition monitoring, mapping and surveillance.

As part of efforts to monitor the nutritional component of the PMGY initiative, the Planning Commission has drawn up in collaboration with the Department of Women and Child Development, a proforma for assessment and reporting of the nutritional status of under-six children. This has been incorporated as a part of the monthly the ICDS reporting format. The Department of Women and Child Development and the Planning Commission have requested the secretaries of the state Departments of Women and Child Development to ensure that the data is compiled district-wise (in two age groups, gender-specific) and reported every month and monitored at the district, state and central levels. The state/central Departments of Women and Child Developments are to monitor the improvement in terms of

— enrolement of children in the 6-36 months age group;

— percentage of children who received complimentary food by six months;

— nutritional status of children in the 6-36 months · age group; and

— fund allocation for nutrition and utilisation of funds provided.

Independent Surveys to Monitor Nutritional Status

The ICMR established the NNMB in 1972 for undertaking:

— data collection on the dietary intakes of families, and individuals belonging to different physiological and age groups, in different states;

— assessing intra-family distribution of food and nutrients;

— generating data on the diet and nutritional status of socially vulnerable groups like the tribals living in the ITDP areas, and the physiologically at-risk population like the elderly and adolescents;

— organising repeat surveys to assess time trends in the diet and nutritional situation.

During the nineties the NNMB has been using the NSSO sampling for their survey in the ten states.

The Food and Nutrition Board of the Department of Women and Child Development conducted a nutrition survey in 1993-94 in 187 districts, the report of which was published in 1998. This was a one-time effort and the sample covered was not derived from a representative sample of the district. The NFHS has undertaken height and weight measurement in a representative sample of children and women at the state-level.

NFHS provides state-level estimates of under-nutrition and over-nutrition at two time points, 1992-93 and 1998-99. Every five years, the National Sample Survey Organisation (NSSO) collects and reports information on expenditure on food at the family level in representative sample population all over the country. The NSSO does not provide information on dietary consumption at the family and individual level and does not assess nutritional status. However, if coupled with the NNMB survey, the NSSO data may provide excellent insights into changing dietary patterns and nutritional status.

Currently it is estimated that only about 20 per cent of the under-six children are weighed in the ICDS blocks. During the Tenth Plan period, all pregnant and lactating women and all under-five children will be weighed at least four times a year to identify under-nourished persons and initiate targeted interventions. Once, a good quality data becomes available at the block and district level on a regular basis, it will be used for:

— building block/district/state level data on prevalence of under-nutrition;

— monitoring ICDS activities for reduction in under-nutrition;

— assessment of the impact of ongoing nutrition interventions;

— planning appropriate mid-course corrections in the ongoing ICDS programme;

— building up a database for nutritional surveillance in vulnerable groups.

During the Tenth Plan, efforts will be made to conduct nutrition surveys in a representative sample of the population in all the states.

Nutrition Surveillance

The nutrition surveillance system (NSS) provides information on under/over nutrition, its spatial distribution, causes, and changes in prevalence/incidence over time, the actions initiated and their impact. Though the National Nutrition Policy recommended the development and establishment of "nutritional surveillance of the country's population especially children and mothers" in the country by the year 2000, the NSS is yet to be developed.

Currently, there are three systems, which provide the essential core information that could be developed into a full-fledged nutrition surveillance during the Tenth Plan period: nutrition monitoring through ICDS system; the NNMB-NSSO databases; and the pilot project on Food Insecurity and Vulnerability Information and Mapping System (FIVIMS) under the Department 359 of Food and Public Distribution.

It is envisaged that the Department of Women and Child Development will ensure an improvement in quality of data being collected by the ICDS functionaries. The NNMB will be expanded to cover all states and carry out regular surveys on dietary consumption, assessment of macro and micro-nutrient nutritional status and morbidity profile; special efforts will be made to cover at-risk groups. FIVIMS will also provide nation-wide data.

Once district-wise data becomes available and problem areas are identified, health and nutrition intervention could be initiated at appropriate levels. Over time, it may be desirable to integrate data on rainfall, food production, food distribution, civil registration and disease surveillance with the nutrition surveillance.

National Nutrition Policy

The National Nutrition Policy had set various goals to be achieved by 2000. All the concerned departments have reviewed the progress achieved and have revised their goals for the Tenth Plan /2010. The goals set in the policy have to be revised in the light of these revised goals. Path Ahead and Goals Set 3.3.149 The Prime Minister, in his Independence Day speech on 15th August, 2001 announced the setting up of a National Nutrition Mission with the following objectives:

— reduction in under-nutrition (CED);

— reduction / elimination of micronutrient deficiencies viz., iron, iodine and Vitamin A;

— reduction in chronic energy deficiency.

The Mission would

— co-ordinate and monitor implementation of the National Nutrition Policy;

— strengthen

— existing programmes;

— research and development;

— nutrition education and IEC;

— relief in natural calamities.

The National Nutrition Mission will be supervised by the National Nutrition Council headed by the Prime Minister.

Strategies for Rapid Reduction of Under Nutrtition

The Tenth Plan envisage a change in strategy to achieve substantial reduction in the severer grades of under-nutrition and health hazards associated with it without massive increase in the cost.

For prevention of under-nutrition, strategy suggested include

— nutrition education through all modes of communication with special focus on inter-personal communication by anganwadi workers and ANMs to promote:

— universal breastfeeding;

— exclusive breastfeeding for first six months;

— continuing breastfeeding up to two years;

— introduction of semi solid supplements from family pot at sixth month;

— giving the complimentary feeds to children at least 4-5 times a day;

— improving intra-familial distribution of food based on needs and providing pre-school children, pregnant and lactating women some more food from the family pot;

— introducing green leafy vegetables at least twice a week in the family meal.

— provide take-home food supplements to children in the 6-36 months age group from BPL families (utilising PMGY funds also) as they cannot consume 300 Kcal food at one sitting at the anganwadi;

— administration of massive dose Vitamin A in April and October to the children at 18, 24, 30 and 36 months by the anganwadi workers under the supervision of the ANMs;

— organise immunisation, maternal and child care at the anganwadi on a fixed date at least once a month so that the health care needs of these vulnerable groups are met;

— the anganwadi workers can keep iron and folic acid tablets and ORS for distribution as and when required in the village and also monitor the regularity of intake;

— promote universal use of iodised salt and organise testing salt for adequacy of iodisation at home level.

The anganwadi workers and the ANMs will be trained by appropriate agencies including Food and Nutrition Board and Home Science and medical colleges so that they learn and communicate the right nutrition and health education messages to the population on a sustained basis. This is a very important but neglected area which does not require any additional financial inputs and could play the most critical role in reducing the prevalence of under nutrition.

For detection and management of undernutrition

— Ensure that all children in the age group of 0-6 years are weighed at least four times in a year and children suffering from grade III and grade IV under-nutrition are identified. Those with grade III and grade IV under- nutrition be provided with double rations (as envisaged in the ICDS guidelines) as take-home food supplements continuously with the instruction that they should be fed these preparations at least four times a day. In addition, appropriate health care should be provided to them by the ANMs and PHC doctors.

— Weigh all pregnant and lactating women, identify those with body weight less than 40 kg and provide them with food grains for the remaining period of pregnancy/lactation or until they cross the cut off point.

— Weigh all adolescent girls at least four times in a year, identify those with weight less than 35 kg and provide foodgrains for the next three months or until they weigh more than 35 kg.

— Organise antenatal and child health clinics in anganwadi by the ANM for screening vulnerable population, early detection and effective treatment of anaemia, Vitamin A deficiency and iodine deficiency disorders. Goals Set for the Tenth Plan

The Tenth Plan has set specific nutrition goals to be achieved by 2007. The major goals are:

— Intensify nutrition and health education to improve infant and child feeding and caring practices so as to:

  — bring down the prevalence of under-weight children under three years from the current level of 47 per cent to 40 per cent;

  — reduce prevalence of severe under-nutrition in children in the 0-6 years age group by 50 per cent.

— reduce prevalence of anaemia by 25% and that of moderate/severe anaemia by 50 per cent;

— eliminate Vitamin Adeficiency as a public health problem; and

— reduce prevalence of IDD in the country to less than 10 percent by 2010.

In view of the massive inter-state/inter-district differences in the availability and access to the nutrition-related services and in nutritional status of the population, the state specific goals to be achieved by 2007 have been evolved based on the current level of these indices and the Tenth Plan goals for the country has been derived from the state specific goals. The progress achieved in terms of the process and impact indicators will be reviewed annually. Midterm review of the progress achieved and the problems faced will enable midcourse corrections. If necessary goals can be reset at the time of the mid-term appraisal.

6

Food Production Challenges

Recent approaches to agricultural development, including food production and food security, have largely failed to reduce the absolute numbers of the food insecure or to ensure environmental sustainability. Whilst global achievements in food production have been impressive in the last 50 years, the global inequalities in food entitlements remain one of the biggest obstacles to achieving food security for all.

There are five contrasting schools of thought on how we should approach these challenges.

— *Environmental pessimists.* This group, with prominent adherents in the official aid circles and the international agricultural research agencies, contends that ecological limits to growth are being approached and will either soon be passed or have already been reached. Following a neo-Malthusian argument, these 'environmental pessimists' claim.that populations continue to grow too rapidly, while yields of major staple crops have declined and will continue to slow, or even fall in future. They argue that, given the current state of knowledge, no new technological breakthroughs are likely; and that some agroecological systems have been too thoroughly degraded to recover. Solving these problems means making population control the first priority

— *Business-as-usual optimists.* This group, with a strong belief in the power of the market, argues that supply will always meet increasing demand, and so recent growth in aggregate food production will continue alongside reductions in population growth. These 'business-as-usual optimists' expect that innovations in biotechnology will sustain the growth in food output. In many countries, however, it is also expected that the area under cultivation will expand dramatically - some estimates put the increase at an extra 79 million hectares in Sub-Saharan Africa alone by 2020

— *Industrialised world to the rescue.* This predominantly northern-based group with ties to the agrochemical industry, asserts that, for a variety of ecological, institutional and political economic reasons, developing countries will never be able to feed themselves. This group insists that the looming food gap will have to be filled by modernised agriculture based in the North. By increasing production in large, mechanised operations, this will force smaller and more 'marginal' farmers to go out of business, so taking the pressure off natural resources, which can then be conserved in protected areas and wilderness reserves. The large producers will then be able to trade their food with those who need it, or have it distributed by international agencies to provide famine relief or food aid. The two remaining groups believe that significant biological yield increases are possible on existing agricultural land. They are, however, fundamentally divided over what is the most appropriate approach to achieve these increases.

— *New modernists.* This group, led by the partnership of the Sasakawa and Global 2000 Foundations, claims that food growth can only come through high-external-input farming, either on existing Green Revolution lands or on the 'high-potential' areas that were missed by the past 30 years of agricultural development. These 'new modernists' argue that farmers simply use too few artificial fertilisers, pesticides, high-yielding seed varieties and other external inputs, which are the only way to improve yields and reduce pressure on natural habitats. They also contend that high-input agriculture is more environmentally sustainable than low-input agriculture, as the latter requires the intensive use of local resources which may be degraded in the process.

— *Sustainable intensification.* This group advances arguments in favour of the sustainable intensification of agricultural production, on the grounds that substantial growth is possible in currently unimproved or degraded areas whilst at the same time protecting or even regenerating natural resources. Those advocating 'sustainable intensification' point to recent empirical evidence from both the North and the South to argue that low-input.(but not necessarily zero-input) agriculture can be highly productive, provided farmers participate fully in all stages of technology development and extension. They maintain that this evidence indicates that changes in the productivity of agricultural and pastoral lands is as much a function of human capacity and ingenuity as it is of biological and physical processes .

The basic challenge for sustainable agriculture is to make better use of available biophysical and human resources. This can be done by minimising the use of external inputs, by optimising the use of internal resources, or by combinations of both. This ensures the efficient and effective use of what is available, and ensures that any improvements will persist, as dependencies on external systems are kept to a reasonable minimum.

Sustainable agriculture seeks the integrated use of a wide range of pest, nutrient, agroforestry, soil and water management technologies. By-products or wastes from one component or enterprise become inputs to another. As natural processes increasingly substitute for external inputs, so the impact on the environment is reduced.

A more sustainable agriculture, therefore, is any system of food or fibre production that systematically pursues the following goals:

— a thorough incorporation of natural processes such as nutrient cycling, nitrogen fixation, and pest-predator relationships;

— a minimisation of the use of external and non-renewable inputs that damage the environment or harm the health of farmers and consumers;

— the participation of farmers and rural people in all processes of problem analysis, technology development, adaptation and extension, and monitoring and evaluation;

— a more equitable access to productive resources and opportunities;

— a greater productive use of local knowledge, practices and resources;

— the incorporation of a diversity of natural resources and enterprises within farms; and

— an increase in self-reliance amongst farmers and rural communities.

It should be emphasised that sustainable agriculture does not represent a return to some form of low-technology, 'backward' or 'traditional' agricultural practices. Instead it implies an incorporation of recent innovations that may originate with scientists, with farmers or both. And it is not just about food production, but about increasing the capacity of rural people to be self-reliant and resilient in the face of change, and about building strong rural organisations and economies.

But precise and absolute definitions of sustainability, and therefore of sustainable agriculture, are impossible. One of the central aims of sustainable agriculture is that the approach should be flexible, and not prescribe a concretely defined set of technologies, practices or policies. This would only serve to restrict the future options of farmers. As conditions change and as knowledge changes, so too must farmers and farming communities. Sustainable agriculture is, therefore, not a simple model or package to be imposed. It is more a process of learning and adaptation.

The Sustainable Agriculture Programme of IIED has examined the extent and impact of sustainable agriculture in a selected number of countries, and used this empirical evidence to estimate sustainable agriculture's potential contribution to global food production. Whilst we were aware that many projects and programmes had improved agricultural yields, these data have never been collated in one place.

The government and non-government programmes and projects included in this analysis share important common characteristics. They have:

— made use of resource-conserving technologies in conjunction with group or collective approaches to agricultural improvement and natural resource management;

— put participatory approaches and farmer-centred activities at the centre of their agenda - hence, these activities are occurring on local people's terms, and so are more likely to persist after the projects and programmes have ended;

— not used subsidies or food-for-work to 'buy' the participation of local people, or to encourage them to adopt particular technologies, and thus improvements are unlikely to fade away or simply disappear at the end of projects or programmes;

— supported the active involvement of women as key producers and facilitators;

— emphasised 'adding value' to agricultural products through agro-processing, marketing, and other off-farm activities. thus creating employment and income-generating opportunities and retaining the surplus in the rural economy.

Two types of transition to sustainable agriculture have been assessed: from modern or conventional high-external input agriculture; and from traditional, rainfed agriculture where cereal yields have largely remained constant over centuries. As these transitions are recent, they provide compelling evidence that similar improvements could occur elsewhere and that they could be repeated on a larger scale .

In the 20 countries of the South (and the total of 63 projects) examined and analysed, there are some 1.93 million households farming 4.1 million hectares with sustainable agriculture technologies and practices. The data in Table 1 do not represent a comprehensive survey of sustainable agriculture in each of the countries. They do illustrate, however, what has been achieved by specific projects and what could be replicated elsewhere. Most of these improvements have occurred in the past ten years. The assumption is that these are representative of what is possible on a wider scale.

It could be argued, however, that they are only successful because they have occurred where there is a combination of the least resistance and most opportunity, although the sheer diversity of approaches and contexts represented undermine such an assertion. Moreover, many of the improvements are occurring in difficult, remote and resource-poor areas that have commonly been assumed in the past to be incapable of producing food surpluses.

This analysis mainly focuses on cereal yields as an important indicator of improved performance. In all of the initiatives assessed, per hectare agricultural productivity has increased - in some cases substantially. These yield improvements differ according to whether agricultural systems are in high-yielding (HY), medium-yielding (MY) and low-yielding (LY) countries. There are currently 56 LY countries, 65 MY countries and 46 HY countries.

Table 1. Impact of sustainable and people-centred agriculture in different agricultural systems

Countries	Number of farming households reported	Number of hectares reported	Dominan crop	Yield Impróvement factor (%)
Rainfed systems				
Brazil	223,000	1,330,000	Maize, Wheat	198 to 246%
Burkina Faso	22,500	37,360	Sorghum/millet	250%
Ethiopia	24,175	21,850	Maize	154%
Guatemala	17,000	17,000	Maize	250%
Honduras	27,000	42,000	Maize	250%
India	307,910	993,410	Sorghum/Millet	288%
Kenya	222,550	250,000	Maize	200%
Mexico	7400	23,500	Coffee	140%
Nepal	3000	1300	Maize, Wheat	164 to 307%
Philippines	850	920	Upland rice	214%
Senegal	200,000	400,000	Sorghum/Millet	300%
Uganda	9426	21,379	Maize	150%
Zambia	6300	6300	Sorghum/Millet	200%
Total	*1,146,111*	*3,257,519*		

Rainfed systems				
Bangladesh	11,025	4772	Rice	110%
China	47,000	12,000	Rice	111%
India	50,000	71,300	Rice	108%
Indonesia	400,000	267,000	Rice	107%
Malaysia	2500	3925	Rice	108%
Philippines	175,000	385,000	Rice	112%
Sri Lanka	100,000	95,350	Rice	117%
Thailand	500	2040	Rice	109%
Vietnam	6600	3540	Rice	108%
Total	**792,625**	**844,927**		
Industrialised Systems				
Germany (integrated)	75,000	200,000	Wheat/Barley	90%
Netherlands (integrated)	500	na	Wheat/Barley	85%
USA (integrated)	40,000	632,000	Wheat/Barley	95%
EU (organic)	50,000	1,200,000	Wheat/Barley	80%
Total	**165,500**	**832,000**		

The greatest increases following a transition to sustainable agriculture are in rainfed agriculture in the lowest yield countries, where the average new yields for wheat, maize and sorghum-millet are of the order of double the yields of conventional or pre-sustainable agriculture. Smaller increases have occurred in the irrigated lands of South East and South Asia, where productivity is already at least three to five times higher than in rainfed lands. Here sustainable agriculture rice yields are slightly more than 10% greater than in conventional or pre-sustainable agriculture.

Table 2. Improvements in cereal yields up to ten years after adoption of sustainable agriculture

	Average current yields (t/ha)	Average high-yield agriculture	Average medium-yield agriculture	Average low-yield agriculture
All Cereals	2.83	102%	166%	212%
Wheat	2.45	95%	210%	220%
Rice	3.05	115%	111%	111%
Maize	4.33	100%	190%	220%
Sorghum-Millet	1.09	95%	265%	265%

In industrialised countries, a shift to sustainable agriculture is expected to bring a decline in productivity, as the production levels are so much higher than in most of Africa, Asia and Latin America. The immediate falls are of the order of 10-20%. The sharp declines in input costs mean, however, that these systems are still as profitable to farmers as the more conventional ones fully dependent on high use of external inputs. In the longer-term (five to ten years), evidence suggests that the yields in sustainable agriculture will rise to former levels. In the

USA, for example, the top 25% of sustainable agriculture farmers have better gross margins and better yields than the top 25% of conventional farmers. There are also variations over time - after conversion to sustainable agriculture in industrialised systems, yields do fall 10-20%; but many farmers find that these return to parity with conventional yields after five years or so, as their knowledge and management skills increase and as the natural capital is rebuilt.

The widespread adoption of sustainable agriculture would have a significant redistributive effect on productive capacity. The currently low and medium yielding countries (which are also the poorest) would benefit more in terms of food production than the high yield countries. Although a useful indication of what can be achieved, these data provide only a partial picture of the improvements that have occurred, or have the potential to occur, through a more sustainable approach to agriculture and rural development.

Sustainable agriculture offers farmers the opportunity to diversify their strategies. For this reason, cereal production may not increase in the short term following the adoption of sustainable agriculture, as many farmers respond to increased yields by diversifying into new crops, so reducing the area under cereals.One pattern is as follows: soon after transition to sustainable agriculture, farmers get excited by the extra productivity; in the following year, everyone is producing so much more that the local market price declines or collapses and producers get poorer returns. In the next year, they reduce the area under cereals, and diversify into new crops. This cycle has been observed in a number of contexts. In Honduras, for example, farmers who used to grow maize exclusively now cultivate upwards of 25 crops per farm;; in Gujarat, India, farmers have diversified away from sorghum/millet based systems to grow many types of vegetables; in Bolivia, upland potato farmers have reduced field sizes (by up to 90%) to save on labour and yet produce the same amount of food. In other cases, farmers have diversified without much change to cereal production. In Taita, Kenya, an NGO reintroduced traditional staples of sweet potato, arrowroot, sugar cane and bananas, together with fruit trees and zero-grazing for livestock, leading to a reduction in food insecurity and an improvement in the nutritional status of the local population. There has been no measurable impact on cereal yields, either positive or negative.

But this is not always the case. There are many examples of food deficit areas such as parts of Ethiopia, Kenya, Uganda, Zimbabwe, Honduras and Guatemala, becoming food surplus areas following adoption of sustainable agriculture. Other factors may have been important, but sustainable agriculture played a key role.

Recent years have seen many efforts to predict the increases in agricultural production needed to achieve global food security over the next quarter to half century. These all conclude that food production will have to increase substantially over the next few decades to feed the increasing global population. But global projections do not necessarily help when it comes to addressing food security at the local level.

What is most commonly omitted is the importance of the 'entitlements' of people and the 'capabilities' these entitlements generate. Food production is not the same as food availability - this is production minus exports, and plus imports. Aggregate availability and the ability to acquire food (ie. food 'entitlements') are also not the same. Whilst food production is undoubtedly among the more important influences in the determination of food entitlements, the connections are complex and many factors are important .

Current levels of agricultural productivity and production say little about potential levels because they are a response largely to present levels of demand and price/market conditions.As Amartya Sen observes:

> Food is produced by ... farmers and others not to demonstrate how much can be grown, but to make economic use of it - to eat, to sell, to exchange. We cannot directly infer how much could have been produced merely by looking at what was actually produced... Food will not be produced beyond the effective demand for it.

Thus, food production is an important part of food security, but not the only part. Some 800 million people currently have completely inadequate consumption levels and access to food. But most of these people, who would otherwise consume more, do not have sufficient incomes to demand more food and cause it to be produced. For poor people, increased demand and increased production are part of the same equation.

If production constraints limit agricultural growth, they act as brakes on both incomes and demand as well as supply. In countries with a heavy dependence on agriculture, progress towards improved food security does depend on making agriculture more productive. This presents us with a paradox. Food security largely depends on access and entitlements to food, which depend on improved incomes for many. If incomes are increased, then more food will be produced. But for many people in many countries, increased income depends on improvements to agriculture.

It is clear that a strategy to enhance rural food security must also focus on creating and supporting linkages which allow increased food production to support healthy rural economies. Agriculture plays a dual role in the abolition of hunger - it produces the food and it can also produce a great many of the jobs needed by households to buy food.

Since agriculture is the world's single largest employer, raising productivity can immediately place additional purchasing power in the hands of the rural poor, who will in turn use the additional income for buying more food and other basic consumer goods. The increased agricultural produce can become raw material for a wide range of agro-based industries and services, stimulating the formation of new enterprises and creating downstream jobs.

Both the 'business-as-usual optimists' and the 'industrialised world to the rescue' lobby make the assumption that developing countries can rely on food imports to ensure their food security. But this may not be possible. The uncertainties of the world food market, the shortage of physical facilities to ship, process and store large volumes of food, foreign exchange constraints and high internal transport costs, all mean that an over-reliance on food imports would be inadvisable in many developing countries. They do not explain how the poor will acquire the purchasing power to buy the food they need. Even if we assume large increases in imports, food security for millions of people in 2020 will still depend on their ability to produce their own food.

The 'environmental pessimists', like the 'optimists', do not account for economic arguments that indicate that current food supply mainly reflects current demand and price conditions. In other words, food will not be produced beyond the effective demand for it. The 'new modernists', in continuing to emphasise food production at all costs, fail to take account of the evidence of the detrimental impacts of high-input agriculture over the past 50 years. It has become clear that not only is this approach failing to improve food security for the most vulnerable groups, it has also been achieved at great environmental and health costs.

Although recent analyses of food security have highlighted the differences between food production and food availability and access, most have failed to address fully the need for social, economic and environmental sustainability in food production. The emphasis on increasing yields has led policy makers to disregard or misunderstand how these approaches may hinder, rather than help, food security in the developing world. Sustainable agriculture offers opportunities to deal with these issues in an integrated way.

The links between sustainable agriculture and food security are summarised in Figure 1. The figure shows how achieving food security depends on ensuring that three key conditions are fulfilled:

— Sustainable food production through the use of regenerative technologies, the full participation of farmers and pastoralists in the processes of planning, research and extension;

— A conserved natural resource base through approaches, practices and technologies that build upon and enhance the health and diversity of available natural resources without depleting them;

— Entitlements or access to food through approaches which strengthen local capacity and build strong and diversified rural economies.

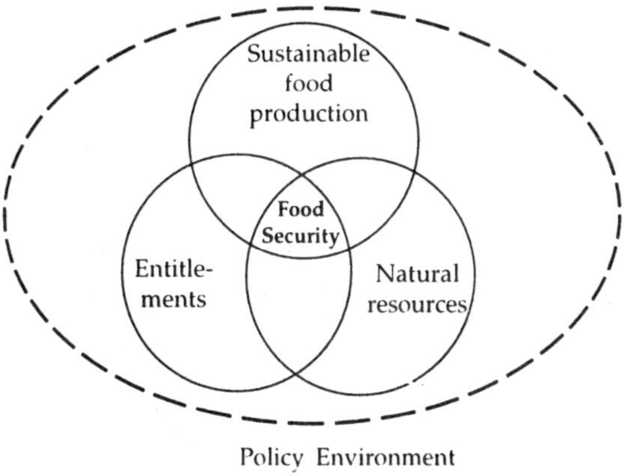

Figure 1. Links between sustainable agriculture and food security

As the model suggests, all these areas are inextricably linked, and the achievement of sustainable food security depends on conditions being met within all three areas. It also shows that meeting these conditions depends on a supportive policy environment.

Improving agricultural productivity through sustainable technologies and practices can go some way toward increasing local food availability. An important theme which emerged in one of IIED's recent surveys is that sustainable agriculture can help to contribute to revitalising and strengthening rural economies, in turn improving many people's ability to acquire food. Some examples included:

— increases in real income and establishing the capacity to save;

— employment creation and the diversification of livelihoods;

— reduced dependence on credit;

— increasing land values and greater investment on farms;

— creation of markets or improved access to markets;

— greater ability to pay school fees, hospital bills, etc.; and

— increasing confidence of people in the productive capacity of their land and in their own abilities.

But sustainable agriculture alone will not be sufficient to meet many people's food security requirements. For a host of reasons, not all rural people are able to produce their own food, and in many areas and for many people, agriculture is not the only, or even the main, source of income.

Even where food supplies are adequate, absence of employment opportunities to provide income to purchase food can result in hunger. In other areas, increasing population pressures have led to the complete absence of free land for development. And of course, while many farmers also migrate seasonally to supplement their incomes, most of them would rather not.

An important lesson drawn from the recent evidence of sustainable agriculture is that it needs to be placed in a wider political and policy context. Strengthening other employment sources, such as small-scale enterprises, cottage industries and small-scale processing units in rural areas can help take pressure off land. This can then mitigate degradation - although this also depends on many other factors, such as land husbandry practices, access to markets, security of tenure, etc. Furthermore, if much of rural consumption depends on non-agrarian incomes and entitlements, then to concentrate exclusively on resource-conserving technologies, participatory research and development approaches and farmer-to-farmer extension will address only part of the problem.

On the basis of these observations, it is clear that a strategy to enhance agricultural production and reduce rural poverty must also aim to promote rurally based non-agrarian incomes. The essence of this would be to find mechanisms to facilitate the retention of surpluses within a region.

Such mechanisms might include new marketing arrangements and the incorporation of a processing stage to develop new forward and backward linkages within the regional agricultural system. Aside from a direct creation of employment in agro-processing, agro-industry and marketing, the resulting positive impact on farmer income would be to create a derived demand for non-agrarian goods and services that could be generated locally.

Finding the institutional mechanisms to make this work will be very difficult, but not necessarily impossible. Identifying and supporting these institutional arrangements, and helping develop the markets for the products being processed should be a central thrust of any broad sustainable agriculture policy cognisant of the realities of regional economic development.

Ashift towards more intensive, sustainable forms of agriculture can make a substantial positive contribution to food security - not only through its ability to contribute to sustainable intensification of production, but also through an emphasis on improving people's ability to acquire food. Food deficit countries appear likely to win the most.

Food exporting countries, such as the USA and those in the EU, will probably see a decline in food production in the short-term, but this is unlikely to be permanent, and financial returns to farmers should remain the same or even be improved, particularly as the levels of direct and indirect subsidies decline.

In the first instance, emphasis should not be placed on agricultural extensification (i.e. bringing more land under production), but on sustainable agricultural intensification. There is no need for agriculture to expand into uncultivated lands, as existing farmlands contain huge potential that is currently being overlooked.

A massive increase in inorganic fertilisers and pesticides is not a necessary condition for feeding the world. In certain agroecological systems, moderate applications of fertilisers will be necessary to ensure the appropriate balance of plant nutrients and minerals in soils. Pesticides will also have a place, but only in so far as they are required in carefully designed and managed integrated pest management programmes.

It also appears that increased food production will not depend on advances in biotechnology. Although biotechnology is expected by many to contribute to agriculture's productivity, and possibly to more environmentally-friendly agriculture, it will make little difference for poor farmers and farmers in low-income food deficit countries. The achievements recorded here all occurred through making the best use of locally-available resources.

Sustainable agriculture represents a capital investment as it helps in natural capital formation. It replenishes the capital stock of soil nutrients, of water resources, and of predators and other beneficial wildlife. Most agriculture today progressively depletes natural and human capital, by removing soil nutrients, organic matter and water, and by diminishing human capacity and skills. Current levels of agricultural productivity are maintained by these processes of asset stripping and under-investment. An investment in approaches and processes that help the transition to sustainable agriculture is an investment both in the current and future capacity to feed the world. A shift to sustainable agriculture will require many different investments, if productivity and environmental sustainability are to be enhanced and if they are to be linked to food security.

There is a need to move beyond the high-external-input modernist approaches to agricultural development and recognise the importance of sustainable agriculture for food security, by:

— Promoting sustainable agriculture and resource-conserving technologies and practices.

— Supporting national policies and strategies for sustainable agriculture.

— Redirecting subsidies and grants towards sustainable technologies and practices.

— Reforming teaching and training establishments to encourage the formal adoption of participatory methods and processes.

— Developing farmer-centred research and extension by supporting farmer-to-farmer exchanges and schemes for farmer training in their own communities.

— Improving rural infrastructure to ensure access to markets with positive price incentives.

— Improving farmers' access to and management of the diversity of wild and cultivated genetic resources.

There is a need to focus on rural social enterprises and surplus retention by:

— Adopting an entitlements perspective that encourages the retention of regional surpluses.

— Focusing on improvements to non-agricultural incomes and off-farm employment.

— Decentralising and devolving authority from governments and aid agencies, while providing local organisations with support to develop their capacity to 'draw down' resources as needed.

— Supporting rural women as producers and facilitators by developing their access to and control of productive resources, including savings and credit, and information.

— Supporting security of tenure for agricultural productivity, especially through indigenous systems, by reasserting community use and management rights to land that build on local rather than centralised systems of property.

— Forming or strengthening farmers' organisations and local users' groups.

— Supporting rural savings and credit provision by avoiding land-tied credit and supporting local savings and credit groups.

Urban Farming: Challenges and Opportunities

In US, current food systems require vast resources for complicated distribution services to move food from where it is raised and processed to reach consumers in cities, with the average supermarket food item in North America travelling 1400 miles. With increasing globalization, the foods now travel even further distances than ever from all over the world.

While many enjoy the advantages of this rich and nutritious array of foods, there are significant social, economic, public health, and environmental costs to the food system. The environmental costs of industrial agriculture include groundwater contamination, soil erosion, and loss of biodiversity. The social and economic costs of a globalized food system include the devastation of rural communities, with subsistence farmers among the poorest people on the planet, and significant levels of hunger amidst plenty, even in the cities of the developed world.

The health costs of this system are seen in epidemic levels of obesity and diet-related diseases. These are some of the hidden costs of the corporate controlled food system. Urban farming is an essential tool that addresses a number of these problems in innovative ways. Environmental stewardship is enhanced through urban agriculture's efforts to green cities.

Economic development and community revitalization are also achieved through urban farming when neighborhoods take new pride in a community garden, when inner-city residents gain the ability to grow and market their own food, when inner-city farmers' markets provide new opportunities for entrepreneurs and commercial farmers.

Individual health and a sense of empowerment and well-being are created when urban dwellers have access to local food and greater control over their own food system. Urban farming takes account of the real cost of food, and the real benefits from local and regional food.

An unacceptable number of Americans, including many children, do not get enough to eat on a daily basis. A USDA document on U.S. food security released in 2000 reports that even in the United States, where food is generally plentiful, safe, nutritious, and relatively inexpensive, 31 million Americans were food insecure in 1999, including approximately 12 million children. Poverty, in all its ramifications, is the root source of much food insecurity.

In 2001, more than 31 million people (11.3% of the population) lived below the poverty line, meaning that if they were a family of four, they earned less than $17,960 each year. People who are living in poverty are likely also to experience food insecurity: children, inner-city residents, single parent female-headed households, people of color, people living with disabilities, the elderly, and farm workers.

Each year in the past decade more and more families reported that they ran out of food and didn't have money to buy more. This represents one in ten households in the United States. Hunger and homelessness rose sharply in major American cities in 2001, according to the Conference of Mayors' 27-City Survey. Requests for emergency food assistance climbed an average of 23 percent and requests for emergency shelter an average of 13 percent in the 27 cities surveyed. Over the same period, resources available for emergency food assistance failed to keep up with demand in most cities.

Food insecurity, whether related to actual food insufficiency, nutritional quality, or anxiety about a future lack of food, affects the quality of life of urban residents in far-reaching ways. Inadequate nutrition is clearly associated with school and work absences, fatigue, and problems with concentration. Hunger and poor nutrition are also linked to the increased incidence and virulence of infectious diseases, many of which- such as TB-are on the rise in US cities.

Furthermore, the lack of a nutritious diet is a well-known risk factor for any number of chronic diseases such as diabetes, hypertension, and heart failure. Even when cash is available to low-income urban residents, food is not always so readily accessible. Many supermarkets have closed or moved from the inner city due to complex market forces related to the increasing impoverishment of their clientele and the deterioration and depopulation of once vibrant communities.

Unfortunately, it is not unusual for many remaining inner-city grocery and convenience stores to hike prices, even on basic foods. "A study in Detroit found that grocery stores near downtown and closer to lower-income neighborhoods charged on average 10 percent more than those on the beltway. Another study of all food stores in three low-income zip codes in Detroit found that only four out of five stores carried a minimal "healthy food basket".

Low-income consumers have less food shopping choices than middle-income consumers across the country: they have fewer retail options, limited transportation options, and often face higher prices at chain supermarkets. Thus ironically, people on limited incomes in cities are likely to pay more for their food than wealthier shoppers in higher income neighborhoods.

The range, freshness, and quality of foods are also often compromised in inner-city groceries, thus further limiting customers' maximal choices for nutritious and affordable meals. As the locus of poverty shifts to urban areas, an expanded urban agriculture program could build community food security by improving the quantity, quality, regularity and nutritional balance of food intake, thereby reducing hunger and improving nutrition.

It provides a more adequate income to the farmers themselves, thereby diminishing their food insecurity. Local fresh vegetables and fruit can have twice the vitamins and essential micro-nutrients available from stale supermarket produce at the same price. Local and regional food is safer and more secure than the products of industrial agriculture that typically travel long distances.

Urban agriculture produces a range of products well matched to the food needs and demands of diverse urban populations, thus assuring them of a more balanced diet. In addition, farming in the city conserves natural resources and contributes to a healthy environment for living.

Urban agriculture in the United States has been enriched by the skills and technologies of immigrant populations, from Japanese market gardeners in California to Italian urban gardeners in the Northeast. In addition, many inner-city communities are rich in social and environmental capital even while they are poor in economic resources. The urban agriculture movement, if it is supported and expanded, can build on this existing, but hitherto neglected or undeveloped expertise, social relationships, and the urban landscape itself.

The regenerative effect of urban agriculture is especially visible when vacant lots are transformed from eyesores-weedy, trash-ridden, dangerous gathering places-into bountiful, beautiful and safe gardens that feed peoples' bodies and souls. With increasing "sprawl" into the suburbs, the last twenty years has seen a common pattern of inner-city neglect in most cities across North America.

Between 1950 and 1990 in the U.S., abandoned lots in inner-city areas remained vacant for between 20 and 30 years in most cities. Failed businesses and homes were bulldozed, leaving relatively inexpensive lots without much economic potential, except, that is, for those lots that have become fruitful examples of urban agriculture.

Even some of the 130,000 to 425,000 contaminated vacant industrial sites, or brownfields, that the General Accounting Office has identified, may be safely converted to agricultural purposes when properly redeveloped. Cities also have other sources of unused land that have been put into food production by advocates of urban agriculture.

For instance, food gardens and orchards have been developed on land surrounding institutions such as schools and hospitals that once contained only landscaped plantings. Portions of city parks have also been converted. While open park spaces are traditionally regarded as recreational and aesthetic but nonproductive, urban agriculture provides an alternative use that is both aesthetic and productive.

Public and private lands in vulnerable areas of the city, such as on steep slopes or flood plains, have been similarly transformed by urban agriculture endeavours using ecologically sound growing practices. Portions of a city's waste stream can be transformed from a problem into a resource for sustainable development through urban agriculture. Urban agriculture reuses its waste and the waste of other sectors to produce food.

For instance, using compost in urban agriculture reduces both the intake and the output in the resources stream, resulting in fewer resources consumed and less pollution. This in turn can make the city more ecologically balanced, and more resourceful. A sustainable future for cities would require a move towards technologies that transform waste into useful products rather than dump it. Urban farming can contribute to this process in several ways: by producing crops for human and livestock consumption, by composting and by processing wastewater for direct production and irrigation.

These features of urban life-unused land and other readily available recycled resources, and community-based agricultural know-how, leadership, and solidarity-can combine in creative ways to bring food to many tables while increasing the quality of urban life. Furthermore, urban agriculture can be an effective arena for the development of economic development through micro- and small businesses. The full scope of urban agriculture appears if the city is seen in its relationships to the urban fringe and the surrounding region.

Urban dwellers want local supplies of food to remain healthful, abundant, and accessible. This is far easier to do when suppliers, distributors, and consumers have the opportunity for more direct local relationships, as with urban and peri-urban agricultural endeavours that provide farm-fresh foods through community-supported agriculture, farmers' markets, restaurants, and educational and other institutions.

Consumers can monitor the accountability of food producers, thus increasing the likelihood that food is raised in sustainable ways that do not harm the earth and the people who grow the food. When consumers purchase locally-grown food, they can vote with their pocketbooks to support horticultural practices and labour relations that are more likely to be sustainable and just. This is unfortunately less likely with foods brought in from outside the urban and regional food system.

In the industrial food distribution system with its hidden subsidies for transportation and energy, food travels on average 1400 miles to reach the consumer. In addition to these complex transportation costs, people are increasingly concerned about food raised and distributed through large-scale industrial systems of corporate food production.

As governmental oversight of food production and processing decreases, public apprehension has increased in regard to a range of food safety problems - from e-coli contamination to the unknown consequences of foods containing genetically modified organisms. Urban agriculture is a significant economic activity, central to the lives of tens of millions of people throughout the world. There is ample evidence here and abroad, that the potential of urban agriculture for food security is very real.

The United Nations Development Program estimates that fifteen percent of food worldwide is grown in cities and this figure could be significantly expanded. Certainly urban agriculture has been an important factor for subsistence among city dwellers caught up in regional conflicts or in the throes of economic readjustment. When transportation lines to the countryside are disrupted or when consumers cannot afford to buy fruits and vegetables, gardens sometimes offer urbanites the only buffer against starvation.

In Russia, food production on large-scale rural farms fell by 40 percent since Soviet times, making the cost of food very high on the new free market. Many Russians have survived through access to dachas (small plots of land given to citizens), which produce 30 percent of the total food grown in the country and 80 percent of the vegetables. Between 1970 and 1990, the number of Moscow families engaged in food production increased from 20 percent to 65 percent. This is one striking example of a powerful shift toward urban agriculture worldwide, especially in response to economic crisis.

While Russia has begun once more to export grain in 2001, small-scale urban growing remains central to people's basic food security. Even in less dire circumstances, urban agriculture presents considerable benefits. For instance, currently 14% of Londoners already grow some food in their gardens. It is estimated that Londoners could produce up to 232,000 tons of fruits and vegetables, or 18% of the population's daily nutritional needs.

In the United States, a 1993 report estimated that one third (696,000) of the 2 million farms are located within metropolitan areas. These farms produced 35% of all crops and livestock sales. At a time when rural farms are going out of business at an unprecedented rate in the U.S., the number of urban and peri-urban farms is actually increasing. In 1998, 15,700 new small farms were registered with state agriculture departments; most of these were located within suburban areas.

People are often surprised about how much produce can be grown on the small plots and acreages usually found in cities. Of course, yields depend on factors such as the weather, the amount of available land, soil conditions, seed species, the availability of a dependable water source, and the gardener's skill. But even given these constraints, the use of intensive methods of growing can maximize the efficiency of small-scale operations, as well as providing much of a household's yearly vegetable needs and nutritional requirements.

Urban commercial gardens using raised beds, soil amendments, and "season extenders" such as row cover and greenhouses produce yields that are generally 13 times more per acre than those of rural farms. This potential is well illustrated by The Food Project in urban and suburban Boston. In addition to vegetables, urban agriculture includes the production of honey (beekeeping), worms for composting and soil amendments, poultry and eggs, fish, and meats such as rabbit, chicken and goat.

There are three broad categories of urban growers who contribute significantly to food security and raise the bulk of food involved in urban agriculture: backyard gardeners, community gardeners, and commercial growers. In actual practice, these categories overlap. For example, community gardeners may sell or barter some of their surplus at the peak of the season, or in another case, suburban backyard growers may decide to move into commercial activity in peri-urban farms.

Moreover, the categories may not encompass the entire range of people involved in urban agriculture. For instance, food is also grown in urban gardens maintained in therapeutic settings such as hospitals, senior citizen programs, drug treatment, and long-term care facilities. In addition, food is raised by children in school programs that incorporate gardening in many facets of the curriculum. These three categories refer to location and purpose, not to who the farmers are.

Urban farmers are as diverse as the population overall. In U.S. urban agriculture, women farmers, immigrant populations, and minorities play significant roles, as they do in urban farming worldwide. Urban backyard gardeners are most apt to grow vegetables, fruits and edible herbs, often along with flowers, in plots around their homes.

The term backyard gardener may be technically a misnomer since some people even garden on their decks, or on their apartment building balconies and rooftops. Good yields can be raised even in the simplest of containers. Backyard gardeners are not only growing plant produce to eat, but also they keep bees for honey and raise fish and small animals at their homes.

In the neighbourhood of Pilsen, the primary entry point for Mexican immigrants into Chicago, six women associated with Heifer International maintain hydroponic aquaculture systems built of recycled materials in their apartments. These systems provide up to 80 pounds of protein per family per year. As many as one quarter of urban households in the United States have gardens.

Many of these urban backyard gardeners are hobbyists who enjoy raising their own food to supplement their diets with seasonal harvests. Surpluses become preserved products and gifts for friends, neighbours, and co-workers. Cultivating hard-to-grow crops is a frequent incentive to garden.

In much of North America, while subsistence is not the immediate goal of such gardeners, in many cases the harvest from a backyard garden has stretched the food budgets of low-income families and their network of relatives and friends. There are indications that many more families would like to garden for this very reason. The Home Gardening Project has installed more than 1400 household gardens in disadvantaged neighborhoods of downtown Portland. New gardeners receive, free of charge, two or three 5' x 8' soil frames filled with organic soil.

In addition, they are given seeds, starts, compost, a trellis, tomato cages, a cookbook, and at least two years of ongoing gardening advice. This program brings all that a low-income family might need-the soil, amendments, wood frame, seeds, and written guidelines for intensive growing-and constructs the garden on site. Bringing in fresh soil without disturbing the existing terrain obviates most concerns about soil quality, fertility, and toxicity.

Urban Agriculture Commercial Growers grow food for sale. Increasing numbers of individuals and organizations are exploring the opportunities offered by producing food in and around cities for market. Repeated agricultural censuses show that U.S. small farms, meaning those less than ten acres, are concentrated in urban counties, except in the Rocky Mountain States. Recent censuses indicate that the number is increasing as urbanization spreads. The suburbanization of cities - and more specifically the loss in density in most cases - facilitates the urban and peri-urban family farm.

A survey by the National Gardening Association finds that there are more than ten million vegetable producers in the United States, with three out of five in urban census tracts. Just as strikingly, commercial urban agriculture produces 40 percent of the total American farm product on ten percent of the agricultural land. These entrepreneurs are responding to, among other trends, the growing desire of urbanites to buy fresh, preferably organically-grown, and nutritious produce grown close to their homes.

More and more urban consumers are also looking for locally produced value-added food products, such as salsa and jams. The growing urban market is also created by the greater ethnic mix of city populations, the increasing abandonment of inner-city areas by large supermarket chains, the phenomenon of urban sprawl, and the fact that Americans are eating much more in restaurants. Consumers are also turning increasingly to local and regional foods, whether in Massachusetts or Oahu.

It is important to emphasize that in the United States - and particularly in its urbanized areas - many a farmer tills the soil and husbands his or her animals, poultry or fish on a part-time basis. In villages and towns, at the fringes of cities and within metropolitan areas, these part-time, small-scale farmers produce for the local market demand first, and secondly for the national market, on the weekend, after a day's work in a non-farm job, and often before dawn.

This kind of part-time farming, while risky, helps families to cover their needs. Items as varied as grass-fed lamb, blooming chrysanthemums, asparagus, culinary herbs, salad greens and ducks, delivered fresh at peak market demand, can cover a family's irregular costs. Part-time urban farming can be reflected in contrasting divisions of household labour. There are households where all active members are active farmers. In other cases, one member of the household is a full-time farmer, with other family members helping occasionally or seasonally. In other cases, none are full-time farmers.

Part-time farming in urban areas is considerably more common than the census reports, since many small-scale farmers, who have another job in the family, do not register as a farm. Typically, for-profit urban farmers are practical, high-energy individuals willing to take advantage of the significantly higher margin the urban farmer can sell to retail, over against the rural farmer. The successful urban farmer must have marketing savvy, and finding niches not served by the corporate food system.

Successful urban farmers can help to address some of the problems with access to food in urban communities. For example, urban agriculture entrepreneurs frequently sell their products at local farmers' markets. According to the USDA, "the number of farmers markets has increased almost 50 percent since 1994." These markets can be a boon to community food security, especially when they are located in low-income urban neighborhoods.

In addition, the next few years may see the expansion of community supported agriculture (CSA) farms onto urban sites. Several CSA's have responded directly to food insecurity issues with experiments in making their shares available to low-income households through such means as outside subsidies. Other urban markets for entrepreneurs are created with initiatives like the USDA Small Farms/School Meals programs that, with sufficient investment and national replication, could eventually reach unmet nutritional needs of schoolchildren.

Similar farm-to-institution programs provide direct marketing opportunities for entrepreneurs to other institutional consumers such as hospitals and prisons. Some commercial growers have opened their fields to gleaning programs after they have harvested their crop for market; these programs provide low-income urban families with opportunities to pick what remains for their own use, increasing local food security.

Many inner-city urban agriculture projects require some form of subsidy-grants or non-profit status to be commercially viable, at least in their initial stages. Yet these same projects have multiple social benefits in terms of job training and community outreach. It is common, for example, to find an urban farming operation where inner-city youth learn a range of job skills that they can later apply elsewhere.

The potential contribution of urban livestock to food security in North America has been supported by the Heifer International (a 56-year old international development organization). Since 1996, this organization has provided assistance to nine community groups in Chicago IL and Milwaukee WI who are raising a variety of livestock for food and sale. One such program is located on Chicago's South Side at the Robert Taylor Homes, the largest public housing project in the United States, with more than 20,000 residents on over 92 acres.

In the midst of this gang-dominated environment, a resident-run youth group has constructed a vermiculture and aquaculture system in the basement of one of the Robert Taylor Homes high-rises where they currently care for Jerry Kaufman and Martin Bailkey, Farming

Inside Cities: Entrepreneurial Urban Agriculture in the United States. In the planting season worm castings are used as a soil additive in their market garden and packaged for sale to city gardeners. Every seven months fish are harvested and eaten by the participating youths' families.

Urban growers may lack the knowledge and skills in production, processing and marketing that bring about successful yields. Resources to solve these problems include:

— Metropolitan areas have Extension services in place

— A number of non-profit urban agriculture projects in cities offer public educational series and on-site demonstrations

— The USDA Community Gardening Coordinator in each state may provide the impetus for supporting urban-based outreach curricula

— Special training activities for trainers have focused on urban agriculture concerns

— Local media have featured columns and shows that highlight information about horticultural tips and small business practices

— School gardening programs at all levels-from pre-school to university - have successfully provided youth with training opportunities

Low-income families spend one-third and more of their income on food. Good-quality fresh food with high levels of vitamins and protein is worth subsidizing. Urban agriculture produce in general costs the same as imported or rural produce, but the challenge is to make sure that this food is made accessible to low-income consumers.

Entrepreneurs and community and backyard gardeners have start-up costs that can be an obstacle to folks on limited incomes. Responses to this problem include:

— Tool banks, including donations of surplus tools, offer gardeners the option of borrowing tools or renting them for a low fee.

— Foundation and government "seed" grants provide much-needed funding for individuals and organizations.

— Banks and government-funded redevelopment plans have provided micro-credit to growers.

— Gardening supply businesses, nurseries, and seed companies donate their wares.

— Community kitchens, offered by churches, schools, and other organizations provide access for food preservation and small-scale value-added production projects.

— Crop or harvest loans, crop insurance, liability insurance, and equipment loans can assist the beginning urban farmer.

Many involved in urban agriculture do not own the land they use to grow food. Without title or three to five year leases, they risk losing their investment when the land is taken for other purposes. Creative solutions to this problem include the following:

— Land trusts successfully secure urban and peri-urban land parcels for agricultural purposes

— Conservation easements are used to delineate environmentally vulnerable lands that then can be used for agriculture

— Communities develop inventories of surplus properties that lead to the inclusion of agriculture in subsequent plans for the land.

— Many urban growers have been able to write medium-to-longer-term leases allowing them to plan for the future

— Many forms of urban agriculture are mobile and/or require little investment, and thus are well suited to shorter-term or more uncertain leases

— Some urban agriculture sites are maintained under usufruct arrangements.

In many climates, food production in cities is seasonal and thus not dependable as a year-round source of food security. Many urban residents have limited knowledge and access to facilities for preserving foods that they grow.

Urban farming, provided it produces, stores and distributes food in an ecologically sound and sustainable manner, can supply much more healthful food than is offered by industrial agriculture and supermarket chains. Fresh fruits and vegetables, free-range poultry, and grass-fed lamb are a source of health for urban consumers, and also respond to concerns regarding excessive use of antibiotics for animals in factory farms, and the inhumane treatment of animals in the dominant food system.

However, there are particular health challenges connected to farming in the city. For example, urban soils can be contaminated with heavy metals such as lead. Measures to counteract this include the following:

- — Raised beds with imported clean soil and compost have been successfully placed on top of questionable soils, enabling farmers to produce healthful food.
- — Lead abatement initiatives have raised public awareness of the problem and removed polluted soils.
- — Using mulch can reduce airborne exposure to questionable soils in some cases.
- — Low-cost soil testing and subsidies have enabled low-income gardeners to know their level of risk and seek appropriate solutions.
- — Phyto-remediation (using plants to take up metals from the soil) has great potential to assist with lead abatement.
- — Sheltered production methods have been used in urban agriculture to avoid contact with the soil and air by providing alternative production sites in contaminated areas (e.g. greenhouses, indoor production, hydroponic growing mediums, etc.)

By incorporating the principles of low-impact development, smart growth, and sustainable urbanization, urban agriculture can contribute to maintaining open space and biodiversity within the urban fabric. A city that promotes urban agriculture can have green space that pays taxes rather than costing taxpayers money. Along with these powerful environmental benefits, there are environmental concerns related to growing food in cities. One of these concerns is that there is little regulation about the use of pesticides used in urban agriculture that may affect food safety. Measures to overcome this problem include:

— Campaigns against pesticide use led by public health professionals, government officials, and the public have led to phasing out the use of some pesticides such as diazinon.

— Extension support for Integrated Pest Management (IPM) has contributed to public awareness of non-chemical and organic alternatives to dangerous pesticides.

— Growing public interest in food safety and ecology has promoted the use of appropriate technologies and approaches such as permaculture.

— Communities can develop regional composting facilities to avert wastes from area landfills.

Bibliography

Beerlandt, H., with J. Serneels, "Manual for a food security diagnosis", K.U. Leuven, *Faculty of Agricultural and Applied Biological Sciences, Working paper* 1996/43, 1997.

Christiaensen, L., and E. Tollens, "Food security: From concept to action—A status quaestionis", K. U. Lueven and B.A.D.C. *research project in the framework of policy preparing research in the field of cooperation in development*, Nr 2, Brussels, 1995.

Chung, K., L. Haddad, J. Ramakrishna, and F. Riely, "Identifying the food insecure: The application of mixed method approaches in India", International Food Policy Research Institute, Washington D.C, 1997.

Clay, E., "Food security: A status review of the literature", *Research Report ESCOR No*. R5911. London: Overseas Development Administration, 1997.

Dercon, S., *Surviving in Developing Countries*, Catholic University Leuven en Oxford University, 1995.

Drèze, J., and A. Sen, *Hunger and Public Action*, Clarendon Press, Oxford, 1989.

Eele, G., R. Hay, and J. Hoddinot,."Household Food Securtiy and Nutrition", in:Demery, L., Ferroni, M., and C., Grootaert, with Wong-Valle, J., *Understanding The Social Effects of Policy Reform*, Washington, D.C., The World Bank, 1993.

FAO (Food and Agriculture Organization), "Guide for the conduct of the constraints analysis component", *Special programme for food security*, Handbook Series, SPFS/DOC/ 18, Rome, 1997.

Maxwell, S., and T. Frankenberger, "Household food security: Concepts, indicators, measurements", *International Fund for Agricultural Development*, Rome, 1992.

Maxwell, D., "Measuring food insecurity: The frequency and severity of "coping strategies." Food Policy", 21: 291–303, 1996.

Riely, F., N. Mock, B. Cogill, L. Bailey, and E. Kenefick, "Food security indicators and framework for use in the monitoring and evaluation of food aid programs", *IMPACT: Food security and nutrition monitoring project*, Arlington, Va., U.S.A, 1995.

______________, and N. Moock, "Inventory of food security impact indicators", *In Food security indicators and framework: A handbook for monitoring and evaluation of food aid programs.* IMPACT, Arlington, Va., U.S.A. Draft, 1995.

Index

CHANGING TRENDS IN HEALTH AND NUTRITION

CHANGING TRENDS IN HEALTH AND NUTRITION

(In 4 Volumes)

Childhood Nutrition and Academic Progress

(Volume 4)

SUJATA K. DASS

ISHA BOOKS
DELHI—110 033

Changing Trends in Health and Nutrition
(Health)

Rs. 3200 (Set in 4 vols.)
Rs. 800 (Each volume)

ISBN: 81-8205-040-5 (Set)
ISBN: 81-8205-044-8 (Vol. 4)

Published in 2004 in India by
Isha Books, D-43, Prithviraj Road
Adarsh Nagar, Delhi-110 033

Lasertypesetting by: Varsha Graphics, Delhi
Printed at: Chawla Offset Press, Delhi

Contents

Preface

Nutrition is vital to all human beings and to the societies that they comprise. Adequately nourished people enjoy optimal growth, health and well-being. Good nutrition during childhood helps to lay the foundation for a healthy adulthood. It strengthens the learning potential and well-being of children. Among well nourished people, acute disease and illness tend to be less frequent, less severe and of shorter duration thus providing increased capacities to perform daily activities. Good nutrition also fosters mental, social and physical well-being throughout life; for instance, by strengthening a positive body image and increasing the sense of personal worth.

Good health and nutrition are needed to achieve one's full educational potential because nutrition affects intellectual development and learning ability. The academic performance and mental ability of pupils with good nutritional status are significantly higher than those of pupils with poor nutritional status, independent of family income, school quality and teacher ability. Schools have been given the mandate and responsibility to enhance all aspects of development and maturation of children and youth under qualified guidance.

Furthermore, schools also provide a setting to introduce nutrition information and technologies to the community and can lead the community in advocating policies and services that promote good nutrition.

The present book is intended to make people aware about the necessity of good nutrition in childhood.

Editor

1

Child Care and Nutrition

"Care" refers to behaviors performed by caregivers that affect nutrient intake, health, and the cognitive and psychosocial development of the child. In order for care behaviors to be exhibited, the caregiver needs sufficient education, time, and support. The provision of these resources can be considered care for the caregiver.

An adaptation of the UNICEF model that incorporates care to the caregiver. Six major categories of resources for care can be identified:

(1) education, knowledge, and beliefs;

(2) health and nutritional status of the caregiver;

(3) mental health, lack of stress, and self-confidence of the caregiver;

(4) autonomy, control of resources, and intrahousehold allocation;

(5) workload and time constraints; and

(6) social support from family members and community.

These aspects are the human and organizational resources identified in the UNICEF model. Education, knowledge, and beliefs represent the capacity of the caregiver to provide appropriate care. The physical and mental health (self-confidence, and lack of stress and depression) of the caregiver represent individual-level factors that facilitate the translation of capacity to behavior. Finally, autonomy, workload, and social support are facilitating conditions in the family and community.

Some of these resource categories have been investigated extensively, whereas others have been investigated primarily in developed countries, or await further investigation.

A Model for Child Care

The extended UNICEF model of child care is a useful framework for assessing the capacity and ability of the caregiver to provide care behaviors. However, a model of child care should include not only an assessment of the caregiver's behavior, but also the behavior of the child, and the characteristics of the environmental context.

All three of these factors play a significant role in the eventual nutritional status of the child. For the past 25 years, psychologists have documented the significant role that children play in the care that they receive. Differences between children, such as endowed healthiness, perceived vulnerability, perceived weight, and even physical attractiveness, affect the behaviors of their caregivers.

The transactional model of care argues that the results or effects of child endowments are a function of a long series of mutual interactions, or transactions, between the developing child and the caregiver, and that these interactions are constantly changing with the changing developmental status of the child.

At the heart of the process is the relationship between the child and the caregiver(s). This affective, or emotional relationship, is a unique and life-long bond between two humans, called an attachment. Healthy development of a child has been found to depend on the development of a secure attachment or a close bond with at least one caregiver during infancy from whom the child received abundant positive attention.

An extensive literature has differentiated attachments into those which are secure and those characterized by insecurity and avoidance of the caregiver in middle-class samples. Attachment can be assessed in a standardized situation and the measure has been used in many different cultures, although there are some questions about the validity of the measurement of attachment across cultures.

Children's nutritional status also has relevance for attachment; Valenzuela in Chile found that children who were undernourished were far less likely to be securely attached, though no causality was established. A critical aspect of quality of care seems to be responsivity to the child's cues, verbalizations, signals, etc. Responsivity does not mean that the caregiver always gives the child what is requested, but that the caregiver's response takes the child's needs and developmental level into account.

Among active and well-nourished children, not acceding to inappropriate demands is an important part of responsivity. Usually, a positive emotional (affective) relationship between caregiver and child will be reflected in warm and responsive caregiving behaviors. However, the lethargic or unresponsive child will have a harder time stimulating responsivity.

The extended UNICEF model can be adapted to include the relationship between child and caregiver(s). The central part of the UNICEF model relating care, nutrient intake, health, and child growth and cognitive development. Eleven specific arrows have been drawn to illustrate the various ways in which the affective relationship between caregiver and child, and the resulting care behaviors, can influence the child's growth, cognitive and psychosocial development, dietary intake, and health status, and how child growth and development may influence care and the affective relationship.

This relationship has been demonstrated in numerous studies, including all three Nutrition Collaborative Research Support Program (CRSP) studies, although the reasons for the linkages are not entirely known. The initial hypothesis of a linkage between energy and protein intake and brain growth has not received unequivocal support, although increasing interest in micronutrient deficiencies may again lead us to a brain model for explaining these effects.

A study in Mexico found that mothers interacted more with better nourished and larger children compared to smaller children. In addition, the lack of responsivity of low birth-weight children has been associated with poorer feeding behaviors by mothers.

Caregivers may be particularly troubled by a child who refuses to eat; feeding difficulties are one of the most common behavioral disturbances of young children reported to pediatricians in industrialized countries. In the United States, 24 percent of two-year-olds and 19 percent of three-year-olds were reported by parents as having problems with feeding.

A number of studies have compared children with non-organic failure to thrive (NOFTT) with normally growing children; many such studies have observed inadequate parent/child interactions among the former group. The causality is difficult to untangle, although one study did find higher incidence of oral-motor difficulties in NOFTT children, suggesting that the child's feeding problems may precipitate poor child/caregiver interactions.

The much higher rate of NOFTT among low birth-weight children also suggests that a child's poor growth may contribute to a problematic caregiver-child relationship or to failure-to-thrive. In the failure to thrive, literature observational studies suggest that mothers of NOFTT children in affluent societies tend to be less attentive to their children and interact and verbalize less, and their children have shorter feeding episodes and intake less food than well-nourished children.

The quality of the relationship of the caregiver to the child may influence health status of the child through health care treatment and seeking of health care. Although direct evidence for this relationship is lacking, the gender differentials in health-seeking behavior frequently reported in the Indian Subcontinent may be examples of caregiver preference influencing health care treatment.

However, without further evidence, it is impossible to determine whether the lower health care seeking is a function of the quality of the relationship or of maternal and family strategies of investment in child care. These arrows illustrate the central role of the affective context of caregiving but much remains to be learned about strategies for changing behavior to enhance child survival, growth, and development.

Indicators of nutritional status may provide a direct measure of the underlying condition of interest or serve as proxy for other factors. They can be divided into those that measure outcomes (such as child weight-for-age), processes or intervening variables, and inputs. This approach has emerged after many years of work on developing indicators for nutritional status. In the case of care, however, the issues of measurement remain to be addressed adequately and the various indicators need to be identified before they are developed at this level.

Cultural differences in caregiving behaviors and resources are often substantial. For example, maternal interaction with children may also vary from culture to culture, as demonstrated by Richman, Miller, and LeVine. They observed that Gusii mothers had a more nurturant attitude towards caregiving at all observed points in time, while American mothers have a more verbal and stimulative attitude towards interaction with their older children.

Developing indicators of care that can be used in different settings is not an easy task. One possible solution may emerge from cross-cultural psychology. Cross-cultural psychologists suggest that there are three theories about cultural differences:

(1) total cultural relativity (every culture has such different functions that one cannot make any judgments across cultures);

(2) absolutism (every culture has the same functions, and the same judgments can be made in every culture, thus culture should not be included in analysis); and

(3) universalism.

The Euro-American women tended to vocalize, some almost continuously, and the infant's response was to wave its arms and legs. The Native American women, on the other hand, used looking and gazing to attract the infant's attention, and the infant returned the gaze. Thus the function of getting children's attention is probably universal, but the appropriate way to do so may vary by culture.

If one simply observed caregiver verbalization, one would have missed the functional equivalence of the two behaviors (vocalization and gaze). Several cross-cultural studies suggest that within-culture differences in many of these behaviors are larger than the between-culture differences, and that what appear initially to be unique and exotic differences between cultures are more similar when better understood.

The existence of important differences both within and between cultures needs to be understood and recognized in defining care behaviors, but the functional equivalence of behaviors should also be recognized. Development of indicators and assessment strategies must include adaptation of functions to the particular context.

For some of the constraints to care, relatively straightforward indicators exist, such as body mass index

(BMI) for women's health status, whereas for others, measures are less well-developed and need to be adapted to the particular cultural context (e.g., stress). Similarly, some care behaviors are relatively well accepted (e.g., hand-washing with soap and water by the caregiver prior to food preparation) and measurable, whereas others are harder to assess (e.g., quality of responsiveness of the caregiver to the child).

Although in each case the variable can be assessed, the cost of doing so might be prohibitive. For some behaviors, cultural variability will be more important than for others. For instance, for psychosocial care, the range of possible adaptive child-rearing methods is likely to be wide, although there may be a set of inappropriate behaviors that could be improved with the reduction of constraints to care. Various quantitative methods have been developed and employed successfully to assess relevant features of psychosocial care.

These include questionnaires or interviews asking parents or caregivers to describe their care practices and/ or their children's typical experiences; "qualitative" rating scales with behaviorally defined scale points to assess broadly stated characteristics of care, following observations in naturalistic or experimental settings; systematic observations of the caregiver and the child in the natural setting, focusing on particular behaviors whose frequencies are reflected in summary scores; and detailed observational coding of ongoing sequences of caregiver-child interaction, aimed at characterizing relevant features of the dyadic relationship.

Many of these strategies for assessing the quality of care in the various research studies require extensive observations and technical methodologies. For the most part, therefore, they are not feasible for practical use in the field as screening procedures. However, some of these approaches to the measurement of care have been, or may be, adapted for practical field use in assessing breakdowns in, or threats to, psychosocial care.

The relevance of these measures in different cultures should always be of concern to investigators. It is important in all such approaches to develop indicators that have meaning and validity across a variety of cultures, although this is a daunting task. A behavior that may appear to be maladaptive to an outside observer may be the norm within a particular culture.

Therefore, it is essential to approach indicators with a healthy skepticism, and to attempt to use a within-culture yardstick-to compare a caregiver with others within her or his own cultural group. The major categories of resources for care identified earlier will be examined in detail to identify the potential indicators that emerge from them:

(1) caregiver education, knowledge, and beliefs;

(2) health and nutritional status of the caregiver;

(3) mental health, lack of stress, and self-confidence of the caregiver;

(4) the caregiver's autonomy and control of resources;

(5) workload and time constraints of the caregiver; and

(6) social support received by the caregiver from family members and the community.

Maternal Education on Child Care

Maternal education is associated with the level of

provision of caring behaviors. Three such examples of caring behaviors are summarized below: breast-feeding, health seeking behaviors, and the level of child-caregiver interactions. The pathways through which maternal education affects care provision behaviors are then discussed. Feeding Practices.

The relationship between maternal education and breast-feeding practices is complex. Education increases both the ability to earn income and the ability to appreciate the importance of caregiving. The former tends to mitigate against breast-feeding, particularly in urban areas, as the caregiver's opportunity cost of time increases. The latter tends to promote caregiving, particularly in supporting workplace environments.

For example, in Israel, mothers with the lowest and highest levels of education engage in long-term breast-feeding. In developing countries, however, the negative effects of breast-feeding tend to predominate. In Brazil, for example, maternal educational levels were strongly correlated with earlier termination of breast-feeding.

In the Philippines, an increase in maternal education by one year is associated with a 36-percent decrease in the probability of exclusive breast-feeding for a six-month-old infant. Maternal education is associated not only with the quantity of breast-feeding (duration, frequency), but also the quality of feeding.

A study conducted in rural Bangladesh found that maternal education is associated with variables that reflect more intense care for their children, i.e., less distraction while feeding, a cleaner feeding environment, and more initiation of child feeding. In the same study, however, more education was associated with less adequate feeding behaviors, such as termination of feeding by the mother more often than by the child, a larger number of bottle feeds per hour, and a fewer number of breast-feeds per hour.

Another caring behavior associated with child health and nutrition is the family's health-seeking behaviors, both preventive health care (immunization, antenatal care for the mother, etc.) as well as health seeking behaviors in the event of morbidity. The effects of education on health care seeking behaviors are well documented; it is becoming increasingly evident that maternal education affects a child's health/nutritional status through its effect on her health care seeking behaviors.

Better educated women are more likely to utilize available health care and community service facilities than women with no education. Observational studies of mother-child interactions of educated and uneducated women have revealed patterns of behavior that reflect a more committed attitude towards child care among educated women.

More educated women were more vocal towards their infants in spite of the fact that infants who grew up to be more vocal themselves would require more attention as toddlers. Richman, Miller, and LeVine find that Mexican mothers with more education are more likely to feed their crying children. The educated mothers were seen to modify their responsive behaviors in relation to the age of the infant, with less educated women continuing to hold their children even with increasing age (10 months); and more educated women displaying more conversational interaction at this age.

The pathways through which maternal education affects care provision behaviors are thought to be (1) the ability to process information, (2) the ability to acquire skills, and (3) the ability to model behavior. Thomas, Strauss, and Henriques and Barrera have reported that it is predominantly through the better knowledge that an educated woman might have that she is able to utilize health care facilities better, keep her environment cleaner, and thereby benefit her children.

They suggest that one of the likely channels through which maternal education affects child height is by improving her acquisition and processing of information (measured as reading newspapers, listening to the radio, and watching television). These indicators explained almost all of the impact of maternal education on child health, but the exact type of "information" that brought about this effect was not identified.

To get at this latter issue, Tucker and Sanjur use the concept of maternal differentiation, a composite variable that incorporates years of education, nutrition knowledge, frequency of reading, and a measure of household productivity. This concept includes evidence of use and retention of information, which they feel is theoretically more coherent than merely using years of schooling as an indicator of maternal character.

"Maternal differentiation" has been found to be positively associated with children's dietary intake and anthropometric status. Barrera proposes that maternal education affects child health by "affecting the productivity of inputs...and lowering the costs of information." Skills acquisition is proposed to be a process through which acquired literacy and language skills make it easier for educated women to build a knowledge base that could guide behavior, as well as learn patterns of behaviors that are useful for participating in modern bureaucracies.

This would allow better utilization of health care services and interactions with doctors and nurses, as well as better compliance with treatment recommendations. The finding that the association between maternal schooling and health care utilization behavior (talking to a doctor) loses significance when controlled for literacy suggests the important role of skills. The theory of "identity acquisition" proposes that it is not literacy alone that determines the behaviors of educated women.

This hypothesis assumes that schooling leads to behavior change through imitation of people in the "modern sector". Another aspect of this theory is that schooling makes women identify with the role of a teacher as well as that of a student. This makes them more amenable to new information and also more interactive in their child care behaviors. That specific caregiving behaviors are affected in different ways by the variables of literacy, skills, and identity. Maternal identity was assessed using maternal appearance and posture as proxy indicators.

Keeping a child clean, a caring behavior, was significantly associated with schooling when controlled for literacy, but not when controlled for identity, suggesting that this behavior was mediated through identity. Clearly, the use of education as an indicator of care is complex, even though some studies reported here demonstrate an enhancement in the quality of caregiving by educated mothers.

The indicators of education used in the literature include literacy status (literate/illiterate), the level of education completed (primary, secondary, etc.), and the number of years of education, as well as indicators of the skills gained from schooling-the ability to read and comprehend written passages, listen and comprehend, and the ability to use decontextualized language.

More testing of the various hypotheses of the pathways of interaction of education and child care may be needed before additional cultural-specific behavioral indicators of education for care are developed. Identifying different behaviors of educated women could also help to develop cultural-specific indicators for the processes through which education affects care.

However, they can be invaluable from the point of view of assessing the sociocultural causes of, and reactions to, malnutrition; infant feeding behaviors that are unique to certain cultures; and beliefs and practices relating to lactation, before embarking on a large-scale survey. The care resource indicators that are expected to emerge from this discussion are the beliefs with respect to breast-feeding, infant feeding, and infant growth.

Cultural beliefs appear to be important in determining the initiation of breast-feeding as well as the termination of breast-feeding. Both of these practices are closely associated with the growth and development of young infants. In a number of developing societies, breast-feeding is a universal practice, which is initiated soon after birth.

In other cultures, particularly in the Indian subcontinent and parts of Southeast Asia, there is a strong belief that colostrum is highly undesirable and prelacteal feeds of sweetened water, goat's milk, or diluted cow's milk are commonly given in the first two-to-three days postpartum.

In a number of studies, the common reasons for cessation of breast-feeding and for weaning onto an adult diet were another pregnancy, perceived breast-milk insufficiency, and/or certain developmental milestones achieved by the child. Perceived breast-milk insufficiency was the most commonly reported reason and the perception of insufficiency was often based on the crying of the infant.

One study has reported that for some, breast-feeding was terminated by the fathers' decision, possibly because of the belief within that culture that breast-feeding mothers should not have intercourse. Another observation from this study was that the quality of breast milk was perceived to change with the age of the child and this affected the choice of a wet nurse.

In Egypt, the timing of the weaning was important from the point of view of minimizing the risk of exposure to the "evil eye" by ensuring no contact with a menstruating woman, a newly-wed woman, etc., at the time of complete weaning. In Ethiopia, the timing of weaning was seen to depend on the season, with the preferable season for weaning being in the winter.

In Egypt, breast-feeding is reported to be associated with responsibility and maturity in a woman, and very young mothers were not expected to breast-feed. The breast milk of mothers who were sad or emotionally disturbed was believed to cause diarrhea in their children. It has been reported that the diet of a mother was believed to be important when she was breast-feeding and in cases where the infant fell ill, the mother was given special foods or drinks so that the breast-fed infant would benefit from it.

The belief that the quality of breast milk is a determinant of the child's health is seen in a number of cultures and often it is the mother who is blamed for an infant's illness, and even treated for it. The fear of "spirits," which could disturb the child, is seen to pervade a number of care-related behaviors in Indonesia; care seems to be taken to keep the child calm during the first few months of life, but once the child is able to sit, it is considered to be less vulnerable to spirits.

The importance of the child's emotional state and contentedness and perception of "emotional maturity" is evident in Gryboski's study in Indonesia, where sibling caregivers are taught to yield to the infant's demands so that the infant is not upset until the child is in late infancy. For instance, infants are fed to induce sleep and calmness in early life, but as the child develops, he/she is not pressed to eat if he/she appears upset and "consent feeding" is the norm rather than force feeding as in the preceding months.

The child's ability to control feeding is believed to come into play after the age of 7 months, as the child is believed to be helpless from birth until 7 months of age. Beliefs regarding complementary feeding have implications for child nutrition since the age at which children are reported to be most vulnerable to growth-faltering is the period between 6 - 18 months, which is the period of transition between breast milk and an adult18 diet.

In Egypt, Harrison et al. have reported that mothers believed that supplementation (after 40 days of full breast-feeding) was necessary to promote growth and "fatness." Mixed feeding was also said to help the mother by reducing the time she would need to breast-feed the child. The belief that breast-feeding is time-consuming is widespread; Cohen et al., in Honduras, report that mothers believed that exclusive breast-feeding (EBF) would take longer even though observational studies showed that breast-feeding and food preparation and serving took the same amount of time as EBF for 4-to-6 months old children.

Many food taboos for young children may limit the types of foods that can be offered. Rabiee and Geissler have reported that in Iran, the introduction of a variety of foods was often delayed, based on the perception that young children could not digest foods that were available to the family (e.g., beans) or that some foods would cause stammering and delayed speech and impair the intellect if introduced before 18 months of age (eggs and cheese, respectively).

This implies that children may not have received adequate amounts of protein- and micronutrient-rich foods until they were 18 months of age. Characteristics of the Child that Affect Decisions about Feeding. Many beliefs about the termination of breast-feeding depend on characteristics of the child and the child's developmental level. Examples related to the initiation and completion of the weaning process include the eruption of teeth, the onset of walking, and a perception that the child was old enough to consume an adult diet. A second factor affecting beliefs is the child's appetite as perceived by the mother.

The recognition of the child's appetite as an indicator of ill-health is seen in many studies. Beliefs about caregiver control of feeding can influence child intake. Dettwyler, in a series of reports from Mali, found that mothers tended to believe that children should control the amount of food ingested, and that the child's hunger or apparent interest in food should determine the amount of food provided to the child.

Perceptions about the child's state of health have also been reported to influence decisions about breast-feeding, particularly duration of breast-feeding. Adair and Popkin have reported that a mother's perception that her infant was small increased the likelihood of her not breast-feeding, even when she had the intent to do so before the birth of the infant.

Conversely, it has also been observed that the perception that the infant was doing well increased the likelihood that breast-feeding would be continued. In Senegal, have reported that small and thin infants were preferentially fed millet-gruel in addition to breast milk, because their mothers perceived the need to feed them something in addition to breast milk.

Beliefs about and behaviors during illness could have implications for child health and nutrition and some information about existing beliefs, in addition to the more easily available information on the use of health care facilities, could prove invaluable in the planning process in these areas. For example, certain illnesses are seen to be a part of the normal development of the child. Some of these illnesses are those that could precipitate malnutrition or aggravate existing situations (e.g., some kinds of diarrhea, upper respiratory tract infections, etc.).

In Pakistan, mothers seldom associate marasmus with consumption of less food; it is more often linked to the influence of spirits or a "bad" person on a child. Similar findings are reported in East Africa, India, Nepal, and Tanganyika, where protein-energy malnutrition was often seen as a result of adultery, breast-feeding while pregnant, or an evil spirit.

Nutritional Status of the Caregiver

The current nutritional situation of women in the developing world indicate that iron deficiency anemia is widespread among pregnant and nonpregnant women in developing countries, with the highest rates in South Asia, using a cutoff of blood levels of hemoglobin less than 12 grams per deciliter. These rates have increased in South Asia and Sub-Saharan Africa over the past decade.

In Egypt, McCullough et al. found a negative association between maternal B6 nutriture and responsiveness to infant vocalizations, as well as less effective maternal responses in cases of infant distress. Chronic energy deficiency, measured using body mass index, has been proposed to have effects on productivity by modifying physical activity patterns. The nutritional status of the mother is also expected to affect her ability to care for children.

The Food and Agriculture Organization of the United Nation/World Health Organization/United Nations University (FAO/WHO/UNU) Joint Consultation on Energy and Protein Requirements has estimated the energy cost of child care activities as 2.2 x basal metabolic rate (BMR), which falls into the category of moderate physical activity.

Child care could be classified as "discretionary activity," which is described as "additional activity outside working hours, the energy requirement to cover which should not be regarded as dispensable as it contributes to the physical and intellectual well-being of the individual, household, or group".

Increased needs to procure food resulted in increased substitution of child care by siblings and other family members. Productivity is also influenced by iron status; supplementation with iron increased women's productivity on tea plantations, farms, and in cotton mills in China.

However, infant behavior is a major component in establishing the affective relationship between mother and child and the effects of maternal nutrition on these behaviors will be examined. Findings from the Egypt CRSP have indicated that maternal intakes of energy and protein from animal sources, iron, and zinc were positively associated with neonatal "habituation" behaviors.

Women between the ages of 15 to 49 spend a significant proportion of their lives in a state of pregnancy and lactation, or both, and the stresses of these periods are expected to lead to a considerable depletion of maternal nutrient levels. The case for improving maternal health and nutrition is stronger than ever before, based on both existing evidence of the effects of maternal health on birth outcomes and emerging evidence of their effect on infant behavior and caregiving.

An atmosphere of psychological and physical violence may have devastating consequences for children's nutritional status, but few investigators have examined the issue. In the United States, a large literature links maternal depression with poor caregiving and problematic outcomes for children.

Depression probably plays a major role in poor caregiving in many developing countries. However, despite reports of high levels of anxiety and depression among women in developing countries studies linking these psychological factors with child caregiving have not been done. A report on the slum improvement project in Bangladesh suggested that "the social isolation of women, coupled with the lack of extended family networks in urban areas, is thought to have negative effects on the mental health of women, which, in turn, is likely to reduce the quality of child care, even when the mother is physically present".

Depression in the United States has been measured by a number of instruments, few of which have been adapted outside of the United States. However, since the most common instruments rely on self-reports and the questions are fairly straightforward, the possibility of adapting the instrument exists. Stress refers to a person's discomfort when exposed to difficult and uncontrollable circumstances, and is one of the characteristics of high risk mothers in the United States.

Stress may also be linked with poorer caregiving. Although there are many measures of stress, one that might be adaptable to different cultural settings is a symptom checklist, such as the Health Opinion Survey, a report of the woman's physical problems in a recent period. Items selected reflect psychosomatic difficulties, such as headaches, feeling tired, unable to eat, or sweating palms.

In the United States, the most dramatic change is death of a spouse, followed by separation from a spouse. Other events include moving to a new area and starting a new form of employment. The degree of intensity of the change can be established for any particular cultural setting, and items can be added or deleted. Other measures of stress may be much more difficult to adapt cross-culturally. The level of confidence of the caregiver is often cited as a critical factor for complementary feeding, particularly for anorexic children, but this relationship has not been tested systematically.

In industrialized countries, the measurement of self-esteem has a long history, and numerous measurements have been developed. These measurements have been found to be associated with a number of outcomes, such as school performance, job success, and test scores, although relationships are not strong. One of the difficulties in adaptation is that the basis for self-esteem probably differs by culture.

A number of studies have suggested that mothers are more likely to allocate resources under their control to children than are fathers, and that the higher percent of income earned by women increases their control over resources. However, working for income does not automatically mean that women control their incomes; in many societies, the income is automatically assumed to be the property of the husband.

Autonomy for women is generally higher in female-headed households, and some studies show that in spite of lower incomes, children in these living situations do better than might have been expected, most likely because intrahousehold distribution practices favored children more in female-headed households than in households headed by men.

In many societies, mothers do not have the authority to make decisions regarding the care and feeding of their young children. These decisions may be made by the child's father or, in many cases, by a mother-in-law or older female in the husband's family. In Jordan, Doan, and Bisharat found that the most significant factor associated with child nutritional status was the degree of autonomy of the mother within the household, even controlling for the woman's age, education, and household size.

Women's time commitments have been recognized as a zero-sum game; no new activities (including new caring behaviors) can be incorporated into their lives unless other activities are replaced. In addition to activities related to child-rearing, women are typically engaged in other time-intensive activities relating to domestic production activities, such as water carrying and fuelwood gathering, and nondomestic production activities, such as agricultural work, informal labor, and formal labor market activities.

A few recent studies have found significant negative associations of work for earnings and child nutritional status. In an evaluation of almost 2,000 rural mothers in India, Abbi et al. found that children of mothers who worked in agricultural labor on their own farms for 5 to 6 hours per day had significantly more malnourished children, regardless of who the alternate caregiver was. However, the women did not have control of their earnings.

Rabiee and Geissler reported significantly lower weight-for-age and higher incidence of diarrhea among Iranian children during the time of seasonal agricultural work, despite the relative wealth of the region. In this case, the caregivers were siblings from 8 to 13 years, and assessments of specific behaviors (e.g., disposal of child wastes) suggested their much lower competence.

The most malnourished children were those who were given sedatives in order to keep them quiet while the mother was working. Gryboski also found negative effects of maternal work in children under a year. Positive effects on either child nutrient intake or nutritional status were found when the work was well paid, when the income was in the hands of the mother, or when the child was over 1 year old.

Variables that appear to be important in examining the roles of time availability and workload for children are (1) the coverage and quality of the alternate caregiving system, (2) child age and characteristics, (3) woman's control of earned income, (4) wage rate of work and flexibility of work, and (5) poverty of the household.

The support provided to the primary caregiver can include explicit child care assistance, information provided to the caregiver, or emotional support provided to the caregiver. One of the most important types of social support is alternate child care. The abilities of the caregiver to provide care may be particularly important for complementary feeding. Engle distinguishes between levels of care needed at various stages of development of the child.

Care by anyone but the mother or a competent adult in the first year of life is associated with higher infant mortality; care needs in the second year of life are still very demanding, although the shortcomings of the caregiver can perhaps be ameliorated by good quality food availability and a healthy and safe environment. By the third year of life, many children are capable of some degree of self care.

The only dimension of quality that has been examined so far is the age of the alternate. Some studies suggest that care by a pre-teen caregiver is associated with lower nutritional status of the child under 2 years, controlling for mother's education and socioeconomic status. To date, the availability of institutional care for very young children is extremely limited in developing countries. However, a number of experimental attempts to provide this kind of care are under way, and some have been able to provide care for the youngest children.

Although there are some cases of female-headed households providing better care for children, the overall trend toward an increasing number of female-headed households, an increasing percentage of women in the labor force, and the increased burden of older family members raises concerns for the burden on the primary caregivers-women. Although men should be more involved with child care as women increase their time in the labor force, this change has been slow, with men still providing far less than an equal share of time in household chores and child care.

Fathers provide a particularly important source of emotional or informational support. There is some evidence that when they contribute a higher percent of their incomes to family budgets, children are better nourished. They may play particularly important roles when there is a tradition of female seclusion, as in Pakistan. Their opinions about child caregiving can have significant effects on decisions about infant feeding, particularly breast-feeding.

Indicators of care provision relate to two dimensions of caring behavior: time spent in those activities (quantity of care), the nature of the activities undertaken (quality of care), or some combination of the two dimensions.

Time spent in child care examines the validity of nonobservational measures of child care time, and discusses the usefulness of time in child care as an indicator. In general, the studies conducted are noncomparable due to different definitions of child care, and different methods of data collection (direct observation, random spot observation, and various recall periods).

If time in child care is to be used as an indicator of care, it should be measured by direct observation, which, in addition to getting accurate measures of time allocation, allows the specific child care activities to be recorded. Whereas measures of the quantity of child care time have been somewhat ambiguously related to child outcomes, measures of quality of time, or of specific behaviors associated with good child care, have been more often associated with positive outcomes.

Child growth has also been associated with observational measures of child-caregiver interaction. Many investigators recommend that the quality of the home environment and the quality of the caregiver-child interaction must be assessed through observational means, even if the observation is brief. The other care behaviors of breast-feeding, food preparation, hygiene, and health seeking and health care will not be discussed here, but these two will serve as models.

Child and caregiver behaviors that could have associations with child nutrient intake can be categorized into (1) adaptation of feeding to the child's characteristics, including psychomotor capabilities (use of finger foods, spoon handling ability, ability to munch or chew) and appetite; (2) the caregiver's ability to feed responsively, including encouragement to eat, offering additional foods, providing second helpings, threats to stimulate eating, timing of feeding, response to poor appetite, and positive or aversive style of interacting; and (3) the feeding situation, including the organization and regularity of the feeding situation, whether the child is supervised and protected while eating, frequency of feeding, with whom the child eats, and distraction during eating events.

Caregivers need to be sure that children are capable of the self-feeding expected of them. However, children also have a drive for independence, and may eat more if they are allowed to use newly learned finger skills to pick up foods. A child's capacity to process food by suckling, sucking, munching, or chewing increases with age.

Children's abilities to hold a spoon, handle a cup, or grasp a piece of solid food also increase with age. Poor child appetite plays a major role in inadequate nutrient intake. Factors that reduce a child's appetite may include a monotonous diet, lack of nutrients needed for appetite (e.g., zinc), illnesses such as fever, diarrhea, malaria, measles, intestinal parasites, chronic malnutrition, sores in the mouth, or anxiety.

These problems are not unique to malnourished children; 24 percent of parents in affluent societies report feeding difficulties with their two-year-old children. Thus the caregiver's ability to deal with child anorexia is significant for child intake. Suggested indicators are lack of appetite and self-feeding-use of finger foods.

Particularly with young children, feeding can be an active process; caregivers can encourage, cajole, offer more helpings, talk to children while eating, model eating behavior, and monitor how much the child eats. In many societies, caregivers are passive feeders, leaving the initiative to eat to children (child control of feeding). At the other extreme are cultural patterns which support caregiver control of eating, characterized by force feeding, continued and even intrusive pressure on children to eat.

In this case, rather than providing an opportunity for interaction and educational enhancement, feeding can become a time of conflict with intrusive, but ineffective, caregiver strategies and high levels of child refusal. Passive feeding may be due to lack of time and energy, or to beliefs that children should not be pressured to eat, that "the stomach knows its limits". Although this belief may seem reasonable, if a child has anorexia or poor appetite, extra encouragement may be necessary for adequate nutrient intake. Anorexic children are difficult to feed.

When anorexia is a problem, caregivers need to actively encourage food consumption. But this means having the time, knowledge, resources, self-confidence and support to encourage anorexic children to eat. In situations in which feeding encouragement is relatively low, increased encouragement of eating has been observed when children are ill or refuse food.

Caregiver understanding of and response to children's hunger cues may be critical for adequate food intake. For example, if caregivers perceive a child's tongue thrust, a typical mouthing response to new food sensations at a particular age, as a food refusal and cease to feed, a child will receive less food. The person who is doing the feeding may influence the child's willingness to eat; often children will refuse food if the preferred caregiver is not present.

Patience and understanding, plus recognizing the child's need to gain familiarity with the caregiver, will increase the chances of successful feeding. Caregiver beliefs about the appropriate level of demand for food by children can result in the shaping of children's behavior to reduce demand for food. If the caregiver feels that a child should learn not to ask for food, or that immediate responses to children's requests for food will represent "spoiling" or inappropriate indulgence of a child, particularly after infancy, the chances of the child achieving adequate intake are lowered, since child demand plays a large role in the amount of food ingested.

Studies comparing failure-to-thrive (FTT) children from normally growing children have found differences in the feeding style of the two groups. In FTT groups, an authoritarian disciplinary approach may override children's internal regulatory system for hunger, and there may be low maternal responsivity and sensitivity to cues. This style may be combined with family isolation, and possibly difficult temperaments or subtle oral/motor feeding problems in the children, leading to a breakdown of the caregiver-child relationship.

Children can be fed on a regular basis each day, sitting in a prescribed place with food easily accessible, or feeding can occur while children wander around, or at the time that the caregiver finds convenient. Children can be easily distracted, particularly if food is difficult to eat (e.g., soup with a spoon that is beyond the child's ability to handle) or not particularly tasty. If supervision of feeding is not adequate, other siblings or even animals may take advantage of a young child's vulnerability to take food away, or food may be spilled on the ground.

Feeding from a common pot may reduce the chances of a younger child getting enough food, and may make it harder for a caregiver to be sure food has been allocated to the youngest child. Studies in developing countries have found associations between specific feeding behaviors, such as location of feeding, organization of the feeding event, use of spoon, with mother's education.

Some study says that more educated mothers had more labor-intensive child care strategies, particularly in selecting a clean and protected location for feeding. Linkages with child nutritional status were not made. Caregivers may not be aware of how much their children eat; one project found that when mothers paid more attention to the quantity children ate, they were surprised by the small amounts, and were willing to increase amounts fed.

When children are fed from a common pot, the amount eaten is not easy to determine. Having a separate bowl for each child can help the caregiver evaluate the quantities eaten. Five types of observational measures have been used to examine child and parent behavior in feeding situations:

(1) observations of time in feeding,

(2) presence or absence of specific feeding behaviors,

(3) quantitative assessments (frequency of specific behaviors) of feeding behaviors,

(4) behavioral ratings (to measure the quality of the caregiver-child interaction), and

(5) structured situation challenge (the caregiver is presented with a new food and her reactions are observed).

The most common assessment technique is to code the presence or absence of child or caregiver behaviors on a series of items that assess the presence or absence of a particular behavior.

In Bangladesh found a number of caregiver behaviors that differed by the mother's education level, adjusting for household education, wealth, child age, birth order, and gender. However, child behavior was not assessed. A study found frequency of feeding to be associated with maternal education.

Frequency of feeding, observed during continuous observations, was associated with child nutritional status for children 18-23 months of age in Kenya. Whereas child demand was associated with child nutritional status, active feeding was not; rather, active feeding was associated with child lack of interest in food, suggesting that caregivers in this situation may feed actively in response to child refusal.

Psychosocial care refers to the provision of affection and warmth, responsivity to the child, and encouragement of autonomy of learning. In this area, as in no other, is the importance of culture central. For example, affection can be shown by physical, visual, and verbal contact with children. Typically, indicators involve the frequency of caregiver behaviors, child behaviors, and child/caregiver interaction patterns are coded.

Behaviors most often assessed are verbalizations of child and caregiver, and looking and touching, although these behaviors will vary by the age of the child. A second technique is to present the caregiver with a task, such as asking her to play with a specific toy with her child, and then rate her behavior on a checklist or to count the number of times an event occurs.

Several studies have suggested that the appearance of a child rated either in a public place, such as the public health clinic or rated over a number of instances in the home may be an indicator of care provision (or lack thereof).

Child Obesity

A large increase in child obesity is occurring and predicts significant ill-health during childhood (including psychological and social consequences), in many cases progressing to numerous serious diseases in adults.

Adult diseases influenced by child obesity include coronary heart disease, stroke and cancer. Child obesity is influenced by many different factors including genetics, dietary intake, physical activity, and prenatal factors.

Food security covers issues of hunger, food quality, food quantity, and cultural appropriateness of foods. Under-nutrition and malnutrition during any period of childhood can lead to impaired cognitive development, increased fatigue, and numerous nutrition related illnesses. The major risk factor for food insecurity in families is low socioeconomic status, especially housing tenure, education, employment, and car ownership, which all impact on the ability to procure and store food.

Iron deficiency is the most common nutrient deficiency found in industrialised countries. It is particularly common among infants and children. The serious effects of iron deficiency include poor growth, increased risk of infection and impaired psychological development. The risk factors for iron deficiency are well understood and they vary depending on the age group.

An optimal calcium intake during childhood and adolescence is required to maximise peak bone mass. Attaining peak bone mass in childhood and adolescence significantly reduces the risk of individuals developing osteoporosis, the debilitating bone disease, later in life. Osteoporosis causes significant death and illness due to wrist and hip fractures.

Providing microbiologically safe food for children is essential to maintain good health. Thousands of children suffer significant illness due to food poisoning each year and some deaths occur. The risk factors for food poisoning are well understood and are related to unsafe handling and food preparation, both in the home and in the food industry.

Appropriate nutrition during childhood is essential for maintaining growth and good health. This section reviews five major areas of nutritional concern relevant to New Zealand children: obesity, food security, iron status, calcium intake, and food safety. Morbidity and mortality. Obesity is a major public health problem in developed and developing countries.

In New Zealand, the National Plan of Action for Nutrition (NPAN) has targets for adult obesity but not for childhood obesity, due to the lack of national prevalence data. The diagnosis of obesity usually involves a measure of weight and height. A measure of body composition such as skinfolds may also be included where practical.

Childhood is a critical period for the initiation of obesity-related ill-health, particularly coronary heart disease. Adolescents are vulnerable to significant cardiovascular risk through abnormal glucose tolerance, hypertension and lipid profile abnormalities. Research from a 55-year follow-up to the Third Harvard Growth Study showed mortality from all causes, coronary heart disease, stroke, and colon cancer was greater in adult males who had been overweight during adolescence than in adult males who had been normal weight adolescents.

Similarly, morbidity was higher in people who had been overweight adolescents compared to people who had been normal-weight adolescents. The study also highlighted the strong tendency for overweight adolescents to remain overweight as adults. Adult obesity is strongly associated with diabetes, high blood pressure, hyperlipidemia, cardiovascular disease, and certain cancers.

While there is little evidence to suggest that overweight preadolescents have a lower self-esteem than normal-weight preadolescents, obesity may have serious psychological and social consequences for some children. Preadolescent children associate overweight body shape with poor social functioning, impaired academic success and reduced health and fitness. Adolescents are strongly socialised to the importance of appearance and weight is critical in the relationship between body image and self-concept.

The phenomenon loosely labelled hunger is now being discussed in a much broader context as food security - a relatively new and evolving concept. Food security is defined as access by all people at all times to the food needed for a healthy life. Existence of adequate quantities of food does not guarantee food security. Achieving food security has three dimensions:

— First, it is necessary to ensure a safe and nutritionally adequate food supply both at the national and household level.

— Second, it is necessary to have a reasonable degree of stability in the supply of food both from one year to the other and during the year.

— Third, and most critically, it is necessary to ensure that each household has physical, social and economic access to enough food to meet its needs.

Obesity in children is often defined as a weight for height, age and sex greater than or equal to the 85th percentile, or triceps skinfold thickness greater than or equal to the 85th percentile. Body mass index (BMI) is also reported frequently in the literature and a child is considered at high risk of being overweight when his/her index is greater than or equal to the 85th percentile, and overweight when his/her index is greater than or equal to the 95th percentile.

Slight differences exist with many other authors recommending the cut off to define overweight for BMI indices to be greater than or equal to the 85th percentile. Research has shown the potential for the misclassification of obesity when North American measures are applied to Australian children, suggesting the importance of developing nation-specific cut-off values.

Our Children's Health that each household must have the knowledge and ability to produce, procure or prepare the food it needs on a sustainable basis. It is also important to encourage the proper distribution of food within the household, among all its members. The International Conference on Nutrition in Rome 1992 identified household food security as a key focus for improving nutrition. Those most at risk of being food-insecure were identified as children, women and the aged.

Childhood hunger indicators have been developed and are being used in the United States. These indicators are composite measures of various aspects of food insufficiency due to constrained resources. While the Ministry of Health has developed indicators of food security for the New Zealand adult population in the 1997 National Nutrition Survey, to date no such measures of food security have been developed for New Zealand children.

Recent research supports the view that under-nutrition during any period of childhood can have detrimental effects on the cognitive development of children and their later productivity as adults. Undernourished children decrease their activity levels and become more apathetic. This in turn affects their social interactions, inquisitiveness and overall cognitive functioning. The majority of international studies on the relationship of birthweight to adult chronic disease report cohorts with birthweights at the lower end of normal having higher prevalence of coronary heart disease, hypertension and diabetes.

Pregnant women who are undernourished are likely to have low birthweight babies. Along with other health risks common to low birthweight babies, these infants are more likely to suffer developmental delays. In the case of very low birthweight infants, permanent cognitive deficiencies associated with smaller head circumference may reflect diminished brain growth.

Research in the United States has shown undernourished children are typically fatigued and uninterested in their social environment. They are also more susceptible to illness and more likely to be absent from school. A significant amount of research has been completed in the United Kingdom which shows diet-related illnesses are more prevalent among vulnerable groups, especially children, pregnant women and older people living in low-income households. Infants in low-income households are less likely to be breast-fed and have a higher prevalence of anaemia.

Toddlers in low-income households have higher intakes of saturated fatty acids and sugars and lower vitamin and mineral intakes. Pregnant women in low-income households have lower energy and nutrient intakes and higher rates of low birthweight babies. United Kingdom studies indicate that young children in persistently poor families have substantial nutritional deficits compared to children from other families. There is an association between long-term measures of income and child nutritional status, whereas, current short-term income measures and child nutritional status do not show any association.

Iron deficiency (ID) is the most common micronutrient deficiency found in the industrialised countries. It is particularly common among infants, women and children. The 1992 International Conference on Nutrition in Rome declared that one of its principal aims was to have ID reduced by one-third by the year 2000. The Ministry of Health has identified research into the prevalence of iron deficiency in at-risk groups, such as infants and children, as a priority.

The debilitating effects of iron deficiency anaemia (IDA) on the health of populations and individuals are well documented. They include poor growth, increased risk of infections and delayed cognitive development. Levels of iron depletion and ID not severe enough to result in anaemia can still cause significant deterioration in health and wellbeing. Iron deficiency has been associated with psychological problems in children. Iron-deficient children exhibit shorter attention spans, lower intelligence and delayed psychomotor development, which in turn affects language development and body balance.

Most research on calcium in children has focused on its role in bone health. Osteoporosis is the reduction in bone mass that increases the susceptibility of bones to fracture. Although the disease predominantly affects post-menopausal women, dietary measures taken during childhood have been demonstrated to help prevent the onset or minimise the severity of osteoporosis later in life.

Osteoporosis is a disease that begins in childhood and adolesence; therefore, prevention must begin in these age groups. Vertebral, femoral and forearm fractures are most commonly associated with osteoporosis. Femoral fractures in particular have a disproportionate frequency in the population in comparison with the age of the population. Femoral fractures cause immediate disability, are characterised by both early and late mortality and cause considerable morbidity.

In New Zealand, in 1994, the mean length of hospital stay for patients with hip fractures was 22.4

days. In the United States it has been suggested that as many as 50 percent of patients suffering a hip fracture will require long-term nursing care. Sixteen percent of people who have hip fractures die within six months.

There are a number of different bacteria associated with significant foodborne illness. The major bacterial causes in New Zealand are Salmonella, Campylobacter, Escherichia coli and Yersinia. Listeria monocytogenes is rare, but very serious when it occurs. New Zealand is witnessing a trend towards an increasing number of notified cases of foodborne illness, ensuring that food safety remains a significant public health issue.

Bacteria associated with significant foodborne illness can produce a range of different symptoms in an infected person. These include cramps, nausea, diarrhoea, vomiting, and fever. More serious complications that are potentially fatal include: dehydration and meningitis. The majority of foodborne illnesses result in 1-5 days of sickness. However, in more vulnerable people such as young children the recovery can be prolonged. Similarly, because children are much smaller than adults, the consequences of food poisoning in a child can be far more serious than that in an adult.

Children may increase the spread of foodborne illness by acting as carriers of the disease. Other food safety issues such as food contaminated with foreign material, pesticide residues, additives, and chemical contaminants have a high public profile, but pose a low risk compared with foodborne illness.

There is considerable anecdotal evidence that New Zealand families, and in particular children, are experiencing a lack of food security. One indicator is the increase in the availability and use of foodbanks. Between 1990 and 1993, the number of Salvation Army foodbanks operating in New Zealand increased ten-fold. A 1995 study of foodbank clients found that most were families with children. Two in every three of these families were single-parent families. Half of the total number of people receiving food parcels were children under the age of 15 years.

In New Zealand, it has been estimated that between 14 and 46 percent of single-parent households are considered to be below the poverty line when income is used as the measure of poverty. The incidence of poverty was highest in households with children, especially those households containing several children.

A recent national school study conducted by the Food and Nutrition Consultancy Service showed that over 20,000 New Zealand school children are perceived by their teachers to be inadequately fed during the school day. Children from regions with a higher proportion of Pacific children and children from large inner city schools were most likely to be rated as inadequately fed.

A number of New Zealand surveys conducted in the 1960s found a high frequency of IDA in infants and children. ID was more prevalent and severe among infants and children. The only community-based study of ID in an ethnically-mixed New Zealand paediatric population in the past 15 years was conducted in 1991-92 in a low socioeconomic population living in Porirua. This was a small, opportunistic sample of children aged 6-36 months and iron deficiency was demonstrated in 24 percent of these children. In a national school-based study of 13-15-year-olds, more girls than boys were found to have an iron intake below 70 percent of the recommended daily intake.

Four percent of boys and 7 percent of girls had an iron intake below 70 percent of the recommended dietary intake (RDI). In a study of third and fourth form girls in Dunedin and Otago, a small number of participants were found to be iron deficient.

Calcium is not widely distributed in the commonly available food groups. As a result, compared to other nutrients, it can be more difficult for people to ensure an adequate dietary intake of calcium. Milk and milk-based foods are the major sources of calcium in the New Zealand diet. These contribute as much as 70 percent of dietary calcium for children.

Sardines are also a good source of calcium and smaller amounts of calcium are found in eggs, green leafy vegetables, legumes, nuts, and wholegrains. However, the bioavailability of calcium from dairy products is significantly higher than from these other sources. In a New Zealand dietary study, 45 percent of girls and 30 percent of boys aged 10-11 years had calcium intakes that fell below 70 percent of the recommended dietary intake.

The notifiable disease system collects some information on the national incidence of foodborne illness. Virtually all cases reported in New Zealand are cases diagnosed and reported by doctors. Not all transmission of food poisoning organisms are foodborne, as many agents may be spread by drinking water and direct personal contact with other cases or infected animals. The most frequently notified foodborne illnesses are those due to Campylobacter and Salmonella species.

The number of notified salmonellosis cases has had a slow rise over the past twenty years. Notifications suggest preschool children are most frequently affected by both diseases. However, the higher number of notifications for preschool children may also reflect the fact that these children are more likely to come to the attention of health professionals than are older children or adults with foodborne illness.

Listeriosis notifications are more rare than other foodborne diseases notified in New Zealand, but they have increased each year for the past 10 years. The notifications for listeriosis between 1990 and 1996 numbered 100. In the first seven months of 1997, listeriosis resulted in the deaths of five unborn New Zealand children.

The two major types of protozoan illness are giardiasis and cryptosporidiosis. Both became notofiable in mid-1996. Large waterborne and foodborne outbreaks of these diseases have been reported overseas. Viral outbreak data suggest that a foodborne viral disease is a significant concern in New Zealand. Probable and confirmed cases of viral outbreak cases total 262 from July 1996 to June 1997, compared with 212 probable and confirmed bacterial outbreak cases.

Notifications do not reveal the true incidence of foodborne illness. It has been estimated that only 10-25 percent of foodborne infections are reported through statutory and voluntary laboratory reports. In comparison to the larger notifications for foodborne diseases, food contaminated with foreign material (glass) ranged between 57-70 cases in the years 1994-96.

While some developed countries now recognise the need to collect data on food insecurity, debate continues over the best ways to collect information on this issue. To date, most information on food insecurity has been collected on adult populations. Data collected on children that may be indicative of food insecurity include measures of iron deficiency and malnutrition.

In North America the prevalence of ID in low-income families declined from 7.8 percent in 1975 to 2.9 percent in 1985. Data from the third National Health and Nutrition Examination Survey 1988-94 shows that for American children aged one to two years the prevalence of ID was nine percent and for IDA the prevalence was 3 percent.

In children aged 3 to 11 years the prevalence of IDA declined to less than 1 percent. ID and IDA are not common in adolescent boys aged 12-15 years (less than 1 percent), yet adolescent girls aged 12-15 years had an ID prevalence of 9 percent, and a further 2 percent had IDA.

The United Kingdom national diet and nutrition survey found that 6 percent of children aged between 2.5 and 3.5 years were anaemic. The 1985 Australian National Dietary Survey of Schoolchildren showed iron deficiency was uncommon among 15-year-old boys, and 9- and 12-year-old girls and boys. However, amongst 15-year-old girls, 20 percent had low serum ferritin levels (less than 12 mg/l), indicating iron deficiency.

Unfortunately, the 1995/96 Australian National Dietary Survey did not collect blood samples, so iron status cannot be determined. Although the exact mechanisms are unclear, a number of prenatal, genetic, familial, and environmental influences are thought to play a hand in the development of obesity. Prenatal risk from in utero over-nutrition (or under-nutrition) may effect the hypothalmic centres responsible for food intake.

In addition, third trimester and postnatal over-nutrition may protect against or promote obesity through changes to adipose cells. Genetic influence is hypothesised to be a complex multifactorial, multigenic gene-gene and gene- environment interaction. The transmission from nuclear families and adoption data suggest heritability levels for obesity of about 20-30 percent. Twin studies have yielded higher estimates of heritability, ranging from 60 to 90 percent.

Obviously, families share more than just genes; they also share the lives of the other family members. However, it is highly likely that the genetic impact of having an obese parent increases the risk of obesity for the child. Family factors combined with genetics produce data that show that a child has an 80 percent chance of obesity if both parents are obese, and a 40 percent chance if one parent is obese.

When neither parent is obese the risk of the child becoming obese reduces to 7 percent Dietary intake is an obvious risk factor for obesity. Research with adults has found a strong association between obesity and the intake of dietary fat, although not total energy intake. The same evidence exists for children. The type of dietary fat that people consume may also be important in determining the development of insulin resistance and altering the disposition of individuals to gain fat.

An increased intake of carbohydrates is believed to aid weight control in adults. Physical activity is believed to be important for weight control. Physical activity is a common complement to dietary management for avoiding weight gain or losing weight because it burns energy and maintains muscle mass. Physical activity favourably alters the distribution of body fat.

Studies conducted overseas have consistently found that, compared to people from higher socioeconomic status groups, people from lower socioeconomic groups are less likely to purchase foods that meet the recommendations of the national dietary guidelines. Lower income is associated with poorer health. Car ownership, housing tenure, education, and employment are all associated with differentials in health.

All of these factors impact on the ability of parents to procure and store food for themselves and their children. In addition, many people on low incomes spend a considerable part of their disposable income on fixed living costs such as accommodation. This leaves relatively little income for spending on food.

Infants older than six months and young children are particularly vulnerable to iron deficiency. This is because iron stores deplete during periods of rapid growth. Other contributing factors are the low iron content of many infant diets and the early use of cow's milk. A milk-based diet provides most of the energy consumed during the first year of life. Therefore, the iron content and bioavailability of various milks is one risk factor to consider for iron status.

Breastfed infants and those consuming mainly iron-fortified formulas are at low risk from iron deficiency. However, those fed non-fortified formulas or cow's milk have a 30-40 percent risk of becoming iron deficient by nine months of age, dependent also on the weaning diet. This risk increases by 12 months old. Breastfed infants without adequate iron from other sources are at risk of becoming iron deficient by six months old.

For boys, the double burden of providing iron for a larger body size and increased erythrocyte mass results in an approximate 25 percent increase in total body iron requirements in the year of peak growth. The iron need of adolescent girls is also high, particularly with the onset of menstruation. Iron requirements increase during pregnancy to a level that exceeds any stores.

Pregnancy during adolescence places young women at especially high risk of iron deficiency. A peak bone mass (PBM) at skeletal maturity is considered the best protection against osteoporosis and subsequent fracture risk later in life. PBM is the maximum level of bone mineral content achieved during young adulthood. Peak bone mass is probably the result of the interaction between endogenous (heredity, endocrine) and exogenous (nutrition, physical activity) factors.

Eighty percent of peak bone mass is thought to be controlled by endogenous factors and 20 percent by exogenous factors. The two strongest exogenous factors are weight-bearing exercise (walking, jogging, aerobics) and dietary calcium. Bone is in a phase of rapid growth and remodelling from birth until about 16 years of age, with bone mass accumulation extending from puberty to the mid-30s.

The most critical period for maximal bone mass formation is during puberty and early adolescence. For females, maximal bone mass formation occurs between nine and 10 years of age, reaching maximum velocity in growth at around 12 years of age. For boys, maximal bone mass occurs at 13 years of age. Bone density at certain sites continues increasing past 17 years of age.

Overseas dietary surveys conducted on children have shown that during the years when an increase in calcium intake is most needed for PBM development, the consumption of milk decreases significantly. The trend seems to be a movement away from drinking milk to drinking increased levels of soft drinks and cordial. Concern that increasing the consumption of milk will lead to an increase in the dietary intake of fat need not be warranted, as there is a wide range of low-fat milks available on the market.

Absorption of calcium may not be sufficient at times of high requirements and its bioavailability from the diet is variable. Calcium is also continuously excreted in urine, faeces and sweat as an obligatory loss. The major determinants of calcium absorption are the amount of calcium in the diet and the vitamin D status of the individual. The presence of lactose in a meal also appears to enhance calcium absorption.

It is assumed that since most New Zealand children spend plenty of time out of doors, even in winter, vitamin D status is likely to be adequate. Encouraging regular exercise and play is also important for bone mineralisation. Several dietary factors affect the bioavailability of calcium. Some foods that contain fibre, oxalic acid and phytic acid inhibit calcium absorption by combining with calcium and forming insoluble complexes which cannot be absorbed by the body.

Milk contains no inhibitory factors. The calcium absorption rate of non-fortified soy milk can be reduced by up to 20 percent, compared with cow's milk, due to the presence of phytate. The dietary calcium:phosphorus ratio is an important factor in calcium bioavailability. A 16:1 ratio appears to be sufficient to achieve a positive calcium balance. Dairy foods have a 36:1 ratio and, therefore, calcium retention is strongly favoured by consuming products containing milk.

The obligatory calcium loss in urine can also be affected by diet. Increased dietary intakes of sodium and protein elevate urinary calcium excretion. However, no study has proven conclusively that high intakes of either sodium or protein have a detrimental effect on bone mass during growth. Sodium intakes should be kept to a minimum by avoiding salty snacks and reducing salt used in food preparation.

Increased urinary calcium excretion occurs when protein levels are high and phosphate intake is low. If phosphate intake increases with protein intake, there is a minimal effect on calcium absorption. Excess dietary fat inhibits calcium absorption by forming an insoluble calcium salt. Excess dietary calcium remains unabsorbed by the body and is excreted in the faeces.

Most raw foods are naturally contaminated with bacteria. Each step between harvesting and the consumer introduces the possibility of further contamination or growth of the naturally occurring bacteria. Food manufacturers, processors, wholesalers, transporters, and retailers all contribute to food safety, and they must have processes in place to reduce and eliminate the risks from these bacteria.

Prevention of foodborne illness depends on education of food handlers in appropriate methods of preparing, cooking and storing food, and in personal hygiene. The World Health Organization has developed 'Ten Golden Rules for Safe Food Preparation', as follows:

1. Choose foods processed for safety.
2. Cook food thoroughly.
3. Eat cooked foods immediately.

4. Store cooked foods carefully.
5. Reheat cooked foods thoroughly.
6. Avoid contact between raw food and cooked food.
7. Wash hands repeatedly.
8. Keep all kitchen surfaces meticulously clean.
9. Protect food from insects, rodents and other animals.
10. Use safe water.

2

Child and Health Education

The well-nourished child is more apt to reach her full potential physically, mentally, and intellectually. Americans today have more health knowledge about nutrition than at any other time in history, yet this knowledge has not translated into proper nutritional behavior for all Americans. Further, although the United States leads the world in food production, many Americans-not just the poor-are malnourished.

Many parents and teachers fail to provide good examples for their children concerning nutritional habits. Nutrition education has been linked as a priority by the U.S. Department of Health and Human services in the 1990 health Objectives for the Nation, as listed by the Surgeon General. The need for nutrition education is crucial.

For example, American elementary school children demonstrate elevated cholesterol levels compared to children from other countries. Studied indicate that sound school nutrition programs can produce positive outcomes. Helping children develop sound nutritional habits should be one of teachers major goals in elementary health instruction.

To accomplish this, teachers must do more than simply provide information. They must counter the impact of television commercials and other sources. Also, they must help children recognize that although the food they eat is strongly influenced by their culture an their lifestyle, they can learn to control these influences.

Teachers must also dispel misconceptions associated with food and nutrition, help children become informed consumers, and develop in them a sense of the importance of nutrition. Every culture has its own food habits and customs. Approached to nutrition are based in part on the food resources available. In Japan, where there is little land available for raising livestock, red meat is not a usual part of the daily diet. Animal protein is supplied instead by fish and other seafood, which abound in the waters around the island nation.

In southern China, as Japan, rice is a staple eaten at every meal. However, in northern China, where rice as in Japan, rice is staple eaten at every meal. However, in northern china, where rice cannot be grown, wheat and millet are substituted for rice.

In Mexico, poorer residents eat beans and corn flour tortillas daily, as was true in Aztec times. This combination of two simple foods provides all essential protein needed for good nutrition. Food customs are also often partly a result of religious ideas. Hindus consume no beef, some Jews eat only kosher foods, and some Buddhists are vegetarians.

Many religious dietary rules were originally based on health considerations. For example, the Jewish and

Islamic prohibitions against eating pork are probably based on the fact that undercooked pork can harbor parasite that cause such diseases in humans as trichinosis. Cooking and eating in class can be a cultural as well as a nutritional experience.

Teachers can explain that different cultural outlooks also influence food customs. Horsemeat is commonly eaten in Frances, but is viewed with disdain in England and other English speaking countries. Milk, which plays such a larger role in American diets, is almost never consumed by adult Chinese, who find the taste and idea of drinking it repellent. Food habits and customs in the United States reflect the multicultural nature of our society.

At one time, there were significant regional differences in cooking and food preferences. Seafood was a major part of the diet on the East coast. Wild game provided much of the meat eaten in the rural Southwest. Today, these regional differences have faded, largely as a result of refrigeration and modern transportation. it is now almost as easy to get fresh fish in Kansas as it is in Massachusetts.

Cultural intermixing has also diminished regional differences, while at the same time expanding the range of dishes commonly eaten, Pasta, for instance, is no longer eaten only by Americans of Italian extraction. Chinese, French, German, Mexican, and Middle Eastern dishes have also become popular. As an affluent, multiethnic nation, we have a greater variety of food and dishes to choose from than almost any other people on earth. This does not mean, however, that American can afford to eat anything they like.

Inflation has influenced the eating habits of all Americans, rich and poor alike—but especially the poor. Those living near or below the poverty level often must subsist on cheap starchy foods, which are filling, if not particularly nutritious. Although economics influences the American diet as it does the diet of every nation, most Americans cannot blame lack of money for poor nutritional habits. Instead, we must look for the reasons in personal preferences and lifestyles.

Personal preference for a food often is formed by reasons that have little or nothing to do with the nourishment that will be provided by that food. The most popular foods eaten by one's subculture and peer group also influence food choices. finally, a food might be chosen because of the way it looks, smells, and tastes. The national lifestyle also influences out nutritional habits.

When the United States was mostly a rural, agrarian society, breakfast was a major meal. The main meal of the day was served at noon. These two meals provided the necessary energy for performing farm labor and chores. Evening dinner was typically a lighter meal. Today, the reverse is true. Most Americans eat a light breakfast, and some skip breakfast entirely.

Lunch is also a light meal, of ten eaten in haste. The largest meal of the day is consumed in the evening, because there is more time to prepare and eat such a meal. Unfortunately, this meal is usually followed by general physical inactivity and then by sleep. This is one reason why so many Americans are overweight.

Also, many overspice their foods, especially with salt and sugar. Others rush through their meals, which reduced the nourishment received from the foods. There is not much that teachers can do to change out hectic national lifestyle. However, they can emphasize the importance of beginning the day with a good breakfast that will provide children with the energy they need for school and studying.

They can also emphasize the value of a balanced, nutritional lunch and a reasonable evening meal. This is not to suggest that teachers should criticize the eating patterns of any child's family, and certainly not any religious dietary restrictions a family might need, but they can be a source of information about sound nutritional practices and encourage students to consider changes in their diet that could lead to sounder nutrition.

For example, teachers should emphasize that snacking on Junk food, such as candy, may spoil a child's appetite for a regular meal as well as contribute to tooth decay. Teacher can also stimulate children's curiosity about trying new dishes that could add needed variety to their diets. The development of positive lifetime eating habits among children is a critical issue.

A parent or teacher should not resort to using a punishment reward system when trying to get a child to eat. nether should each mealtime become a war zone. The following suggestions may help in establishing the proper habits for children:

— Don't force the issue introduce children at an early age to new foods, and your child determine the portion at first. If the child does not like a specific food at first, try to prepare it in different ways:

— Create a calm environment this can be helpful whether at home or in the school cafeteria. Even when cafeteria schedules are rushed try to make mealtime relaxing. Also, praise the child when he tries an unpopular food:

— Make snacks count—Most children have a metabolism level that burns calories quickly: therefore many of them get hungry between meals. Try to think of snacktimes as mini meals. Offer variety of nutritious snacks and have then available so the child will consider it as convenient to choose the nutritious snack as the "junk" snack. Also, these snacks should be limited so as not to interrupt regular meals.

Food is one of the delights of every civilization. Preparation of some dished in many cultures is an art. Eating a fine meal is an aesthetic experience, not just fulfillment of nutritional requirements, but even the simplest dish can provide great pleasure. Teachers can use this positive approach in presenting nutritional concepts. Too often nutrition is taught as a grim and dry subject, divorced from the human perspective.

Food's most basic function is to provide nutrients to the body. Nutrients are the substances in food needed to support life functions. One vital way in which this is accomplished is by providing energy that the body needs. This energy, produced as a by product of food consumption, is measured in calories. A calorie is defined as the amount of heat energy required to raise the temperature of one kilogram of water one degree Celsius.

All foods have specific caloric values, and a given among of food will produce a certain number of calories when broken down by the body. They number of calories needed by the body daily depends on two factor:

(1) the individual's basal metabolism and

(2) the amount of energy expanded in daily activities.

Basal metabolism is the minimum amount of heat produced by the body when at rest. This heat, among other things, is necessary to maintain a normal body temperature. The amount of energy expended by an individual varies, depending on the activities of the individual. Thus, someone who engages in heavy physical labor each day needs more calories than someone who works in an office.

Young children need fewer calories per day then active adults, because of the difference in body sizes. Although caloric requirements differ with age, basal metabolism, and daily activities, the Food Agricultural Organization of the United nations recommends a daily minimum intake for adult of 2,650 calories. However, more than half the people in the world exist on fewer than 2,200 calories per day.

Carbohydrates are found in food as monosaccharide, disaccharides, and polysaccharides. The monosaccharides are glucose, galactose, and fructose. The disaccharides are sucrose, lactose an maltose. Many adults, especially those of Oriental and back ancestry, suffer from lactose intolerance.

In other words, undigested lactose is not absorbed and remains in the gastrointestinal tract, resulting in bloating, a large amount of gas, and abdominal cramping. This malady can be treated through a diet that includes high protein, high carbohydrate, low to moderate fat, and high calories.

The polysaccharides are comprised of many glucose molecules and are the following: (1) glycogen, (2) cellulose, and (3) starch. Carbohydrates are broken down into glucose, and the metabolism of carbohydrates produces energy. Four calories are produced per gram of carbohydrates. If carbohydrates are not abundant in the diet, protein and fat have to be metabolized to produce needed energy.

Carbohydrates must be constantly replenish in the blood, either by eating or by breaking down glycogen stored in the liver and muscles. Carbohydrates are important in a child's diet and should comprise approximately 58% of total calorie intake. Foods rich in carbohydrates include rice, spaghetti noodles, bread, breakfast cereals, and potatoes.

Many vegetables, fruits and fruit juices also contain some carbohydrates. Although candy and cookies are good sources of carbohydrates, the refined sugar they contain contributes to tooth decay and gum disease and does not provide additional nutrients. If food such as milk, fruit, and vegetables are eaten, the individual should brush and floss after the meal. If he cannot brush immediately after meal, he should at least rinse out his mouth with water.

Brushing the flossing before bedtime are especially important in reducing tooth decay. Fruits, vegetables, and juices make healthier snacks. Protein means "to come first". This suggests that proteins are essential nutrients. No organism can live and almost no biological process can take place without protein. A protein molecule is composed of smaller structures called amino acids.

Some amino acids are termed essential, which means they must be provided by the diet, and some are termed nonessential, which means they are synthesized by the body. These amino acids are building blocks necessary for several body functions. Proteins are present in every cell, in enzymes, and in body secretions.

Proteins provide calories but also serve other important and complex functions. They are important components of DNA and RNA molecules, which determine individuals genetic makeup. Also, proteins help build new cells and tissues in growing children, maintain tissues that are already built, and play a role in the manufacture of blood, enzymes, hormones, and human milk.

Further, antibodies, which combat infection, are synthesized from proteins in response to infectious agents. Proteins provide four calories per gram. Protein should comprise about 12% of a child's total caloric intake. Most children require approximately 60 grams of protein daily. Milk and meat products are excellent sources of protein.

Poultry is another good source of this essential nutrient. If a person eats a vegetarian diet, enough protein must be ingested to support normal growth and development, especially in children. This is called complementary protein ingestion, a dietary strategy which ensures that each food supplies some amino acides that the others lack. for example, peanut protein is combined with wheat, oats, corn rice, or coconut, and soy protein is combined with corn, wheat, rye, or sesame.

Non meat sources of protein include soybeans, dried beans, and nuts. Central grains, vegetables , and fruits contain vegetable protein, which must be augmented by other protein sources, as in the tortilla and beans example mentioned earlier. Fats, or lipids, are the most concentrated source of calories we ingest.

Fasts provide nine calories per gram, as compared with four for proteins and carbohydrates. There are two types of fatty acids : saturated and unsaturated. The dietary sources of saturated fatty acids are animal fat, beef, butter, chicken eggs, and whole milk. Unsaturated fats are found in vegetable oils, such as corn, olive, soybean, peanut, and safflower. The more saturated a fat is, the harder it is at room temperature.

Polyunsaturated fats, such as linoleic acid, can reduce serum cholesterol levels. Fats are an important part of our diets. Their vital role is sometimes overlooked because of the association of fats with cardiovascular problems. However, fats serve several vital functions. The energy they provide spares protein for tissue synthesis.

Fats also serve as carriers of the fat soluble vitamins A, D, E, and K. As food, they provide satiety, because the rate at which a meal is emptied from the stomach is related to the fat content. The higher the fat content, the slower the food empties from the stomach. Fats are an important part of all cells, membrane structure in the body, and tissues. Additionally, fats provide protection in the adipose tissue just under the skin. This layer of adipose tissue also helps in maintaining the body temperature at a constant level despite changes in the environment temperature.

Similarly, fats provide a layer of protective shock absorbing tissue between the kidneys, reproductive organs, and other organs. They also provide padding for the cheeks, palms of the hand, and balls of the feet. Finally, fast make foods more appetizing and flavorful. Fats should comprise 30% of total caloric intake . These fats should be equally divided among polyunsaturated, saturated, and monounsaturated fats.

The major food sources of fat are animal and vegetable fats, such as butter, cream, lard, and salad dressings. Olives and nuts also have a significant fat content. An issue closely related to ingestion of fats, obesity, and health risks is blood cholesterol levels. Cholesterol is a vital part of the body, but too much of it can result in health risks. Cholesterol is a waxy, fatlike substance found mainly in the liver, kidneys, and brain.

Most of the cholesterol is transported through the body as lipoprotein. There are different forms of lipoprotein, and they are classified by their density. The most important forms of lipoprotein, and they are classified by their density. The most important forms of lipoprotein are low density lipoprotein cholesterol (LDL) and the high density lipoprotein cholesterol (HDL). High levels of LDL indicate a cardiovascular risk.

Many blood tests will provide only a total blood cholesterol reading, but a more important factor is the ratio of total cholesterol to HDL. The smaller the ration, the less the cardiovascular risk. Even though some foods might be labeled truthfully as containing no cholesterol, these foods might be high in saturated fats which will cause the body to produce more blood cholesterol.

Although the body produces more cholesterol than is ingested through foods, the blood cholesterol level can be positively altered through a healthy diet. Generally, foods of animal origin, such as eggs and organ meats, should be increased. These foods will increase the amount of fiber in the diet, which will aid in digestion, increase intestinal motility, and possibly further lower cardiovascular risk.

High fiber diets are also beneficial in preventing constipation, obesity, hypoglycemia, and high levels of cholesterol in the blood. In considering nutrition, water is often overlooked, but it is second only to oxygen in importance to body functioning. A person can survive longer without food than water; there can be no life without water. Water is an essential component of body structure. It also acts as a solvent for minerals and other physiologically important compounds. In the body, it transports nutrients to and waste products from the cells.

Further, water helps regulate the body temperature. Water comes from fluids and solids in the diet and is also produced by the metabilizing of energy nutrients within the tissues. The amount of activity and the climate are important factors influencing the amount of water a person needs. Because children usually participate in more physical activities, they perspire more and therefore need more water than many adults.

Water is also list through exhaled air. The recommended daily intake is the equivalent of six to eight glasses of water. Much of this is gained from solid foods. The body needs organic compounds, such as carbohydrates, fats, and proteins for proper nutrition, but it also needs inorganic materials, such as minerals. These inorganic elements are present in the body in small amounts, but they play a vital role in nutrition.

The major minerals needed by the body are calcium, phosphorus, potassium, sulfur, sodium, chlorine and magnesium. Food sources for these major minerals are:

- Calcium—milk, cheese, sardines, salmon, green vegetables
- Phosphorus—milk, cheese, lean meat

— Potassium—oranges, bananas, dried fruits

— Sulfur—eggs, poultry, fish

— Sodium—table salt, beef, eggs, cheese

— Chlorine—table salt, meat

— Magnesium—green vegetables, whole grains

Other mineral elements, known as trace elements and required in lesser amounts, are iron, zinc, selenium, magnesium copper, iodine, fluorine, chromium, molybdenum, and cobalt. Minerals function in the body in several ways. After the organic compounds have been oxidized, minerals remain to from actual body parts. For example, calcium, magnesium and phosphours are components of the bones and teeth.

Minerals also act as regulators and are necessary to certain body functions. For example, minerals contribute to the water and electrolyte balance of the body and are important in the functioning of the transmission of nerve impulses. Minerals contribute to the osmotic pressure of the transmission of nerve impulses. Minerals contribute to the osmotic pressure of body fluids and to the maintenance of neutrality—the acid base balance of the blood and body tissues.

For example, elevated levels of sodium are associated with high blood pressure an cardiovascular disease. Socium can be restricted through the diet by eliminating table salt, using sodium free salt substitutes, drinking low salt milk, and using vegetable salts as spices. A lack of essential minerals can cause malnutrition. For example, iron deficiency anemia is a major health problem in the United states and Canada and even more so in the rest of the World.

Children deprived of iron show a lack of motivation and less ability to work and play. This deficiency occurs most frequently in infants, adolescent males, and females during child bearing years. No group of nutrients has captured the imagination of the public more than vitamins. Vitamins were discovered fairly recently, when physicians sought the cause of several diseases such as scurvy.

They concluded that the chemical compounds called vitamins can make a great deal of difference to health. These vitamin related discoveries have led people to equate good nutrition with vitamins. The normal recommended daily allowances (RDA) for vitamins is sufficient for optimal health. Megadoses of vitamins sometimes result in impaired physical health.

The enrichment of food with vitamins and the use of vitamins as diet supplements are commonplace in our country. Vitamins are organic compounds that must be provided by the diet because the body is not able to synthesize them in the required amounts. Vitamins foster growth, promote the ability to produce healthy offspring, maintain health, aid in the normal function of the appetite and digestive tract, and help the body's resistance to bacterial infections.

Thiamin is necessary for carbohydrate metabolism. It aids in the release of energy from food. Riboflavin helps body cells use oxygen, promotes tissue repaid, and helps the nervous system function properly. Niacin is essential to growth: without niacin, thiamine and riboflavin could not function properly in the body. Pantothenic acid helps increase vitality and influences glandular functions.

Pyridoxine is necessary for healthy teeth and gums and helps maintain normal body cholesterol. Further, it aids in the production of antibodies. Cobalamin works in conjunction with folic acid and iron to build normal blood cells and prevent pernicious anemia. folic acid aids in the proper growth and reproduction of blood cells and contributes to health skin. biotin is necessary for the proper utilization of fats, carbohydrates, and protein.

Biotin also helps produce antibodies. Vitamins sometimes serve as catalysts for important body functions. They are required only in small amounts and are vital to nourishment. They are unlike minerals, however, in that they do not become part of the body, as calcium does in the teeth and bones. Food sources for some of the vitamins are:

- A—liver, whole milk, butter, dark green leafy vegetables.
- C—Citrus fruits, broccoli, tomatoes, potatoes.
- D—Eggs, liver, fortified milk.
- E—margarine, salad dressing.
- K—egg yolk, liver, milk, cabbage.
- Thiamin (B1)—pork, beef, liver eggs, fish, whole grains, legumes.
- Riboflavin (B2)—milk, green vegetables, cereals.
- Pyridoxine (B6)—pork, milk, eggs, legumes.
- B12—seafood, meats, eggs, milk.
- Niacin—milk, eggs, fish, poultry.
- Folacin—spinach, asparagus, broccoli, kidney beans.
- Biotin—milk, liver, mushrooms, legumes.

About 50 different nutrients are needed to maintain. No food contain all the nutrients needed, not even milk, which is highly regarded in our society. Therefore, a variety of foods are required to satisfy nutritional needs. One way to assure this variety and to establish a balanced diet is to select each day from the types of foods identified by the Institute of Home Economics of the United States Department of Agriculture.

Fruits are usually good sources of vitamin C, vitamin A, and fiber, Citrus fruits are especially good sources of vitamin C. One to two servings daily, each about equal in size to an orange, are recommended. Vegetables are usually good sources of vitamin A. vitamin C, and fiber. Vegetables are low in calories if served without added fat. Deep green, leafy vegetables like spinach, kale, collard greens, mustard greens, and broccoli are high in vitamin A, vitamin C, and calcium.

Problems concerned with food have been a part of human life from the earliest times. In past ages, crop failures have to led to famine and war. Even today, starvation kills hundred of thousands of children and adults in very poor nations each year. Although there is also poverty in the United States, few children actually face the threat of starvation. Unfortunately, this does not mean that our nation does not have food problems.

In the United States, malnutrition due to undernutrition is most likely to occur in infants, children, and adolescents, when nutritional requirements for tissue growth and development are high. Undernutrition may inhabit growth, delay nutrition, limit physical activity, and interference with learning. The cause of undernutrition are many; poverty and lack of nutrition education are two major factors.

Psychological factors can also lead to undernutrition. Hurried meals in haphazard settings may be deleterious because of the type and amount of food as well as how the food is eaten. The noise and confusion that often accompany rushed meals can affect proper digestion. An improper concept of one's nutritional state can bring on health problems such as anorexia nervosa. This condition should be considered a psychological disorder more than a simple eating disorder. This condition, which can begin as early as 10 years of age, is one in which the person perceives herself as overweight even when body weight is extremely low.

Anorexia lose more than 25% of their total body weight. Girls are more affected than boys by anorexia nervosa, but the incidence among males is increasing. Girls and boys are equally affected by anorexia athletica, in which the young person reduces fatness for optimal athletic performance. The anorexic person controls weight by severely restricting food intake and exercising to extremes. This condition results in severe physical problems, including death in extreme circumstances.

The anorexic sometimes suffers from a low self-image due to a feeling of incompetence, so he becomes consumed with losing weight to demonstrate to himself and others that he is in total control. Therefore, if a friend, parent, or teacher admonishes the anorexic for looking too thin, the anorexic may take this as a compliment, for it means others are aware of his disciplined approach to weight loss.

Psychological counseling and family therapy are needed to correct some anorexic cases. A related disorder is bulimia, in which a person eats large quantities of food during short periods of time and attempts to control weight by self-induced vomiting or laxative use. Bulimia is thought to result from a lack of self-esteem and desire to become an "ideal" woman.

A research has shown that hunger definitely has an effect on learning behaviour. Hunger increases nervousness, irritability, and disinterest in a learning situation. Children who are hungry will demonstrate a lack of interest in what is being taught and an inability to concentrate. Hunger and malnutrition lead to weakness and illness. A variety of avitaminoses can result form malnutrition.

A child's development and brain function can be severely affected by hunger. Malnourished children are also more suspectable to infections, which can further lead to impaired growth. Teachers should provide accurate information concerning nutrition and teach children how to make wise decision in order to help prevent undernourishment among students.

They need to emphasize the importance of eating a good breakfast and lunch, as well as encourage sociability among students when they are eating. Teachers can help the students enjoy the taste, smell, color, and texture of food and thereby increase in it. In addition, teachers have an excellent chance to be exemplary role models by eating the right foods in the right way while at school.

The number of overweight children is increasing. Further, there is an increasing number of extremely obese children. Weight reduction demands self-discipline and commitment. An overweight individual must accept personal responsibility for the condition. If an emotional problem is the cause, that problem must be treated first to ensure long-lasting success at weight control because the overweight condition is only a symptom of a deeper problem.

Teachers can also educate obese and overweight students about proper nutrition and encourage physical activity. To nurture the emotional health of the obese student, teachers need to offer security and acceptance without pitying or overprotecting the child. Being supportive will produce much better results than constant harassment or criticism. Trying to reduce the child's anxiety while helping build self-esteem and independence is also important.

Obese individuals may understand the need to diet but may want to do so as painlessly as possible. Such individuals are vulnerable to fad diets advertised to help a person lose weight quickly. Some of these fad diets are restricted in variety, expensive, unless, and sometimes even detrimental to health. Most fad diets are directed at adults, rather than children, of course, but children are impressionable. It is important to put these diets into proper perspective.

The fact is that most people who are overweight do not need to read a book on what to eat to lose weight. Simply eating somewhat less of everything will usually produce results, if the diet is followed conscientiously. In emphasizing sound nutrition to students, teachers need to make sure that the learning opportunities they provide are interesting and personalized Students should be taught to help themselves make responsible food choices.

Many times school lunches are criticized for being bland and lacking in nutrition. A 1987 study of school foods found significantly more total fat and sodium than is recommended. The goals of school lunches are to:

1. Provide one third of the child's RDA
2. Serve a minimum of five times with minimum portions

3. Use resources provided by the government
4. Appeal to students—if the school offers vending machines with other choices, however, the student will choose this instead of the school lunch
5. Break even financially—a major problem because most school systems operate on a limited budget.

During the secondary school period, pupils are undergoing those important physiological changes and emotional adjustments incident to adolescence. The pupil is less ready to accept the dictates of authority. This means that he must make a readjustment of relations with the parent in the home. He is less willing to follow the health practices that have been prescribed by the school.

He is increasingly interested in participation in selecting areas and planning the program of study in health. He is a nonconformist who is likely to reject a program of behaviour reflected in the health rules of earlier years until he realizes more keenly that these same practices are demanded for athletic success, for social approval, and for employment.

Health supervision in connection with athletics becomes more important; personality maladjustments are more numerous and more serious. Perhaps the greatest disadvantage in the health program of the secondary school as compared with that of the elementary school arises from departmentalization. The teacher is less an alter parens, interested in the whole child, and confining his attention to 30 children or less. The secondary school teacher is a "subject" teacher, meeting scores of children every day.

The pupil has no one to whom he can turn for advice as readily as the elementary school pupil turns to his classroom teacher. The "homeroom" teacher has an opportunity to develop teacher-pupil health relationships: but too often he is more of an attendance officer and record-keeper for the pupils assigned to sit in his room while waiting for academic class sessions.

At best he can make a considerable contribution to health attitudes and practices. The secondary school is an institution of limitless diversities-diversities in the kind of schools and in the study programs followered by different groups and diversities among the pupils themselves. Planning a health program is a complex task. Most elementary school pupils now continue through high school.

The importance of the secondary school in preoccupational training is increasing. Both the youths who take a job and establish a home directly after high school and the large number of young people going on to junior college and to college must be considered in planning the high school health program.

The different kinds of schools and the varied types of curricula make it impossible to set up a single model high school program in health education. Each pupil is in the hands of many teachers, and interrelation-ships in health subject matter must be definitely arranged by the teachers of different departmentalized subjects. Cooperative planning for both indirect health learnings and direct health instruction is needed. This planning is often done by a faculty health committee.

In small schools, such a committee may consist of only the principal, the health, teacher, and one or two other persons. In any case, all of the teachers who include some health instruction in their subjects need to be members of such a committee. Teachers of biology and other basic sciences, social sciences, home economics, and physical education would ordinarily be included.

The committee may include representatives from school health personnel, such as physician, nurse and director of the lunchroom. In addition to laying out the program of direct health instruction, a committee of such broad membership can plan for health education in connection with health services and school sanitation, and for other activities involving health and health education.

It may initiate special school-wide health projects or campaigns. Home and School cooperation is usually less intimate in the secondary school. Teachers are not so likely to visit the home, but parents come in contact with health programs through the physician and the nurse and through visits to school exhibitions where health instruction and physical education are demonstrated.

School nurses, health educators, and guidance counselors have a direct relationship with the home in their work with individual students. At least one, and preferably two, health examinations should be provided at the junior-senior high school level. Here is an opportunity to give most welcome health guidance. In some cities pupils are encouraged to secure examinations from the family physician, bringing to school the doctor's report on a standard form. The nurse, the health coordinator, the physical educator, and the homeroom teacher have important responsibilities in securing the correction of physical defects.

It is desirable that cumulative health records be continued in use in the high school. The opportunities for incidental health teaching involved in communicable disease control, school sanitation, school health services, and the hygienic regimen have been discussed elsewhere.

Every member of the school staff-not merely the health specialist-has a responsibility to help make the school day a sound health-learning experience for the student. There are certain special activities involving cooperative effort which are not commonly found in the elementary school but with which the high school health education program may be profitably interrelated.

High school newspapers can contribute to the health program by publishing health news and timely information. A special health column may be developed in which health information, slogans, and answers to health questions are included. There may be occasional editorials on health activities.

In addition, the student council and the teachers of hygiene, home economics, and physical education cooperate with the lunchroom by encouraging the selection of desirable food and by developing an appreciation of the scientific and efficient service which the lunchroom renders.

They encourage the use of the school lunchroom in preference to less desirable eating places in the vicinity of the school. In the lunchroom, specially desirable combinations are promoted by low prices and catchy names. Candy may be kept off the counter, at least until after the whole line has gone through. Special foods, like fruit, milk, salad, and whole-grain bread, are sold at very attractive prices.

Food trays may occasionally be checked by a nutritionist or by seniors in home economics and "A-!" cards placed on trays carrying a well-balanced lunch. Lunch suggestions may be shown on a poster. The promotion or serving of a standard lunch is not entirely popular, but it can provide a lunch of good dietary balance. Weighing and measuring take place less frequently than in the elementary school.

Interest in growth has, to a considerable degree, been supplanted by interest in athletic accomplishment and personal appearance. Some pupils of high school age, especially girls, prefer not to increase in weight and indulge in injudicious dieting frequently injurious to health. The homeroom is now the place where the beginnings of a communicable disease or lapses in personal appearance can be observed.

The homeroom teacher is on the alert to detect pupils showing signs of illness and refer them promptly to the doctor or nurse. Teachers should also refer to the health counselor, nurse, or doctor any pupils whose continuing health status appears to be unsatisfactory.

In the secondary school, many students need expert health counseling in physical and mental health and in social adjustment. In the early years of junior high school, students are going through the physical changes of pubescence. They are adjusting to a new type of school schedule. Parental and social relationships may become strained. In the senior high school, there are problems of future career, athletic achievement, and mating, as well as departures from normal health. Physical examination of the high school student is a place for wise health counseling by the physician.

In many schools, there is also a plan for systematic counseling which is carried out by the health teacher, the teacher of physical education for girls, the director of physical education for boys, the school nurse, or some other person. Basic to such counseling is the interview, the preparation and conduct of which deserves special consideration.

In the departmentalized program for the junior and senior high school, health knowledge is presented (1) through health instruction introduced into other subjects and (2) through health courses. Health instruction through other subjects.

Through the planning of the previously mentioned faculty health committee to strengthen interrelationships and avoid undesirable duplication, various subjects can make important contributions to health education. Home economics commonly provides important and valuable instruction for girls in the field of health, including units of instruction upon such topics as laundering; food preservation; menu planning; individual menus; cleanliness in the kitchen; the sanitary condition of stores and markets; the care of clothing; the nature of textiles and weaves; the relation of clothing to the weather; the selection and use of different types of clothing, shoes, stockings, footwear, and underwear, care of the scalp and the hair; the use of cosmetics; the care of the home; the selection of food; and making meals attractive.

In some school systems home nursing and child care are taught in connection with the work of the home economic department. General science and separate courses in physics, chemistry, and biology contribute to health education through the discussion of air and its relation to health; safe drinking water and its health values, specific problems of pollution, the effect of weather upon health, ventilation and heating, sunlight, chemical elements in the human body, the nature of light and vision, sound and hearing, kinds of plants and their relation to the well-being of man, animals as a source of food and as a source of disease, and selected problems in sanitation.

The percentage of high school students who take biology is not large, but those who do take this subject learn much about life processes and their relationship to health. The student studies growth, nutrition, respiration, movement, fatigue, reproduction, and responses to stimuli.

Physical education makes an important contribution to both health and health education. Stamina, neuromuscular coordination, and good body mechanics are developed. The desire for athletic achievement is an outstanding motivating force and stimulus in the development of sound health practices.

The teacher of physical education finds many opportunities for giving needed health advice to individual students. Helpful learning experiences develop with reference to the importance of exercise, group leadership, and the wholesome use of leisure time.

The importance of adequate nutrition to athletic capacity and the dangers of alcohol, tobacco, and narcotics are pointed out. Safety relationships are effectively taught in relation to the different sports.

The contributions to health by art and music have already been described. Foreign languages are related to health through occasional health topics that arise in connection with reading and study. Mathematics may use health material as data for graphs, percentages, space requirements in dwellings, or tax rates for health purposes.

Manual arts contribute to health education by requiring clean hands and materials, proper clothing, correct posture, good ventilation, safety precautions, and habits of concentration and industry. Most subjects of instruction in the high school can make some contribution to health, and in every course due consideration should be given to mental and physical health in developing the schedules and methods of instruction. Health courses, Direct health instruction must vary in different high schools because problems, teacher training, and educational resources vary.

Good health teaching is adapted to the maturity of the student. It has a scientific approach and separates health facts from health fallacies, establishing sound basic knowledge for individual health guidance. It involves pupil planning and pupil action. There are plenty of challenging health problems.

Students make surveys of sanitation, visit the activities of official and voluntary health advertising, community recreation, child guidance programs, and any number of other health-related activities. Health teaching is directed toward the development of sound concepts, attitudes, and behaviour and is not limited to the memorizing of health facts. The scope of health education is broad. The Joint Committee report on Health Education suggests the following ten major subject areas:

(1) the human body:

(2) the balanced regimen:

(3) mental health;

(4) preparation for marriage, family life, and child care;

(5) communicable and non communicable diseases;

(6) consumer health education;

(7) accident prevention and emergency care;

(8) protection from hazards of poisons, drugs, and narcotics;

(9) community health; and

(10) health careers.

The health teacher needs a good background in personal and community health, communicable disease, school hygiene, educational psychology, modern teaching technique, and secondary education, with a good understanding of the programs of physical education, home economics, student counseling, first aid, and health service. The big high schools can us of the full time of a teacher in health courses.

In the smaller high schools the teacher must teach some other subject, such as for example, biology, or physical education. Adequate teaching facilities include a classroom providing an instructional area with furniture which can be arranged for individual or group work, a demonstration desk at the front of the room storage space for supplies and apparatus, bulletin board display areas, and source materials in the form of supplementary printed mater, charts, films and models.

The office of the teacher or a small conference room is needed for regular hours set aside for health conselling. Practices and opinions have varied with respect to the grade distribution, course organization, and time allotment of health teaching in the secondary school.

One procedure has been to teach health one period a week throughout the secondary school on the basis that the student would have a continuing stimulus toward more healthful living. Another procedure has been to make the health course a part of the course in physical education and to have the class meet for health education once or twice a week.

In some cases a teacher of physical education will be the health teacher, but experience indicates that the health course should be an entity in itself. Another procedure has been to try to put all of the health teaching into the science course. There is too much health subject matter to be presented through incidental teaching or as an occasional science unit.

Where health is taught by the science teacher, therefore, experience has led to the grouping of health units together into a health course which represented the instruction in science for a semester. Authoritative opinion now supports the policy of concentrating health instruction into courses which meet four or five times a week and insisting upon one such course in the eighth or ninth grade and another in the eleventh or twelfth grade.

The minimum time allotment for the junior high school health course should be a daily period for at least two semesters, during the seventh, eighth, or ninth grades. The minimum time allotment for the health course in the senior high school should be a daily period for at least two semesters. preferably during the eleventh or twelfth grades. health courses should receive credit equal to that given for courses in other areas.

Health courses should be given in regular classrooms, adequately equipped. The classes should be comparable in size to those in other subject matter areas. Home nursing is often taught by a school nurse with the required preparation in health education, as a separate subject or unit of instruction in the program of ninth or tenth grade girls. The intensive health problem course given in grade 11 or 12 deals with all the major health problems of effective living. It is adapted to the current health needs of the students; but it also recognizes that these young people are soon to be confronted with new health problems as they become workers, citizens, and parents.

There is an increasing demand for instruction that is related in a practical way to the after-school life of boys and girls whose formal education terminates with the senior high school The value of practical health instruction in enabling a boy or girl to secure and hold a job is being increasingly appreciated. Employers desire young people of good health and good personal appearance.

They also wish the employee to possess the poise, emotional balance, and social adjustment that accompany good mental health. The following statement is quoted from Planning for Health Education in Schools, published jointly by the United Nations Educational Scientific and Cultural organization and the World Health Organization. It may be helpful to curriculum committees to see a list of the subjects of instruction found in secondary school health curricula.

The scope of the different topics varies and the sub-topics listed below the distributed differently in different outlines. The following pages do not suggest what should be taught in secondary schools or any specific country, district or community. The choice will be based upon the important health problems and health needs of the students involved, upon the available time and facilities and upon the belief and practices which may need to be changed.

The digestive system, the circulatory system, the sense organs, the nervous system, the excretory system, the skin, physiological development related to adolescence, growth patterns individual differences. Food and growth, food groups, food values, adequate diet, food selection, the handling and care of food, preservation of foods, habits of eating.

Exercise and rest, sleep, study, relaxation, recreation, the use of leisure time, values of physical activity, individual health needs, daily schedule. Emotions, understanding one's self, personality, getting along with others at home and at school, accepting reality, interrelationship o physical emotional, and social factors, personal appearance grooming posture.

Health examinations correcting defects, alcohol, tobacco, narcotics, dental care, care of the sense organs, dangers of self-medication. Most curricula emphasize the importance of the family, the relationships within the family, the care of the children, and the care of the sick. Differences in instruction are found in what is taught regarding maturation, sex hygiene, population growth, boy and girl relationships, and social customs of engagement and marriage.

In some countries rather extensive instruction is given in those matters, in other countries very little in given. Safety at home and at school, sage transportation, safe recreation, bicycles, steps in the prevention of accidents. Individual health needs, sleep and rest, recreation, exercise, body mechanics, study, daily schedule, grooming, dress.

Family living, child care, heredity and eugenics, choosing a mate, preparing for marriage, marriage and the establishment of a home, housing, medical care for the family, planned parenthood. dental services, needs and costs of health maintenance. Consideration of venereal diseases, respiratory diseases, other common communicable diseases, and such organic diseases as cancer, heart disease, diabetes, and mental illness.

Nutritional needs, metabolism, vitamins, carbohydrates, fats proteins meal planning, food values, nutritional deficiencies and diseases, school gardens and the cultivation of desirable foods, food conservation, food preservation, food adulteration, food sanitation, food additives, digestive hygiene and digestive disorders, diarrhea and other intestinal infections, indigestion, colitis, appendicitis.

Expenditures for health, adequate health care, fads, quackery, consumer protection and truth in the adverting of health products, sources of information about health, distribution of health expenses, insurance against sickness and accidents the evaluation of advertising appeals. Water supply, waste disposal, drug control, radiation, air pollution, insect control, rat control, governmental health agencies, voluntary health agencies individual responsibility for community health.

Drug dependence, habituation, addiction, dangerous drugs and their effects, alcohol and alcoholism, injurious effects of smoking. Consideration of such professions as medicine, public health, dentistry, social work, nursing teaching, nutrition, dietetics, hospital administration, occupational therapy, physical education, medical records, medical illustration, radiological technology, therapeutic recreation, dental laboratory assistant, histologic technology, and public health or hospital laboratory services.

A good lecture presents information efficiently and quickly. The higher the educational level, the more effectively it can be used; but even at the college level, a series of lectures is usually supplemented by discussion and quiz sections. In the secondary school, the teacher gives few full-period lectures, but he commonly talks to the class at some length in introducing or summarizing a unit of study or in presenting a demonstration or in outlining an experiment. A lecture does not have to be any given length. Lincoln's Gettysburg Address was a talk of about 3 minutes.

The teacher commonly gives three or four short "lectures" interspersed with discussion in a class period. These presentations need careful planning. The quality of a lecture-type presentation is so important to its acceptance by the student and its contribution to learning that some thought may be given to the method of making it as useful as possible.

There is an old saying that the lecturer should tell his audience what he is going to tell them; tell them; then tell them what he has told them. In other words, the lecturer should have an attention getting beginning, with an introduction, telling what he is going to try to do and how he expects to do it. The basic framework o the lecture should be simple, with a few main points. Visual materials should be drawn upon when they are useful.

The teacher's appearance before the class is important. Impressions are derived from the manner in which he stands and walks, his muscular tensions, his eye movements, his gestures, his voice, and his inflections. There is an unlimited number of possible special projects of interest to secondary school students, including surveys and special investigations in the community and in the library.

Surveys may be made of student interests in health, of accident hazards, of sanitary conditions, of dental health, of voluntary health agencies in the community, of clinic and hospital facilities, of morbidity and mortality rates. Investigations which can be carried out in the library include a study of state laws and regulations regarding safety in hunting or boating, problems of world population growth, and activities of international health agencies.

Careful advance planning is needed with the students and with the host establishment to make sure that the trip is not merely an excursion or an outing. At its best, the field trip allows the community to serve as a laboratory in which the student clarifies his concepts, gains skill in observation, and learns how to report observations clearly and accurately. Profitable visitations are made to health departments, public health laboratories, hospitals and clinics, food procession plants, museums, traffic courts, and many other places.

Stimulating enrichment in the study of some health topics can be brought to high school students by members of the health professions and representatives of health-related occupations, speaking at a school assembly or to students enrolled in health classes. The contribution of such speakers in integrated into the program of study and in not substituted for units of work on important themes.

The speaker should be advised as to the age group, what will be expected of him, and the exact time and place of meeting. From the health department, the health officer himself may be available to present public health programs or special health problems of the community. The public health educator may discuss health education campaigns with the adult population.

The sanitary engineer or director of sanitation and the director of public health nursing may help with health problems in their respective fields. The country medical society and country dental society are usually ready to provide speakers on special medical and dental topics, such as mental health, alcoholism, the dangers of drugs, narcotics and self-medication, dental caries, and the fluoridation of water supplies.

An industrial physician may discuss health in industry. A nutritionist may discuss weight control, special diets, and the relation of nutrition to general health. The police chief may discuss safety ordinances; a beautician may discuss beauty practices: a milk inspector may discuss the sanitary control of the milk supply.

In larger communities, voluntary health agencies can supply experts in their special interests, such as tuberculosis, diabetes, arthritis, epilepsy, safety, first aid, and home nursing. In the legislative activity of cities, states, and nations, regulations, standards, codes, and laws and set according to the same basic procedures.

In the health class, a small group may be assigned the task of drafting a proposals and presenting it to the class as a whole for class discussion. This procedure might be used, for example, in the development of standards for safety and courtesy in driving an automobile, hygienic standards for athletic training, daily dietary requirements,m the responsibility of the citizen for public health, training requirements for baby sitters, standards for unitary housing, safety practices in bathing and swimming, requirements of an ideal recreation, desirable procedures in consumer hygiene, the control of quackery of the criteria of emotional maturity.

Health Education Curriculum

Many school administrators have not yet reached a clear understanding of the nature of a health-education programme that develops habits and attitudes along with its health information. Some confuse such a programme with a physical-education programme of big-muscle activity. Other feel that if they have school doctors and school nurses, the children will receive health training from them. Others think that individual teachers can do a splendid piece of work without a health-education curriculum. The benefits of a definite health-education curriculum are these:

— It makes clear to the teacher that the administrator in charge of the school expects health education to be a part of the school programme.

— It makes clear to the teacher what is expected at the grade level where he is at work. It gives him specific objectives. It avoids the same programme for an individual child in two or three successive grades.

— It provides the necessary class time.

— It gives the teacher suggestions and methods for developing the work.

— It suggested methods of measuring results.

There are three different methods for developing a health education curriculum. The first method is through experimentation by an individual or a small group of people working together over a period of several years. This method was used in the city of Malden where the writer, with the assistance of a special supervisor of health education, developed a curriculum during a period of about ten years.

The teachers participated in the testing of various health-education procedures in the different grades. They contributed, developed, and tested many original ideas. The feature that distinguishes this procedure from the two to be mentioned below is the actual experimentation in all grades by one individual, as contrasted with the observation of work in different grades by a director of health education or by general supervisors.

The second method, which is in complete contrast to the first, is the familiar one in which the school system concerned makes little or no original contribution. Everybody knows of curricula that are of the scissors-and-paste variety. Probably these are not altogether to be scorned. We cannot expect every school system to prepare its own curriculum in spite of the fact that new life and interest will be produced thereby if it involves teacher cooperation.

Many communities will take the best that has been produced in other places and adapt it to the needs without an extensive curriculum-building process. It is probably better to do this unless adequate time, thought, and skill for curriculum-making can be provided. This is, in effect, the procedure followed when a city uses the state course of study.

The third, and more common, method is the construction of a curriculum by committee activity. To some extent this method draws upon both of the other two, because the members of the committees have experience to bring to their work and use published materials from all good available sources. Committees must include experts in the field of health and in the various field of education. They should also include experts in teaching at the different grade levels.

For that reason it is usually customary to have a central committee and a committee of teachers from each grade. On the central committee the school administration should be represented by the superintendent or an assistant superintendent or supervisor. A principal may also be included.

The various special health services - medical service, nursing, perhaps the dental services, and the fields of physical education and nutrition - should also be represented. If there is a department of psychology and a department of research in the school system, persons from these departments should be on the committee. Professional leadership for the whole programme of wok should rest upon the best qualified expert in health education available.

The science of hygiene and public health is in a position to state certain needs common to practically all children. The other possible procedure is to gather direct information concerning the needs of the children and adults in the community. Both procedures are useful. In the study of the specific situation, it is well worth while for the health expert to review the causes of health in the community and to determine in relation to each of these what habits, knowledge, and attitudes would be helpful in prevention.

In many school systems the teacher does not know what medical service is rendered by the school medical staff. Many teachers do not dare to open the windows in their schoolrooms, no matter how high the temperature goes, because of the wrath of the janitor. There should be, and there usually is, some approved procedure by which the teacher can get relief from an overheated classroom. Such provisions should be clearly stated in the course of study, which is in the hands of every teacher.

Toward the end of the nineteenth century some new ideas were introduced into school curricula. This resulted from a feeling on the part of certain individuals that the evil effect of alcoholic beverages should be taught. They also felt there should be a greater emphasis on the hygienic aspects of living. As a result, these concepts became an important part of health teaching, especially in colleges. This emphasis continued until the early twentieth century.

Then, the impact of World Wars I and II gave health education the impetus it needed to become firmly imbedded as an important part of the school programme. The public became aroused, for example, by the number of defects discovered in young men through selective service examinations. There has been an increased emphasis on the school health programme because of this public concern. Results of this emphasis have included passing state laws, developing courses of study publishing many textbooks dealing with health education, and providing for the training of special teachers in this area.

Today, there is increased recognition that health education can play a very important role in helping to make individuals aware of their responsibility for not only their own health but also that of others. Health is rapidly being regarded as "everybody's business." It has been pointed out that this chapter is primarily concerned with health education. It is interested in those knowledges, attitudes, and practices essential to good health.

School health services and healthful school living are also important. The success of a school health programme is dependent upon the successful functioning and coordination of all three. Health education can play an important part in motivating children in the development of healthful habits and attitudes. Superstitions and fads can be proved unsound as a result of developing an attitude of appreciation for scientifically accurate knowledge.

Such an attitude recognizes the importance of consulting qualified medical persons in regard to health matters, the dangers of self-diagnosis and self-medication, the need to distinguish between fact and fallacy, and the importance of obtaining health information from authoritative sources. The manner in which health education is administered will vary with the local situation.

In many schools it is placed in such areas as physical education, science, and home economics. In other schools it is a separate area by itself. In the larger schools especially, it seems important to have a separate health education department with full-time personnel who have been trained in the area of health education.

Such an administrative arrangement is conducive to good interrelationships between the school and public health agencies, to the development of a school health council, and to a well-coordinated and well-integrated school health programme. In smaller and medium-sized schools where inadequate budgets made it impossible to have full-time health educators, physical education personnel or others closely related and interested in the area of school health may be charged with this important responsibility.

In many cases, with pressure for winning teams, the class instruction programme is neglected. School administrators should recognize that health education is a very important part of the school offering. As such, it should not be placed just anywhere in the school structure and assigned to that person who happens to have a little training in this particular area, or whose interests and teaching load make it feasible.

It should be given only to qualified persons and should receive ample time and facilities to make it effective. Every school, regardless of size, should have someone on its staff assigned to coordinate the various aspects of the school health programme. In larger schools this might be a full-time position.

In smaller schools it could be the principal, physical education teacher, or some qualified staff member who has interest and responsibility in this area. The school health educator, according to the Committee on Terminology, is "a person specially qualified to serve as a teacher, consultant, coordinator, or supervision of health education in an individual school or a school system."

Health coordination, according to this same committee, is "the process of developing relationships within the school health programmes which contribute to harmonious action in the solution of problems relating to pupil health." A health coordinator can render valuable service in seeing that a well-rounded health programme exists.

Health instruction can be more carefully planned. In addition to the direct health teaching, there can also be provision for the correlation and integration of health instruction with many subject-matter areas. Resource materials can be provided for classroom and other teachers involved in health-teaching. School and community relationships can be developed. The total school health programme can be guided to function as an integrated whole.

Every school administrator should recognize the importance of the position and designate a person qualified for such a responsibility. The administration of the health education programme should also include a school health council or committee. The school health council, according to the committee on terminology, is "a representative group of persons recognized for the purposes of study, planning, and action aimed at the identification and solution of school health problems."

There is considerable knowledge and information that may be taught in health education. While all the literature that is available in such forms as textbooks, resource books, pamphlets, and promotional material it is important that content be selected with care. At the present time there is little uniformity in the content of health education courses being taught in the schools throughout the country. Content areas in health education should be selected on the basis of many pertinent factors. These include the interests and needs of children in any given locality; attitudes, understandings, and behaviour of any particular group; type of community in which the school is located; resources available; and the philosophy of the school and community.

Health knowledge is important and can be justified only as the pupils apply it to their own lives and the lives of individuals around them. Problems that affect them personally must be selected in preference to detailed information on general health. There is no one course of study or general health format that may be stated as being the best. Although the basic health needs of all individuals are similar in some aspects, the application of specific facts and information will be governed by the local situation. It has been pointed out that content areas in health education should be selected, to a certain degree, on the basis of the needs and interests of the children being served.

The American Association of School Administrators suggests seven ways in which this vital information may be obtained.

— First, interests and needs may be determined through an analysis of health records, which every school should keep in a cumulative manner and which certain such valuable information as the result of health appraisal and health counselling.

— Second, the teacher's observation offers some indication of interests, desires, and health problems.

— Third, tests of knowledge, attitudes, and habits uncover superstitions and other health problems, together with the accuracy of the health knowledge possessed by the student.

— Fourth, conferences with parents, teachers, and pupils reveal many health interests and needs.

— Fifth, a student-interest survey will offer an indication of the interests in the field of health, as the students themselves see them.

— Sixth, a study of current literature concerned with scientific information in the field of health is essential. New knowledge and new health problems are revealed each day through experimentation and research on the part of the medical and other professions.

— Finally, a study of the health of the community is imperative, in order to know the health problems that are peculiar to the local setting with its own industrial, housing, sanitation, water supply, and other problems which characterize it.

Although the specific course of study will vary from community to community it is still necessary to recognize that the basic health needs of children and the general content areas of health education are similar. To a great degree, what takes place is the specific adaptation of these general areas to the local situations. It seems important for the general information of the reader to point out some of the basic health needs of children and also the general health, content areas, as listed by the leaders in the field.

There are many health needs that are common to children at various age levels, although they may manifest themselves differently. She lists and discusses eleven basic health needs with which those interested in health education should be concerned. These are:

— food and eating,

— elimination of body wastes.

— exercise and play,

— sleep and rest,

— eyes and ears,

— teeth,

— posture

— illnesses and disease,

— accidents and injuries.

— emotional adjustments, and

— sex adjustments.

The fact that some of these problems are more pronounced in certain communities, and possibly restricted to some population groups, together with the fact that some education might tend to stimulate curiosity, are reasons put forth for not including them in courses of study. On the other hand, instruction in regard to the ill effects of narcotics and alcohol is required by law in many states. Furthermore, it is felt that if children and youth are provided with the facts, intelligent instruction in these subjects will act as a preventive measure.

In the area of sex education, it is believed that the term "sex education" creates opposition among many parents and church groups and consequently should not be used. If it is introduced in the natural process of instruction without undue emphasis, much good can be done. Some of the best thinking in the fields emphasize the fact that the nature of the instruction will depend upon the local situation.

Where a narcotics or alcohol problem exists, there should be provision in the school curricula for the presentation of sociological, physiological, and psychological facts, as well as the legal aspects of such a problem. Students should understand these facts and be guided intelligently in making the right decisions and establishing a sound standard of values.

Health education is not the only area in which discussions of sex, narcotics and alcohol should take place. Social studies, biology, general science, physical education, and other classes also have a responsibility. Many phases of these subjects logically fit into certain aspects of these courses. Teachers most appreciate the importance of such instruction and the need for dealing with these subjects objectively on the basic of the facts. It is not necessary for the teacher to take a definite stand and act in the capacity of a minister preaching on the subject.

Instead, if students obtain the necessary facts through research or some other methods and then interpret them intelligently, the right answers will be clear. The students make their own decisions, not on the basis of the teacher's position but on the basis of the facts which they have collected. In regard to sex education, the emphasis should be more on the moral and sociological aspects rather than only on the biological aspects.

The end result should be to have students recognize what is desirable behaviour and what constitutes high moral standards rather than only to become acquainted with a body of factual knowledge such as that concerned with the reproductive organs. Students should be taught to live the finest type of lives possible. Sex education should not be a separate course but should be included and discussed in every course where its various aspects arise during regular discussions.

Parents and representative community groups should be consulted and asked to participate in any discussions relative to the planning for instruction in this area. It is very important to have well-trained and qualified teachers handling such instruction. Health education at the elementary level is aimed primarily at having the child develop good health habits and health attitudes, and live happily, healthfully, and safely. This is achieved in great measure by adapting good health practices to the regular routine of school and home living, rather than by dispensing technical, factual knowledge concerning health.

The type of health programme offered should be adapted to the child's level and planned in accordance with his or her interests and needs. It should also be remembered that health education is a continuous process and cannot be compartmentalized within a definite subject area or within a class period.

It embraces all the activities and subjects that are a part of the child's life. It is difficult to prescribe the amount of time that should be devoted to the teaching of health on the elementary level because the needs and interests of pupils vary. However, the amount of time devoted to health education should be equal to the other major areas of the curriculum. At the primary grade level the emphasis should be more on the child and his daily routine as affected by certain health practices and attitudes. His various routines and associations at school and at home form the basis for the health emphasis.

The importance of a healthful classroom environment is stressed. Such items as cleanliness, eating, use of lavatories, safety, and good mental hygiene are brought out as the child plays, eats, and performs those many experiences which are common to all youngsters of his age. In the upper elementary years the values of certain health practices are brought out. A planed progression in instruction is developed.

Although there is still stress on the actual practices and attitude concerned with the daily routines and associations, more factual information is incorporated to form the basis for such habits. Furthermore, more and ore responsibility is placed on the child for his own self-direction and self-control. The utilization of trips and textbooks which point up the value of healthful living, interesting and inspiring stories, visual aids, class discussions, and projects can become a part of the experiences of each child so that the need for certain behaviour is dramatically and effectively stamped upon his mind and total being.

Since health experiences should be based on the needs and interests of the child, the wise teacher will utilize various means of obtaining accurate information about these needs and interests. Such techniques as talks with parents and pupils, observations of children under various situations, a perusal of health records, a study of the home environment and community together with scientific measuring devices that have been developed to determine health knowledge and attitudes will be utilized. According to the American Association of School Administrators' Twentieth Yearbook, the health problems that confront and interest children in the primary grades include such topics as:

1. growth and health,
2. nutrition,
3. elimination,

4. exercise, relaxation, rest, sleep;
5. personal hygiene,
6. prevention and control of disease,
7. care of eyes and ears,
8. medical and dental attention,
9. emotional and social adjustment, and
10. safety.

These various subjects would of course be adapted to the child at the primary school age. At the intermediate level the health problems would cover many of the same topics with information and experiences being adapted to the level of this child. These topics include.

1. growth and health,
2. nutrition,
3. exercise, relaxation, rest, and sleep,
4. personal hygiene,
5. care of eyes and ears, and
6. prevention and control of disease.

The classroom teacher is the key school person involved in the health of the elementary school child. The organization of the school with the self-contained classroom enables her to continually observe the pupils and to note deviations from normal. Continuous contact with the same children over a long period of time also makes it possible for her to know a great deal about their physical, social, emotional, and mental health.

She can help them develop the right knowledge, attitudes, and practices. Some of the responsibilities which fall to the classroom teacher in regard to the health of her pupils require that she do the following:

— Possess an understanding of what constitutes a well-rounded school health programme and the teacher's part in it.

— Meet with the school physician, nurse, and others in order to determine how she can best contribute to the total health programme.

— Become acquainted with the parents and homes of her students. Establish parent-school cooperation.

— Discover the health needs and interests of her pupils.

— Organize health teaching units which are meaningful and in terms of the health needs and interests of her students.

— See that children needing special care are referred to proper places for help.

— Be versed in first-aid procedures.

— Participate in work of the school health council. If none exists, interpret the need for one.

— Provide an environment for children while at school which is conductive to healthful living.

— Continually be on the alert for children with deviations from normal behaviour and signs of communicable diseases.

— Provide experiences for living healthfully at school.

— Help pupils assume an increasing responsibility for their own health as well as the health of others.

— Set an example for the child of what constitutes healthful living.

— Motivate the child to be well and happy.

— Be present at health examination of pupils and contribute in any way which is helpful to physician in charge.

— Follow through in cooperation with nurse to see that remediable health defects are corrected.

— Interpret the school health programme to the community and enlist its support in solving health problems.

— Provide a well-rounded class physical education programme.

— Help supervise various activities which directly affect health, i.e. school lunch, rest periods, etc.,

— Become familiar with teaching aids and school and community resources for enhancing the health programme.

— Be aware of the individual differences of pupils.

Schools should play a key part in adult education programmes through the facilities, staff, and other resources at their disposal. They should cooperate fully with the many official and voluntary health agencies, and other interested community groups, in the furtherance of health objectives. Adult education programmes in the area of health should be designed to discover community health problems, understand the health needs of children, and understand school health programmes. The health of school children is a most important consideration for educators, parents, physicians, and others who desire to develop a fit populace.

A good school health service programme is an essential in the achievement of this goal. Without satisfactory health services, the health of school children cannot be adequately developed maintained and projected. The history of health services shows that in early schools the stress was mainly on providing sanitary facilities and a clean environment. This was accomplished through a system of inspections and procedures. As more thinking has been given to this subject, however, there has been increased attention focused on those measures essential to the maintenance and improvement of the child's health.

As a result, physicians, dentists, and other specialists have become more closely related in the schools. In turn, this has meant better detection of health defects, a more complete follow-through to insure the correction of such defects, more adequate means for preventing and controlling communicable disease, an increased realization of the potentialities of the medical examination as an educational tool, and more attention the to the eyes, throat, ears, nose, and teeth.

As the need fro better health services are recognized by the public at large, state laws were passed to provide these services. These laws required such procedures as periodic medical examinations and regular checking of vision and hearing. They also stressed the need for school nurses, who trained not only in their particular area but also in the field of education.

The child who is a "suspect" in regard to some communicable disease should immediately be isolated from the group. This is the rule of thumb that should be followed. Isolating a child does not constitute diagnosis. The details and procedures followed in each school regarding isolation should be in writing and clearly understood by all concerned.

The school is responsible for providing each child with the necessary protection and care. The school acts in loco parent is and it is assumed that the child will receive the same care and protection during the hours of school that he normally would receive at home. Children often become sick or injured during school hours. Therefore, the school must provide the necessary attention until this can be undertaken by the parents.

3

Health Education: Controlling HIV/AIDS Transmission to Children

By the end of 2001, over 40 million people were living with HIV/AIDS, nearly 25 million people had died of AIDS, and more than 15.6 million children under the age of 15 had lost their mother or both parents. As well as the human tragedy, the epidemic has a profound impact on growth and poverty: the United Nations Programme on HIV/AIDS estimates a loss of more than 20 percent of gross domestic product in the worst-affected countries by 2020.

The epidemic's grip on Africa has been by far the deadliest, but no part of the world is immune. The epidemic is on the upswing globally, spreading fastest in Eastern Europe, but also rising in the Caribbean. Data from Asia warn against complacency: national prevalence rates are currently low, but in some countries are similar to those in West Africa that are now recognized to be at the beginning of an epidemic, while India is second only to South Africa in the number of people currently infected.

Most devastating and far-reaching, perhaps, is the epidemic's impact on education systems. HIV/AIDS is draining the supply of education, eroding its quality, weakening demand and access, drying up countries' pools of skilled workers, and increasing the sector's costs. The full scope of the epidemic's impact on education becomes apparent when viewed in the context of the formidable challenges already confronting the sector.

More than 113 million school-age children are out of school in developing countries, two-thirds of them girls. Of those who enter school, one out of four drops out before attaining literacy. At least 55 of the poorest countries seem unlikely to achieve EFA by 2015, and 31 of these countries are also among the 36 worst-affected by HIV/AIDS. The time for business-as-usual is past.

No country can afford not to act. The worst-affected countries need to arrest the epidemic's ravages and protect future generations, while low-prevalence countries need to recognize the speed with which complacency can lead to crisis and the tremendous opportunity for saving lives and financial resources through prevention.

Countries need to accelerate their efforts toward achieving EFA goals, both because of the importance of education for a country's viability and because of the critical role it can play in preventing HIV/AIDS. Education is a major engine of economic and social development. It drives a country's future.

Economic prosperity and the reduction of global poverty cannot be accomplished unless all children in all countries have access to, and can complete, a primary education of adequate quality. It is pivotal to the achievement of several of the Millennium Development Goals, adopted unanimously by 189 countries in September 2000.

Education has powerful poverty-reducing synergies: one year of schooling for women lowers fertility by about 10 percent, while one or two years of schooling for mothers reduces child mortality by 15 percent. Education is a proven means to prevent HIV/AIDS. It has been proven to provide protection against HIV infection.

A general basic education has an important preventive impact. It can equip children and youth to make healthy decisions concerning their own lives, bring about long-term healthy behaviors, and give people the opportunity for economic independence and hope.

It is among the most powerful tools for reducing girls' vulnerability. Girls' education can go far in slowing and reversing the spread of HIV by contributing to female economic independence, delayed marriage, family planning, and work outside the home. It offers a ready-made infrastructure for delivering HIV/AIDS prevention efforts to large numbers of the uninfected population-schoolchildren-as well as youth, who in many countries are the age group most at risk.

It is highly cost-effective as a prevention mechanism, because the school system brings together students, teachers, parents, and the community, and preventing AIDS through education avoids the major AIDS-related costs of health care and additional education supply. Full speed ahead on EFA goals is vital. A general basic education-and not merely instruction on prevention-is among the strongest weapons against the HIV/AIDS epidemic.

An urgent, strategic, and education-centered response by countries and their partners is of utmost importance. HIV/AIDS has an impact on the supply of education. While reliable data are limited, there is little doubt that the epidemic is seriously damaging the quantity and quality of education.

Africa in particular appears to be experiencing sharp increases in mortality rates among teachers and administrators at all levels of education. Even where teachers are present, they may be sick and ineffective, or poorly qualified as schools either make do with whoever is available, or cut corners on training. There is also an impact on the demand for education.

For most countries, increases in the school-age population are expected. While the school-age population will be smaller than in the absence of AIDS, it will nonetheless continue to grow. Estimates by the U.S. Bureau of Census suggest that only 6 of the 26 countries worst affected by AIDS will show an actual reduction in the school-age population by 2015.

In some countries, but not all, there is evidence of lower enrollment and higher dropout rates among orphans, perhaps particularly at the secondary and tertiary levels. Although the evidence is still unclear, the epidemic may reduce girls' access to education at all levels. Girls are highly vulnerable to contracting AIDS because of social, cultural, economic, and physiological reasons, and compared with boys are more often retained at home.

The World Bank has estimated the cost of achieving EFA by 2015 in low-income countries. As part of these analyses, a preliminary estimate has been made of the additional costs of achieving EFA that might be attributable to the impact of HIV/AIDS on education systems. HIV/AIDS is estimated to add between US$450 million and US$550 million per year to the cost of achieving EFA in the 33 African countries studied.

This implies that HIV/AIDS increases the total EFA external financing gap for these countries by about one-third. HIV/AIDS increases education sector costs. On the supply side, budgets are having to accommodate higher teacher hiring and training costs to replace teachers who have died of AIDS, as well as the payment of full salaries to sick teachers who are absent and additional salary costs for substitute teachers.

Zambia has estimated the epidemic's financial burden on the supply of teachers to amount to some US$25 million between 2000 and 2010, and Mozambique's estimate is about twice as much. Neither estimate includes demand-side costs, yet efforts to reach orphans and other vulnerable children are a rapidly growing new expenditure, especially in the worst-affected countries.

Providing a basic education to children-while ensuring equal opportunities for girls-is among the most promising directions in responding to the AIDS epidemic. Supporting children, especially girls, to complete their secondary education is also a powerful tool in mitigating the circumstances that put youth at risk.

Countries that have emphasized access as well as the quality of learning and sought innovative responses to long-standing constraints have seen the greatest advances. Projecting the future needs of the education sector is an essential part of education planning.

For the worst-affected countries there is an immediate need to protect and replace teachers; for all countries there is a longer-term need to ensure the stability and quality of supply. School-based prevention programs. Reproductive health programs begin in primary schools, with the aim of reaching students before they begin sexual activity, but must continue through all levels of education.

The Focusing Resources on Effective School Health (FRESH) framework, which aims to focus resources on effective school health, was created by a partnership among the United Nations Educational, Scientific, and Cultural Organization; the World Health Organization; the United Nations Children's Fund; the World Bank; and others to provide a unified approach to school health. Skills-based health education.

Information about sex and HIV is insufficient by itself to bring about low-risk behaviors, but must be linked with the development of interpersonal and other skills, such as critical and creative thinking, decisionmaking, and self-awareness, as well as with the development of the knowledge, attitudes, and values needed to make sound health-related decisions.

Peer education and focus on youth. A powerful means to influence youth, peer education by respected students or other youth of the same age can help develop healthy behaviors and practices. Support for orphans and out-of-school youth. The burgeoning numbers of these disad-vantaged children, and the lack of understanding of the constraints on their education, pose an enormous new challenge for which no tested solutions are available.

The combination of little experience and weak data is potentially explosive and urgently needs attention.

Innovation, cross-sectoral efforts, and information sharing to learn lessons quickly are essential to ensure that these children obtain a basic education. Multimedia campaigns.

Countries can create support for and understanding of education sector HIV/AIDS prevention activities and promote community support by using communication strategies to reach large numbers of people through multiple channels: prime time television series, radio dramas, booklets, and other materials.

The success of the approaches described here depends heavily on strong collaboration and partnership across sectors, across stakeholders within a country (communities, families, government, the private sector, and nongovernmental organizations), and with and across international agencies. A broad strategic response rooted in education-and set within a national, multisectoral context-is essential for all countries.

Responses to the HIV/AIDS epidemic have too often been piecemeal, small-scale, health-focused, and weakly integrated into related efforts. Strong political commitment is key to addressing such shortcomings. Particularly in low-prevalence countries, governments will need to recognize early on that complacency can be disastrous. The following three elements are central to an effective strategy:

— *Define objectives and targeted outcomes*: The starting point for an effective response is thus the affirmation of EFA goals and the express recognition that the education sector could be fortified to become a country's strongest weapon against HIV/AIDS, or, failing that, its worst victim, reversing decades of hard-won gains. Ensuring that children, especially girls, complete their secondary education is key to mitigating the circumstances that place youth at risk. Equally important is the need to establish key outcomes that can be monitored.

— *Expand the knowledge base*: A prerequisite for effective action is an adequate knowledge base to inform the development of immediate and long-term responses. Success will hinge on a strategy tailored to national circumstances. This step involves estimating the impact of HIV/AIDS on education supply and demand and on prospects for achieving EFA goals.

— *Identify appropriate actions, informed by a stocktaking process*: It urges the development of a country-specific action program comprising measures drawn from a menu of promising approaches. Priorities of universal relevance are educating girls, delivering prevention messages to teachers and students at all levels, and ensuring that the supply of education is adequate in quality and quantity in relation to expected demand.

Countries will have to establish not only that need exists, but also that resources are being effectively used and producing results. Policy reforms aimed at improving educational quality-and that help keep children in school-also serve to substan-tially lower countries' costs of achieving EFA and preventing HIV/AIDS. The World Bank is a long-standing partner in the efforts of the poorest countries to educate their people, and is the largest external source of financing for education and for HIV/AIDS activities worldwide.

The Bank is committed to supporting the world in an education-centered fight against AIDS, an objective that resonates strongly with its mission of poverty reduction. This fits squarely within the Bank's strategic framework, which emphasizes support for investment in people and progress toward the Millennium Development Goals.

The Bank's work in education is centered on two priorities:

— The first is EFA, which includes the objectives of universal primary education and gender equity in schooling.

— Second, the Bank's strategy for education recognizes that EFA is a first step along the continuum of lifelong learning to provide education for the knowledge economy, which is crucial to the development of skills and competencies that will strengthen national competitiveness in the global arena.

An urgent challenge is to integrate HIV/AIDS issues into the Bank's dual-focused support, as has most recently voiced by the Group of Eight Task Force on Education, established in 2001 to accelerate progress on EFA. For the Bank, this directive implies helping countries to pursue overall education goals more vigorously while factoring in the epidemic's impact, and to ensure adequate education aimed specifically at HIV/AIDS prevention.

The broad principles that underlie all Bank support for education are as follows:

— *Scaling up successful approaches*: The Bank is working with partners to support countries throughout Africa in assessing the impact of HIV/AIDS on their education systems and planning an appropriate response using the Education and HIV/AIDS (Ed-

SIDA/AIDS) approach, and to implement skills-based school health programs based on the FRESH framework.

— *Mobilizing resources*: The Bank is reinforcing political commitment for EFA, both as an end in itself and as an important weapon in fighting AIDS. There is a need to increase both the overall level of external support and the share of resources allocated to education.

The Bank is currently financing 143 education projects implemented in 78 countries, reflecting investments of US$9.7 billion. During the last five years, new commitments for girls' education projects have averaged nearly 60 percent of total primary and secondary education lending.

The Bank supports countries in modifying existing projects and in ensuring that new EFA and girls' education projects include a specific response to HIV/AIDS wherever relevant. All social sector projects may support education, and there is a specific aim to increase support for orphans and other vulnerable children.

A total of US$36 billion in debt savings has been committed to 24 countries, where social spending is now projected to increase by some US$2.2 billion per year. Early indications are that some 40 percent of these extra resources will be directed to education and 25 percent to health. The multisectoral Multicountry HIV/AIDS Program for Africa has committed US$462.5 million to 12 countries, and a similar initiative has made US$53.5 million available to Caribbean countries.

The Bank is helping countries to draw on worldwide and regional best practice and to undertake analytical work to ensure sound approaches and effective use of resources, and is evaluating the impact of education system approaches across several countries. Expanding and consolidating Web-based "gateways" is another priority.

The Bank is also working with partners to develop a sourcebook that brings together best practice on school-based prevention methods. Urgent priorities include assessing the impact of education responses to the AIDS epidemic and finding solutions to the challenges orphans and other vulnerable children face.

The Bank is a founding member of UNAIDS and a member of the United Nations Interagency Working Group on schools and education, a partnership that facilitates countries' development of strategic plans for HIV/AIDS prevention and impact management in education systems. The development and implementation of the FRESH framework and the Ed-SIDA/AIDS model are examples of the importance of partnerships in the fight against AIDS.

On EFA, the Bank is taking the lead in working with various partners to analyze the policy and resource gaps for meeting the goals and for assessing the impact of HIV/AIDS on the cost of achieving EFA. The Bank recognizes the need for innovative and flexible responses, in particular, for the worst-affected countries and the most vulnerable groups, such as orphans and youth.

Schools are the primary institutions able to reach the great majority of children and young people, while also having an impact at the community level. With the growing recognition that attitudes and beliefs are formed early in life, more reproductive health programs are being implemented in primary schools with the aim of reaching students before they become sexually active and, in many cases, drop out of school.

Schools also have the benefit of staff equipped with the tools of teaching and learning, and in many developing countries teachers assume an important role in the community, while also serving as role models to many adolescents. In addition, schools may often be the only place where adolescents can obtain accurate information on repro-ductive health.

A study in Vietnam, for example, found teenagers complaining that discussions with adults about HIV/ AIDS often focused on morality rather than on the practicalities of prevention. School-based reproductive health programs vary greatly between and within countries. Programs could include one or more of these elements: family life or life skills education, sex education, HIV/AIDS education, and school-based health services.

With the spread of AIDS long-standing taboos on sex education are beginning to be relaxed. According to some researchers, most countries are seeking to develop school-based AIDS education as part of their wider public education strategies. In Zimbabwe subjects once avoided are now discussed frankly in the context of HIV/AIDS prevention.

In Trinidad and Tobago a survey of youths showing gross misinformation about AIDS prevention led to the rec-ommendation to add a comprehensive HIV/AIDS education program to secondary school curricula. Knowledge about how HIV/AIDS is transmitted can be embedded in the science curriculum. In countries where the curriculum is already overloaded, integrating new themes into existing subjects may be more effective than adding new ones.

The issues surrounding HIV/AIDS can also be addressed in civics, social studies, and "moral education" curricula. Recognizing and respecting diversity, and respecting and valuing all people as full individuals, can be powerful antidotes to the stigmatization of people affected and infected by HIV/AIDS.

4

School-based Health and Nutrition

In March 1990, in Jomtien, Thailand, for the World Conference on Education for All: Meeting Basic Learning Needs. Its goal was to 'launch a renewed worldwide initiative to meet the basic learning needs of all children, youth and adults and to reverse the serious decline in basic education'. The conference organizers chose a different approach: rather than focus on the traditional issues of how to provide school buildings, textbooks, and teachers, they decided to address the process of learning and the needs of the learners.

Health and nutrition were included as important contributors to the success of both the learner and the learning process. In preparation for the round table, 'School Performance, Nutrition and Health' at the Conference, UNESCO published a key document - Malnutrition and Infection in the Classroom -which presented the relationship between the status of children's nutrition and health and their performance in school.

In 1998, UNICEF estimated that out of 625 million children of primary school age, 79% were in school. The vast majority was receiving some basic education. It is also estimated that 70% of children in the developing world complete at least four years of schooling. Therefore, a school's potential to affect the health status and learning ability of an enormous number of the world's children stands before us. There are far more teachers than nurses or health-care workers in most countries.

The teaching corps around the world can deliver many health promotion and health service interventions easily and effectively, with benefits to the teachers themselves as well. They called for an expanded vision of basic education, one that recognized that 'education does not work in a vacuum or in isolation from other factors that have a bearing on society'.

Ultimately, the 1990 World Declaration of EFA and its articles recognized the relationship among health, education, and health/nutrition policies and programmes, stating that 'education can help ensure a safer, healthier, more prosperous and environmentally sound world' and 'learning does not take place in isolation. Societies must ensure that all learners receive the nutrition, health care, and general physical and emotional support they need in order to participate actively in and benefit from education'.

Conference participants addressed the link between health and education. For example, UNESCO and the World Food Programme organized a round table on 'School Performance, Nutrition and Health'. The participants concluded that to learn effectively, children need good health. Further, they asserted that malnutrition and poor health may be important factors in low school enrolment, absenteeism, poor classroom performance, and early school dropout.

Curriculum development must be based on the health needs of the different age groups and take into consideration the socio-cultural background of the schoolchildren. Curriculum development committees must include parents and community leaders. Personal and social development must, along with intellectual development, be given due weight in schools in order to foster values, attitudes, and behaviour conducive to health and well-being.

The teaching of school health education requires teacher preparation, guidelines, teacher learning material and curriculum support. Teacher training institutions must revise their courses in the light of this need. Team training of all categories of school personnel, including the health, administrative, and general staff, is recommended for a comprehensive school health programme.

The pivotal role of teachers in promoting health in the school and community needs to be given high priority. The support of teacher associations must be sought to increase the health awareness of teachers and encourage them to assume responsibility for being role models for health in the school and community.

Although the round tables on school health and education gave strong and clear guidance for improving school health programmes as a means of achieving education for all. Furthermore, no specific goals for school health and nutrition or indicators were established for the decade 1990-2000. In the decade since EFA, many publications and studies have elaborated on the link between learning and health status.

A WHO report states, 'As long ago as 1950 it has been noted that nutritional deficiencies and poor health in primary-school-age children are among the causes of low school enrolment, high absenteeism, early dropout, and poor classroom performance.

Health is thus a key factor in school entry as well as continued participation and attainment in school. Moreover, education that provides children with basic academic skills and specific knowledge, attitudes, and skills related to health is vital to their physical, psychological, and social well-being. This is not only true in the short term; such education lays the foundation for a child's healthy development through adolescence and across the entire lifespan'.

Nutritional deficiencies (protein-energy malnutrition, iron, Vitamin A, and iodine deficiency) and health problems such as helminth infections (especially schistosomiasis and infections with roundworm and other intestinal parasites) and malaria affect school participation and learning. A 1990 analysis of nine studies on the relationship between nutritional anthropometric indicators and school indicators showed that better nutritional status was consistently linked to higher cognitive test scores or better school performance.

Violence, unintentional injuries, suicidal tendencies and related lifestyle behaviours, such as the use of alcohol and other drugs, interfere with the learning process. Children exposed to violence may become highly aggressive, use psychoactive substances, or show other dysfunctional ways of dealing with anxiety.

This behaviour, in turn, may reduce attendance at school, impair concentration, and detrimentally affect cognitive development. Sexual behaviours, especially unprotected sex that results in HIV infection, other sexually transmitted diseases, and unwanted or too-early pregnancies, affect both students' and teachers' participation in education. These behaviours place at risk students who have successfully reached secondary school.

Too-early pregnancies negatively affect the education of young girls, who often must drop out of school. HIV/AIDS has already had a devastating impact on children in sub-Saharan Africa, where over 90% of all AIDS orphans live - most of them will never complete a basic education. It is important that most of these issues be addressed effectively through health, hygiene and nutrition policies and programmes for students and staff.

School-based nutrition and health interventions can improve academic performance. Students' health and nutrition status affects their enrolment, retention, and absenteeism. Multiple co-ordinated strategies produce a greater effect than individual strategies, but multiple strategies for any one audience must be targeted carefully. Evidence from around the world shows that treating nutritional and health conditions in school can improve academic performance. For example, some school food programmes have shown marked effects on attendance and school performance.

In Benin, children in schools with food services scored significantly higher on second-grade tests than did those in schools without food services. In Jamaica, providing breakfast to primary-school students significantly increased attendance and arithmetic scores.

In the United States, low-income children scored significantly lower in achievement tests than higher-income children before they participated in a school breakfast programme. Once children were in the programme, their scores improved more than the scores of non-participants.

Nutritional interventions such as micronutrient supplements and the treatment of intestinal worms have also proved to increase students' attention, cognitive problem-solving, and test scores. Research by the Ghana Partnership for Child Development showed that iron supplements - which could be effectively administered by teachers - lead to a very significant improvement in school performance for a period of up to six months.

In Malawi, when the diets of primary-school children were supplemented with iron as well as iodine, the gain in IQ scores was greater than with iodine supplements alone. Pollitt concluded that iron-deficient anaemic children showed lower aptitude when they first enrolled in school. However, this disadvantage disappeared once the children became iron-replete (e.g. through school-based supplementation).

In the West Indies, a single chemotherapy treatment for whipworm infection given to children at school, without nutritional supplements or improvements in education, improved the children's learning capacity to the point that their test scores matched those of children who were not infected.

Height and weight for age are typical markers for entering school, and children not tall or heavy enough might be denied access. Thus, children in good health are more likely to start school at the developmentally appropriate age. 'For example, in Nepal, a study found that the probability of attending school was 5% for stunted children and 27% for children of normal nutritional status'.

In Ghana, malnourished children entered school at a later age and completed fewer years of school than better-nourished children. School feeding programmes have been shown to lower absenteeism and dropout rates. A recent evaluation of a school feeding programme in Burkina Faso found that school food services were associated with regular attendance, consistently lower repeat rates, lower dropout rates, and higher success rates in national examinations, especially for girls.

In Malawi, a small pilot school-feeding programme over a three-month period led to a 5% increase in enrolment and up to a 35% improvement in attendance. In the Dominican Republic, up to 25% of children - especially those from rural areas and girls - dropped out of school during a period without a school feeding programme. Regular school attendance is one of the essential means of improving health. The school itself - through its culture, organization, and management; the quality of its physical and social environment; its curricula and teaching and learning methods; and the manner in which students' progress is assessed - has a direct effect on self-esteem, educational achievement, and therefore the health of students and staff.

Multiple years of schooling and the acquisition of literacy in several domains make it more likely that a person will be able to safeguard his or her health through living circumstances, earning power, access to health services, and general quality of life. Even a few years of schooling, evidence suggests, are associated with important changes of economic value in individual skills.

Schooling pays off with higher incomes and a healthier workforce.

Education can reduce social and gender inequities. Poor health at school age is often connected with poverty and gender. School health programmes have the potential to reduce inequities in society and to begin to break the cycle of poverty. 'Poor children with the worst health have the most to gain from school-based health and nutrition programs and the most to gain educationally.

During the twentieth century, 'education, skills and other knowledge have become crucial determinants of a person's and a nation's productivity. The primary determinant of a country's standard of living is how well it succeeds in developing and utilizing the skills, knowledge, health, and habits of its population'.

One major reason given for the dramatic differences in economic development between East Asia and Africa, for example, is the significantly higher level of investment that East Asia has made in the education and health care of its citizens. Thus, investments in education can have both short- and long-term benefits to an individual's health and the productivity of nations.

Girls, in particular, are likely to benefit: educated girls are likely to delay their first pregnancy and have fewer and healthier children. For example, data from thirteen African countries between 1975 and 1985 showed that a 10% increase in female literacy rates yielded a 10% reduction in child death rates. Schools are also places where girls' nutritional and reproductive health can be addressed early, thereby preventing later problems.

In Tamil Nadu, 'a school feeding programme attracted more girls to attend school and improved the attendance of those already in school. In addition to benefiting educationally, these girls had the opportunity to learn about family planning. As a result they had fewer children when they reached child-bearing age'.

The health of teachers is an important factor in the learning process. Teachers are the key to both education and health promotion in schools. They are caretakers of both the school and the students. Their health is thus critical to the achievement of EFA. While teachers must be trained about health matters affecting students, they also need training about taking care of their own health.

Inevitably, the physical and mental health of the staff affects students directly through the quality of teaching and the attributes of the school's psychosocial environment. Attending to teachers' health interests can motivate them to address students' health needs as well. Some studies of the effectiveness of health promotion programmes for school staff have shown that they decrease touchers' absenteeism and improve both their morale and the quality of classroom instruction.

Teachers who have participated in school health programmes reported improved attitudes towards their personal health and increased perceptions of general well-being. Other studies found that the school personnel's knowledge of and behaviours concerning health were positively affected. One staff programme in the United States demonstrated reductions in body weight, resting pulse rate, serum cholesterol level, and blood pressure.

Money invested in the prevention of health problems through the schools can save societal costs of treating disease. A recent study in the United States estimated that every US dollar invested in schools on effective tobacco education saves $18.80 in the cost of addressing problems caused by tobacco use; every US dollar spent on education for preventing alcohol and other drug abuse saves $5.69; and every US dollar spent on eduction to prevent early and unprotected sexual behaviour saves $5.10.

A 1993 World Bank analysis determined that a basic public-health package with five central elements could reduce the burden of disease for a relatively modest per capita cost. Extensive analyses of disease-control priorities have established that school-based treatments of children are exceptionally cost-effective.

For example, school nutrition and health programmes have been estimated to cost only $20 to $34 per disability-adjusted life year (DALY) gained, and school-based tobacco and alcohol prevention programmes cost $35 to $55 per DALY gained. Improving School Performance in the Developing World through Better Health and Nutrition, offers evidence that treating diseases prevalent in the school-age population can help to interrupt the transmission of disease to the surrounding community.

For example, on the Caribbean Island of Montserrat, more than 90% of schoolchildren aged 4 to 12 were treated at four-month intervals for two and a-half months with an antiworm drug. Infection rates declined to almost zero. While less than 4% of adults in the community received treatment during the same time, their rate of infection declined an almost equal amount because of reduced transmission from the school-age children.

Multiple co-ordinated strategies produce a greater effect than individual strategies, but multiple strategies for any one audience must be targeted carefully. Strategies for school health programmes at both the national and local level have, for the most part, been singular in their approach. However, research continues to show the positive impact of multiple and targeted co-ordinated strategies.

For example, a curriculum combined with youth community service is more effective in reducing risk behaviours such as fighting, early sexual behaviour, and substance use than a curriculum alone. Policies for tobacco-free schools, combined with a skills-based curriculum on tobacco prevention, are more effective than the curriculum alone.

In 1994 the Ghana Partnership for Child Development implemented a programme to treat parasitic infections in children through many schools in the Volta region. The programme used a combination of strategies, including clinical treatment, teacher and administrator training, and classroom education. Programme planners must then choose between providing a variety of strategies for a given population or focusing on a smaller number of activities.

The National Structured Evaluation of Alcohol and Drug Abuse Prevention in the United States undertook an analysis of more than 300 community-based substance abuse prevention initiatives. The researchers concluded that projects that attempted to offer more than three or four types of activity to a single adolescent population were generally ineffective. The study concluded that 'comprehensive prevention depends more on selecting appropriate activities and services for each population served than on trying to provide a wide variety of activities and services.

There may be an effective limit to the variety of activities that should be provided at a given time to a single population, beyond which the addition of a greater variety of activities adds little to measured effects of the prevention efforts'. The implication for school-based prevention is that planners need to select and target a few strategies to promote health, and to address the most serious health threats.

Health education aims not only to improve pupils' interest in health, their ability to relate what they learn to their own lives, and their understanding of basic ideas about health, but also to apply what they learn to the lives of their families and friends. To do so, health learning must emphasize skills development over simple information sharing, and provide opportunities for students to practice healthy behaviours or to address the conditions that promote health both personally and collectively.

Skills-based health education, including life skills, and interactive teaching methods have been shown to promote healthy lifestyles and reduce risk behaviours. A meta-analysis of 207 school-based drug-prevention programmes grouped the approaches to prevention into nine categories. Programmes were also grouped according to whether they used interactive methods or not.

The study concluded that 'the most successful of the interactive programs are the comprehensive life skills programs that incorporate the refusal skills offered in the social influences programs and add many general life skills such as assertiveness, coping, communication skills, etc.

Skills-based health education and life skills have been shown to reduce the chances that young people will engage in delinquent behaviour and interpersonal violence; the use of alcohol, tobacco, and other drugs; high-risk sexual activity that can result in pregnancy or STD or HIV infections; emotional disorders; and bullying.

Training for school personnel is an important aspect of school health-promotion programmes. Studies show that training teachers how to use a health-education curriculum improves its implementation. Similarly, an evaluation of the Teenage Health Teaching Modules (THTM) curriculum, using skills-based approaches for health education in grades 7 to 12 in the United States, showed that training teachers before using the curriculum positively affected teachers' self-reported feeling of preparedness and had positive effects on both curriculum implementation and student outcomes.

Students in health education classes taught by trained teachers scored significantly higher on health knowledge and attitude scores, and, at the senior high-school level, were also more able to curb self-reported use of illegal drugs, than those covering the same material with untrained teachers. Training teachers has the added value of gaining their commitment and support, as well as their understanding of a specific curriculum and its supporting policies and programme—all important factors for successful implementation.

The effect on education of health issues, such as safe water and sanitation, helminth infections and nutrition, and lifestyle behaviours associated with STDs, HIV/AIDS, and alcohol, tobacco and other drugs are highlighted, and evidence is given that schools can address these issues effectively. Improvements in education will not succeed if we do not simultaneously pay attention to the healthy development of both students and staff in schools.

The record of the past decade affirms that the world community can translate its highest aspirations for children into effective programmes. If the past is indeed a prelude to the future, we can say with confidence that the pace in responding to the learning and health needs of children greatly accelerates once consensus has been achieved on policies and programmes that work.

Major leaders and change agents in the field must come together around a common framework, relevant to the education sector. Such a framework should be part of a larger effort to improve the general quality of the schools and the education children receive. The creation of frameworks in the past decade contributed enormously to driving the school health agenda forward. Frameworks have increased creativity, generated experimentation, and inspired a broad range of research and programme activities.

At this juncture, however, we run the risk of allowing the proliferation of so many frameworks to diffuse human and financial resources and to confuse those who are ready to take action. A shared framework should drive an action agenda that:

1) promotes healthy development and focuses on the most serious and common health threats through the co-ordinated implementation of core components of a school health and nutrition programme in schools everywhere;

2) sets specific, quantifiable goals for the agenda;

3) applies lessons learned from the past decade on how best to implement the core components; and

4) establishes indicators to monitor the implementation and effectiveness of the core components in countries and schools worldwide.

A shared framework must view the school as a dynamic system in which people can effect change to promote health and learning and which focuses not only on children but also on staff, teachers, parents and community members, and links to health services. To be successful, school health, hygiene and nutrition efforts must be led by educators, supported and assisted by health professionals, and made an integral part of the efforts to improve education through policies and goals.

School health and nutrition efforts can have a powerful effect on improving the status of schools (through efforts by schools and communities) as well as of education (through policies and goals). Much of the power of school health programmes lies in their ability to mobilize schools and communities around the improvement in educational quality and outcomes for their children.

Educators must be convinced that such programmes are practical and feasible, yield results, are beneficial to staff and students, and advance learning. It is equally important that leaders relate the efforts to the social and economic agenda in gaining support. Recruiting a small but highly influential group of well-known and respected international educators to champion the school health agenda would be valuable.

Experiments have taken place at the world, regional, and national levels to bring the education and health sectors together. Where successful, these collaborations have created a common language, provided unique contributions for sharing and learning, and leveraged resources. However, sustaining the collaboration is difficult. It is also important to identify and use the unique roles of various participants.

Collaboration does not mean that everyone does the same thing, but that each sector makes its own unique contribution to common goals. Successful collaboration must identify the most relevant role for the educator, the health worker, and the parent and community member. More must be done to sustain emerging networks for collaboration, providing professional development, resources, and materials to increase their capacity and to sustain energy and commitment in the face of obstacles.

More investment is needed for health services that children and adolescents can reach easily, without stigma. More health services should be located in or near schools and staffed with people trained to work with youth. Young people all over the world need health services, particularly those that are 'youth-friendly'.

Traditional health services must move beyond medical treatment to preventive services and early intervention and accommodate the particular needs of young people (e.g. for emotional support, confidentiality and accessibility). Access to information as well as sustained support to use it (e.g. professional development, technical co-operation, and mentoring) must be improved for education and health workers.

There is a need for ongoing professional development and technical know-how for education and health workers about how to identify, select, and implement the most effective strategies for their needs. A creative use of the Internet and on-line training must be applied to the field of school health and nutrition on a global scale. Multiple targeted and co-ordinated strategies are needed to improve desired behaviour patterns and health outcomes.

Research in public health, the foundation of most approaches to school health, has demonstrated that multiple strategies co-ordinated to address a few common goals are more effective in producing desired behaviour changes and health outcomes than single-track approaches. Such strategies may include co-ordinated policy, supportive environments, community action, personal skills, and health services targeted to a few selected conditions.

While there has been tremendous progress since Jomtien, it is impossible to tell the full story of what has happened globally without common indicators of progress. Such indicators could provide information about national capacities and infrastructure to implement school health programmes.

Measures could include the availability of school policies and budgets with line items dedicated to health, mechanisms for collaboration, and the health-related training of teachers and health workers. Beyond measures of capacity, indicators of children's health status could include height and weight data, rates of anaemia and other micronutrient deficiency diseases, and number of meals or fruit and vegetable servings per day.

At the national and local level, too, more and better programme planning and evaluation tools are necessary. Model programmes should be developed for different levels of investment, because countries vary in what they can afford. In many countries, people who are very poor and disenfranchised have reported that their participation in addressing health issues in schools has made a difference to their lives. The opportunity to have a voice and role in creating change to improve the quality of life for their children, themselves, and their community has transformed their world.

With the participation of all - the education and health sectors, parents, teachers, and community members - people everywhere can make gradual improvements in their quality of life. As we consider the changes that policy-makers, practitioners, and citizens can bring about in the future, it is good to reflect on developments in the past.

International collaboration in school health has a history of more than 120 years. In the 1800s, school health became an issue when compulsory education laws were enforced in Europe. In 1880, the Third International Congress on Education in Brussels addressed school hygiene as one of the plenary topics.

Through each decade of the 1900s, the agenda of international school health conferences included such topics as school construction and furniture, medical inspection in schools, individual health records, physical education and training, the hygiene of dormitories, the prevention of contagious diseases in schools, and hygiene for teachers, students, and families.

Following a 1946 survey of ministries of education, the International Bureau of Education of UNESCO prepared recommendations to improve the teaching of health in primary schools, with the goal of making it a genuine part of education. By 1967, all of the ninety-four countries replying to a second survey indicated that some form of health education was compulsory in primary schools and was often integrated into other subject areas, such as science education.

Nevertheless, the report recognized that not all schools were effectively assisting children in adopting positive attitudes and behaviours about safeguarding their own health and that of others. From the 1960s until the mid-1980s, international conferences and publications in the field of school health were less evident. This decline of attention at the international level was consequential because international leadership and advocacy can be catalytic for national and local efforts.

However, during this same period when school health was less visible on the international stage, the developing world was making considerable progress on another front: increasing the survival rates of children from birth to 5 years of age. In 1960, only five of every six children born (83%) lived to their first birthday.

By 1991, at least 12 of every 13 children born (92%) were expected to reach that landmark. The success of the Child Survival movement meant that more and more children were going to enter school. By the end of the 1980s, a number of international organizations renewed their interest in school health and nutrition programmes around the globe.

UNESCO was one of the first United Nations agencies to address the area of school health and nutrition. In the 1980s, UNESCO initiated the Nutrition Education Series and held various technical meetings on this topic. Also, the Council on Europe, the European

Commission, and the WHO Regional Office in Copenhagen were beginning to discuss a broader concept of school health. These groups looked at all aspects of the school as a system and a setting in which health could be promoted by those in it.

In the United States, with the support of the Centres for Disease Control and Prevention, and backed by the evaluations of several major school health education programmes, the concept of a comprehensive school health programme with eight components became more widely understood and implemented.

While there was growing recognition of the need to address the health status of young people to maximize learning leading up to Jomtien. School health efforts in 1990 can be characterized in the following ways:

1. Health initiatives in schools focused primarily on disease prevention.
2. There was confusion about the concept and definition of school health.
3. Single, uncoordinated intervention strategies dominated.
4. Few formal mechanisms for multisectoral collaboration were in place.
5. Didactic, topic-by-topic teaching was the typical approach to health education.
6. Evidence of the effectiveness of interventions was not well known or disseminated.
7. Few tools were available to guide assessment and strategic planning.
8. Few donors earmarked school health programmes as a priority for funding.

Many school health efforts aimed to improve hygiene, prevent the spread of infections, treat specific health conditions, and provide screening or medical examinations. Many countries also expanded their efforts to incorporate health topics into national curricula.

Both the services and curricular work tended to emphasize specific disease prevention more than health promotion. For example, in 1987 Pakistan initiated a School Health Services Programme and recommended in its five-year plan that all children have a complete medical check-up when they enter school and a comprehensive quarterly check-up as long as they remain in school.

Pakistan's subsequent five-year plan recommended that the programme be reoriented towards developing healthy lifestyles among schoolchildren, thus recognizing the need for a more comprehensive and lifestyle-oriented approach. In 1990 Namibian schools provided immunization, physical examinations, and a limited amount of information on 'health matters'.

There was confusion about the concept and definition of school health. As Donald Bundy of the World Bank commented, 'There was considerable confusion about the definition of school health and nutrition in 1990. There was even more confusion over whether the goal was to improve health, or to improve education through improved health'.

Anna-Maria Hoffmann-Barthes of UNESCO commented, 'Health education, unlike other subjects in the curriculum, is one with a history of involvement by people from outside the education system, frequently health professionals. The risks of such "outside ownership" and subsequent lack of co-operation between the education and health sectors are numerous.

Education professionals have often shown a certain disinterest in health issues; health professionals invited to teach the subject typically lack understanding of the pedagogy necessary for skill development and behaviour change and the effective implementation of school health education programmes'.

In 1990 health and education professionals usually defined school health and nutrition as either health curriculum or health services, but seldom as the integration of the two. While the importance of linking health instruction to services and other components was often discussed, there was no unifying concept to galvanize all the participants to work together for a truly global effort.

Experience has shown that a powerful concept can create enthusiasm and motivate policy-makers and practitioners to implement new ideas. And, as David Rivett of the European Network of Health-Promoting Schools said, 'It has been critical for us in Europe to have a concept or framework in place first.

In 1990, at the international level, there was no single, clear definition or framework across all the agencies to guide their direction and activity. In the early 1990s a few more integrated concepts began to appear. However, no matter what concept was used, school health and nutrition were often regarded as separate and apart from the mission of basic education.

School health advocates often found themselves frustrated and unable to convince educators of the importance and interdependence of health and education.

Manyschool health efforts involved curricula that were not complemented by policies or a supportive school environment. For example, teaching about the dangers of tobacco took place in schools in which students and faculty were allowed to smoke.

Similarly, health services treated conditions like intestinal worms, but often without complementary improvements in sanitation and safe water or educational messages to prevent re-infection. Seldom were approaches comprehensive, that is, uniting policy with instruction, services and the school environment to reinforce one another in targeting specific health and educational outcomes.

There may also have been a health education programme in the same school, but it was not co-ordinated with any other component of a school health programme. The water and sanitation effort was not accompanied by any reinforcing education strategy and there was no evaluation of academic outcomes. There was no look at whether the provision of these services increased enrolment (especially of girls) or general use of the facilities by students or community members'.

Too often there has been a vertical approach to a problem such as malaria. For example, medical personnel will arrive at a school with the view that 'malaria is your problem and this is what you must do to treat it'. There has been little attempt to gain community participation and support for the intervention. Therefore its acceptance and success are limited. On the other hand, multiple strategies that are co-ordinated to address a few common goals have proved effective.

In the United States, for example, Project Northland is a school/community substance-abuse prevention programme that includes planned parental involvement, peer-led skills-building sessions, community policy change and enforcement, all designed to test the efficacy of a multilevel, multistrategy, multiyear intervention programme for youth. After three years, an evaluation demonstrated that the percentage of students who reported alcohol use in the previous month and week was significantly lower in the intervention group at the end of eighth grade than in the reference group.

In 1990 there were few cross-sectoral mechanisms in place at the international, regional, national, or local levels. These mechanisms provide a way for partners to unite around common goals, co-ordinate and leverage valuable resources, provide a forum for learning, and exchange technical expertise.

However, the education sector typically handled health instruction while the health sector addressed services, with few linkages between the two. Agencies responsible for water, sanitation, and the school's physical structure have usually acted independently of the other sectors. Given the effectiveness of targeting multiple strategies to improve children's health and learning, collaboration is necessary across sectors (education, public health, medicine, environmental services) and between agencies with common goals and interests (governmental and non-governmental agencies, national and international organizations).

The lack of such important structural mechanisms to expedite policy development and programme implementation, combined with confusion about a unifying concept, was the most critical obstacle to progress in the field. Without such structures, it is difficult at any level to harness the multidisciplinary expertise and resources necessary to achieve school health goals. Most school health education programmes have been concerned with providing information on specific topics, not with building skills.

A review of curricula from the early 1990s reveals that they typically provided information about ten topics, almost all about physical health or specific diseases, rather than building skills to practice healthy overall behaviour. Sexuality was usually omitted, as was any attention to emotional or mental health; violence and suicide were not regarded as public health issues. A review of school health education in Europe in 1991 reported, 'There is general agreement in Europe over the range of health issues which need to be addressed in schools.

There has been a tendency, however, for school health education to be dominated by single health issues - particularly drugs and AIDS - which has inhibited the wholehearted adoption of the holistic healthy lifestyle approach necessary for a balanced and convincing programme in schools'. While several innovative skills-based or life skills curricula were developed during the 1980s, the primary teaching method continued to be the didactic lecture.

It has now been well documented that the teaching methods with the strongest likelihood of producing change in the health behaviour of students are interactive learning strategies or experiential learning. Many in the field recognized the child-to-child approach as an outstanding programme in health education at the time of EFA. Begun in London, the child-to-child approach focused on teaching older children to deliver health messages to their younger siblings through interactive methods.

Gradually, the approach expanded to prepare children to promote good health among their peers, families, and communities. Child-to-child placed young people in an active teaching role. Evidence of the effectiveness of interventions was not well known or disseminated. Few evaluations were made of the effectiveness of health education curricula or any other school health initiative. Those that did exist were disseminated primarily to health education professionals rather than to the mainstream education sector or to professionals in the public health or medical arenas.

Similarly, research about health service interventions was published primarily in journals aimed at the medical, nutrition, or public health sectors. There were few opportunities for the two important audiences of educators and health workers to learn together about the important link between health and education. By 1990 a new body of research was emerging concerning the impact of health interventions on the status of health and on cognition and learning outcomes.

Planning in public health, education, and organizational development often begins with the collection of data to define the problem and the assets or strengths to address it. From there, planners can set measurable goals and objectives, then define action steps and milestones to measure progress. In 1990 few, if any, assessment and strategic planning tools were available for education policy-makers and programme planners to collect and use data to plan policies, programmes, and interventions in an integrated and complementary manner designed for the health needs of children and adolescents in school.

Thus, educators in particular had little information about the strengths and limitations of the many parts of a school health programme that could have guided them in selecting and developing effective intervention strategies. In addition, there was limited information about the costs associated with implementing specific interventions.

Few donors earmarked school health programmes as a priority for funding. Many workers in the field share the general perception that it was difficult to find departments within United Nations agencies and international non-governmental organizations with a brief that included school health programmes. It was also difficult to find donors who had made it a priority to fund international efforts to improve school health programmes. The field of school health and nutrition has progressed considerably over the past decade.

A major accomplishment since the World Conference on Education for All in Jomtien has been the development of conceptual frameworks or unifying principles for school health policies and programmes. These frameworks have also served as a catalyst to mobilize partnerships across sectors at all levels. In addition to the frameworks developed by United Nations agencies and a few other international organizations, significant and noteworthy activity was also conducted by frontline grassroots organizations in the past decade.

Frameworks developed in the 1990s include the concept of the Health-Promoting School; the Child-Friendly School (UNICEF); the Basic Cost-Effective Public Health Package; and Active Learning Capacity. One framework, FRESH (Focusing Resources on Effective School Health (WHO, UNICEF, UNESCO, World Bank), was launched jointly at the EFA Conference in Senegal in April 2000.

The concept of the health-promoting school (HPS) started in Europe. It is based on public health theory and builds on the Ottawa Charter of Health Promotion, which recognized that 'health is created and lived by people within the settings of their everyday life; where they learn, work, play and love. Health is created by caring for oneself and others, by being able to make decisions and have control over one's life and circumstances, and by ensuring that the society one lives in creates conditions that allow the attainment of health by all its members'.

The WHO Regional Office for Europe, the Council of Europe, and the European Commission first widely promoted the HPS concept. The aim was to achieve healthy lifestyles for the total school population by developing environments conducive to the promotion of health. The HPS concept extended beyond school health education to a broader array of complementary interventions. The earliest descriptions of the HPS, then called the 'Healthy School', were developed during the first major conference of all the European nations on school health promotion in Scotland in 1986.

A Health-Promoting School:

— Strives to improve the health of school personnel, families, and community members as well as students.

— Fosters health and learning with all the measures at its disposal.

— Engages health and education officials, teachers, teachers' unions, students, parents, health providers, and community leaders in efforts to make the school a healthy place.

— Strives to provide a healthy environment, school health education, and school health services along with school/ community projects and outreach, health promotion programmes for staff, nutrition and food safety programmes, opportunities for physical education and recreation, and programmes for counselling, social support, and mental health promotion.

Based on the Jomtien documents and a number of other developments in the field of children's rights, UNICEF has recently developed a framework of rights-based, child-friendly education systems and schools that are characterized by being 'healthy for children, effective with children, protective of children, and involved with families and communities and children'. This framework builds on the proclamation at the Jomtien Conference that 'education is a fundamental right for all people, women and men, of all ages, throughout our world'.

Referring to health, the declaration went on to say that 'education can help ensure a safer, healthier, more prosperous and environmentally sound world'. UNICEF's framework was also inspired by the Convention on the Rights of the Child, held in 1989, which set the stage by acknowledging that children's rights require special protection for the purpose of the general improvement of their conditions and for their development and education.

UNICEF's framework broadly defines core components that characterize a child-friendly school, each component incorporating factors concerning education, health, and human rights. In a child-friendly school:

— The school is a significant personal and social environment in the lives of its students.

— A child-friendly school ensures every child an environment that is physically safe, emotionally secure, and psychologically enabling.

— Teachers are the single most important factor in creating an effective and inclusive classroom.

— Child-friendly schools are teacher-friendly, supporting, encouraging, and they facilitate teachers towards being motivated, capable, self-confident, and consistently available.

— Children are natural learners, but the capacity to learn can be undermined and sometimes destroyed.

— A child-friendly school recognizes, encourages, and supports children's growing capacities as learners by providing a school culture, teaching behaviours, and curriculum content that are focused on learning and the learner.

— The ability of a school to be and to call itself child-friendly is directly linked to the support, participation, and collaboration it receives from families.

— Child-friendly schools have a key role to play in ensuring that children's rights are reflected throughout the education system, just as education systems must ensure that schools have the resources to act on behalf of all children.

The rights of children as articulated in the CRC are indivisible. They all apply, all of the time, to all children. Schools and education systems have a role in ensuring that children's rights are reflected throughout a country's governance community. Child-friendly schools aim to develop a learning environment in which children are motivated and able to learn. Staff members are friendly and welcoming to children and attend to all their health and safety needs. WHO supports the framework of the child-friendly school by helping schools become 'health-promoting' as an essential step towards becoming 'child-friendly'.

The concept that schools are in a position to deliver a basic package of health services to students has been widely acknowledged during the 1990s. The appropriate level of services for the schools to offer depends on each country's operational and financial resources. A 1993 World Bank analysis concluded that most regions of the world could greatly benefit by implementing a limited package of five cost-effective public-health elements.

The five elements are:

i) an extended programme on immunization;

ii) school health programmes to treat worm infections and micronutrient deficiencies and to provide health education;

iii) programmes to increase public knowledge about family planning and nutrition, self-care or indications for seeking care, and vector control and disease surveillance activities;

iv) programmes to reduce the consumption of tobacco, alcohol, and other drugs;

v) AIDS-prevention programmes with a strong component on other sexually transmitted diseases.

The WHO Expert Committee on Comprehensive School Health Education and Promotion commented on this basic package that '[al]though school health programmes are explicitly mentioned in only one of the above elements, for a large portion of the world's population, schools could efficiently provide all five elements of the recommended package'. The Partnership for Child Development, UNICEF, the World Bank, and other agencies have used this framework to guide programme development in countries around the world.

In the state of São Paulo, Brazil, a World Bank loan is helping to provide a broad range of school-based services including feeding programmes, health and nutrition screening of schoolchildren, nutrition and health education in the school curriculum, and school-based programmes for iron and vitamin A supplementation. A more limited package' of services with low-cost, easy to implement interventions is applied in Guinea, where almost no prior nutrition and health programmes for school-age children existed.

The elements of a school-based health package in Guinea initially include a deworming programme and iron and iodine supplementation, accompanied by education in health and hygiene. Carefully monitored school-based health and nutrition programmes implemented by the Partnership for Child Development in Ghana, the United Republic of Tanzania, India, and Indonesia have now shown that the education sector is capable of delivering a simple health package to large numbers of schoolchildren without the creation of specific infrastructures.

These experiences suggest that the school system can contribute to health delivery as long as the package is simple, demands little school time, and is perceived as being appropriate to local needs.

In the early 1990s, in support of the mission to achieve Education for All, Beryl Levinger of EDC wrote for USAID and UNDP about the need to concentrate on improving a child's 'active learning capacity' (ALC). Consistent with theories in education and the social sciences, she defined ALC as 'the child's ability to interact with and take optimal advantage of the full complement of resources offered by any formal or informal learning environment'.

The importance of this definition lies in its belief that to maximize learning, a child must be psychologically, emotionally, and physically well, able to concentrate on and participate actively in the learning process, able to pay attention and concentrate on tasks, and missing only a few days of school for illness or other reasons.

The ALC framework focuses on improving the quality of life of the child as one of the most important factors in achieving the goals of Education for All. This framework includes three primary variables: health and nutrition status, hunger level, and psychosocial support. Health and nutrition status refers to both current and prior physical or mental conditions, such as height for age, sensory abilities, nutritional status, and helminthic infections that influence a child's ability to take optimal advantage of learning resources and opportunities.

Temporary hunger, especially if a child is malnourished, contributes to a child's distractibility, inattentiveness to environmental stimuli, and adaptive behaviours of passivity and inactivity, all of which impinge on the development of a child's ALC. Psychosocial support encompasses the degree to which parents, caretakers, community leaders, and other significant adults, community institutions, as well as values and norms encourage a child's independence and inquisitiveness and support expectations that favour overall learning as well as formal schooling.

Three variables are considered secondary in determining active learning capacity: prior learning experience, a child's learning receptiveness, and a child's aptitude for learning. Prior learning experience refers to a child's exposure to formal and informal situations conducive to acquiring new knowledge and skills, such as pre-school programmes.

Learning receptiveness refers to a child's motivation and attention, which are influenced by health status and hunger level, as well as by the quality of the child/ caretaker relationship. Aptitude relates to the time a child needs to learn a particular task, attend to stimuli, and concentrate. The ALC framework represents a dynamic portrayal of the complex interplay among the determinants of educational outcomes, capturing the high degree of influence that health, nutrition, sensory impairment, and temporary hunger exert on the quality of the child and hence on the child's learning outcomes.

This framework was used widely by the South African Active Learning Network, a group of NGOs, to develop materials, protocols, and broker links between the health and education sectors. Many of the Network's activities were designed to promote the ALC model or to further its application. Importance of frameworks in collaboration. Some of the most important lessons learned in recent years are the need for multisectoral collaboration and co-operation in order to move towards the health and educational goals of Education for All.

'Indicators of a favourable policy setting include a demonstrated ability to secure interministerial co-operation; a co-ordinated, intersectoral approach to human development; a history of support for community-based health and education programs; and a commitment at the highest political levels to programs that address questions of equity as well as growth'.

For example, during the past decade, the World Bank coordinated information to enhance the quality of school health and nutrition programmes through its International School Health Initiative. Its experiences of good practice suggest that school-based health and nutrition programmes should be simple and locally relevant.

The FRESH Framework: a concerted effort to focus resources on effective school health. A framework proposed jointly by WHO, UNICEF, UNESCO, and the World Bank suggests that there is a core group of cost-effective components that could form the basis for intensified and joint action. These agencies are now developing a partnership for Focusing Resources on Effective School Health (FRESH), launched at the Education for All Conference in Senegal in April 2000.

Each component of the framework stresses that a young person's health is one of the many important factors that must be adequately addressed to achieve any country's educational goals. School health is an investment in a country's future and in the capacity of its people to thrive economically and as a society'.

Health policies in schools, including policies for skills-based health education and the provision of some health services, can help promote the overall health, hygiene, and nutrition of children. Good health policies should also ensure a safe and secure physical environment and a positive psychosocial environment and should address issues such as the abuse of students, sexual harassment, school violence, and bullying.

By guaranteeing the continued education of pregnant schoolgirls and young mothers, school health policies will help promote inclusion and equity in the school environment. Policies that help to prevent and reduce harassment by other students, and even by teachers, also combat the reasons why girls withdraw or are withdrawn from schools.

Policies regarding the health practices of teachers and students can reinforce health education by requiring that teachers do not smoke at school and thus act as positive role models for their students. The process of developing and agreeing on policies draws attention to these issues. The policies are best developed by involving many levels, including the national level, and teachers, children, and parents at the school level.

Safe water and sanitation facilities are the realistic goal in most countries to ensure that all schools have access to clean water and sanitation. Without clean water and adequate sanitation, hygiene education is meaningless. The school environment may even damage the health and nutritional status of its children if it increases their exposure to hazards such as infectious diseases carried by the water supply.

By providing clean water and sanitation, schools can reinforce the health and hygiene messages and act as an example to both students and the wider community. This in turn can lead to a demand from the community for similar facilities. Sound construction policies will help ensure that facilities address issues such as gender access and privacy.

Separate facilities for girls, particularly adolescents, are important in reducing dropout at menstruation and even before. Sound maintenance policies will help ensure the continuing safe use of these facilities.

Health in this context extends beyond the physical to include psychosocial and environmental health issues. The development of attitudes towards gender equity and respect between girls and boys and the development of specific skills, such as dealing with peer pressure, are central to both an effective skills-based health education and positive psychosocial environments. With these skills, individuals are more likely to adopt and sustain a healthy lifestyle during their schooling and for the rest of their lives.

Schools can effectively deliver some health and nutrition services as long as the services are simple, safe, and familiar and address problems that are prevalent and recognized as important in the community. If these criteria are met, then the community sees the teacher and school more positively, and teachers see themselves as playing important roles.

For example, micronutrient deficiencies and worm infections may be effectively dealt with by infrequent (half-yearly or annual) oral treatment; changing the timing of meals or providing a snack to address short-term hunger during the school day - an important constraint on learning - can contribute to school performance; and providing spectacles will allow some children to participate in class fully for the first time.

Within this framework, these four components are intended to be supported by effective partnerships between teachers and health workers, effective community partnerships, and pupil awareness and participation.

Several major global trends over the past decade have dramatically influenced the scope and direction of school health work:

1. The AIDS pandemic stimulated a new demand and urgency for school health.
2. There was a gradual move from individual to multiple strategies and to integrated and co-ordinated approaches to school health programmes.
3. New mechanisms have emerged for multisectoral collaboration.
4. Student and community participation has been an important factor in promoting school health.
5. Skills-based methods for health education have gained recognition and greater use.
6. The documentation and dissemination of evidence of effectiveness have increased.
7. New tools have been tested for assessment, planning and monitoring.
8. Donor recognition of the field and investment have both increased.
9. International conferences have addressed school health.
10. Various barriers still exist that can hinder progress towards effective and sustained school health and nutrition interventions.

A defining characteristic of the 1990s has been the influence of the HIV/AIDS pandemic on school health policies and programmes. Many children have been orphaned and many teachers and students are dying. While this pandemic closed the school door to many children and teachers affected directly or indirectly by it, it also opened many doors to school health programmes.

Because education to increase protective behaviours is one of the few measures available to prevent HIV, and because prevention ideally should begin before the onset of sexual activity or alcohol and drug use, schools became a very important setting for delivering life-saving interventions to children and adolescents worldwide. As educators and health workers began to plan and implement school-based efforts to prevent HIV infection, many in the field were asking which strategies would be most likely to motivate people to adopt protective behaviours.

Such questioning, in the face of the threat of HIV infection, led to reviews of lessons learned from health education, sex education, family life, and reproductive health education; increased calls for the implementation and improvement of such programmes; the innovative use of skills-based methods; the cross-fertilization of ideas and strategies among experts; and the involvement of young people in designing and delivering programmes.

UNESCO, for example, launched a global Programme of Education for the Prevention of AIDS, which focuses on integrating HIV/AIDS education into school curricula. Its main goal is to put in place large national programmes that draw on the experiences of other projects and programmes. UNESCO's resource centres disseminate numerous materials and documents on HIV/AIDS education, along with seminars and training for ministerial staff and teachers.

Since Jomtien, the following types of activity illustrate how the complex and sensitive issues surrounding HIV/AIDS served as an impetus for strengthening national, regional, and international efforts to improve health through schools.

In Zimbabwe, which has one of the highest rates of AIDS cases on the African continent, the Ministry of Education and Culture initiated an AIDS Action Programme targeting students and teachers in grades 4 to 7. More than 2,000 teachers have been trained to use not only specified AIDS educational materials, but also participatory life skills methods.

National programmes fostered by UNICEF and focusing on life skills have strengthened school health efforts by helping teachers to explore their own attitudes and values about health, to establish an open and positive classroom climate, to place education about HIV/AIDS in the context of a general programme on health, personal development, and living skills, and to use positive approaches that emphasize an awareness of values, assertiveness, and other relationship skills.

In 1993, participants in the Inter-Country Consultative Meeting on Comprehensive School Health Education, convened by the WHO Regional Office for South-East Asia, recommended that in view of the physical, social, and psychological needs of children, adolescents, and youth and the emerging health problems, comprehensive school health education be given the status of a separate subject in the school curriculum, in addition to being integrated into other relevant subject areas.

In 1995, EI, WHO, UNESCO and UNAIDS, in collaboration with CDC and EDC, created an alliance to increase the interest and involvement of teachers' unions in HIV/AIDS prevention and in strengthening school health programmes. In July 1998, at the EI Second World Congress, teachers' unions from around the world adopted a resolution on Health Promotion and School Health.

Establish or develop contacts with parents and health professionals at the local or national level. Commit themselves, especially in the framework of the Health-Promoting School, to make the school a healthy place that offers a reliable infrastructure to guarantee protection from diseases, violence, and harmful substances. Such actions show an increased recognition of the need for and value of working collaboratively to address HIV/AIDS while also improving school-based efforts that address other issues affecting health and learning.

During the 1990s, frameworks evolved that included multiple strategies - rather than individual approaches - to promote health and nutrition through schools. For example, WHO's Health-Promoting School model and its supporting tools involve various participants at the school level to foster health and learning with all the measures at their disposal.

In UNICEF's Child-Friendly Schools Framework, the school culture, teaching behaviours, and curricula content are all conducive to learning and learners. In the United States, the book Health Is Academic outlines the concept and components of co-ordinated school health programmes. It was developed by EDC, with funding by CDC/DASH, and reviewed by more than 300 professionals before it was published in 1998.

The tendency towards more integrated and co-ordinated approaches to school health is likely to continue and will balance content from traditional disciplines. Health education can be co-ordinated with or integrated into other subjects such as science, technology, physical education, home economics, and social studies. There are some notable examples of implementing co-ordinated school health initiatives with multiple strategies, which can both inspire and guide the field in the decade to come.

During the 1990s it became increasingly apparent that in order for schools to improve health, international, national, provincial, and local agencies, education and health professionals and parents and communities will need to work together on behalf of young people. A recent survey of donors and agencies found that 'there is a move towards inter-agency school health planning, monitoring and evaluation, particularly in the UN.

This reflects a move by the UN system and bilaterals towards a sector-wide approach to funding, and away from a project approach'. For example, a situation analysis that includes assessments of adolescents' needs and responses was developed as an inter-agency activity by UNDP, UNESCO, UNFPA, WHO, and PCD and has been evaluated by WHO in Ghana, Zimbabwe, Botswana, Uganda, and Kenya.

The World Bank's International School Health Initiative has helped to create global partnerships that focus on a common school health agenda. Agencies and donors have also expressed interest in a school health website and mailing list, as is currently being developed by PCD with the World Bank, which will provide a vehicle for greater collaboration. The Partnership for

Child Development (PCD) as established programmes that emphasize the development of national collaborations as a part of locally managed programmes, the core of which is the essential partnership between the health and education sectors.

A major new global partner is Education International. Established in 1993, EI represents more than 25 million teachers and workers in the education sector, and more than 250 teachers' unions in 150 countries are affiliated with EI. EI has adopted resolutions to promote health and nutrition for its membership and has also participated extensively with WHO, UNAIDS, UNESCO, and HHD/EDC in providing professional development on health promotion for members and HIV prevention initiatives.

Regionally, networks of persons responsible for school health from both the education and health sectors have been created to share experience and foster collaboration across sectors. One of these networks is the European Network of Health-Promoting Schools, a consolidating initiative between the health and education sectors.

WHO's Mega Country Health Promotion Network serves as a new mechanism to foster co-operation between the ministries of education and health in the eleven most populous countries, which face the common problem of size. In the E-9 Initiative, sponsored by UNESCO, UNICEF, and UNFPA, leaders of the nine most populous developing countries pledged to universalize primary education and reduce illiteracy in their respective countries.

During the 1990s, many publications and actions have recognized and strongly supported youth and community involvement as important for effective school health and nutrition programmes. WHO's Adolescent Health Programme concluded that youth involvement ensures project relevance, acceptability, dedication to project objectives, long-term effectiveness, and personal development for the young participants.

The European Network of Health-Promoting Schools (ENHPS) has published many case studies that show how students have been involved in planning, implementing, and evaluating various school projects. In Gandrup School in Denmark, students have been involved in planning. The pupils, who claimed that they learn more when they are able to influence the choice of subjects, discussed the WHO definition of health and then identified conditions they wished to change in their school life, the community, or their own lives.

In a school in Finland, students were actively involved in the evaluation of a school democracy project in which they evaluate themselves, their actions, and their progress twice a year. 'This is important to the young people because they can compare themselves with the prevailing norms and then decide themselves in which ways they want to improve or change.' Feedback from teachers, pupils, and others has proved that this project is worth continuing.

Family and community involvement has also been strongly supported during the past decade. A recent UN study included community and family involvement as a vital factor for 'programmes that work'. Community members must be recognized as central actors rather than as passive beneficiaries.

In the United Republic of Tanzania, for example, severe malnutrition disappeared during a programme featuring growth monitoring in the community. Active community participation has also played an increasingly prominent role in effective collaboration. An extensive analysis of the progress in the development of education in Africa found that 'the role of communities as providers of education is becoming more complex and more substantive. . . . Communities are becoming involved in matters previously regarded as within the domain of professionals and ministries. In Ghana, communities 'revealed not only their interest inalleviating the health and nutrition problems of their school-age children but also a willingness to help pay for these services'.

Interactive methods, which give young people in the classroom the opportunities to practise these skills with regard to important health issues, are the most critical factor in achieving success. Increasingly, schools are giving priority to teaching life skills. Numerous products have emerged to support skills-based approaches. Many countries have carried out skills-based health education projects. Uganda launched a very well-planned, comprehensive school health initiative.

Along with creating a network of health educators at the district level for health education activities, skills-based health education was integrated into the basic science curriculum and also became part of the examination process. The past ten years have seen an explosion in the number of documents published by international organizations to report on the effects of single interventions, such as treatments for intestinal worms or nutritional deficits to reduce health problems and improve learning.

One of the greatest innovations of the past decade is the use of the World Wide Web for global knowledge sharing. The Web, relatively untapped for school health in 1990, is broadly disseminating evidence of the best practices worldwide in timely and cost-effective ways.

During the past decade, many major international conferences have brought together important leaders and change agents and gained international attention. School health issues were addressed in various contexts as part of these conferences. Various barriers still exist that can hinder progress towards effective and sustained school health and nutrition interventions.

Despite the encouraging global trends of the past decade, barriers, controversies, and missed opportunities continue to impede the implementation and effectiveness of school programmes at the national and local level. Significant work is still needed to make the hope of a health-promoting and child-friendly school a reality for most schools.

The deterioration of the initial positive effects of many school health interventions owing to unsupportive conditions in the school and its surrounding environment (e.g. the availability of drugs, tobacco, and alcohol; messages in the media that contradict messages promoted at school). Many schools still exemplify unhealthy living, where teachers and sometimes students smoke, where the only food choices are unhealthy, dirt is prevalent, and harassment is unchecked.

There is an urgency and opportunity to use the knowledge, momentum and international commitment gained since Jomtien to tackle the operational challenges that impede progress within countries and within schools. To overcome these barriers, strong and genuine partnerships at all levels - i.e. between different sectors, between governmental and non-governmental agencies, between teachers and health workers, between school and parents and the larger community - are critical to successful school programmes.

Progress in school health and nutrition has varied dramatically across regions and nations. In Central and Eastern Europe, many of the formal mechanisms that were in place in 1990 providing social services to young people, including those through the education system, have deteriorated. This change occurred when the communist system fell apart and with it the numerous structures that were reaching out to young people.

5

Effective School Health

UNICEF estimates that more than 90% of the world's children are now surviving beyond the age of 5 years. As a result there are now more children of school age and a higher proportion of children attending school than ever before. Despite the improvements in survival of school-aged children, there is still a major burden of disease and ill health among this group, particularly in areas such as poor nutrition and intestinal parasitic diseases.

This burden of ill health compromises the children's development, school attendance and ability to take advantage of what may be their only opportunity to obtain a formal education. Improving the health and learning of school children through school-based health and nutrition programmes is not a new concept. Many countries have school health programmes, and many agencies have decades of experience.

An interagency initiative (Focusing Resources on Effective School Health - FRESH), that includes WHO,

UNICEF, UNESCO and the World Bank, has identified a core group of activities, each already recommended by the participating agencies, that captures the best practices from programme experiences. This core group of activities consists of health-related school policies; provision of safe water and sanitation; skills based health education and school based health and nutrition services.

Focusing initially on these activities will allow concerted action by the participating agencies, and will ensure consistent advice to country programmes and projects. Because of the simplicity of this approach, it will increase the number of countries able to implement school health components of child-friendly school reforms, and help ensure that these programmes go to scale.

It also serves to highlight areas that are still of great concern. These include the problems of HIV/AIDS infection and that of girls' access to education. APPROACH - 1997 SURVEY The original survey was commissioned by the Scientific Coordinating Centre of the Partnership for Child Development (PCD), based in the University of Oxford, England. The main objective of this work was the preparation of a synopsis of donor support for school-based health and nutrition initiatives. The information was collected over a three-week period using telephone, fax, email and the web site. These media provide a useful introduction to the subject but fall short of providing a comprehensive overview.

The World Health Organization is the UN agency that is the coordinating authority for international health work. In 1996, WHO launched the Global School Health Initiative (GSHI) which aims to increase the number of schools that can be called "health promoting" schools

(HPS). A HPS is defined as a school that "constantly strengthens its capacity as a healthy setting for living, learning and working".

Within WHO this initiative is coordinated by a multi-sectoral working group that incorporates expertise in mental health and Life Skills Training (LST), health and nutrition, physical environments etc. Some 22 WHO divisions are relevant to school health strategy, and 8 of these are represented in a coordinating group. WHO also collaborates with other UN organisations and with the World Bank.

WHO is a cosponsor of PCD. Four broad strategies have been identified to help schools become health promoting:

— Building capacity to advocate for improved school health programmes

— Mobilising resources for developing Health Promoting Schools

— Strengthening national capacities

— Research to improve school health programmes

This initiative emphasises the need to harness existing resources that exist at country, community and school level whilst also assisting governments to advocate for increased funds for HPS. The focus therefore is on influencing government policy through advocacy and the longer term sustainability of the initiative. To date, a broad range of advocacy orientated activities have been implemented under the auspices of WHO.

Although all seven WHO regional offices are actively involved in supporting this initiative, they are at various stages of development and employ different entry points to HPS depending on the regional location. In Fujian, China, for example, WHO have been supporting a project for de-worming since 1996 as an entry point to the development of HPS. A pilot study was undertaken to demonstrate the benefits of de-worming and health education.

In addition, the HPS project has become a trigger for activities that improved the physical environment through mobilising local government and community funds. These improvements included tree planting, extending the school buildings, increased numbers of toilets and taps for handwashing and other general environmental improvements.

WHO has also supported research on school based health services through the Task Force for Healthy School Children, within WHO/Special Programme for Research and Training in Tropical Diseases (TDR). This Task Force, within which PCD was represented, undertook enabling research on school based health service delivery, and field tested the UNICEF-led inter-agency Situation Analysis in Africa.

The Division of Control of Tropical Disease (CTD) has conducted school based deworming activities in Zanzibar, Seychelles, Oman and Mauritius and has worked with World Bank projects in West Africa (Guinea, Mauritania, Mali) to design school based health service delivery of anthelmintics. The Division is currently establishing a formal collaboration with the World Bank to support school based deworming projects.

WHO has set a target of 75% coverage with regular anthelmintic treatment of school-age children in countries where helminth infections are a public health problem.

The Partnership for Child Development is also part of the network aiming for this goal in year 2010. Other sector work on school health is also underway. For example, a general survey of the role of the school environment on child health has been completed.

An interagency evaluation of life skills training in schools is being planned. Regional offices are also actively pursuing their own programmes in this area. For example, the Pan American Health Organisation has a well established network of health promoting schools in the Americas. Schools are also the basis of health delivery for the 'PEPIN' disease control initiative that is active in Nicaragua, El Salvador, Guatemala and Honduras, and is currently expanding to 12 other countries. In October 1997, the World Bank and PAHO launched a joint initiative to promote school health and nutrition programmes in the Americas.

PAN AMERICAN HEALTH ORGANIZATION (PAHO) is an international public health agency with more than 90 years of experience in working to improve the health and living standards of the countries of the Americas. It serves as the specialised organization for health of the Inter-American System. It also serves as the Regional Office for the Americas of the World Health Organization.

PAHO works in all the countries of the region of the Americas, including the Caribbean. They have offices (called Representations) in 29 countries, each with a health promotion consultant who works directly with the Ministry of health and Education, as well as NGOs and teacher training colleges to strengthen school health programmes in the context of the Health Promoting Schools Initiative (HPSI).

PAHO's policy towards the school-age child is to promote the development of life skills, in the context of the HPSI, as well as to provide early detection, preventing services and primary health care through the schools and the health service structure in each country. The HPSI is a school based health promotion strategy, supporting through technical cooperation.

Most of PAHO's work is in advocacy to strengthen school policies and programs that go beyond traditional screening and school feeding programs, to integrate health promotion activities, especially life skills and to establish risk factor surveillance as a school based research activity. The HPSI strategy includes the following components:

— Needs assessment to identify strengths and weaknesses in school health programs.

— Review of policy and programs, with establishment or strengthening of joint commissions to coordinate school health activities between Health and Education sectors.

— Review and up-date of school health curriculum.

— Review and up-date of teacher training programs.

— Establishment of life skills education.

— Establishment of youth risk behaviour surveillance.

— Evaluation of health promoting capacity of schools.

Based on the results of a needs assessment, the HPSI integrates health requirements and interventions into a comprehensive strategy. Other programs in PAHO deal with specific issues, such as HIV/AIDS, helminth infection (Division of Disease Prevention and Control), nutrition education guidelines and micronutrient supplementation (Food and Nutrition Program), water and sanitation (Health and Environment Division).

PAHO and the World Bank established a Partnership to support school health programs in 1997, and in the context of this partnership have prepared joint documents and are in the process of preparing a joint publication on the school health situation in LAC, including case studies to highlight some good practices in depth.

Food and Agricultural Organisation (FAO)'s approach towards the health of school aged children is guided by the resolutions approved at the International Conference on Nutrition in December 1992 and further reconfirmed at the World Food Summit in 1996. FAO's current focus is on consolidating and expanding a programme on Nutrition Education in Primary Schools (NEPS), initiated in collaboration with the Netherlands Nutrition Center. This programme evolved from a survey in 55 countries Worldwide, which revealed the need for nutrition-related materials in primary schools and for teacher training in the use of these materials.

The NEPS programme of FAO aims at promoting interest in school-based nutrition education and assisting developing countries in the planning of such activities in primary schools. The English version of the two main documents of the NEPS programme, a "Handbook for National Curriculum Planners" and a "Planning Guide for Intermediaries and Teachers" will be available early in 2000.

The curriculum for a preparatory course for professionals, who will become facilitators of the planning process with teachers, has also been developed and will be tested in the first quarter of 2000. The next step is to utilise these materials to assist countries in developing their own nutrition education programmes and to prepare teaching and learning materials on nutrition for children between the ages of six and fourteen.

These materials will have to be appropriate to the local food and nutrition situation and to the level of detail and institutional capacity of the country of concern. For example, some countries may wish to incorporate nutrition education into the education curriculum while others will want to use the materials in a less structured way. By simultaneously addressing pupils, teachers, school personnel, parents and the community—an approach the NEPS programme is emphasising—it is possible to accelerate improvement in both the learning and living environments of the students.

FAO's strategy on nutrition education in schools fits well within the concept of health promoting schools as defined by World Health Organization (WHO). Accordingly, FAO is actively collaborating in the world-wide School Health Initiative, promoted by the WHO and its respective regional networks for health promoting schools.

World Food Programme (WFP) is concerned with two main areas in relation to school health: school feeding programmes and a micronutrient and health programme. These form part of the WFP's 'Food-for-Growth' objectives, with projects that target needy people at the most criticaltimes of their lives: babies, school children, pregnant and breast feeding women and the elderly.

WFP has a long-standing role in support of School Feeding Programmes (SFP) and supports around 60 programmes today. SFPs are increasingly targeted at poor countries and poor population groups within these countries: by the end of 1997 90% of WFP resources were to be directed at low-income food deficit countries.

SFPs are justified on the basis that they contribute to improvements in school enrolment and attendance rates, improvements in children's capacity to concentrate and assimilate information by alleviating short-term hunger and because they reduce the prevalence of some micronutrient deficiencies through the provision of fortified foods (Vitamin A, iron and iodine).

Increasingly, school-based de-worming programmes are being integrated into SFPs. Training of ministerial government staff, teachers and health staff at the peripheral level enables them to take responsibility for drug distribution. WFP, in collaboration with WHO, has completed the production of a "Health and Nutrition Manual for School Feeding Programmes". WFP is also coordinating the Women's Health and Nutrition Facility (WHNF), a programme funded by CIDA.

WHNF started in 1996 and is targeted at 15 low-income countries reaching over 900,000 women and 2.2 million children, including the school-aged child. Fortified foods, and specific micronutrients (depending on country needs) along with de-worming tablets are targeted to the most vulnerable in the population and at the most vulnerable stages in their life. As one of five key activity areas WFP focuses on projects that promote trade-offs in favour of education for girls and women. When supply of food is short and household income is low, girls' education often suffers, with a decrease in school attendance.

Along with 'traditional' school feeding programmes, WFP advocates the wider use of an approach tested in Malawi, Morocco, Niger, Pakistan and Yemen, which involves provision of a ration of food to the family when the daughter attends school, rather than assisting by feeding the child at school.

United Nations Children's Fund (UNICEF)'s medium-term strategy for 1996-2001 has identified women and young people as two main priority groups. Their policy is to help meet the basic rights and expand opportunities of children aged 0 to 18 within the framework of the 1989 UN Convention of the Rights of the Child, the 1990 World Summit for Children and the 1990 World Conference "Education for All" (EFA).

In addition, UNICEF's mandate is to support WHO and UNESCO policies and develop common strategies that address school health and the joint UN Programme on AIDS, which improves coverage and quality of school-based life skills/AIDS programmes. They also work within the Framework for Girls Education and take guidance from the Notebook on Programming for Young People's Health and Development.

UNICEF's Programme Priorities for 1998-2000 target key World Summit for Children goals, such as increased immunization coverage and improved access to education, in countries where progress is most needed. UNICEF is also part of the joint WHO Roll Back Malaria Campaign. UNICEF has been involved with school health programmes for many years and collaborates with a number of agencies including the World Bank, WHO, UNESCO and UNFPA.

Recently UNICEF has worked in some depth with several countries on school health programme policy.

Currently UNICEF supports a range of school health programmes in the following areas:

— Water, Sanitation and Hygiene programmes for schools in many countries (e.g. Uganda, Vietnam, and West Africa). These include health education courses in primary schools that focus on hygiene and the environment, provision of facilities for safe water, latrines, handwashing and garbage disposal.

— Life skills/AIDS programmes in schools including curriculum training (e.g. Zimbabwe, Thailand, Caribbean, Uganda, and Sri Lanka).

— Child-to-Child and extra-curricular activities for the whole community, with NGOs, for example: World Scout Federation, Red Cross and Red Cross Crescent Societies.

— Health and Nutrition services including the provision of micronutrients, anthelminthics and malaria tablets as part of UNICEF's overall strategy.

— Situation Analysis including adolescents' needs and responses. This was developed as an inter-agency (UNDP, UNESCO, UNFPA, WHO) activity, with PCD, and has been evaluated (by WHO) in Ghana, Zimbabwe, Botswana, Uganda and Kenya.

UNICEF is also currently developing ideas for a package of school based interventions that have the scope for sustainable national adaptation. Currently this package has four components as follows:

— *School Policies*: the focus will be country specific but should include protecting children against physical/ sexual abuse, protecting the rights of pregnant schoolgirls, protecting the rights of children who are disabled or are living with HIV/AIDS, and avoiding tobacco and substance abuse.

— *Skills-based health education/Life Skills Training*: ensuring school children get the skills as well as the information they need (for everything from preventing HIV/AIDS to contributing to civil society), in a way that fosters an interactive relationship between teachers and school children.

— *Water , Sanitation and Hygiene Promotion*: which should be linked to environmental issues and the hygiene component of health education. Schools could possibly act as a central point for community managed water programmes.

— *Specific medical/nutrition interventions*: there are a number of interventions that can be safely and simply implemented by teachers including the regular treatment of helminth infections, micronutrient supplementation (iron, vitamin A and iodine) and possibly, in selected areas, malaria treatment and tetracycline for the treatment of trachoma. Four programme principles have been identified to support these four interventions:

— *Strengthening partnerships/linkages*: between schools and communities/ parents, between education and the health sector including water and environmental health and between teachers and health workers.

— *Capacity building*: supporting the work teachers are already doing rather than overwhelming them; this includes the provision of training and the production of materials.

— *Sustainability*: seeking long term programmes, although not necessarily independent of external support.

— *Children's participation*: programmes which respond to needs recognised by the beneficiaries, and involving them actively in implementation.

Many UNICEF country programmes are already supporting elements of the package outlined above. For example in Punjab Province, Pakistan, UNICEF supports the Government Education Department in an integrated water, sanitation and hygiene education project in primary schools (IWSHEP).

The IWSHEP aims to increase access to water and sanitation facilities (through the provision of hand pumps and construction of latrines) in primary schools for girls; to promote hygiene practices and improved health among school-aged children and to strengthen the capacity of the Education Department by improving in-service teacher training which includes a hygiene-education component.

Additional support is targeted at NGO elementary schools to promote personal hygiene awareness and environmental sanitation among primary school children. School children and teachers provide an effective channel for education and appropriate training materials have been developed. About 8000 teachers were trained under the project in 1994. In Zimbabwe, UNICEF supports a LST/AIDS programme that is now under the Ministry of Education.

In 1992 UNICEF gave US$350,000 for the hire of local staff and programme start-up after which a fundraising campaign with local donors led to the raising of US$4 million of supplementary funding for 2 years. The programme supports weekly (compulsory) lessons on life skills and HIV/AIDS in all schools for children from grade 4 (9-10 years of age).

Teacher and student manuals are provided which are appropriate for the grade level, which address relationships, growing-up, life skills and health. Self-esteem and assertion are positively encouraged and concrete ways of responding to negative peer pressure are role-played at school.

Children undertake community-based projects that explore drug use, coping with HIV/AIDS and responsibilities of husbands and wives. Whilst many UNICEF country programmes are supporting school health initiatives, these have not yet been adequately tried and tested in order to be formalised within the organisation. It is anticipated that a select number of countries will be identified to pilot the package outlined above and explore the various programming implications before UNICEF formerly adopts the approach as a broad-based strategy.

In addition to school based programmes, UNICEF are also considering the more difficult area of reaching children in crises, as well as street children and working children, who are often not attending schools and whose health and nutrition are often most compromised. Work is also underway to examine options for improving the nutritional status of adolescents.

United Nations Educational, Scientific and Cultural Organisation (UNESCO) has a longstanding commitment to promote health and quality of life of all people and was one of the first UN organisations to undertake sector work on school health and nutrition. Ever since its establishment, various UNESCO programmes and projects have encompassed topics in relation to school health. In the late 1980s, revised definitions of school health served as a basis for a theory for a comprehensive approach to school health, as well as the comprehension that poor health and malnutrition lead to lowered school enrolment, educational wastage and poor classroom performance.

This was notably reflected in the World Declaration on Education for All and Framework of Action adopted in 1990. UNESCO plays a number of roles in relation to school health, covering the domains of healthy school environments, health education and delivery of school health services. Promoting safe and supportive environments for development of teaching and learning is an integral part of UNESCO's action. This includes assistance, for example, in providing comfortable and functional classrooms, adequate sanitary conditions at schools, a broad and balanced curriculum or caring interactions between and amongst staff and pupils.

Several programmes and projects of UNESCO concern the teaching and learning of health. Health and nutrition education is promoted in collaboration notably with WHO within the framework of the global school health initiative; however, co-operation with other relevant agencies such as UNICEF, World Bank or FAO is also being fostered. Current activities include national and sub-regional health education projects, teacher training and material development.

Health education issues are also mainstreamed throughout the education system, notably within the context of science and technology education, based as they are on similar aims and pedagogical principles providing knowledge and skills to improve the present and future well-being of all. UNESCO is also fostering the integration of specific health issues such as HIV/AIDS education, prevention of drug abuse, population education and reproductive health in numerous programmes world-wide in collaboration with UNAIDS, UNDCP, UNFPA, Education International and others.

In the field of school health services, UNESCO provides technical support for WFP School Feeding Programmes. This includes assistance with the appraisal of new programmes, management reviews, the evaluation of existing SFPs and the development of manuals on different aspects of design and implementation of SFPs.

United Nations Drug Control Programme (UNDCP) works in collaboration with other UN (and non-UN) agencies and organisations to support a number of programmes aimed at drug abuse prevention in young people. An example of UNDCP support is the project 'Young People in Crisis', implemented by UNICEF, UNDCP and other UN agencies, intergovernmental and non-governmental organisations. The project aims at meeting the health and developmental need of young people, focusing on prevention and reduction of the abuse of drugs, within the context of a comprehensive approach to the health and development of young people.

UNDCP supported projects include those aimed at both in-school and out-of-school young people. Practices used in the projects include peer counselling and education, employed in preventive education and awareness campaigns, as well as the use of alternative activities such as theatre, performance arts and sport. UNFPA also supports HIV/AIDS prevention activities for youth and adolescents in approximately 95 countries within the global strategy of the Joint United Nations

Programme on HIV/AIDS (UNAIDS) which became operational in 1996.

The main focus of UNFPA's activities is at the country level where the AIDS prevention activities are integrated into ongoing programmes and projects in reproductive health. Collaboration with NGOs in undertaking HIV/AIDS prevention activities is an integral part of most country programmes. An important objective of many UNFPA programmes is to strengthen the ability of developing countries to carry out the Programme of Action of the International Conference on Population Development (ICPD), agreed by all countries at the conference in 1994.

United Nations Programme on HIV/AIDS (UNAIDS) was launched in 1996 and seeks to coordinate global - especially UN - strategy on HIV/AIDS prevention, research and advocacy. Co-sponsors include WHO, UNFPA, UNDP, UNESCO, UNICEF, UNDCP and the World Bank. UNAIDS concentrates on working with all UN Agencies and otherpartners to comprehensively integrate action on HIV/AIDS. The three areas of focus in UNAIDS activities are:

— Facilitation of broad action

— Advocacy

— Identification of best practice in responding to HIV/AIDS

UNAIDS also acts as an information resource and can provide access to a range of useful materials including; the Best Practice collection, epidemiological information and evaluated materials. There has been a specific focus on school-based activities, and one of the inter-agency working groups deals only with this topic.

The major aim of this group is to promote life skills and Information, Education and Communication about HIV/AIDS programmes through schools. Although UNAIDS does not have a specific policy towards the school-aged child as such, UNAIDS publishes a range of items that refer to HIV/AIDS prevention for the school-aged child.

UNAIDS supports school-based health programmes by facilitating and advocating for action, rather than outright funding. UNAIDS plans and works with UN and other Agencies to advocate for greater attention to HIV prevention. UNAIDS is involved in mobilising partners at the country level, and assisting with technical expertise, as well as developing or attracting the necessary material and human resources to implement programs. In addition, the World Aids Campaign has focused on young people for several years.

International Atomic Energy Agency (IAEA) has a mandate to enlarge the contribution of atomic energy to health (and peace and prosperity) throughout the world. Specifically, IAEA supports a Human Health Programme, which includes a nutrition and health-related environmental studies sub-programme.

Projects supported under this sub-programme include "applied human nutrition assessment and research using nuclear and isotopic techniques" which aims to demonstrate the practical use of nuclear and isotopic techniques as tools for improving nutrition monitoring and for identifying effective food and nutrition strategies in developing countries. During 1997, the IAEA supported co-ordinated research in 33 developing countries and technical co-operation in 9 countries.

The World Bank is now giving greater emphasis to social sector approaches which are child-centred, which target poverty and which are responsive to client country needs. School based health and nutrition programmes contribute to this new approach, and are endorsed in the Health, Nutrition and Population Sector Strategy and are in the current draft of the Education Sector Strategy. Africa Region has a School Health and Nutrition Affinity Group and an articulated strategy.

Latin America and the Caribbean Region also has a strategy paper, and has launched a joint initiative with the Pan American Health Organisation to undertake operations and sector work in the Region. The World Bank is seeking to coordinate information on school health and nutrition approaches through an International School Health Initiative based in the Human Development Network. This seeks to enhance the quality of school health and nutrition programmes by:

— Providing access to expert advice, particularly in and from client countries.

— Providing a clearing house for examples of good practice.

— Developing practical toolkits for implementation, based on actual experience. o= Making quality information available through the Internet, the World Bank intranet and the World Bank Advisory Services.

— Building partnerships with governments and international agencies, institutions and NGOs.

— Assisting task teams to prepare school health components for World Bank projects.

The World Bank has established collaborations in order to promote quality technical input into programme design. The Bank has a formal partnership with PAHO in Latin American Countries (LAC), and is in dialogue with WHO on technical support for Africa. Within the UN system, partnerships are being developed with UNICEF, UNAIDS and WFP, amongst others. Partnerships are also being created with bilaterals.

For example, USAID are co-sponsors of the International School Health Initiative, and DFID, UK, are co-sponsors of sector work on the out of school child. The Bank is also developing partnerships with NGOs, for example Save the Children Federation, USA, and is a co-sponsor of the Partnership for Child Development and the Micronutrient Initiative. The rationale for World Bank interest in school health and nutrition programmes includes the following issues:

— There are more school-age children, and more in school, than ever before.

— School children are neglected by most health systems.

— Freedom from disease promotes intellectual as well as physical development.

— Healthy children get maximum benefit from their only opportunity for education.

— The benefits are greatest for the most disadvantaged - the girl child, the malnourished and the poor.

— The combination of an accessible population and an extensive trained workforce of teachers keep financial costs to a minimum.

— Builds on the investment in early child development, and builds the basics for appropriate social behaviour in adolescence.

In terms of World Bank Human Development strategy, school-based health and nutrition programmes should be simple and locally relevant, and should not overload already overstretched teachers or the curriculum. The following items might usefully contribute to such programmes:

— Life Skills Training and IEC - as part of a strategy to promote healthy lifestyles, and avoid violence, substance abuse, HIV/AIDS and teenage pregnancy.

— Health Services - as part of the Primary Health Care system, and providing screening for sight and hearing, simple health interventions (deworming, first aid) and referral.

— School Snacks - which are fortified with micronutrients and provided early in the school day.

— Exemplary School Environment - which supports health education messages about hygiene and sanitation.

— Equitable School Health Policies - that ensure the rights of school children.

— Strategies Beyond the School - that use the school as a community centre to provide services to out of school children.

Inter-American Development Bank (IADB), the oldest and largest regional multilateral development institution, was established in 1959 to help accelerate economic and social development in Latin America and the Caribbean. The Bank's operations cover the entire spectrum of economic and social development, including public health and education.

Current lending priorities include the areas of poverty reduction, social equity, modernisation and integration. IADB has an established record in supporting school-based health and nutrition projects.

Asian Development Bank (ADB) emphasises its strategic objective of promoting human development by expanding investments in the critical sectors of education, health and nutrition, water supply and sanitation. School health programmes supported by the ADB include:

—Nepal: Assistance to Primary School Feeding, in collaboration with WHO and bilateral donors. The project aims to enhance learning capacity by alleviating short-term hunger and to reduce the prevalence and intensity of intestinal parasites by deworming.

— Kyrgyz Republic: Community-Based Early Childhood Development. This projects includes a package of nutrition interventions such as community - and-school level growth monitoring and food supplementation interventions to address micronutrient and protein/energy deficiencies.

— Pakistan: Primary School Quality Improvement. This project includes the provision of free textbooks, incentives to keep girls in school and special courses in nutrition and life skills. It also provides interventions to upgrade shelterless schools.

Canadian International Development Agency (CIDA) is a lead donor in the area of nutrition programming. Since 1992, CIDA has contributed over $87 million to nutrition projects of which $78 million have been focused on micronutrients. An additional $120 million has been contributed to integrated projects which combine nutrition with health, basic education and income generation activities.

CIDA is a founding member of the Micronutrient Initiative (MI) which has a grant of approximately $53 million and is supported by IDRC, UNDP, UNICEF, USAID and the World Bank. Although CIDA's budget is not exclusively channelled through the school system, examples of CIDA programmes that affect the school-aged child include:

— Funding to WFP for school feeding/health programmes and through the Women's Health Facility.

— The MI South Asia Programme which aims to eliminate iodine and vitamin A deficiency and reduce iron deficiency in women in Bangladesh, India, Nepal and Pakistan by the year 2000.

— The Ecuador Iodine Deficiency Disorder (IDD) Programme which has implemented a school-based IDD monitoring system where school children bring samples of salt to school to test for iodine in class using low-cost rapid tests.

— A School Feeding Programme in Haiti implemented by a French-Canadian NGO costing $1.6 million which started in 1998.

CIDA recognises the link between girls' education wider health issues, and that discrimination against the education of girls is an important area to address in many countries. "Women's education, especially the number of years of schooling, is closely related to reduction of child mortality and morbidity, improvement of family health and nutrition, and decline in population growth."

Danish International Development Assistance (DANIDA) do not have a defined strategy for support towards school based health programmes although they are supporting other agencies through their bilateral programme. For example funding to UNICEF in Uganda for school based health education activities. Members of the education and health sector in DANIDA have discussed the need for school-based health and nutrition programming on a number of occasions but constraints on time and finances have prevented them from taking this further.

Although DANIDA's water and sanitation strategy, "Water, Sanitation and Hygiene (WASH)" does not refer to schoolchildren directly, DANIDA supports the provision of water supplies to primary schools within their rural water supplies programmes in developing countries. The health education component of their water strategy, which incorporates messages about hygiene behaviour and water-related diseases also, targets primary schools.

Department for International Development, U.K. (DFID) do not have a current policy which refers specifically to the school aged child although they have supported a range of projects and programmes which directly benefit this group. Support to SCF in South America for an HIV/AIDS programme which works with adolescents within schools and a programme that supports professionals (school teachers, health workers) in detecting and providing follow-up to individual cases of child abuse.

In India, DFID have supported a large programme in Andhra Pradesh aimed at improving the health of school children by reorganising and strengthening existing school health services. The programme, costing more than UKPDS 4 million over a five-year period has recently been terminated for diverse reasons. Also in India DFID provides funding for the School Health Action and training Programme (SeHAT) Programme and its expansion into Delhi centre.

Norwegian Agency for Development Co-operation (NORAD) does not have a particular policy focus for school-aged children but does support the education sectors in many developing countries in basic educationprogrammes, including teacher training greater access to education for girls and construction of schools.

Under this programme, which targets children from first to fourth grade in primary school, 18 new schools were built and 76 teachers trained in 1998. The programme also includes providing water supplies and digging hygienic latrines on school sites, with associated education in hygiene and simple health precautions.

NORAD are currently supporting a School Nutrition Programme (SNP) in Sindh, Pakistan which is implemented with co-operation from the Government of Sindh and Aga Khan University along with NGOs. The SNP is a pilot programme that supports school feeding in schools in four rural districts. Initiated in 1994 the programme reaches around 12,000 beneficiaries and supports the following objectives:

— Increase enrolment, retention and regular attendance of children, especially girls, in school

— Improve the nutritional status of primary school children and their siblings o= Improve student achievement

— Increase parental and community awareness of the importance of child nutrition and education

— Explore possibilities for community involvement at the school level in improving education and nutrition

— Explore the possibilities for implementing SNP through NGOs.

The SNP supports participatory training for PTAs and NGOs to enable them to take increasing responsibility for the programme and thus ensure its long-term sustainability. PTAs are responsible for dealing with the funds, food purchasing and in some areas, food preparation. The formation and commitment of the PTAs is viewed as a particular strength of the programme.

The SNP is being expanded into additional districts and is being considered as an approach for replication in Nepal. The impact of the SNP has recently been evaluated which suggests that whilst the nutritional status of children has improved along with the school enrolment and retention rates, there has also been a decline in educational achievement. The latter may be due to the programme demands on parents and children time.

Swedish International Development Agency (SIDA) has no special policy with respect to the health and nutrition of the school aged child but supports basic education and education reform. Within their education reform programme, SIDA supports, and intend to increase their support for, curriculum development work relating to HIV/AIDS education such as the production of materials, teacher training and the use of popular theatre media etc to reduce risk behaviour.

They consider school-based programmes to be most effective if integrated with other curriculum content i.e. health education, social science and biology. They are working closely with governments as well as international organisations (UNAIDS and UNICEF) and NGOs. They also support UNESCO's resource centre for HIV/AIDS education and UNESCO's regional training programme for HIV/AIDS education. The importance of sexual and reproductive health is acknowledged by SIDA in its "Strategy for Promotion of Sexual and Reproductive Health and Rights in Development Cooperation".

SIDA sees peer education programmes as particularly important in this area. An emphasis on gender equality is also seen as important. SIDA and NORAD are co-funding an African Medical Research Foundation (AMREF) project "Regional Adolescent Sexual and Reproductive Health (ASHR) Project" with components in Kenya, Tanzania, Uganda and Ethiopia. The project aims to "achieve an improved and maintained health status of adolescents in the region through healthy sexual relations and behaviour, reduced exposure to STD/HIV, unwanted pregnancy and increased access to effective services".

Youth both in and out of school are targeted as well as service providers, teachers, parents and community elders. In the broader area of child health in general, SIDA places emphasis on preventive measures (e.g. immunisation) and on the integrated management of childhood illness.

United States Agency for International Development (USAID) is the United States federal government agency that implements America's foreign economic and humanitarian assistance programs. USAID's Africa

Bureau has formulated a school health position paper that emphasises the same program elements and rationale as that of the World Bank.

USAID support large school-based health programs that deliver health interventions such as deworming and micronutrient supplementation across Africa. Many of these programs are in various stages of evaluation. USAID also support smaller school health activities such as latrine construction, community based nutrition grants, school gardens and borehole drilling within USAID and UNICEF sponsored programmes in Africa.

ActionAid works in countries in Africa and Asia and Latin America. 60% of their income is provided by child sponsors who regularly contribute to projects. Other sources of income include appeals, grants from the UK National Lottery Charity Board and Comic Relief. Support is given in a number of areas such as: emergency relief projects; health -particularly maternal and child; education - including adult literacy, increasing access to education, renovating and building schools; water and sanitation; HIV/AIDS prevention.

Over the last fifteen years, The Aga Khan Foundation (AKF) has supported various programmes in the area of health education, particularly in six countries: India, Tanzania (Zanzibar), Pakistan, Uganda, Kenya and, most recently, Tajikistan. AKF also supported the Child-to-Child Trust in the United Kingdom during its early years.

The AKF-funded health education projects have usually followed the Child-to-Child approach, aiming to increase the knowledge and practices of good health promoting behaviours in school-aged children: i.e.,

Informed children pass on key health messages and practices to their peers and younger children and also share the information with their families and the wider community. When AKF developed its Education Programme, it included attention to the importance of early childhood development and school improvement at primary and secondary levels.

AKF supports programmes which recognize that children are part of a family and wider community which influence, and are influenced by, them (the children). The average duration of AKF funding for education projects is six years. This has generally been enough time to experiment with a curriculum model and make changes, develop training and support materials, begin to disseminate the results, and assist the project in becoming self-sufficient. For example, one of the first Child-to-Child projects in Delhi, India become the basis for a national health education programme sponsored by the government.

American Jewish World Service (AJWS) founded in 1985, AJWS provides non-sectarian humanitarian assistance to disadvantaged people in Africa, Asia, Latin America, the Middle East, Russia and Ukraine. Working in partnership with local grassroots NGOs, AJWS supports and implements small-scale international development projects.

Although Healthlink Worldwide has no formal policy or guidelines on school health, they support school-based health programmes through both programming and funding. The main focus of Healthlink Worldwide's support for school age children is in the area of health education, producing educational materials for use by school children, and using innovative approaches for training teachers in the use of these materials.

The emphasis is on general health and nutrition, although this may include educational and promotional work in areas such as HIV/AIDS, water and sanitation. Healthlink Worldwide is supporting the Municipal Corporation of Delhi and Bombay Municipal Corporation, through an NGO called SEARCH New Delhi to implement one large programme in India that focuses on primary schools in Delhi and Bombay called the School Health Action and Training Project (SeHAT).

SeHAT received funding from, DFID, European Union, UK National Lottery Charity Fund, Stanley Thomas Johnson Foundation and the Aga Khan Foundation. Initially Healthlink Worldwide and the School Health Services in Delhi ran a pilot programme in selected low-income schools for four years, developing methods and materials for incorporating health topics into the curriculum.

These include communicable diseases, sanitation, nutrition and personal cleanliness as well as other health-related behaviour including tobacco, safety and pollution. Government policy informs the programme approach: a re-orientation of teaching methodology away from traditional didactic techniques and towards child-centred, activity based teaching that fosters informed choice and a teacher-led, curriculum oriented approach to health education in schools.

Evaluation of the pilot found that there had been a marked increase in awareness of health issues, up-take of programme issues such as self-care, improvements in oral hygiene and a marked involvement by teachers and parents in the programme. SeHAT is well monitored and most recently evaluated in 1997. Currently the programme covers a total of 850 primary schools, reaching approximately 68,000 children.

Healthlink Worldwide is currently exploring ways of incorporating malaria education and control into health promoting schools in Sub Saharan Africa, in collaboration with theMalaria Consortium, the London School of Tropical Medicine and the Liverpool School of Tropical Medicine. Other plans include collaboration with the Child to Child Trust in a project working with families affected by HIV/AIDS in Kenya and Uganda, involving both school age children and development of children under five.

CARE has a number of program areas that affect school-aged children, these include:

— *Education*: promoting literacy, numeracy, and school attendance, especially among girls.

— *Food Security*: including school feeding.

— *Health and Population:* encompassing promotion of AIDS awareness and prevention, children's health, water and sanitation.

CARE integrates reproductive health efforts with other programmes, including girls' education, water and sanitation, microenterprise and children's health. CARE supports a range of school health and nutrition projects through its education and health programmes.

Catholic Fund for Overseas Development (CAFOD)'s current guidelines are not to support formal education. Recently, however, they are reconsidering their policy on this as Asian and African governments are increasingly requesting assistance in the education sector (including health and nutrition). This has prompted an analysis of the issues in CAFOD who have been developing a database of existing education-based programmes, which is now nearing completion.

CAFOD support a range of small programmes in Africa and Asia (usually through partners) that affect the school age child but are not school-based. Examples include support for orphans of AIDS victims through the provision of school fees and education materials; youth programmes which include health components, for example HIV/AIDS education and life skills training.

A food frequency questionnaire and a nutrition knowledge test were administered to all students before and after the intervention. The results indicate that the experimental group significantly increased their intake of fruits and vegetables and showed a significant increase in nutrition knowledge compared to the control group.

Catholic Relief Services (CRS) is currently implementing/supporting education programming in approximately 25 countries in Africa, Asia, Europe/ Balkans, Latin America, and the Caribbean. Of these, approximately 15 country programs are implementing health/hygiene/nutrition (HHN) programming within schools or nonformal education settings. Twelve of these 15 are carrying out school feeding programs.

Of the school feeding programs, most (Burkina Faso, Ghana, Liberia, Sierra Leone, Benin, Sudan, Haiti, India) are being funded primarily by USAID's Food for Peace office. Another three are funded by the European Community (Pakistan, Egypt, Armenia), and one (Mali) is funded by World Food Programme. In addition, Egypt is implementing a nonformal education program for adolescent girls which has a large health education component, funded by CEDPA (Centre for Education, Development, & Population Activities).

Child to Child Trust (CtC) support child centred approaches to health education through:

— Design and distribution of health education materials which are used by children, teachers and health workers.

— Advice and assistance to health education workers in planning, implementing and evaluating projects using the Child-to Child approach.

— Coordinating a Worldwide information network for people and projects around the world who use the Child-to-Child approach.

The school based approach is undertaken in-line with the WHO Global Initiative and emphasises what poorer schools can realistically do to improve the health of school children within the framework of existing resources and without the exploitation of children or the over-burdening of the teachers. Priority areas for the Child-to-Child Trust are:

— Helping children who live in difficult circumstances, for example those who live in refugee camps, children affected by war, and children with disabilities.

— Improving health promotion in schools, involving children in spreading good health ideas and practices to families, out-of-school children and the wider community.

— Supporting the development of local Child-to-Child resource units and networks. In the Mpika District of Zambia, CtC have started a new initiative, funded by Comic Relief, to develop strategies for implementing inclusive education (IE).

CtC run an annual course in London, 'Planning Health Promotion in Schools' and have published a book, Health Promotion in Our Schools, which is a practical guide for those who wish to develop 'Health Action' schools. In Pakistan, a five year pilot project entitled Health Action Schools Pilot Project has been initiated to develop prototypes for 'Health Action' schools and is funded by the Aga Khan Foundation and SCF UK.

The project, which is located in contrasting socio-economic areas (urban, rural and mixed urban/rural) supports the development of training and support networks for schools endeavouring to become 'Health Action' schools and has an operational research component to identify changes in health awareness, health behaviour and education performance among the school children.

In Kenya, a CtC project has been implemented through which it is hoped that major policy changes will occur, especially the inclusion of health education as a separate curriculum subject in primary education. The programme, based on a three-year plan supports the dissemination of CtC; training for those working for 'Health Action' schools, production of materials, and teacher training in CtC. Funding is provided by DANIDA.

CtC resource units and networks have been developed to promote and encourage Child-to- Child activities in the Arab world, Central and South America, East and West Africa and India.

Christian Aid (CA) works in over 60 countries throughout the world. It runs emergency appeals for areas in crisis (In recent years for Rwanda, Montserrat, Sierra Leone and former Yugoslavia). It campaigns for fair trade and an end to Third World Debt and has highlighted issues 'such as the child sex industry in southeast Asia and child labour in Pakistan. CA projects fall into three main categories in relation to school-age children and health:

—Educating children on health issues through the existing school system. An example of this support is the 'Molo Songololo' project in South Africa which works with school-age children on children's rights and the promotion of equity among all races to promote a more equal society. Molo publish a magazine that is read by more than 50,000 children and teachers. Also in South Africa, CA supports the African and Educational Puppetry Production (AREPP) which focuses on HIV/AIDS awareness, children's empowerment which tackles issues around child abuse. These productions are performed throughout SA in urban and rural schools.

In Jamaica, CA support an AIDS awareness project, which support school-based workshops and work with youth groups. In Kenya, CA support the Kenya Tourism Concern project which works in schools to sensitise children on the issues relating to tourism and child prostitution.

Establishing alternative education establishments where health education forms part of the curriculum. CA works in situations where the school system is inadequate (e.g. because of political unrest, government cuts etc.) and therefore supports community efforts to provide education and LST to children who would otherwise not receive any education. An example of this is the S-Corner project in Jamaica that involved the establishment of a college in a very poor area of Kingston experiencing gang violence and a high dropout rate from schooling. The educational programme includes health education and LST.

Community-based work which addresses both children's education and health as part of an overall community development strategy. CA support a range of community based projects that assist children who are forced to work in the day to obtain night-time schooling (e.g. in India and Tibet) and therefore help them break away from the destructive poverty cycle which often leads to child-labour.

Danish Bilharziasis Laboratory (DBL) is an independent research institution affiliated to the Ministry of Foreign Affairs/ DANIDA, Denmark, and the University of Copenhagen. The core funding is from DANIDA, but a substantial part of the research is externally funded. DBL has the double aim of strengthening research capacity and carrying out applied research, through extensive course activities and collaborative research projects. DBL main activities take place in a number of sub-Saharan African countries with the main emphasis on Uganda, Kenya, Tanzania, Zimbabwe and Ghana.

In terms of school health, DBL is deeply involved in school based research projects in Kenya (Kenyan-Danish Health Research Project - KEDAHR) and Tanzania (The Pangani Project). The various projects are primarily research projects which aim at improving and developing school health programmes rather than providing services as such. Furthermore, DBL is, or has been, involved in school health projects in Malawi, Northern Tanzania, Eastern Uganda and the Coastal Province of Kenya.

From 1982 to the present, a significant increase in USAID and private funding has allowed Helen Keller Internationa (HKI) to accelerate its program development and expand in to new countries in Africa and South America. All partnerships are developed with the expectation of eventual HKI withdrawal based on a turnover of responsibility within a given period.

The primary goal of HKI programs has become upgrading local and indigenous skills in areas of service delivery, program design and implementation, evaluation, and operations research. Helen Keller International specialises in the programmes that address Nutrition (especially Vitamin A and micronutrient deficiencies), Onchocerciasis, Trachoma, Eye care and Education and rehabilitation of the blind.

Oxfam is currently running a campaign in education. The campaign on education is aimed at achieving national and international policy changes to contribute to the goal of universal primary education by 2015. Oxfam has education programmes in several countries in Africa, South Asia and Latin America. The aim is to scale up these programmes as part of Oxfam contribution to the education for all objective.

Although there is no specific health aspect at present, these programmes are building a framework where health education could be introduced in the future. Oxfam are also interested in collaborating with other organisations in the delivery of school health interventions. In Angola and Kosova Oxfam have been running programmes for refurbishing schools, that include incorporating water and sanitation facilities, with hygiene education.

Partnership for Child Development (PCD) was set up in 1992 to undertake operations research on school health programmes. The Partnership is involved in research, technical advice and support in some 50 countries throughout the world. The Partnership tests and evaluates simple, low cost school health programmes in several countries at an operationally realistic scale, involving between 50,000 and 3 million children in widely scattered sites throughout the world.

The Peace Corps was established in the USA in 1961. It is a voluntary organisation with approximately 155,00 volunteers working on development projects in 134 countries around the world. 40% of volunteers work in education and 18% in health. Both these fields include projects with school health components. Peace Corps education projects often seek to improve education for women and girls. They include primary education projects with a particular focus on health education and awareness.

Health Extension volunteers aim to raise consciousness in communities about the need for health education. They may also assist in the training of trainers for peer education about STDs/AIDS. An example of a Peace Corps program in the area of AIDS prevention is the 'Teach English Prevent AIDS' program in Cameroon, which involves the teaching of English in Francophone schools, using health education about HIV/AIDS prevention.

Water and Sanitation Extension Volunteers serve in a broad range of water/sanitation projects and hygiene education activities. This includes constructing wells, tapping springs and building latrines; improving facilities for storing potable water and doing community outreach to heighten awareness of water, sanitation and health issues.

Plan International (PLAN) is one of the world's largest child-focused development organisations. PLAN has five main inter-related "Domain and Programme Principles":

— Growing up Healthy

— Learning

— Habitat

— Livelihood

— Building Relations.

PLAN currently runs programmes in 42 countries. PLAN's Growing up Healthy Domain is concerned with the physical and mental health of children, that of adults who care for them, and the children's emotional and social well being. Within this domain, interventions supported by PLAN, addressing the health and development of the school age children, include:

— School and community based health and nutrition education: Child-to-child, health clubs, peer support groups.

— Promotion of good nutrition: Prevention and control of micronutrient deficiency, school meals and school gardens.

— Promotion of school medical services in collaboration with the Ministry of Health: Control of intestinal parasites and other infectious diseases which affect the health of the school-age child, dental health, early detection and correction of visual and hearing impairments.

— Promotion of personal hygiene.

— Prevention of neglect, abuse and exploitation.

— Life skills training.

PLAN also support programmes concerned with the health and development of adolescents (including life skills, sexual and reproductive health), health and development of children with special needs and those with disabilities. PLAN's advisory groups believe that the child-to-child approach is an effective option in health education. PLAN also encourages the Growing up Healthy and Learning Domains to collaborate with each other to promote the inclusion of health topics in school curricula.

Save the Children Federation, USA (SC/US) has made the policy decision to establish school health and nutrition as a programming priority. In a 1998 strategy paper, SCF, USA identifies a four-part defined core for school health, targeted at primary school attendees through their schools. The core school health programme consists of: parasite control (especially intestinal helminths); micronutrient supplementation (e.g. iron, iodine. Vitamin A); child-centred active learning; "Life skills - skills for life", including areas such as health education, reproductive health and decision-making.

SC/US has mobilised private resources to enhance agency capacity and initiate and plan pilot programs to serve as models for school-based health and nutrition activities. These model programmes can be shared with other countries, donors and interested parties to learn from and serve as a basis for sharing ideas. They have successfully used this "living university" approach to expand their nutrition programmes from small pilots to countrywide 'to-scale' programmes.

In April, 2000, WHO, UNESCO, UNICEF, and the World Bank jointly organized a strategy session at the World Education Forum in Dakar, Senegal. The strategy session was aimed at raising the education sector's awareness of the value of implementing an effective school health, hygiene and nutrition programme as one of its major strategies to achieve Education for All.

Interactive radio instruction (IRI), a methodology developed to turn a typically one-way technology into a tool for active learning in and outside the classroom, continues to be an attractive educational strategy in developing countries after almost 30 years. The original model for IRI math, created in Nicaragua by a team from Stanford University in the early 1970s, sought to combine the low cost and high reach of the radio medium and a clear understanding of how people learn.

Since that time, 20 countries around the world have developed IRI programs for a variety of subjects, audiences, and learning environments, many of which have been sustained for up to 10 years and counting. The methodology has been expanded and adapted to include different levels of math, science, health, English, Spanish and Portuguese, environmental education, early childhood development, and adult basic education for learners of all ages.

In each case, the series has been designed specifically by local specialists to be engaging and to meet learning objectives in that country. After three decades, interest in IRI does not seem to be waning. In Guinea, IRI has gone to scale on an unprecedented level in West Africa to reach students and teachers on a national level. The Guinean IRI series is integrated with teacher development initiatives and is used in almost all primary schools across the nation, with 880,000 students.

In Zambia, a new IRI series is being developed that reaches out to students who otherwise would be without schools, and have become increasingly vulnerable due to poverty and the HIV/AIDs. This example shows how IRI can be used effectively to overcome obstacles of access in Africa and to increase the chances that students can receive an education.

IRI is distinct from most other forms of distance education because its primary goal has been improvement of educational quality. Unlike many distance learning efforts that are designed primarily to address access issues, IRI began as a tool to use in the classroom to counteract inadequate teacher training, poor achievement among learners, and few resources.

While IRI has demonstrated that it can be used to expand access and increase equity in both formal and nonformal educational settings, it retains a development strategy and methodology that require that active learning, attention to pedagogy, and formative evaluation included in the design.

The IRI methodology is also different in that it requires that learners stop and react to questions and exercises through verbal response to radio characters, group work, and physical and intellectual activities while the program is on the air. For both teacher and student, the lesson becomes an immediate hands-on and experiential guide. Short pauses are provided throughout the lessons, after questions and during exercises, to ensure that students have the time to think and respond adequately.

Interaction also is encouraged within the learning environment between teacher and learners as they work together to conduct short experiments, perform activities, and solve problems using local resources and imaginative situations and stories. The pedagogy of IRI is more deliberate than active learning alone. IRI series guide learners through the learning process with activities related to measurable learning objectives.

Educational content is organized and distributed across lessons so that learning is built on previous knowledge, and new learners can understand more easily the subject being taught. Activities and problems are modeled first by radio characters so the teacher and learners have an idea of the process they are undertaking and the skills and support that may be required.

All of these elements are knit together through story lines, music, characterization, and other attributes available through the audio medium. IRI programs cater specifically to the audience and the situation where they will be used. Thus, one of the most important aspects of the design is its reliance on audience research, participation, and field-level formative evaluation to ensure that lessons are engaging and relevant and that learners can achieve the educational objectives.

The attraction of the IRI approach can be attributed at least partially to well-evaluated projects that have demonstrated greater learning gains for students using IRI programs than students in control groups not using IRI programs.

In most cases, students show progressively greater achievement increases over time. In South Africa, for example, students who received fewer than 33 English in Action lessons improved by 6.7%, students who received between 34 and 66 lessons improved by 13%, and students who received more than 66 programs improved by 24%.

In Zambia, interactive radio instruction now shows that IRI also can help to increase access to education for children who are without schools and teachers and who are increasing vulnerable due to the effects of HIV/AIDs and poverty. IRI is delivering basic education to out-of-school children, especially orphans and other vulnerable children, in community learning centres.

IRI is a collaborative effort among communities, churches, nongovernmental organizations (NGOs), the Ministry of Education's Educational Broadcast Services (EBS), the Peace Corps, and the Education Development Centre. EBS develops and broadcasts the programs and develops supplementary materials such as mentor's guides, and the Ministry of Education trains mentors in its District Resource Centres and provides supervision/ monitoring at participating learning centres.

Communities, churches, schools (both government and community), and NGOs provide the learning centre venues, mentor(s) to facilitate the radio broadcasts, radio receivers, a blackboard, and some locally made materials. Communities also mobilize out-of-school children to attend the learning centres each day.

The Education Development Centre (EDC) has trained EBS writers and producers and assisted EBS to develop a training of trainers program for Ministry of Education resource centre staff who, in turn, train mentors to run the community-based learning centres.

The Republic of Guinea, a former French colony on the West African coast, provides an example of how a multichannel learning approach and IRI can and do improve instruction on a nationwide scale. In Guinea, school enrolment has been at best around 40% (and closer to 30% for girls), and dropout, particularly female dropout, is frequent, and repetition rampant.

Even for those who attain grade 6 (about 35% of those who start primary school), more than half fail the state exam that allows them to graduate to the seventh grade. The Guinean curriculum is not strikingly different from or more difficult than the curriculum used by neigh-boring nations with higher enrolment and retention rates.

This suggests that it is not what is being taught in Guinea, but, rather the organization of the learning processor the flow of what happens in the classroom-that has to be addressed to provide children with better access to the concepts and topics that make up the Guinean curriculum.

In addition, Guinean classrooms are often devoid of any instructional aids. In general, they are undecorated, tin-roofed spaces where teachers, who must instruct between 50 and 80 students, have nothing other than a blackboard and chalk, and the children have only a blank book and a pen. Such problems are nationwide, so the EDC needed to devise a program that would reach the roughly 22,000 primary teachers in need of support and in-service training.

Both face-to-face training and materials focus on widening the channel of teacher-student communication to permit two-way communication (teacher-student and student- teacher). Once teachers are able to accept student input along the teacher-student communication channel, they are better able, for example, to perceive the abilities of their female students and better able to call on those abilities in organizing student-student communication.

Teacher training and other recurrent costs stay relatively consistent over time after the development stage, and then vary, depending on how much training is integrated into the program, the subject being taught, and the special circumstances of the country. Other recurrent costs include airtime, distribution of simple supplementary print materials (such as one-page worksheets inserted into local newspapers or distributed at the beginning of the year), batteries and radios, and maintaining a management system or unit focused on IRI.

IRI is also different from many other educational strategies because of the wide reach of the radio broadcasts. As a result, increasing the number of learners increases the cost very little. In contrast, most other interventions with high variable costs require a proportional number of new school facilities, textbooks, or teachers as additional learners are added.

In an IRI project, these extra factors do not influence the cost of the program dramatically, and, because the primary products- radio programs-are broadcast, the cost per learner decreases proportionally with any increase in users. Governments using IRI projects have experimented with various cost-sharing and income-generation schemes to pay for recurrent costs.

In addition, most IRI projects are sustained at least partially through partnerships between ministries of education and ministries of communication and broadcasting. Most cost analyses of IRI programs have incorporated these factors into their design and project per student costs over time using the underlying principle that the cost of development is offset when more learners use the programs.

6

Child Nutrition: An Essential Element of Academic Progress

A Health-Promoting School contributes to improve environmental conditions, such as technical and societal issues in the school, community and family, might not be ideal and affect the extent to which nutrition interventions can be implemented by fostering nutrition-related interventions even in a less healthful environment.

Healthy nutrition takes many forms and is understood differently in different countries and among different cultures. In general, healthy nutrition should be an integral part of daily life that contributes to the physiological, mental and social well-being of individuals. It is the combined effect of food, health and care.

Nutritional well-being is determined by consuming safe food as part of an appropriate and balanced diet that contains adequate amounts of nutrients in relation to bodily requirements. The health and lifestyle of an individual influences the extent to which food contributes to good social, mental and physical well-being.

Care is shown by providing time, attention and support in the household and the community to meet the food and health needs of the child and other family members. Furthermore, social ties are validated and maintained by the exchange of food since offering food is associated with offering love, affection and friendship.

Malnutrition is any physical condition resulting either from an inappropriate or inadequate diet, such as a diet that either provides too much or too little of necessary nutrients, or from a physical inability to absorb or metabolize nutrients. Malnutrition can be related to various factors, such as infections which lead to poor appetite and malabsorption, poverty, and lack of access to food, sanitation and/or health services. Malnutrition negatively affects the quality of life and learning as well as death and disease status.

Malnutrition includes overnutrition and nutritional deficiencies as well as undernutrition which impair health, intellectual activity, adaptive behaviour, education, productivity and well-being, and can induce death. Nutrition interventions are policies, services, learning experiences and other actions implemented by schools, individuals or groups to make healthy nutrition a way of daily life. Nutrition interventions are designed to promote health and decrease the risk of disease.

In a Health-Promoting School, nutrition interventions are integrated into all aspects of the school and community life, such as the physical and psychosocial environment; a wide variety of educational opportunities; school/community projects; school health services; health promotion for school staff; counselling and social support programmes; physical exercise, recreation and sport; and food programmes.

Nutrition is vital to all human beings and to the societies that they comprise. Adequately nourished people enjoy optimal growth, health and well-being. Girls in particular benefit from good nutrition as their health status and eating habits have a major impact on pregnancy, lactation and nourishment of their children.

While over 800 million people are estimated to lack access to food to meet their daily basic needs for energy and protein, more than 3 billion people are deficient in essential micronutrients such as iodine, vitamin A and iron. Many forms of malnutrition exceed the worldwide incidence of most other diseases. For instance, more than half of the 12.2 million deaths every year of children under the age of 5 in developing countries are associated with malnutrition.

Thus, efforts are needed to make healthy nutrition accessible for everyone, everywhere and at all times. Schools provide the most effective and efficient way to reach large portions of the population, including young people, school personnel, families and community members. Students can be reached at influential stages in their lives, during childhood and adolescence when lifelong nutritional patterns are formed. Children at every successive year from the earliest grade through secondary school can be addressed.

Schools have been given the mandate and responsibility to enhance all aspects of development and maturation of children and youth under qualified guidance. Furthermore, schools also provide a setting to introduce nutrition information and technologies to the community and can lead the community in advocating policies and services that promote good nutrition.

Good nutrition strengthens the learning potential and well-being of children Good health and nutrition are needed to achieve one's full educational potential because nutrition affects intellectual development and learning ability. Multiple studies report significant findings between the nutritional status and cognitive test scores or school performance.

Consistently, children with more adequate diets score higher on tests of factual knowledge than those with less adequate nutrition. For instance, studies in Honduras, Kenya and the Philippines show that the academic performance and mental ability of pupils with good nutritional status are significantly higher than those of pupils with poor.nutritional status, independent of family income, school quality and teacher ability.

Good nutrition in early life enables healthy adulthood and ageing Among well nourished people, acute disease and illness tend to be less frequent, less severe and of shorter duration thus providing increased capacities to perform daily activities. Good nutrition also fosters mental, social and physical well-being throughout life; for instance, by strengthening a positive body image and increasing the sense of personal worth.

Healthy nutrition can also contribute to a more comfortable life by helping young people to develop healthy teeth and gums. Thus, good nutrition during childhood helps to lay the foundation for a healthy adulthood. A healthy diet can also contribute to more mobility in older age. For instance, it is likely that youth is a unique time to acquire the strongest possible bones to decrease the risk of osteoporosis in old age.

Diets rich in calcium can help build stronger bones while diets rich in protein and salt increase the chances of losing bone density later in life. Thus, it is important to enable children to establish or reinforce personal skills, healthy perceptions and useful knowledge in nutrition to promote their own health and the health of those they care for. It is beneficial to teach persons healthy eating patterns when they are young since eating patterns are established early in life and are difficult to change once they are developed during youth.

Many of the problems of childbirth, such as haemorrhage, infection and obstructed labour, can be reduced in severity by adequate nutrition earlier in life. For instance, small stature, which may be related to undernutrition, is a well-known risk factor for obstructed labour. Anaemia, which can result from inadequate intake of iron-rich foods, lack of iron supplements or parasite infection, is known to cause about one-fifth of maternal deaths during pregnancy and childbirth.

Women's social roles can also be enhanced through nutrition interventions in areas where women primarily perform the role of preparing food for their families. Increases in women's nutritional knowledge help ensure better preparation, preservation, handling and distribution of foods. Increased capacity to handle their responsibilities can, in turn, enhance women's social and economic status.

Thus, ensuring schooling with effective nutrition interventions for young girls can be one of the most important and effective means of improving women's nutrition and health status because of the associated effects on health, fertility and social development.

Healthy nutrition contributes to decreasing the risks of today's leading health problems Studies show that early indicators of chronic disease begin in youth. For instance, avoiding obesity in childhood and youth is important because once attained, obesity tends to continue in adulthood, contributing to chronic diseases. Furthermore, the hardening of arteries and high blood cholesterol levels, which make a major contribution to coronary heart.disease, are influenced by nutrition and lifestyle.

Thus, adequate nutrition and physical activity are likely to have long-term health benefits in reducing the growing number of diet-related, non-communicable diseases. Obesity in infants, children and adults is a major problem worldwide. The prevalence of obesity in adults is 10% to 25% in most countries of Western Europe, 20% to 25% in some countries in the Americas, up to 40% in some countries in Eastern Europe, and more than 50% in some countries in the Western Pacific.

Obesity rates, which are doubling every 5-10 years in many parts of the world, are placing significant additional financial burdens on health systems to deal with the resulting problems. Obesity will eventually lead to chronic disorders such as diabetes, high blood pressure, high cholesterol levels, hardening of arteries and some forms of cancer.

Obesity also leads to acute consequences of chronic disorders including strokes and heart attacks. Reducing caloric intake and increasing physical activity help decrease the risk of obesity. Cardiovascular Diseases include coronary heart disease which is a major cause of adult death. The risk of cardiovascular disease can be decreased by healthy eating, especially by consuming a low fat diet.

Cancer accounts for 25% of all deaths in developed countries. It has been suggested that practicable dietary means could reduce cancer deaths by as much as 35%. Eating a diet that contains plenty of fruit and vegetables in general can significantly reduce the risk of cancer. Eating Disorders present serious threats to adolescents' health and can lead to death.

Psychological counselling, medical treatment and dietary advice can help to prevent and treat eating disorders. Nutrition education has been shown to have a significant effect in fostering healthful eating habits. Thus, schools can contribute to reducing these nutrition-related problems by integrating nutrition interventions into a comprehensive approach to school health, as illustrated by the Health-Promoting School.

Adequate nutrition is necessary for children to become fit and productive adults, capable of fulfilling their responsibilities in life. People who are well-nourished and educated are clearly more productive and consequently improve their own income as well as their contribution to the national economy.

For instance, improvements in health and well-being of women and their families through better nutrition contribute to reducing their financial burdens and time constraints. Gained time and resources can be used for income-generating and productive activities or for participating in educational, health or social engagements from which women and their families can benefit.

Furthermore, implementing essential public health programmes, including nutrition and health education and micronutrient supplementation, have been estimated to reduce a considerable amount of the disease burden in low- and middle-income countries. For example, using conservative assumptions, the benefits of investing in school feeding will far exceed the costs even though this is one of the most expensive possible nutrition interventions.

In addition, nutrition interventions can contribute to reducing the substantial health care costs for nutrition-related chronic diseases and for productivity losses due to nutrition-related health problems. Malnutrition weakens the learning potential and well-being of children The education of millions of children throughout the world is being held back by malnutrition. Malnutrition in early childhood can affect school aptitudes, time of school enrolment, concentration and attentiveness.

Undernourishment also impairs the ability to concentrate, learn and attend school regularly. A child who is malnourished and subsequently suffering from poor health cannot adequately take advantage of instructional and learning materials. Thus, good nutrition is needed to strengthen the learning potential of children, to enable them to learn effectively and maximize investments in education.

Malnutrition causes death and impairs the growth and development of millions of children Malnutrition is a major factor in 54% of deaths to children under the age of 5 in the developing world. Moreover, 83% of these deaths are attributable to mild-to-moderate, rather than severe, malnutrition. Malnutrition disrupts growth and weakens the mental development of children, leading to less fit and productive adults.

Protein-energy malnutrition (PEM) affects about 200 million children worldwide under the age of 5. The actual numbers of protein-energy malnourished children has recently risen in Africa and South-East Asia. Protein-deficient children do not grow at their genetic potential. They also have an increased risk of severe consequences from common childhood infections.

Current and prior protein-energy malnutrition has been shown to result in poor retention of factual knowledge, poor school attendance and poor school performance. Iron deficiency affects approximately 2 000 million people in developed and developing countries. Iron deficiency anaemia in infants and children can retard physical growth and delay cognitive development as well as increase susceptibility to infection.

Furthermore, it impairs the reproductive function of women, which puts the lives of both women and their babies at risk. Vitamin A deficiency puts over 250 million children worldwide at risk of blindness. Every year up to one half of a million children become partly or totally blind. Two-thirds of these children die within a few months of going blind. Even moderate levels of deficiency can lead to stunted growth, increased susceptibility and severity of infections and higher death rates.

Vitamin A deficiency is the single greatest cause of preventable childhood blindness. Iodine deficiency is estimated to affect over 800 million people worldwide. Over 40 million people are affected by some degree of iodine deficiency-related brain damage. In later infancy and childhood, iodine deficiency causes mental retardation, delayed motor development, growth failure, stunting, speech and hearing defects.

Iodine deficiency is the single most common preventable cause of mental retardation and brain damage in children. All of these consequences of malnutrition compromise children's attendance and performance at school. They can be reduced by school-based interventions. Also, educating parents, parents-to-be and other family and community members as well as providing resources to correct deficiencies will help decrease the risk of developing these conditions.

Nutrition interventions improve children's health, learning potential and school attendance Good health and nutrition are needed for concentration, regular school attendance and optimum class performance. Existing research makes a convincing case that nutrition and health interventions will improve school performance.

For instance, studies in multiple countries show that the academic performance and mental ability of pupils with good nutritional status are significantly higher than those of pupils with poor nutritional status. This and other evidence of the positive impact of good nutrition has been so convincing that the United Nations Sub-Committee on Nutrition recommends health and nutrition programmes among efforts to increase school enrolment and learning.

Schools are vitally important settings through which to promote good nutrition and provide nutrition interventions Schools offer more effective, efficient and equal opportunities than any other setting to promote health and healthy eating. They reach young people at a critical age of development in which lifestyles, including eating patterns, are developed, tested and adapted in schools and through social interactions between students, teachers, parents and others.

Especially, lower grade levels provide excellent opportunities because eating habits are formed early in life. In addition, schools have the potential to reach not only students but also staff, teachers, parents and community members, including young people not attending school.

A Health-Promoting School provides a means to develop and manage nutrition interventions in cooperation with parents and students. Schools are an ideal setting to promote health and healthy nutrition for several reasons:

— Schools reach a high proportion of children and adolescents.

— Schools provide opportunities to practice healthy eating and food safety.

— Schools can teach students how to resist unhealthy social pressures since eating is a socially learned behaviour that is influenced by social pressures.

— Skilled personnel are available to provide follow-up and guidance-after appropriate training of students, teachers and other service personnel.

— Evaluations show that school-based nutrition education can improve eating behaviours of young persons.

Evidence for many years has supported that well-managed nutrition education programmes can, at relatively low cost, bring about behaviour changes that contribute to improved nutritional well-being. For instance, studies in the United States have documented that carefully designed and implemented comprehensive health education curricula can prevent certain adverse health behaviours, including dietary patterns that cause disease.

Students in behaviourally based health and nutrition education programmes have shown significant favourable changes in blood cholesterol, blood pressure and body fat. Thus, a focus on behaviour is considered a key determinant in the success of nutrition education programmes. Additionally, school feeding programmes increase food availability to schoolchildren who need adequate food while promoting long-term development through support and education.

Schools can provide interventions to improve nutrition in ways that are highly cost-effective Cost-effective interventions in schools can prevent or greatly reduce health problems and consequences of malnutrition and foster the positive effects of nutrition. Compared with various public health approaches, school health programmes that provide safe and low-cost health service interventions, such as screening and health education, are shown by research to be one of the most cost-effective investments a nation can make to improve health.

Furthermore, among the most cost-effective investments in health are programmes that include expanded micronutrient supplementation and increased knowledge about nutrition. Illustratively, a nutrition education programme in Indonesia which was based on behavioural change showed a considerably greater impact at notably lower cost than other types of interventions to which it was compared.

Education and healthy nutrition for girls have a positive impact on the health of families Improving and expanding educational opportunities for girls is one of the best health and social investments. Improvements to girls' health will in turn improve the health of their children and families because women generally have a major responsibility to care for others within the household.

This generally involves household management, food preparation, cleaning duties, obtaining health care, education and supervision of children, all of which can have a significant impact on health. Furthermore, educated girls are healthier than girls with no or little education. Educated girls and women seek appropriate prenatal care, give birth to healthier babies and bring them home to healthier environments.

Malnourished mothers tend to have low birth weight babies, thus perpetuating the problem of malnutrition and ill health from one generation to the next. For instance, a child's aptitude for formal education may be in jeopardy even prior to school enrolment if the mother suffered from maternal iodine deficiency during pregnancy. Thus, educating young mothers and mothers-to-be is one of the best ways of ensuring the nutritional future of the next generation.

In addition, the school system may be particularly useful in trying to supplement the diet of girls before puberty to ensure the remaining growth potential is fully achieved during this critical stage. Nutrition interventions in schools benefit the entire community School health education about good nutrition also serves as a means to inform families and other community members about ways to promote well-being and prevent malnutrition.

For instance, educating children about good eating habits has the potential to enhance the nutrition and health status of their younger siblings whom they may take care of as well as of other family members that learn concomitantly with their children. In addition, involving parents in nutrition interventions at the elementary school level has been shown to enhance the eating behaviour of both students and parents.

Some studies shows that school health education interventions can be considerably strengthened by complementary community-wide strategies. Thus, schools can be the centre for community enhancement projects that include programmes to improve the health and nutritional status of the community. Schools also provide a setting to introduce new health information and technologies to the community.

For instance, the establishment of school canteens offering healthy food choices and practising good food safety is a way to demonstrate how to improve facilities in communities. Furthermore, partnerships between schools, organizations and businesses can benefit both the school and the community, if the partnership is mutually beneficial.

Nutrition can be an entry point for building a school's capacity to plan and implement a wide range of health promotion strategies and interventions that will respond to identified needs and contribute to both health and education. Once nutrition is recognized as a priority for both education and health, the next step is to plan the interventions. This can be done by determining which strategies will have the most significant influence on health, education and development and how such interventions can be integrated with other health promotion efforts for maximum results.

Interventions should enable students, parents, teachers and community members to make healthy decisions, practice healthy behaviours and create conditions conducive to health. This section describes important steps that should be considered in planning healthy nutrition as an essential element of a Health-Promoting School.

Steps include establishing or involving a school health team and a community advisory committee, conducting a situation analysis, obtaining political and community commitments, establishing supportive school health policies and setting objectives.

Health-Promoting Schools involve members of the school and community in planning programmes that respond to their needs and that can be maintained with available resources and commitments. Two important groups that should be involved in the planning process are a school health team and a community advisory committee. A Health-Promoting School should have a designated team to coordinate and monitor health promotion policies and activities.

Since schools should implement programmes that respond to important and relevant community needs, it is essential to involve students, parents, teachers and school management from the beginning in the planning process. When young people are involved early, they can help develop and plan a programme that responds to their specific needs and concerns.

Parents and teachers can help ensure that programmes are developed in a culturally appropriate manner. Active participation also builds a sense of ownership of the programme, which enhances its sustainability and support. Since teachers and other school staff play a key role in carrying out health promotion interventions, their participation is important to ensure that interventions are developed with consideration to what they know and what they can do to establish healthy nutrition as an essential element of a Health-Promoting School.

Potential members of the school health team include: teachers, administrators, students, parents and school-based service providers, such as members of food services and health services. A school health team needs to be designated with responsibility and given time and authority to lead and oversee health promotion efforts in the school. A healthy nutrition task force within that group can be responsible for planning, designing and evaluating efforts to achieve healthy nutrition.

Potential partners from outside the school include: representatives of local government, community residents, businesses, vendors, media, community youth agencies, nongovernmental organizations, social service providers, health service providers, sports figures and religious leaders. Subsequently, this committee can also address other health promotion issues.

To facilitate the efforts of the school health team, the community advisory committee, or selected advisors, can help determine local needs and resources, disseminate information about health and healthy nutrition, build support across the community, encourage community involvement, help to obtain resources and funding for health and nutrition interventions, and reinforce learning experiences provided in school. The committee should include men and women with a diversity of skills who are influential in the community or district, interested in health promotion and healthy nutrition, able to mobilize support and connections, and represent the community's geographical areas as well as economic, social, ethnic and religious makeup.

The community advisory committee and the school health team should work together in planning health promotion efforts and in coordinating the various components of a Health-Promoting School, such as health education, health services, community and family involvement, etc., so that all aspects of health promotion work together for health and healthy nutrition.

Various quantitative and qualitative information is needed for planning health promotion and nutrition interventions and for establishing a baseline for evaluation. Quantitative information includes numbers and scores while qualitative information includes perceptions and feelings. The following information can help determine local needs concerning nutrition:

— Current health and nutritional status at national, regional, local and/or school level and how well it corresponds with relevant guidelines. This data should include the proportion of persons who are affected by malnutrition and infections and how severely they are affected.

— Knowledge, attitudes, beliefs, values, behaviours and conditions related to health and nutrition, eating patterns and food customs. For example, people might not know which foods are nutritious; poorly prepared food may influence a student's attitude about food that may be highly nutritious; local beliefs or superstitions may prevent people from eating certain foods; people might choose to ignore conditions of malnutrition because they have been with them for generations; or people might not be familiar with precautions to safely preserve food. This information is crucial to design effective health promotion strategies because values, beliefs and attitudes positively or negatively influence behaviours and conditions associated with nutrition and health. Without information about these helping or hindering forces, educational interventions are not likely to be targeted to the most relevant factors that contribute to health or malnutrition in the community and thus are unlikely to achieve the desired result.

— Available resources in the school and community. This includes determining which specific personnel and financial resources and services are available. Assessments should include the nature and extent of existing programmes, either through the school or community, that might help in implementing health promotion and nutrition interventions, such as deworming, oral hygiene or sport programmes. Knowing this information allows the school health team to draw on available resources for implementing new programmes or improving existing ones.

Nutrition interventions in a Health-Promoting School are most successful when a wide range of individuals and groups support the programme and become involved in it. It is important in the early stages to secure the acceptance and support of government officials, community and business leaders, educators, parents, students and the community in general.

The success of efforts to create a Health-Promoting School relies also on the extent to which people in the community are aware of and willing to support health promotion efforts. Schools need to receive input from parents and community members regarding the design, delivery, content and assessment of school health promotion, so as to respond to their concerns and to attain their commitment.

Family and community members should be involved very early; for instance, through community group meetings, parent-teacher associations, formal presentations, open houses, civic clubs and religious centres. Commitment and support of many parties on various levels is needed to share expertise, facilities and resources. Partnerships of representative individuals, groups and organizations from numerous sectors, such as nongovernment, education, health, business, agriculture, communication, recreation, voluntary service and religion can demonstrate and provide commitment, resources and support for health promotion and nutrition interventions.

Supportive school policies provide an essential framework that guides schools in planning, implementing and evaluating efforts to promote health and healthy nutrition. School policies are brief documents that promote a clear set of school norms regarding health and nutrition. They incorporate input from all relevant constituents of the school community: students, teachers, parents, staff, administrators, food service personnel, nurses and counsellors.

Policies need to meet national and local needs and standards and should be adapted to the health concerns, food preferences and dietary practices of different ethnic and cultural groups represented at school. Policies that support collaboration and coordination between the health, education, food and agricultural sectors of the government and between the school and the community are encouraged.

Written policies should guarantee nutrition and other health interventions for all levels of schooling, starting in the earliest grade and continuing through the last grade. Policies should address all components of a Health-Promoting School that will be modified, such as education about nutrition, food choices at the school canteen, feeding programmes, family involvement and food handling procedures.

Especially important are regulations about a Health-Promoting School's environment and about health education. For instance, school policies should guarantee adequate sanitation, a pleasant eating environment and collaboration with vendors as well as provision of teacher training, learning materials and a curriculum for nutrition and health education. Regulations, rules and protocols that ensure:

— students, parents, teachers and other school personnel are involved in planning of health promotion and nutrition interventions; for instance, through their participation on the school health team.

— the community advisory committee meets periodically to sustain coordination between school and community.

— the school curriculum includes education about nutrition as part of a sequential, comprehensive school health education programme, as an integral part of other relevant subject areas or, ideally, as a combination of both.

— teachers and other school personnel receive ongoing training about nutrition and food safety.

— all school facilities and events, including cafeterias, snack bars, rewards, staff meetings, parents' meetings and special events serve nutritious food, based on local, district and/or national guidelines.

— parents are educated about the value of healthy meals and food safety practices and about their role as reinforcers and motivators of concepts and knowledge for better eating and learning.

— school health services offer screening for conditions of malnutrition among students (where relevant) and report the results to teachers, parents and community members.

Using the information gathered in the situation analysis, the school health team, in collaboration with the community advisory committee, can develop a vision for change and an action plan. This provides a basis for formulating goals and objectives for health promotion and nutrition interventions. Goals and objectives are necessary to make clear what the interventions should achieve.

Nutrition intervention goals of a Health-Promoting School should aim at:

— gaining the full health and educational potential of food and nutrition sources for students and other members of the school, family and community.

— applying the school's full organizational potential to improve the nutritional status of students, staff, families and community members.

— laying a foundation of lifelong healthy eating based on favourable experiences, sufficient skills and confidence in one's capacity to practice a healthy lifestyle.

Components of a Health Promoting School

A Health-Promoting School strives to use the school's full organizational capacity to improve the health of students, school personnel, families and community members. Such a school offers many opportunities to promote nutrition as an essential element for the attainment of health. Nutrition interventions can serve as an entry point for the development or enhancement of policies, planning groups and various components which serve as a framework for a Health-Promoting School. These components include, but are not limited to:

— School health education - Community and family involvement and outreach

— Healthy school environment- Physical exercise, recreation and sport

— School health services - Counselling and social support

— Nutrition and food programmes - Health promotion for school staff.

The effectiveness of interventions integrated into each of the above components is influenced by the extent to which they are supported by a variety of people, policies and trained staff. The effectiveness is also influenced by the extent to which interventions in each of these components combine with other health promotion efforts to complement and reinforce each other. Not all schools will have the resources to integrate nutrition interventions into all of the components at one time.

Therefore, each school has to establish its own priorities, in collaboration with all parties concerned, to decide the extent to which the components should be addressed. A Health-Promoting School enables students, parents, teachers and community members to work together to make such decisions. It is more important to start with small changes that are possible than to wait until resources become available to address all of these components simultaneously.

The primary goals of school health education are to help individuals adopt behaviours and to create conditions that are conducive to health. Thus, the clear and precise delineation of behaviours and conditions specifically relevant to healthy nutrition is essential for the development of effective school health education efforts.

Close collaboration between education, health and food officials; the school health team; the community advisory committee; and other school and community members is necessary to identify the nutrition-related behaviours and conditions relevant to health in each community.

School health education is designed to help students acquire the knowledge, attitudes, beliefs and skills which are needed to make informed decisions, practice healthy behaviours and create conditions that are conducive to health. Knowledge provides a factual background on which to base decisions, such as knowledge about the relationship of eating and health and about planning for healthy nutrition using assessments and nutritional guidelines.

In a Health-Promoting School, school health education about nutrition addresses food, its preparation and its consumption as an essential positive and enjoyable aspect of life. A Health-Promoting School provides opportunities for students to practice important skills, such as decision-making about food choices. To be relevant to student needs, learning experiences should be related to food preferences and other motivational factors that guide students to improve their nutrition and that of their family and community.

School health education about nutrition should also teach that lifestyle influences a person's food requirements. In a Health-Promoting School, curricula are also designed to address the emotional and socio-cultural aspects of healthy eating along with informational and skill-building learning experiences. School health education should be provided as a planned sequential course of instruction from the primary through the secondary levels, addressing the physical, mental, emotional and social dimensions of health. It can be taught as a specific subject, as part of other subjects, or ideally, as a combination of both.

Thus, health education about nutrition should be an important part of a school health curriculum; integrated into such subject areas as science, home economics, mathematics, and agriculture; as well as included in the school's extracurricular activities. Nutrition education will enhance the overall framework of a Health-Promoting School if it is integrated into other school health components, such as physical activity and health promotion for staff, as well as in the school health education component.

Education about nutrition should be combined with efforts addressing other health issues, such as reproductive health, life skills, and alcohol and drug use prevention, so that the learning experiences will complement and reinforce each other. Linking these issues can be accomplished by organizing them into a school health education curriculum and coordinating.the simultaneous or sequential presentation of related topics in different classes.

Linkages of health and nutrition issues and other relevant topics can also be facilitated by co-teaching, sharing teaching resources, referring students to related lessons and involving students from different classes in group activities. Curricula for nutrition and other health-related issues may be available through governmental and nongovernmental agencies and organizations, universities or teachers' unions.

Educational methods such as lectures, discussions, debates, role-plays and audio-visual aids should be designed or selected to increase knowledge, build positive attitudes and values, dispel myths, increase skills and provide support for the development of healthy lifestyles. They need to be appropriate for the developmental level of students.

For example, a lecture is an effective way to increase knowledge but is less effective in influencing beliefs and building skills. Discussions, debates and carefully prepared written materials can be more effective than a lecture in dispelling local myths. Practice sessions, such as cooking nutritious recipes and growing food in a school garden, can be more effective than lectures, discussions, debates and written materials in building skills.

A diversity of instructional strategies is essential to effective curriculum development. In selecting information to convey to students about nutrition, scientific terms and details are considered less important than practical and basic information that will enable students to make healthy food choices and to prepare foods safely.

For example, it is more essential for a student to know how to prepare a healthy meal than to learn the exact grams of nutrients in different foods. Students are more likely to adopt healthy eating patterns when they learn about these behaviours through enjoyable and participatory activities that emphasize the positive aspects of healthy eating in a context of what is relevant and important to students.

Students should have repeated opportunities to taste and choose a variety of foods with high nutritional value. They should have learning opportunities to acquire knowledge, attitudes and skills that they can apply in school, at home and in the community. An action-oriented learning process should also help students recognise the importance of socialization during meal times and of making appropriate choices and decisions about health and nutrition.

Teacher training, both pre-service and in-service, is an important factor in a successful school health education programme. Teacher training should sensitise them to the concept of health promotion in schools. All teachers need to receive training and accurate information to effectively address health and nutrition in their content area. Education and training should inspire and equip teachers with knowledge and skills to make a curriculum exciting in order to encourage students to build healthy eating practices and to make nutritious food choices.

Teachers who are primarily responsible for nutrition education should receive specific and relevant training in implementing a selected curriculum. This training should address content and teaching strategies. Since nutrition education involves influencing attitudes, beliefs and skills, as well as knowledge to promote healthy behaviours and conditions, teachers must be trained to use a wide variety of teaching methods.

Environment for Healthy School

The school's environment plays a significant role in determining whether interventions to promote health and healthy nutrition will be effective and sustainable. Thus, students should have access to food of high nutritional value and to the support of persons around them to develop and maintain a healthy diet.

A Health-Promoting School provides a safe and healthy environment that presents a realistic and attractive range of health choices to encourage a healthy lifestyle. It also helps students and others develop their physical, psychological and social potential. In a Health-Promoting School, the physical and psychosocial school environment should be consistent with and reinforce other health promotion efforts.

The physical environment includes the school building, classrooms, eating facilities, water and foods provided at school and the surroundings in which the school is situated. The condition of the physical environment can have a powerful effect on reinforcing or contradicting health education and nutrition interventions in the school. The following nutrition-related aspects of a healthy physical environment can be integrated into a Health-Promoting School, supported by related school health policies:

— *Sanitation*: In schools, the presence of clean water, safe food and sanitary facilities as well as proper waste collection and disposal are essential to good health and nutrition. Adequate sanitation contributes to reducing the risk for food-borne and other infections related to health and nutrition.

— *Healthy food choices*: A Health-Promoting School promotes and provides appropriate healthy and high quality foods and meals to offer opportunities for healthy choices.

— *Pleasant eating environment*: A pleasant eating environment in a Health-Promoting School provides sufficient space and comfortable surroundings for socializing during meal times and for enjoyment of food, which in turn enhance mental, social and physical health.

— *Outside vendors*: Efforts to create a health-conducive environment should also include food vendors that may be present on or near the school property, who provide an important source of food for students. Schools should strive to gain cooperation with vendors to offer nutritious food choices to encourage the school's health promotion efforts.

— *Special facilities*: A Health-Promoting School may also have facilities to carry out practical nutrition-related activities, such as food preparation, food experiments and growing food.

For creating a healthy physical school environment, food services and food safety are key factors that must be addressed. School food services need to be integrated into and coordinated with health and nutrition education and with other components of the Health-Promoting School to reinforce messages on healthy eating and ensure consistent nutrition support. The school cafeteria provides a place for students to practice healthy eating.

Therefore, the school canteen needs to offer a variety of healthy food choices and limit the availability of food with low nutritional value to help students apply skills taught in the classroom. The food supply at the school canteen should be based on national or regional dietary guidelines if these are applicable to children. In addition to offering nutritious food choices, food service personnel can also be involved in other components of a Health-Promoting School.

Some examples of how the activities of food service personnel can contribute to the development of a Health-Promoting School include:

- visiting classrooms and explaining how they make sure meals meet the standards of the dietary guidelines
- inviting classes to visit the cafeteria kitchen and learn how to prepare healthy meals
- involving students in planning the school menu and preparing recipes
- offering foods that reinforce classroom lessons (e.g. whole wheat bread to reinforce a lesson on dietary fibre)

— posting in the cafeteria, or where children eat, information and guidance about nutrition and its value to health

— displaying nutrition information about available foods

— giving students opportunities to practice food analysis and selection skilis learned in the classroom.

It is important that environmental conditions in schools ensure a safe food supply. Such conditions are supported by clean and safe water and food, safe means of waste disposal, good standards of hygiene, cleanliness, tidiness and adequate ventilation. These efforts should be reinforced through personnel at school. Applying rules for safe food preparation is also essential for students, teachers and service providers.

Environmental efforts to ensure food safety should support instructional content on the same subject. While each school should follow the regulations and standards established by their respective government concerning food safety, WHO has developed the following general Golden Rules for Safe Food Preparation:

1. Choose foods processed for safety.
2. Cook food thoroughly.
3. Eat cooked foods immediately.
4. Store cooked foods carefully.
5. Reheat cooked foods thoroughly.
6. Avoid contact between raw foods and cooked foods.
7. Wash hands repeatedly with soap and water.
8. Keep all kitchen surfaces meticulously clean.

9. Protect foods from insects, rodents and other animals.

10. Use safe water.

The psychosocial environment relates to social and mental conditions which affect education and health. This incorporates the cultural norms and expectations regarding food and eating patterns as expressed by friends, parents and school personnel. A Health-Promoting School provides an ambience which respects the individual and fosters confidence in healthy choices and enjoyment of food.

The following aspects of a healthy psychosocial environment should be integrated into a Health-Promoting School:

— *Support*: The psychosocial environment should support health-conducive perceptions and actions of all who live, work and learn in the school. It should be consistent with other health-promoting interventions in the school and classroom. For instance, the friendliness and support of school staff as well as community members involved in school projects can contribute to psychosocial support. Such support can help build confidence and self-esteem with regard to healthy eating practices.

— *Teacher role models*: One aspect of the school's psychosocial environment is the important role that teachers play as adult role models and as mentors. For instance, teachers can encourage students to follow a healthy way of life by demonstrating healthy eating.

— *Peer reinforcement*: Another aspect is students' influence on peers. Students can provide positive reinforcement to their peers by advising and reminding each other of healthy eating habits. This requires that schools provide students with sufficient time to eat and socialize.

School health services help to prevent, reduce, monitor or treat important health problems or conditions as well as foster health and well-being. In a Health-Promoting School, health services work in partnership with and are provided for students, school personnel, families and community members. They should be coordinated with other services and activities at school and in the community to utilise the potential of specialist resources to provide advice and support for health promotion and nutrition interventions.

Schools and communities need to consider what preventive and treatment services are best provided at school sites and avoid duplicating services available in the community that would easily be accessible for students and school personnel. Models for providing school health services vary tremendously, not only from developed to developing countries but also among and within nations themselves.

School health services can consist of a teacher designated to be responsible for first aid, a trained school nurse or a school health team. Such staff contribute to the well-being of students, faculty and community through caring for individuals' health and nutritional status. Their roles can include screening for indicators of malnutrition and health status, providing treatments such as micronutrient supplements and parasite medications, referring to appropriate nutritional and other services, and supplying health and nutrition information to teachers and students to help them make healthy decisions and to educate others about healthy nutrition.

Institutions of higher education that train medical professionals and paraprofessionals or nongovernmental organizations may provide training for school health service providers. Screening and diagnosis of health and nutritional status, including conditions of malnutrition, can play an important role in planning efforts to enhance health or influence unhealthy eating habits.

Nutritional screening can include food consumption surveys, which are compared to food guidelines, as well as measurements of body weight and height, which are compared to a subject's age and sex. In addition, blood tests can be used to diagnose micronutrient deficiencies, such as iron deficiency anaemia and indicators of nutrition-related chronic diseases, such as high blood cholesterol.

School health services can also provide information about where to obtain nutritious food, dietary guidelines and other appropriate services. A summary of screening results can also be referred to the school health team, teachers and parent associations to inform them about the current situation and to assist in planning.

Programmes for Food and Nutrition

Children who are not adequately nourished are more likely to be absent from school, less likely to concentrate and perform well and more likely to be susceptible to infections. Therefore, a Health-Promoting School should integrate efforts to ensure students' nutritional adequacy into a variety of its health promotion interventions.

School feeding programmes are one example of interventions aiming at increasing food availability while promoting healthy eating. These programmes might provide breakfast, lunch and/or snacks at reduced price or free of charge, providing calories, protein and micronutrients to schoolchildren without adequate food. Feeding programmes have been shown to increase weight and in some cases also school attendance and achievement.

The composition of provided meals in terms of food items and nutritional value has been shown to play a role in educational achievement. For instance, research with elementary and high school students in Chile showed improvements in educational accomplishments with more frequent consumption of dairy products and with more nutrient intake, in particular protein and calcium.

Diets deficient in essential vitamins and minerals can have an enormous health impact. Thus, micronutrient supplementation is another example of nutrition interventions to prevent specific deficiency diseases in individuals and to promote well-being. This intervention method supplies micronutrients separately from the normal diet. Children who receive supplements must obtain them regularly; therefore, schools are an appropriate place to distribute them.

Micronutrient supplements can be given orally or by injection. These supplements may include vitamin A capsules to prevent blindness, iron tablets to prevent anaemia and iodized oil or iodized salt to prevent goitre and mental retardation. Ample evidence exists of the value of treating micronutrient deficiencies resulting in improved performance at school or work and reduced burden of illness, disability and death.

Family and community members can be involved in Health-Promoting Schools in various ways:

— Taking part in planning and decision-making; for instance, participating in the school health team or community advisory committee.

— Participating in activities and services offered through schools; for instance, attending projects to gain specific health and nutritional knowledge and skills, such as in exhibitions, photo expositions, concerts, drama, community-wide entertainment, festivals and health fairs.

— Providing support and resources; for instance, supplying financial or material donations, being guest speakers or providing specialist services related to health and nutrition. Nutritionists from the community can offer nutritional assessments for students and parents, and supermarkets and farms can offer healthy food.

— Advocating for health; for instance, knowledge and skills acquired in a school/community project can be used by community and family members to take communal actions that will result in sustainable healthy eating practices.

The family and community also provide a setting for students to understand, practice and share what they learn about health and nutrition in the classroom. They have the potential to support and reinforce nutrition education and health promotion. Thus, it is essential that school staff, parents and community members work together in order to create conditions that allow the maximum attainment of health by all its members.

Students are most likely to adopt healthy eating patterns if they receive consistent information and support through multiple channels, such as parents, peers, teachers, community members and media. Thus, a Health-Promoting School should strengthen community links and involve parents and the wider community as much as possible.

Health-Promoting Schools should closely collaborate with parents so that children are less likely to experience inconsistencies between suggestions and practices at home and at school. Thus, establishing dynamic, positive and productive links with families is an important part of a Health-Promoting School. Connections with parents can be established, for instance, during a school health fair to which parents are invited, a health-related workshop for parents, a parent-teacher meeting or a parent's visit to relevant food services at school or in the community.

Parents and other caregivers play an important role in their child's life in their roles as nurturer, teacher, disciplinarian, role model and supervisor since parents control most of the food choices available at home. Therefore, it is essential that they understand and reinforce what the Health-Promoting School seeks to achieve. The school can provide parents and family members with information, resources and skills about important principles of healthy nutrition in an effort to enhance and extend the programme in the student's home.

Improving parents' eating habits may be one of the most effective ways to promote healthy eating for their children as parents create conditions at home that are conducive or not conducive to healthy nutrition. At the elementary school level, involving parents in nutrition-related learning experiences such as games, take-home activities and meals in school, is especially effective in enhancing the eating behaviours of both the students and the parents. Thus, parent involvement should begin early.

Cooperation and coordination between the school health programme and the community is likely to be most successful where there are dynamic, positive and productive school/community links. Schools and communities can benefit from partnerships with local businesses and representatives from agencies and organizations, such as local health departments, farmers' organizations, youth-serving agencies and local retailers.

For instance, the school can utilise the potential of specialist services in the community for advice and support in nutrition and health matters and can actively involve community nutritionists and community health services at school. Commercial organisations and businesses can offer health-related and relevant visits to their stores, advice on healthy choices or donations in support of nutrition programmes.

Constructive collaboration is especially important with national and local food businesses, supermarkets, restaurants and food vendors in an effort to gain their support for healthy nutrition and to involve them in supplying food with high nutritional value. Partnerships may involve communication among organisations and schools, cooperation of jointly scheduled activities, coordination of resources and collaboration under a mutually agreed mission.

Role of mass media

Mass media can encourage new behaviours. They can be used on a national and local scale as well as in classrooms for health promotion and nutrition interventions. Mass media include radio, television, signboards, posters, calendars, comics, photo novels, newspapers, magazines, booklets, leaflets, audiovisual materials and traditional communication forms such as dance troupes.

For instance, nutritional radio, television quiz programmes for schoolchildren and crossword puzzles in children's newspapers have been utilised to promote health and nutrition. Some materials can be distributed through more than one channel or can be used with different target groups: a nutrition teacher with a cassette recorder can play the same programme at the village well that can be broadcast over radio or discussed in class.

Multimedia approaches that combine face-to-face and mass channels are appropriate for nutrition education because nutrition is relevant to everyone and different channels are necessary for different phases in the learning process. Food advertising is also a pervasive and influential aspect of the media. Children have to be taught to recognize the purposes of advertising strategies such as those which provide important information and those solely promoting a particular product.

Children also need to learn to recognize that some advertising may not be supportive of good nutrition. If advertising sources are involved in school/community efforts, they can also be helpful in informing people about facts of good nutrition. It is important that materials targeted towards children with dietary information and advice are consistent with official health standards and guidelines.

Eating a healthy diet does not in itself guarantee good health. A healthy diet is however an important part of a healthy lifestyle that also includes physical exercise, not using tobacco in any form, not drinking alcoholic beverages in excess and not abusing drugs. All of these issues should thus be addressed by a Health-Promoting School in an organized and complementary manner.

The importance of addressing lifestyle holistically is clearly illustrated in the linkage between nutrition and active living. Physical exercise, recreation and sport help individuals.acquire and maintain physical fitness and serve as a healthy means of self-expression and social development. Expending energy in physical exercise and sport balances the intake of energy from food, especially in regions that do not incorporate physical activity into daily living through farming, herding animals, walking long distances or other activities.

Thus, physical activity and nutrition must be addressed in a complementary manner when integrated into the components of a Health-Promoting School. Nutrition interventions should stress that all children and adults should have the opportunity to attain the healthful benefits of exercise, games, dance, sport or an active lifestyle.

In regions where overnutrition is prevalent, efforts to promote physical activity and sport should stress the benefits of reducing the risk of obesity and related disorders since negative health consequences of overweight and obesity are likely to be more serious in sedentary than in active obese people. Thus, physical exercise and sport, together with healthy nutrition, can help reduce the effects of age and chronic disease on heart, lungs and muscles; reduce fatigue, mild anxiety and depression; and diminish the loss of bone calcium while creating vigour, stamina and other fundamental requirements for well-being.

Additionally, recreation activities and healthy nutrition can restore strength and spirits after school and work. Ball games, dances or other recreational events can be supportive of good health and offer nutritious food. In a Health-Promoting School, personnel, community members and families can participate together in planning and implementing such activities which in turn strengthen community spirit.

Maintaining and supporting the mental health of students and staff should also be addressed in a Health-Promoting School in a manner which complements and supports nutritional and physical health. An individual's psychological well-being, including self-esteem and self-confidence, is critical in maintaining physical health and the ability to make healthy decisions and avoid risk behaviours.

Thus, school counselling programmes and actions to provide social support are important components of a Health-Promoting School that can help students, school personnel and families in coping with difficulties, adjustments, growth and development. Personal feelings and emotions influence food choices.

For children and adults to thrive they not only need an appropriate diet and body image but also care and nurturing. Care is the provision of time, attention, support and skills that can help meet individuals' physical, mental and social needs. A supportive psychosocial environment within the school can provide a buffering effect on transitions or stressful life events experienced by students and others.

For instance, social and emotional support can.be provided during meals by any member of the school community for individuals who are changing their eating behaviour. Social support can also strengthen students to resist social pressures to eat food of low nutritional value since eating is influenced by social forces. Thus, care and support services can enhance nutrition interventions by encouraging students and others to make appropriate choices about their diet, promoting self-esteem and supporting students' efforts to fulfill their physical, psychological and social potential.

A Health-Promoting School aims at promoting healthy lifestyles among all who study, work and use the school. Thus, strategies to promote health and nutrition should become an integral part of a Health-Promoting School; for instance, as part of in-service training. School health promotion programmes for staff are intended to increase their interest in health and help them acquire healthy lifestyles.

Examples for nutritional health promotion include printed materials from national or local organizations, healthy meals and guidelines provided by the school cafeteria, and workshops for staff members held by community nutritionists or others. There are several reasons why health promotion for school personnel is important. First, healthy employees are better able to fulfill their responsibilities.

Thus, health promotion activities should help them assess and improve their own eating practices. Second, teachers and school personnel need to be aware of and responsible for the messages they give as role models to students and others. Third, school personnel can help identify policies and practices that are needed in order to support health and well-being in a Health-Promoting School.

Health and Nutrition of School Children

An understanding and awareness of the heavy burden of malnutrition and disease among school-age children is growing although until recently there have been relatively few large scale surveys that document levels of morbidity in any detail. While a better picture of the health and nutrition status of this age group is being built, the true extent of the burden of ill health and malnutrition is still not fully known.

The main nutritional problems facing the school-age child include stunting, underweight, anaemia and iodine deficiency and, on the basis of information from recent surveys, vitamin A deficiency. In countries experiencing the 'nutrition transition', overweight and obesity are increasing problems in the school-age child.

The main health problems facing school-age children are malaria, helminth infections, diarrhoeal diseases, respiratory infections and the direct and indirect effects of HIV/AIDS. Much of the disease burden derives from the poor environmental conditions in which children live including exposure to biological, chemical and physical hazards in the environment and a lack of resources essential for human health.

Malnutrition refers to disorders resulting from an inadequate diet or from failure to absorb or assimilate dietary elements. Stunting (low height-for-age) is a physical indicator of chronic or long term malnutrition and is often linked to poor mental development. Stunting is a cumulative process of poor growth that primarily occurs before the age of three years and is not easily reversed.

This infers that these first years of life provide a window of opportunity for effective nutritional programming. Underweight (low weight-for-age) is an indicator of both chronic and acute undernutrition. Wasting (low weight-for-height) is an indicator of acute undernutrition.

The Africa region has the highest estimated prevalence of stunting and has the lowest rate of improvement. In East Africa sub-region, rates of stunting are increasing. The prevalence of stunting in Asia is also high, particularly in South Central Asia, although rates of stunting continue to improve throughout this region. In Latin America and the Caribbean, the prevalence of stunting is significantly lower than the other two regions and is improving, except in the Central America sub-region.

For preschool children, the prevalence of underweight and wasting follow similar regional patterns to the prevalence of stunting. Estimates for prevalence of underweight pre-school children in different regions of Africa in the year 2000 range from 14 to 36.5% underweight; Asia 28.9 to 43.6% and Latin America and the Caribbean 3.2 to 15.4%. Although estimates of prevalence of wasting are not available for all sub-regions, overall estimates for wasting in preschool children by region are available for 1995: Africa 9.6%, Asia 10.4% and Latin America and the Caribbean 2.9%.

Children stunted at school-age are likely to have been exposed to poor nutrition since early childhood and that the degree of stunting tends to increase throughout the school-age years. However, children can exhibit catch-up growth if their environment improves . This suggests that interventions in school-age children can supplement efforts in the preschool years to reduce levels of stunting and related effects on children's health and education.

Underweight among school-age children, like stunting, can reflect a broad range of insults such as prenatal undernutrition, deficiencies of macro- and micronutrients, infection and, possibly, inadequate attention by caregivers. Wasting, which reflects acute malnutrition, is not as common as either stunting or underweight in school-age children.

Nevertheless, wasting rates can change rapidly in situations of acute food crisis, with school-age children, adolescents in particular, becoming severely malnourished in such situations. Recent studies on school-age children have shed new information on stunting, wasting and underweight for this age group:

— one of the largest studies of anthropometric status of rural school children in low income countries (Ghana, Tanzania, Indonesia, Vietnam and India) found the overall prevalence of stunting and underweight to be high in all five countries, ranging from 48 to 56% for stunting and from 34 to 62% for underweight. Second, in all countries there was a trend for z-scores for height-for-age and weight-for-age to decrease with age, thus as children got older they became progressively shorter relative to the reference population. Third, the boys in most countries tended to be more stunted than girls and in all countries boys were more underweight than girls

— a longitudinal study of changes in height and weight of school-age children on Pemba Island, Zanzibar showed the prevalence of stunting increased with age

(14% prevalence in seven year olds increasing to 83% in 13 year olds) and peaked in girls at age 12 then declined when they entered their pubertal growth spurt. In boys, however, the prevalence of stunting rose steadily up to age 13 years and then slowly declined. Boys accumulated a height deficit of 11.9cm and girls a height deficit of 8.5cm compared to the reference population

— a recent cross sectional survey of the nutritional status of adolescent boys and girls in Bangladesh found that 67% of adolescents were thin and 48% were stunted. Whereas, thinness was found to decline in prevalence with age from 95% at age 10 years to 12% at age 17 years, the prevalence of stunting increased from 34% at age ten years to 65% at age 17 years.

— a study in Brazil of the gender differences in growth of school-age children suffering from helminth infections found that 21% of school-age children were stunted and 13% were underweight. Both indices of nutritional status worsened as the study population got older, particularly for boys. The later onset of puberty and the growth-spurt in boys was controlled for in the growth data analysis, but boys remained significantly more malnourished than girls .

— in a recent prospective cohort study of school-age children in Bangladesh, diarrhoea was found to retard weight gain and slow linear growth, although respiratory infections did not have the same effect

— another study from an impoverished rural area of Guatemala that had recently benefited from a poverty alleviation programme, identified sanitation and housing conditions as risk factors for growth faltering in school-age children. Adult women's body mass index was also identified as a risk factor for stunting in school-age children

The evidence suggests that boys are more likely to be stunted and underweight than girls, and in some countries, more likely to be wasted than girls . This may be due to a bias in the school population. It is also suggested that it could reflect delayed onset of puberty. Overall, height deficits have declined in both boys and girls, although the overall height deficit in boys was found to be greater than for girls in each period studied.

Whilst growth can be improved during the childhood period, growth improvements observed in studies of one year or less duration have been disappointing . Longer-term interventions need to be conducted to determine if gains in growth can be sustained long enough to become significant.

From the mid-90s several studies have focused on the health status on out-of-school children. One study in Ghana compared the health of enrolled and non-enrolled children in primary school and showed that there were considerable differences between enrolled and non-enrolled children . Non-enrolled children of both sexes were significantly smaller in height than enrolled children of the same age range. Just over half (51%) of children aged six to seven years who were not enrolled in primary school were stunted in comparison with only 19% who were enrolled in school.

It is likely that many of the chronic health problems encountered in the six to seven year old children studied are the product of disease and poor nutrition before they enrolled in school. Important questions are raised from these studies that reflect the need for more information on the patterns and determinants of growth in this age group.

— First, it is important to identify whether the height deficits accrued during the primary school years are made up through longer pubertal growth and at what stage boys and girls stop growing in height.

— Second, the functional implications of linear growth retardation in school-age children needs to be more clearly understood.

— Third, the question as to what extent school-age stunting is preventable through school-based interventions needs to be addressed .

The studies of the effect of undernutrition on cognitive ability although not entirely conclusive, indicate that chronic undernutrition is associated with lower achievement levels in school children. Recent studies have found: that severe stunting in the first two years of life is strongly associated with lower test scores in school-age children.

However, deficits in children's scores were smaller at older ages, suggesting that adverse effects may decline over time. In addition, lower test scores were related to later enrolment, increased absenteeism and repetition of school years among stunted children.

Nutritional anaemia, particularly deficiencies of iron, iodine, and vitamin A are major problems for school-age children in low income countries. It has been shown that such deficiencies can negatively impact on growth, increase susceptibility to infection and also impair the mental development and learning ability of school children.

Iron deficiency (ID) is the most common nutritional disorder in the world and is estimated to affect more than 2b people of whom 1.2b suffer from iron deficiency anaemia (IDA). Insufficient intake of iron rich foods is the major cause of ID. It can also be caused by parasitic infections (particularly hookworm and malaria) and deficiencies of other nutrients .

There is little evidence to suggest any recent decrease in the prevalence of anaemia . It is estimated that 53% or 210m school-age children suffer from IDA . The highest prevalence is reported in Asia followed by Africa. Recent studies and surveys have tried to capture the prevalence of IDA in school children:

A survey of nearly 14,000 rural school children in Africa and Asia, the prevalence of IDA was more than 40% in five African countries (Mali, Tanzania, Mozambique, Ghana, and Malawi) amongst children aged 7-11 years and in four African countries amongst children aged 12-14 years. In the two Asian countries studied, the overall prevalence of IDA was found to be considerably lower than in Africa.

Children aged 7-11 years were found to have lower mean haemoglobin concentrations, while IDA was found to be more common in the older age group. Girls were also found to have lower haemoglobin concentrations than boys, although the overall prevalence of IDA was higher in boys, particularly in the 12-13 year age group. An association between late enrollment in school, as compared to enrolling closer to the correct age, and a higher prevalence of anaemia was also found.

A study of 1,210 primary school girls aged 7-14, in Riyadh, Saudia Arabia, an anaemia level of 55.4% was found. The highest level (71.4%) was found among 14 year-old girls. Another study of adolescent males and females in Bangladesh, extremely high levels of anaemia were identified in both females (98%) and males. At age 17, 100% of females were anaemic. A survey of 6,486 adolescent students (12-15 years) in East Java, Indonesia, anaemia levels of over 25% in girls, 24% in pre-pubertal boys and 12% in pubertal boys were detected. Higher levels of anaemia were found among adolescents of lower socio-economic status. In this study as well, puberty increased the risk of anaemia among girls .

In Thailand, large differences were found between school children with anaemia and/or iron deficiency and iron replete children in their performance on a Thai language test and a test of general reasoning ability, yet not in arithmetic scores. Soemantri found smaller differences between Indonesian school children with IDA and iron replete children in their performance on a range of school exams, although the children did not differ in a test of concentration.

The main focus of IDA reduction programmes has been young children and women of reproductive age. Recent studies have emphasized the high prevalence of iron deficiency and anaemia in school-age children. This has resulted in an increased programmatic response for this age. However, there is conflicting evidence concerning the beneficial effect of iron supplementation on growth in children. Some studies have shown that daily supplementation improves growth and appetite, while others have not found any beneficial growth response.

In recent years, a number of studies have suggested that weekly iron supplementation is as effective as daily supplementation in raising haemoglobin levels, however, there is a still a need to further assess the effectiveness of weekly supplements under programme conditions to ensure that compliance is achieved. A study of school children in Bolivia suggest that iron supplementation for five days per week is as effective as weekly supplementation over the course of 16 weeks.

One of the few studies from Africa that has examined the impact of weekly supplementation with 400mg of ferrous sulphate for four months on the iron status and growth of adolescent schoolgirls found a significant increase in serum ferritin levels in the group receiving iron supplements a study of reducing anaemia in adolescent schoolgirls in Peru tested both daily and intermittent iron supplementation over a 17 week period.

It was found that while both supplementation schedules resulted in improved iron status, daily supplementation resulted in the greatest increase in haemoglobin concentration and significantly reduced the prevalence of anaemia an experimental community trial was conducted to observe the effect of a communication programme on compliance with weekly iron supplementation in urban Tanzanian adolescent schoolgirls. A total of 237 girls, aged 14-17 were randomly recruited from five schools.

Iodine deficiency affects an estimated 1.6b people worldwide and estimated 60m school-age children. The consequences of iodine deficiency include severe mental retardation, goitre (a condition involving the enlargement of the thyroid gland and a disruption of normal thyroid production), hypothyroidism, abortion, stillbirths and low birthweight and mild forms of motor and cognitive deficits.

Recent studies in school-age children have found very high levels of goitre and iodine deficiency. School-age children are often the target population of IDD assessments because of their physiological vulnerability and their accessibility. Recent studies of IDD in school children have been carried out in Egypt, Swaziland and South Africa.

Overall prevalence rates of between 35 and 70% have been found indicating a severe public health problem in each of areas studied. In Calcutta, India, after having implemented a universal iodized salt programme for several years, a monitoring survey reported 23% of male school children and 32% of female school were moderately to severely iodine deficient

Iodine deficiency is the leading cause of preventable intellectual impairment worldwide. A number of studies comparing children living in iodine-deficient areas with those living in iodine sufficient areas have found that the iodine deficient children have poorer levels of cognitive development and school achievement.

Observational studies carried out over the past 30 years, have found that school-age children living in iodine-deficient areas have lower IQs and poorer cognitive and motor function than school-age children living in iodine-sufficient areas. In a study of school-age children suffering from mild and moderate iodine deficiency in Bangladesh, it was found that hypothyroid children performed worse than normal children in reading and spelling .

A study of the association between hypothyroidism and cognitive and motor function and school achievement in Bangladeshi school-age children found that the hypothyroid children performed worse in reading and spelling than non-hypothyroid children. These differences were observed after controlling for biological, socio-cultural and socio-economic conditions.

In audition it was found that stimulation and the availability of materials were also significantly associated with improved reading, spelling and mathematics. This study concluded that children suffer a range of disadvantages in addition to iodine deficiency and if they are to benefit fully from education, a comprehensive approach to their health and nutrition problems is needed.

In Benin, a randomized control trial was implemented on an iodine-deficient population of 196 school children. Due to the availability of iodized salt to the study population during the intervention, participant results were split post hoc based on improved iodine status measured in urine samples. Results indicate that children with improvements in urinary iodine status (from capsules or iodized salt) had significantly better test scores, particularly on tests of abstract reasoning and verbal fluency compared to children without improvements in iodine status.

As the tests included time limits for response, these findings may indicate an improvement in the level and or speed of task performance. These results may indicate a "catch-up" effect as well. The group of children whose urinary iodine concentrations were unchanged during the intervention showed less progress even though their iodine status was, on average, better than the improved group both initially and at the end of the study.

Universal iodization of salt is seen as the permanent and sustainable solution to the global IDD problem. Iodization of salt is the preferred approach for supplementation in iodine deficient populations. It is now mandatory for manufactured salt to be iodized in most countries, however, this does not guarantee the elimination or reduction of IDD.

In many countries a persistence of goitre in school children is being observed despite near universal iodized salt consumption. In areas where iodized salt is not available and where the prompt correction of IDD is urgent, iodized oil can be administered to school children inexpensively and simply, maintaining iodine levels for a period of twelve months.

In Guatemala where the purchase of iodized salt has been problematic, IDD education through schools has been piloted. It was found that a participatory education module appeared to result in an increase in the purchase of iodized salt at the household level . In South Africa, where mandatory iodization of salt was introduced in 1995, a study of the effects on school children in an endemically goitrous area after one year found that iodine deficiency was virtually eradicated.

In China, a randomized clinical trial was implemented comparing iodine interventions in 205 school children aged 8-10 with low to moderate levels of iodine deficiency.

Vitamin A Deficiency (VAD) causes impaired immune function, increased severity of some infections and an increased risk of mortality from infectious diseases and is widely recognized as an important cause of blindness in children. It is estimated that 85m school-age children are at increased risk of acute respiratory and other infections because they are deficient in vitamin A . VAD also affects iron metabolism so that with any iron supplements taken, subsequent improvement in iron status may be limited when vitamin A status is low.

School-age children have not been considered an 'at-risk' group for VAD in the past. Little is known about the occurrence or effects of VAD in this age group. However, the small number of recent studies conducted, suggest that VAD is a public health problem in school-age children.

In Bangladesh, which achieves vitamin A supplement coverage of over 90% in underfives, evidence suggests that VAD may be a larger problem among school-age children than pre-school children. VAD studies in Bangladesh noted that although the extent of clinically evident VAD among school-age and adolescent children has decreased slightly in the last two decades, it remains a significant problem, with deficiency levels higher in boys than girls.

A recent assessment of the vitamin A status of school children in Tanzania, Ghana, Indonesia and Vietnam found that that VAD was a severe public health problem in Tanzania (30% deficient in vitamin A), a moderate problem in Ghana and a mild problem in Indonesia and Vietnam according to WHO criteria. In Cameroon, a study of the relationship of the effect of the parasite, Onchocerca volvulus on plasma vitamin A levels in 261 school children reported sub-clinical vitamin A deficiency in over 80% of the children.

Children with onchocerciasis had significantly lower vitamin A concentrations in their plasma compared to children without infections. A recent study of the prevalence of vitamin A deficiency in northern Ethiopia among 824 school-age children reported a xeropthalmia rate of 5.8%. Serum retinol concentrations were deficient in 8.4 and low in 51.1% of the children. A significant difference was noted between sexes only in vitamin A reserves; girls had significantly lower vitamin A reserve than boys.

Food-based approaches, including fortification, are the preferred long term strategy to prevent VAD. However, for the short term, providing vitamin A supplements, multiple micronutrient supplements or vitamin A fortified foods to school-age children may be effective strategies to prevent VAD in this population.

In the Philippines, a randomized double-blind, controlled trial evaluating the effect of a vitamin-A fortified wheat flour bun was implemented with 835 children ages 6-13 attending four rural schools. The children in the experimental group consumed buns five days a week for 30 weeks fortified with 33% of the RDA for vitamin A. Results were stratified based on initial serum retinol levels.

The children with marginal- to-low initial serum retinol levels significantly improved their vitamin A status with daily consumption of vitamin A-fortified buns. These results suggest that fortified foods can improve vitamin A status in deficient school-age children.

Single micronutrient deficiencies seldom occur in isolation, but instead, interact and tend to cluster. For example, iron deficiency and VAD often coexist in the same populations (see below). Providing vitamin A supplementation can both improve vitamin A status, as well as, iron metabolism in deficient populations. Further, vitamin A food fortification programmes produce similar results. School-age children, like most populations in low income countries, suffer from multiple micronutrient deficiencies.

In one study in China, children supplemented with zinc and other micronutrients had the largest improvements in growth and cognitive function; growth unproved with micronutrient supplementation, but showed little change with only zinc supplementation. These results are consistent with other studies and suggest that deficiencies of other micronutrients can suppress the growth response after zinc repletion.

In a recent study of the relationship between vitamin A, iron status and helminth infection among Bangladeshi school children, children with low serum retinol levels had significantly lower ferritin and haemoglobin levels that those with higher serum retinol levels. Although vitamin A supplementation increased haemoglobin levels and growth parameters significantly, the group of children who received the combined vitamin A and iron supplements had the greatest improvements compared with the placebo group in all indicators. The low cost and simplicity of this study suggest that vitamin A and iron supplementation have a role in the prevention of IDA and growth retardation.

Giving micronutrient deficient school children in South Africa biscuits fortified with iron, iodine and beta-carotene has been shown to significantly improve their micronutrient status. The prevalence of low serum retinol concentrations decreased from 39.1% to 12.2 %, anaemia declined from 27.8% to 13.9% and low urinary iodine concentrations declined from 97.5% to 5.4%. The biscuit was given in the morning for a period of 215 days at a cost of just US$0.7 per child, per school year.

In a case-control study of 66 school children (aged 10-12) in India, those identified as deficient in iron and vitamin A were fed biscuits made with cauliflower leaf powder (a source of iron and vitamin A) for a period of four months. After the intervention, the experimental group had significantly higher haemoglobin and serum retinol levels. Initially 27.27% of children in the experimental group had normal nutritional status compared to 42.42% post intervention.

There was a significant treatment effect of vitamin A on serum retinol levels, as well as, a suggested additive effect between vitamin A fortification and de-worming, i.e. vitamin A supplementation with de-worming had a greater effect on vitamin A status than vitamin A fortification alone. At baseline 34.7% of the children were vitamin A deficient and 15.5% were anaemic. Significant cognitive treatment effects were not found in either of the groups that received biscuits fortified with multiple micronutrients.

Overweight

Overweight and obesity is becoming increasingly prevalent in low income countries where improvements in socioeconomic conditions and rapid urbanization are causing a 'nutrition transition'. A rapid shift in the composition of diet (higher fat and lower carbohydrate), reduced activity patterns and a subsequent shift in body composition characterize this transition.

Countries undergoing a 'nutrition transition' have high levels of stunting, which is believed to be a risk factor for obesity. This may be explained by the relationship of stunting to undernutrition. Evidence from animal and human studies suggests that with malnutrition in utero and in early life, endocrine development may be affected, resulting in hormonal alterations and a predisposition to metabolic disorders and obesity. It is suggested that the increased risk of obesity among stunted children will lead to considerable problems with obesity in children in low income countries over the coming decades .

Although there is a growing body of data on obesity and overweight in this age group, few data are available on the true extent of overweight among school-age children in low income countries. Nationally representative data are lacking and few countries have repeated surveys, thus trend data are limited. Furthermore, there are methodological concerns, the use and interpretation of weight-for-height indices based on children from the US has been questioned in populations with significant levels of stunting .

In 1995, an estimated 17.6m children in the low income countries were overweight . The overall prevalence of overweight in the pre-school population is low, at 3.3%. Available data suggest that the problem of obesity begins in preschool children, becoming more evident among school-age children . In Sub-Saharan Africa and in South Asia obesity is rare. However, in the more developed countries of Latin America, the Middle East, Central Eastern Europe, the Commonwealth

Independent States and North Africa, obesity is as prevalent as in the United States.

Northern Africa and Central America, areas undergoing rapid nutrition transitions, have both problems of stunting and overweight among children. In school-age children, the following has been observed:

— in Chile, 20.7% of school-age children were reported to be overweight and 13.5% obese in 1995

— a study of school-age children (and pre-school-age) in four countries undergoing the nutrition transition (Russia, China, Brazil and South Africa) found that the prevalence of child overweight ranged from 10.5% to 25.6%. Boys in Russia have an overweight prevalence comparable with boys in the US. Stunting is also common in these countries affecting between 9% and 30% of all children and a significant association was found between stunting and overweight status in all four countries

— from China, urban-rural combined data comparing the level of overweight school children from 1991 to 1995 indicate increases of 6 to 9.8% for boys and 5 and 7.6% for girls over this time period. Increases in dietary fat intake and lower levels of physical activity have been attributed to the increasing levels of obesity

— in a study of nutritional status of Kuwaiti elementary school children (6-10 years old) the level of obesity was significantly higher for boys than girls. Stunting was found to be higher in boys as well, 9.5% compared to 4.6% in girls. In comparing results of this study (1995) to a previous study (1985), obesity levels have increased significantly from 12.9% to

21.9% (above the 95 percentile weight-for-height) . In the US, 13% of similarly aged children (6 -11 years old) were above the 95 percentile. These results indicate that Kuwaiti school children have a higher prevalence of obesity than US school children

— in a study of an urban low-income population in Brazil, although wasting (10.2%) was the most prevalent form of malnutrition, adolescent girls had stunting levels of 11% and an obesity rate of 5.5%. Girls suffered more from stunting and overweight/ obesity than boys did. These results suggest that improved living conditions in urban areas in populations 'adapted' to chronic food shortages may increase the susceptibility to obesity

— a representative study of 10 to 13 year old school children from both private and public schools in the urban area of San Jose, Costa Rica found that the prevalence of overweight was similar in both groups, with 31% overweight (85 to 94 percentile BMI reference curves). These findings suggest that overweight is equally a problem among children from lower income families as among children from families with higher incomes

— in a cross sectional study of school children 9 to 16 years old from a low to middle income town in the Mexico City area, found that 24% of the children were obese. Television viewing was associated with an increased risk for obesity, a 12% greater risk for each additional hour of daily TV viewing was estimated. Participating in physical activity, particularly vigorous physical activity was found to protect against obesity ; and

— a longitudinal study of 2,252 primary and secondary school children in Hat Yai, a urban area in Thailand, found that overweight in males increased from 12.4% in 1992 to 21% in 1997, however, the percentage of overweight in females decreased from 15.2% to 12.6%. Over the 5-year period of the study, children who were overweight during childhood were 12 times more likely to be overweight during adolescence than their non-overweight classmates. A family history of obesity, a monthly income greater than 5,000 baht, a low exercise level and one or more parents with high a BMI level were associated with overweight tracking.

Short Term Hunger and School Nutrition Programmes (SNP)

There is increasing evidence of the negative consequences for children suffering from short term hunger, particularly in children who are not fed before going to school. Children who are hungry are more likely to have difficulty concentrating and performing complex tasks, even if otherwise well nourished . In recent years there has been some doubt about the value of stand-alone school feeding programmes in terms of their impact on either nutrition of education. However, the value when implemented in the right context should not be underestimated.

In 2000, a School Feeding/Food for Education stakeholders meeting brought together top practitioners and experts from USAID, USDA, the World Bank, UNICEF and other organizations who either administer or implement SNPs , who reviewed the current situation. In

India, school children participating in a SNP were also provided with treatment for geohelminths. This resulted in a reduction in helminth infection from 71% to 40% with minimal additional costs.

Another recent study (case-control) evaluated the impact of a mid day meal (MDM) programme in 60 primary schools in India. It reported significantly higher enrollment, attendance, and retention rates with reduced dropout rates among MDM programme children.

The poor, particularly children in low income countries, carry the greatest burden of morbidity and mortality. Much of this burden results from hazards within their homes or their immediate environment . High levels of malnutrition, and its known synergistic relationship exacerbate their vulnerability to disease particularly diarrhoeal disease, helminth infections, acute respiratory infections (ARIs) and malaria.

For the urban poor in low income countries, there is a double jeopardy as they find themselves exposed to both "traditional" diseases of poor sanitation and overcrowding and the "modern" diseases of chronic heart and lung disease. School-age children living in poor urban areas are also at a high risk of injury from road traffic accidents.

For children in low income countries, many of the health problems of childhood are associated with lack of clean water and poor sanitation. Diarrhoea is the passage of loose or liquid stools, more frequently than is normal for the individual. It is primarily a symptom of intestinal infection, cased by a wide range of viral, bacterial and parasitic organisms.

One of the most common means of infection is through water contaminated with human faeces. If severe or persistent, the fluid loss and dehydration associated with diarrhoea may be life threatening, especially in infants and young children, the malnourished, or people with impaired immunity.

The total global number of diarrhoeal episodes may be as high as 4000m. WHO estimates that 3.3m children die from intestinal infections such as cholera, typhoid or infectious hepatitis every year. The total number of diarrhoeal episodes may be as high as 4000m. Most of the diarrhoeal disease burden occurs in children in developing countries, with under-fives at greatest risk.

Approximately 90% of the diarrhoeal disease burden is related to environmental factors of poor sanitation and lack of access to clean water and safe food.

Hygiene promotion in schools is a primary intervention because of the potential high risk of disease transmission if facilities are either nonexistent, in a poor state of repair or incorrectly used. In addition, studies show that school-age children can provide effective links with their peers (child to child) and the wider community in communicating important hygiene messages as well as promoting improved sanitation.

Encouraging safer behaviour through participatory hygiene promotion has been shown to be more effective than traditional didactic measures, especially when linked with parallel efforts promoting hygienic behaviour, safe water and sanitation projects within in the community . In many schools, facilities are either poor or absent.

The aim of any school sanitation, hygiene and water programme is to combine hardware and 'software'. The former revolves around the construction of facilities and their subsequent maintenance and use, while the latter focuses on necessary and appropriate learning experiences to encourage safe practice at school, home and throughout later life.

As well as assisting with the construction, maintenance and cleaning of facilities in the school environment, studies reveal that promoting latrine construction through school children can be a successful medium for promoting construction in the wider community.

Hygiene promotion is now seen as an intrinsic element of any water and sanitation initiative and, in the context of school health, is now a central focus for school sanitation and hygiene programme . This approach has the following key elements:

— the safe, efficient and hygienic disposal of faeces, particularly child faeces

— the safe, efficient and hygienic management of water from extraction, through transport and storage to use (particularly for drinking and hand-washing); and

— the regular and effective use of water (with a scouring agent like soap or ash) for hand-washing after contact with stools .

These three are generally considered to be the most important behavioural domains because they carry the greatest potential risk both on a personal and a communal level. There is increasing recognition of the importance of promoting safe hygiene behaviour among school children not simply because of its importance in the immediate school environment but also because of the communication opportunities and potential influence on the family and future families .

In addition to the obvious health benefits and timesavings (particularly affecting young school-age girls), such programmes can also have an influence on school enrollment and attendance. The lack of adequate, separate sanitary facilities in schools is one of the main factors preventing girls from attending school, particularly when menstruating.

In Bangladesh, a school sanitation programme increased girls' enrollment by 11%, a level that is beyond the reach of conventional educational reform. Parasitic helminth infections are a major public health problem throughout the world with over a quarter of the world's population infected with one or more of the most common of these parasites:

- roundworm (Ascaris lumbricoides),
- whipworm (Trichuris trichiura) and
- hookworm (Necator americanus and Ancylostoma duode-nale); and
- the schistosomes: Schistosoma haematobium (urinary)

Infection with intestinal worms is by a simple faecal-oral route. Infection with schistosomes is through contact with contaminated water (e.g. wading, bathing or swimming in ponds, rivers or lakes) that also contains fresh water snails that act as intermediate hosts. Prevalence of these infections rises to a maximum in childhood and settles to a stable asymptote in the adult population.

However, for the age-intensity (or worm burden) profile, there is a marked convexity, such that it is the school-age child who has the most intense infections (the greatest worm burden). As morbidity is directly related to the intensity of infection, it follows that it is this age group who is particularly susceptible.

As numbers of worms build up over time, many of the health problems caused by these worms are chronic and can be long lasting. In addition polyparasitism is a common occurrence; children may be infected concurrently with several parasite species . Children with chronic worm infections and large numbers of worms may be stunted and underweight, which can lead to long term retardation of mental and physical development, even death in severe cases.

Worms can also contribute to malnutrition through inappetance and malabsorption and aneamia through loss of blood. The most significant infection causing blood loss is hookworm infection. This may be caused by blood lose at the site of feeding; exacerbation of bleeding by the secretion of an anticoagulant; interference of uptake of iron in the duodenum; impaired appetite (with moderate to heavy infections).

The school-age child, but also pregnant women and preschool children, are most at risk from hookworm-attributable anaemia. Many studies have focused on the comparison of the prevalence and intensity of schistosomiasis between enrolled and non-enrolled children.

Recent studies of the effect of de-worming on growth have, as with previous studies, reported varied impact. Research suggests helminth infection suppress children's appetites and that treatment results in weight gains. However, improved height gains have not consistently occurred in treatment trials. The intensity of infection, the regularity and duration of treatment and nutritional status have all been identified as important factors that influence programme impact.

Overall the growth and nutritional deficits caused by these infections have been shown to be reversible through appropriate treatment.

- in Guatemala, school children who were given two treatments for very high levels of Ascaris infection (91%) were found to have modest increases in weight gain 6 months after the initial treatment
- a more recent evaluation study from East Africa into the effect of a school-based de-worming programme on growth after one year found that linear growth improved in children who received twice or thrice yearly treatment.

Malaria is probably the world's most important parasitic infectious disease, occurring in tropical and sub-tropical countries. It is caused by four species of Plas-modium parasite; P. falciparum, P. vivax, P. ovale and P. malariae. Several species of Anopheles mosquito can act as the definitive host, and it is transmitted via the bite of infected female mosquitoes, which breed in fresh (or occasionally brackish) water. The symptoms of malaria include fever, chills, headache, nausea, muscle aches, tiredness, vomiting, diarrhoea, anaemia and jaundice.

In severe cases, it can also cause convulsions, coma, severe anaemia and kidney failure. Globally the malaria situation is serious and worsening with mortality ranging between 1.5-2.7m and morbidity 300-500m annually. Although malaria affects 40% of the world's population, 90% of the burden is in Africa.

Most studies to date have focused primarily upon preschool children estimating that over 75% of all-age malaria mortality is experienced by this age group . In contrast there are few empirical studies on mortality in school-aged children. However, recent preliminary estimates suggest mortality among school-aged children is between 5-14% lower than among younger children. This implies that malaria may still account for 10-20% of all-cause deaths among school-age children.

School children who have not acquired exposure-driven immunity may be at particularly high risk of severe and fatal consequences when exposed to the disease in unstable transmission areas. However, these risks are balanced by the low, and often very seasonal, exposure to the parasite. Pregnant schoolgirls are also a particular high-risk group . Malaria is also an important cause of morbidity, but again, data is lacking, although recent data suggests that the risk of morbidity declines rapidly with age.

Malaria can cause iron deficiency and anaemia. However, the effect of malaria on iron metabolism and anaemia is not fully understood, particularly in endemic areas where large numbers of school-age children are affected but are asymptomatic. The prevalence of anaemia increased when higher numbers of Plasmodium species were detected; and the prevalence of anaemia increased with the complexity and extent of Plasmodium species . These results suggest that low-level plasmodial infections also contribute to anaemia.

Malaria accounts for between less than 3% and 8% of all reasons of absenteeism. However, of preventable medical causes of absenteeism malaria counts for a significant 13-50% of school days missed per annum. Under the assumption that each malaria attack contributes two to five days absence from school, it is estimated that malaria is responsible for 4-10m school days lost.

The evidence also suggests that brain insult, as a consequence of cerebral malaria, in early childhood may have an effect on a child's cognitive and learning ability; residual neurological sequelae of 1-5% of children infected early in life. The priority age group for malaria control is younger than school-age children .

However, WHO and the World Bank are working with the Roll Back Malaria Partnership to identify an effective, operational response to the issue of malaria control in school-age children. Some interventions may be inappropriate for the school child.

However, school-based malaria prevention programmes are a good example of how schools can make a contribution to community health. It is suggested that children can be important agents for change in malaria control programmes. The promotion, by schools, of prompt and effective presumptive treatment provides an affordable control option.

Skills based health education can give children the ability to recognize the signs and symptoms of malaria, to recognize the need to seek treatment, and to differentiate symptomatic from curative treatment. Skills based health education through schools can also help promote a community wide understanding of malaria with particular emphasis on the need for community based control measures such as the use of impregnated bed nets.

Schools can serve as a focus for synchronised impregnation of bed nets and distribution . Human Immunodeficiency Virus (HIV)/Acquired Immune

Deficiency Syndrome (AIDS) and School-Age Children Approximately 40m people throughout the world are now living with HIV/AIDS (with 70% of these people living in sub-Saharan Africa), including almost 3m children under the age of 15.

The impact and repercussions of this global epidemic in every sphere of people's lives is now becoming apparent. HIV is a retrovirus that attacks and weakens the immune system. Although an infected person may look and feel well for many years, as their immune system weakens they become unable to fight infection and become more vulnerable to a range of serious diseases, such as tuberculosis, pneumonia and cancer, and to opportunistic infections (such as fungal infections) that would not normally affect people with healthy immune systems.

AIDS is the term used for the group of health problems, such as weight loss, various infections, tumours and other health problems associated with HIV infection. HIV is contracted and spread through sexual contact (unprotected vaginal or anal sex); direct inoculation of with infected blood (e.g. through contaminated needles) and from an HIV positive mother to her child.

Throughout the world, HIV infection prevalence is lowest in the 5 to 14 year old age group, and AIDS mortality does not have its primary effect on school-age children. The majority of children dying of AIDS are young children who have contracted the disease from mother-child transmission. An estimated 3.8m children have been infected with HIV since the epidemic began, and more than two-thirds have died. UNAIDS estimates that in 2001, 800,000 children under the age of 15 became newly infected with HIV, and that 580,000 children under the age of 15 died of AIDS, the vast majority of them in Sub-Saharan Africa .

HIV/AIDS for social, cultural, economic, and even physiological reasons. A lack of education increases this vulnerability, due to inequalities in status, power, and access to resources. Many girls and young women find that they have little choice and control over decisions about sex, and may be exposed to unprotected sex, often with older men. This may be in exchange for gifts, money or favours, or as a result of abuse, including by teachers.

Effects of HIV/AIDS

The relatively low prevalence of HIV/AIDS in school-age children means that the direct effects of AIDS related illness in this age group constitute a relatively small proportion of the total burden of disease. In contrast, the indirect effects are enormous. Children may suffer both physically, socially and psychologically through death or illness of members of their family - including parents.

In countries with the highest prevalence of HIV/ AIDS, the concentration of AIDS in the working age adult population means that there are fewer adults to care for the increasing population of orphans and vulnerable children. This situation includes countries such as Botswana - where one in three adults are infected, Zimbabwe - where it is one in four, and countries such as Zambia and South Africa - where 20% of adults are infected.

One of the greatest impacts of the AIDS epidemic is on the children orphaned by AIDS. Before AIDS, an estimated 2% of children in Africa were orphans. Today, the proportion has risen to almost 15% of children in some African countries. It is estimated that 50% of these children were orphaned by AIDS. Over 13m children under the age of 15 have lost their mother or both parents to AIDS, most of them in sub-Saharan Africa.

Orphans are amongst the most vulnerable people in society. They suffer the trauma of seeing one or both parents becoming ill and dying from AIDS. Many will have to change home several times as they move to live with other family members or relatives, who may themselves become ill and die. They also run a greater risk of becoming stunted and malnourished and may miss out on schooling, due to lack of funds.

HIV/AIDS does not affect only households with children orphaned by AIDS; it also affects the children living with HIV-positive parents or relatives. This group of children serves as an indicator for the future orphan burden. The exact number is unknown and most countries have no estimates. Like the children who have lost their mothers or both parents, this group of children may be discriminated against, may lack basic health care and education, may experience physical and psychosocial stress, and may have little or no social and economic support.

The children are frequently young: the mean age of orphaning is only 6.2 years . They are also often forced to take on responsibilities far beyond their years, not only caring for other siblings but also for their parents - the people who they look to for love and support. An adult who has AIDS requires increasing help with everyday activities (which is expected from the child), but also suffers from frequent opportunistic infections such as uncontrollable episodes of diarrhoea, in conjunction with the slow debilitating effects of the HIV itself.

Following are the five key strategies for supporting orphans and other children affected by HIV/ AIDS:

1. strengthen and support the capacity of families to protect and care for their children
2. mobilize and strengthen community-based responses
3. strengthen the capacity of children and young people to meet their own needs
4. ensure that governments develop appropriate policies, including legal and programmatic frameworks, as well as essential services for most vulnerable children; and
5. raise awareness within societies to create an environment that enables support for children affected by HIV/AIDS .

For school-age children, especially vulnerable children, finding strategies to keep them in school, or to reach them in out of school situations, is one of the key lines in defence against HIV/AIDS, especially for girls. By remaining in education, girls may have the opportunity to reduce the social and economic vulnerability that exposes them to the higher risk of contracting HIV.

The major obstacles currently limiting orphans and other vulnerable children's access to education are: lack of finances; increased family responsibilities; discrimination, stigma and trauma; scepticism about the value of primary education and poor educational quality.

In some countries programmes have been initiated by local and international NGOs to help subsidize individual children or groups of children, often by linking them with sponsors or a sponsorship organisation. Countries including Zambia, Zimbabwe, Malawi and South Africa currently have such schemes, helping to increase access to school for some of the most vulnerable children, who are currently excluded for financial reasons.

Besides the problems of adequate food, health care and education, an area that is too frequently neglected is the emotional distress of children living with a parent who is terminally ill, or who have lost one or both parents.

Schools are the main institutions able to reach a large number of children and young people, with the support and involvement of the local community. Schools have the opportunity to reach children before they become sexually active, and while they are open to adopting healthy ways of behaving and protecting themselves from infection.

Schools can serve as the forum where adolescents can obtain accurate information on reproductive health and HIV/AIDS, together with the skills and support needed to help them protect themselves from infection. However, at present there is still little hard evidence that school HIV/AIDS prevention programmes that fail to adopt the skills-based approach have a major impact on sexual behaviour.

In many countries, school-based reproductive health and HIV/AIDS education is often used as part of a wider strategy of community and national HIV/AIDS prevention programmes, and may be most effective in this context, especially when a skills-based approach is utilized.

Skills-based health education, including HIV/AIDS prevention, aims to help children develop the knowledge, altitudes, values, and skills- including interpersonal skills, critical and creative thinking, decision-making, and self awareness -needed to make sound health-related and social decisions.

The UNAIDS Interagency Task Team (IATT) for HIV/AIDS is an initiative that seeks to share experiences among countries in sub-Saharan Africa with the intent to promote Education for All (EFA) and the Millennium Development Goals (MDG) . Improving the health and learning of school children through school-based nutrition and health programmes is not a new concept. However, many early programmes have been characterized as being heavily focused on disease prevention, being uncoordinated, lacking integration and poorly evaluated and disseminated.

Most importantly, the traditional school nutrition and health programmes have been based in the better off schools and in urban centres. This situation appears to be rapidly improving as new policies and partnerships are being formulated which help ensure that programmes are socially progressive and specifically target the poor, girls and the most disadvantaged children.

This change in perspective is timely as countries and agencies seek to achieve Education for All (EFA) by 2015, and address the Millennium Development Goals (MDG) of Universal Basic Education and Gender Equality in Education Access. If every girl and boy is to be able to complete a basic education of good quality, then school nutrition and health programmes are essential to ensure that the poorest children, who suffer the most malnutrition and ill health, are also able to attend school.

In order to operationalize an effective response, education sectors need to develop an infrastructure and policy context for improving the nutrition and health of school children. A major step forward was taken when a framework to Focus Resources on Effective School Health (FRESH) was developed by UNESCO, WHO, UNICEF, Education International and the World Bank and launched at the World Education Forum in Dakar in April 2000.

The FRESH framework provides the context for effective implementation of access to health and nutrition services within school health programmes. School based health and nutrition services, such as food for education, micronutrient supplementation and deworming, are most effective when they are supported by other strategies. These strategies include policies to provide a nondiscriminatory safe and secure environment, provision of safe water and sanitation, effective referral to external health service providers and links with the community.

The FRESH framework provides this context by positioning access to health and nutrition services among four core components that should be made available together for all schools:

— health related school policies

— safe water and sanitation

— skills based health and nutrition education

— access to health and nutrition services

These core components of the FRESH framework require school-community partnerships as the supporting strategies for the success of school health and nutrition programmes. These include effective partnerships between the health and education sectors, teachers and health workers, schools and community groups and between the pupils and those responsible for implementing school health and nutrition programmes.

WHO and of the "child friendly" schools of UNICEF, as well as of many other global efforts to make schools effective, healthy, hygienic and safe. The FRESH framework specifically addresses the need for nutrition and health services in schools. School-based nutrition and health services are effective and cost-efficient provided that the services are simple, safe and familiar, and address problems that are prevalent and recognized as important within the community.

For example, improving meal timing or providing snacks can address student hunger during school, which seriously constrains learning and contributes to poor school performance. Similarly, semiannual or annual oral treatments can be an effective means of addressing micronutrient deficiencies and worm infections. With treatment of worms, micronutrient supplementation is a cost-effective and simple method of reducing certain vitamin deficiencies in school-age children.

School officials delivering simple health services in schools can easily correct these basic, yet pervasive, health deficiencies. Technical documents have been produced by the agency partners in support of the FRESH framework, including:

— rationales for the four core FRESH activities

— a School Health Toolkit for teachers and programme implementers; and

— FRESH and its role in the Achievement of Education for All.

As a result of concerted action by the participating agencies, national programmes using the FRESH framework have now been adopted by over 20 countries in sub-Saharan Africa, ultimately benefiting a target population of 45m school age children. These school nutrition and health programmes provide an infrastructure and a context for the education sector to deliver a wide range of specific interventions.

The 54 World Health Assembly's resolution set a global target of scaling up intervention to regularly treat 75% of school-age children (398m) at risk by 2010. To achieve this goal, WHO has taken the lead in developing a broad partnership that promotes the in-corporation of deworming of school-age children into existing institutions and programmes, for both the education and health sectors.

The Partnership for Parasite Control (PPC) was launched in 2001, with the aim of mobilizing resources and promoting new synergy among public and private efforts for the control of soil-transmitted helminths and schistosomiasis at the global and national levels. Working with the World Food Programme (WFP), the Canadian International Development Agency and the World Bank, WHO in 2001 trained representatives of the ministries of health and education of 21 countries, and deworming programmes have already begun in 19 of the 41 endemic countries in Africa.

An initiative of the HIV/AIDS affected countries and the UNAIDS IATT for HIV/AIDS and Education calls for a multi-partner effort from countries, development partners, civil society and the private sector to promote high level understanding and leadership, and the development of effective national responses across the education sector . The initiative seeks to share experiences among countries in sub-Saharan Africa, and has two main objectives:

— First, to promote EFA and the MDG, which will ensure that every girl and boy has access to quality education despite the impact of HIV/AIDS on the education system.

— Second, to strengthen the capacity of the education sector to respond with timely actions to prevent students and teachers from being infected with HIV.

Food security is too often formulated as food production, and little attention is given to determining whether agricultural activities contribute to alleviating hunger and improving overall nutritional status. As well as, nutrition is too often seen as a health issue, focusing on biomedical interventions that emphasize supplementation and fortification over food-based strategies linked to agricultural production.

Moreover, both agriculture and nutrition communities tend to overlook the importance of gender analysis in their work. If hunger-related interventions do not address the different challenges men and women face as producers and caregivers, the interventions will have a limited effect. In the Agriculture and Nutrition Advantage Project, each country team includes representatives from the agriculture and nutrition sectors and a gender expert.

They have developed Plans of Action that will compile existing evidence or generate new evidence that demonstrates how to operationalize the links between agriculture and nutrition, with value added by gender analysis. They will use that evidence to advocate for changes in policies, resource allocations and programmatic approaches that bring agriculture and nutrition closer together. Teams will partner with communities and other relevant agents to influence key decision-makers in government, the private sector, donor organizations, and implementing agencies.

For example, the Nigerian team has conducted a nationally representative food and nutrition survey. Based on the findings, it will pinpoint geographic areas with the potential to reduce malnutrition through interventions that apply agriculture, nutrition and gender strategies.

In Uganda, the project will incorporate the Ugandan Gov-ernment's decentralized structure, the new Plan for the Modernization of Agriculture (PMA), and the National Agricultural Advisory Service (NAADS) as a framework. The team will work with farmer groups and other community-based organizations (the lowest point of the decentralized system) to demand support from the NAADS for gender-sensitive agriculture and nutrition interventions.

The goal is to identify factors that make the bottom-up demand-side work and advocate for including nutrition as a crosscutting theme in the PMA. The ICRW/IFPRI team is doing similar work with the intent of influencing key decision-makers in development agencies, such as the World Bank and USAID.

Its advocacy objectives focus on tripling resources for gender-sensitive, agriculture-nutrition activities, and on persuading donors to hire nutritionists in their agriculture programs. It also aims to persuade key development practitioners to adopt practices that embody a gender-sensitive approach linking agriculture and nutrition to cut hunger.

An IFPRI study in Mozambique, Nigeria and Uganda will identify institutional factors that inhibit or promote links between agriculture and nutrition, including the use of gender analysis in the design, implementation and evaluation of policies and programs.

Brazilian Civil Society launches National Human Rights´ Rapporteur Programme. The Brazilian Platform on Economic, Social and Cultural Human Rights (PDHESC- Brasil), in partnership with United Nations Volunteer Programme (UNV) and the Brazilian Sate Secretariat on Human Rights, launched the National Economic, Social and Cultural Human Rights Rapporteur Programme in July 2002.

The UN thematic Human Rights Rapporteurs´s Programme inspired it and Brazil the first country in the world to adopt such a programme. Civil society organizations and human rights defenders expect that it contributes to the full realization of human rights in Brazil.

From October 2002 to December 2003, six national rappor-teurs will address the following themes: education; environment; adequate food, water and rural land; health; housing; and work. A tripartite committee chose the rapporteurs after a broad consultation with Brazilian society. The rapporteurs are not remunerated, but is provided with a full-time assistant from the UNV programme and travel money for two investigative missions.

Further support will be provided by the civil society organization hosting the rapporteur. The rapporteur's mandate includes the prerogative to carry out in situ investigative missions, to collect and investigate violation claims, to present violation claims at regional and national public hearings, and to elaborate independent analytical and propositive reports, incorporating gender, ethnic, racial and generational issues.

The resulting reports will be presented to the National Human Rights Organizations Forum, to the National Human Rights Conference, held annually in the National Congress, to the National Council for the Protection of the Human Person, to the Inter-American Human Rights Commission, and to the UN Human Rights Commission.

Child Health and Nutrition Research Initiative (CHNRI) is an international coalition of partners from universities, NGOs, foundations, international agencies, bilateral donors and research institutes established to improve child health and nutrition. The concept underlying CHNRI was developed as a result of several meetings convened by the Global Forum for Health Research in Geneva.

In order to achieve its goal, CHNRI engages in a number of activities, including: identifying priority research topics from the domains determining a child's well being, generating knowledge related to priority research topics, and strengthening the capacity of research networks responsible for implementation in child health and nutrition research in low and middle income countries.

CHNRI held a parallel session at Forum 6 in Arusha, Tanzania, between 12-15 November 2002. At the session, the three principal investigators conducting regional profiling and priority setting exercises in Latin America, Africa, and Asia presented their interim results and final steps to complete this mapping exercise. Each group will submit a final report by April 2003, which will detail the state of child health and nutrition research in their respected regions.

International Atomic Energy Agency (IAEA)

Impact on ageing on human energy, macro- and micronutrient metabolism and requirements By the year 2025 there will be 1.2b elderly people in the world, 60% of them in developing countries. In this context, the activities of the International Dietary Consultative Group are increasingly focusing on the health and nutrition problems of the elderly.

Large shifts occur in dietary patterns- mainly in energy metabolism- as populations become older. Even small increases in physical activity and/or small weight losses can have considerable metabolic effects (e.g. lowering the incidence of glucose intolerance). The impact of weight loss or gain on the overall health of ageing subjects in relation to the incidence of morbidity and mortality is attracting more research attention.

An earlier coordinated research project (CRP) on the application of nuclear techniques in the prevention of degenerative diseases (e.g. obesity, non-insulin dependent diabetes, and coronary heart diseases) in ageing and a technical co-operation (TC) project using isotopes in the evaluation of nutrition intervention programmes, have contributed to an understanding of several methodological issues related to the use of doubly labelled water (DLW).

Intrauterine growth retardation (IUGR)

IUGR, a condition where foetal growth has been constrained, is the main cause of low birthweight (LBW) in developing countries. Most LBW in industrialized countries is due to preterm birth. Approximately 30m infants born every year in developing countries suffer from IUGR. Stable isotopes are invaluable in nutrition research since there is virtually no health risk involved in their use. They are preferred for work in humans, especially for target populations, such as infants and pregnant women.

The tracer dilution technique using 2 H20 is the only appropriate reference technique to evaluate the nutritional status for these target populations in their own environment.

International Centre for Research on Women (ICWR)

ICRW has been invited by the World Bank to serve as the Secretariat for a new initiative on nutrition and gender issues. The World Bank Development Grant Facility has provided seed funding for this initiative. Research findings suggest that to eliminate malnutrition over the long-term, interventions need to consider the important underlying gender issues, which constrain women's capabilities.

Many poor women lack the authority to make decisions about household resources that could enhance nutritional status. For example, women may be forced to marry during their adolescent years leading to early pregnancy, poorer birth outcomes, and poorer micronutrient status. Studies also indicate that where women have more capabilities and are more empowered, nutrition outcomes such as maternal and child nutrition are improved.

It is plausible then, that improving the status of women could lead to improved pregnancy outcomes, and thus should help break the inter-generational cycle of malnutrition. To achieve this, programmes designed to tackle malnutrition need to intervene at key points in the life cycle, including adolescence. The Secretariat will partner with a local hub in West Africa and later one in South Asia in an innovative and cross-sectoral approach among the nutrition, gender and development arenas.

Overall, the programme aims to gain an understanding of how nutrition programmes can be enhanced by integrating a gender focus and how to enhance women's roles, decision-making capabilities, and control over resources to improve nutrition outcomes. Specifically, the use of action research will shed light on how to break the cycle of malnutrition by addressing the causes of poor foetal growth and low birthweight by focusing on results, and by developing new models for cross-sectoral collaboration.

International Food Policy Research Institute (IFPRI)

Household food security is an important dimension of well-being. However, obtaining detailed data on food security status - such as 24-hour recall data on food intake or acquisition for every member of a household -is time consuming and expensive. It also requires a high level of technical skill both in data collection and analysis.

IFPRI has conducted research to determine whether household-level dietary diversity (HDD) could act as an alternative indicator of food security. The analysis from ten data sets encompassed both low and middle-income countries, rural and urban sectors, seasonal data, and data on energy acquisition obtained using both seven-day recall on food consumption and 24-hour individual intake data.

International Fund for Agricultural Development (IFAD)

Launching a new training tool for impact assessment in rural development projects. IFAD, the Italian National Institute for Research on Food and Nutrition (INRAN) and the Government of Guinea have begun distributing a training video entitled: Benchmark Assessment of Impact Indicators. The video illustrates how to plan and implement a benchmark assessment of selected impact indicators in the context of rural development projects.

The indicators covered are directly linked to the Millennium Development Goals (MDGs) such as:

— prevalence of malnutrition in underfive years (underweight, chronic and acute)

— access to safe water supply

— access to adequate sanitation

— female literacy

The video is designed as a practical guide to help non-specialists become familiar with the basic concepts involved in benchmark assessments, and to provide step-by-step examples from an assessment carried out in Guinea. The first major distribution took place in October 2002, at an implementation workshop for 50 IFAD-supported projects in West and Central Africa, involving project managers, government representatives and other partners from countries throughout the region.

If poor childhood nutrition and health does in fact hurt education and the acquisition of skills, it could be central to understanding the intergenerational transmission of poverty in less developed countries. The relationship is also critically important for poor country policymakers and donors, who need to allocate limited education and health budget among many competing priorities.

Yet many existing non-experimental studies exploring the impact of poor nutrition on education are difficult to interpret due to the possibility of omitted variable bias. In particular, unobserved household socioeconomic variation, parental investments in children, and child genetic endowments may all affect both child nutrition and education, generating a spurious correlation between them.

Approximately 68 percent of children in the sample were anemic and 24 percent suffered from intestinal helminth (worm) infections at baseline. Anemia and intestinal worm infections are among the world's most widespread health problems, especially for children. The pre-schools in the study were randomly divided into three groups, and the schools were gradually phased into the program as it expanded over the course of two years.

The NGO Pratham Delhi has established an extensive network of pre-schools (balwadis) in the underprivileged communities of South Shahdara (in eastern Delhi), ten to twenty year old "resettlement colonies" that have absorbed large population in-flows during Delhi's relentless recent expansion. The children in Pratham Delhi balwadis are two to six years old, typically come from families of poor migrant laborers, and are at high risk of anemia and other nutritional deficiencies.

Pre-school teachers are young women who live in these communities, and the pre-schools usually take place in their homes; thus when a teacher moves, marries, or obtains full-time employment, the pre-school may close, and this leads to considerable "turn-over" in the pre-schools an issues we return to below.

The pre-schools' main goal is to teach the children basic literacy and numeracy schools, and to avoid delayed enrollment in primary school - a major problem in this setting - and as part of this they have also included a nutrition and health intervention administered every three months at "health camps" and in the pre-schools. The pre-school health intervention consists of 32 mg of elemental iron, and 400mg of albendazole, taken at the health camp.

Following WHO recommendations, pre-school teachers in treatment schools were instructed to administer daily iron doses for 30 school days following each health camp, to children attending the preschool that day. Both treatment and comparison school children also receive 200,000 I.U. of Vitamin A (at alternate health camps), and thus the treatment effect estimates should be interpreted as the impact of iron and deworming in addition to Vitamin A supplementation, relative to Vitamin A supplementation alone; note that Vitamin A may promote the absorption of iron.

The World Health Organization (WHO) defines anemia in children 6 to 60 months of age at hemoglobin concentrations below 11.0 g/dL and 69.4 percent of children in the baseline balwadi population met this standard. Moreover, over seven percent of sample children were severely anemic (< 7.0 g/dL) and 41 percent moderately anemic (7.0-9.9 g/dL).

Iron deficiency anemia leads to weakness and poor physical growth, and to a compromised immune system, decreasing the ability to fight infections and increasing morbidity; it is also hypothesized that cognitive performance is impaired and psychomotor development delayed. We also find that measured child anemia rates from the 1998-1999 Indian National Family Health Survey (NFHS) are extremely similar to our figures: in the NFHS Delhi sample, 69 percent of the children aged 6-35 months old were anemic, of whom four percent were severely anemic and 43 percent had moderate anemia, thus our population of balwadi children appears largely representative of the Delhi population, in terms of anemia.

Fully 24 percent of the balwadi children sample has some sort of helminth infection , mainly roundworm (19 percent prevalence), although some children were also infected with hookworm, Hymenolipis nana, and threadworm. Worm infections lead to poor child health. For instance, roundworm (Ascaris lumbricoides) infections can cause protein energy malnutrition and growth stunting, abdominal pain and general weakness and lethargy.

Hookworm causes diarrhea, abdominal pain, weight loss and iron deficiency anemia. The WHO has recommended mass deworming treatment in populations where anemia is prevalent and helminths infect at least 20 percent of the population. Z-scores reflect the difference from the mean of a reference healthy U.S. child (of a particular sex and age) in terms of standard deviations. Weight-for-height reflects wasting (acute undernutrition), weight-for -age reflects being underweight (chronic and acute undernutrition), and height-for-age reflects stunting (chronic undernutrition).

The population is mainly composed of individuals whose original home lies outside of Delhi (75.8 percent of the sample), many of whom are recent migrants and of which the majority are from Uttar Pradesh (54.4 percent). Only 20 percent of the population has lived in their current household for fifteen or more years, further evidence on the largely transient nature of the population in these poor "resettlement colonies". A significant share of this population (21 percent) is Muslim, compared to the NFHS, which reports that only 8 percent of Delhi household heads are Muslim.

Bibliography

Ainsworth, M., K. Beegle, and G. Koda, "The Impact of Adult Mortality on Primary School Enrollment in Northwestern Tanzania", *Background paper for the Africa Development Forum 2000*, Addis Ababa, Ethiopia, UNAIDS, Geneva, 2001.

Badcock-Walters, P., "The Impact of HIV/AIDS on Education in KwaZulu Natal", *KZNDEC Provincial Education Development Unit*, Durban, South Africa, 2001.

Bakaki, P., "The Orphan Study Activity in Uganda", *A report submitted to the Nutrition and Early Childhood Development Project*, Ministry of Health, Kampala, Uganda, 2001.

Barnet, E., K. de Koning, and V. Francis, "Health and HIV/AIDS Education in Primary and Secondary Schools in Africa and Asia", *Education Research no.* 14, 1995.

Bennel, P., "Improving Youth Livelihoods in Sub-Saharan Africa", *A Review of Policies and Programmes with Particular Reference to the Link between Sexual Behaviour and Economic Well-Being*, USAID, Washington, D.C, 2000.

Bocage, C., "Presentation on Project Lifestyle, FAO/ILSI Workshop on Food-based Dietary Guidelines and Nutrition Education for the Caribbean", Bridgetown, Barbados, Food and Agriculture Organization,1999.

Bundy, D. A. P., Guyatt, H. L., "Global Distribution of Parasitic Worm Infections", Paris, UNESCO, 1989.

______________,"Schools for Health: Focus on Health, Education and the School-age Child", Parasitology Today, 1994.

______________, Mcguire, J.; Hall, A., Dolan, C., "School Based Health and Nutrition Programmes", *A Survey of Donor and Agency Support*, 1998.

Connolly, M., "Principles to Guide Programming for Orphans and Other Vulnerable Children", Draft, *UNICEF, Child Protection Section*, New York, 2001.

Carrin, G, Hollmeyer, H, Jones, J, Everad, M, Ron, A, Savioli, L, Sen-Hai, Y. et al., "School Health Insurance as a Vehicle for Health-Promoting Schools", 1999.

Cerqueira, M. T., "Health-Promoting Schools in the Americas", *World Health, Vol.* 49, No. 4, pp. 12–13, 1996.

Chinpah, V., "Handbook on Monitoring Learning Achievement: Towards Capacity Building", Paris, UNESCO, 1997.

Cooper, K. J., "Worldwide Effort Focuses on Educating 'the Girl-Child'", *Seattle Times*, 21 February 1999.

Foster, G., and J. Williamson, "A Review of Current Literature on the Impact of HIV/AIDS on Children in Sub-Saharan Africa", *AIDS 2000* 14(suppl 3): S275–S284, 2001.

Gachuhi, D., "The Impact of HIV/AIDS on Education Systems in the Eastern and Southern Africa Region and the Response of Education Systems to HIV/AIDS: Life Skills Programs", *Paper prepared for UNICEF presentation at the Sub-Saharan Africa Conference on EFA 2000*, Johannesburg, South Africa, December 6–10, 1999.

Index